Principles of Biomedical Ethics

Principles of Biomedical Ethics

FOURTH EDITION

Tom L. Beauchamp
James F. Childress

New York   Oxford
OXFORD UNIVERSITY PRESS
1994

Oxford University Press

Oxford   New York   Toronto
Delhi   Bombay   Calcutta   Madras   Karachi
Kuala Lumpur   Singapore   Hong Kong   Tokyo
Nairobi   Dar es Salaam   Cape Town
Melbourne   Auckland   Madrid

and associated companies in
Berlin   Ibadan

Published by Oxford University Press, Inc.,
198 Madison Avenue, New York, New York 10016-4314

Oxford is a registered trademark of Oxford University Press

Library of Congress Cataloging-in-Publication Data
Beauchamp, Tom L.
Principles of biomedical ethics -
Tom L. Beauchamp, James F. Childress.—4th ed.
p. cm.   Includes bibliographical references and index.
ISBN 0-19-508536-1.—ISBN 0-19-508537-X (pbk.)
1. Medical ethics.   I. Childress, James F.   II. Title.
[DNLM: 1. Ethics, Medical.]
R724.B36   1994
174'.2—dc20   93-24390

9 8 7 6 5 4 3

Printed in the United States of America
on acid-free paper

To
Georgia, Ruth, and Don

I can no other answer make but thanks,
And thanks, and ever thanks.

Twelfth Night

Preface to the Fourth Edition

Biomedical ethics was a young field when the first edition of this book went to press in late 1977. Immense changes occurred in the field's literature between the first edition and the present, fourth edition. Although major changes have appeared in all editions after the first, this edition includes more significant changes than any other.

Readers will notice particularly far-reaching changes in Chapters 1, 2, and 8, which contain our main views in ethical theory. In Chapter 1, entirely new sections have been added on Method, Justification, and Truth; Specifying and Balancing Principles; and The Place of Principles. In Chapter 2, new sections have been developed on Liberal Individualism, Communitarianism, The Ethics of Care, Casuistry, and Principle-Based, Common-Morality Theories. In Chapter 8, new sections appear on Virtues in Professional Roles, Four Focal Virtues, and Moral Excellence. In other chapters, major sections have been added on The Justification of Assistance in Dying, The Value and Quality of Life, and Rationing through Priorities in the Health Care Budget. Many substantive changes also appear in sections that are not new to this edition. For example, in the Fair Opportunity section of Chapter 6, we have added a subsection on Distributing Health Care on the Basis of Gender and Race.

Despite these changes, the book retains its previous chapter structure and characteristic perspectives on major issues. Most of the chapter and sectional headings have also been retained from the third edition.

Because of the concentration on theory in the first two chapters, some readers may prefer to read the chapters devoted to various principles (Chapters 3–6), rules (Chapter 7), and virtues (Chapter 8) before exploring our approaches to theory and method.

We have also altered the way we present cases in this edition. More complete versions of the relevant cases are now found in the text, rather than the appendix. Thus, although the appendix of cases is now smaller, more discussion of cases is provided throughout the text.

We have received many helpful suggestions for improvements in the previous edition from students, colleagues, health professionals, and teachers who use the book. We owe special thanks in this edition to David DeGrazia and Henry Richardson for their assessments of new sections in Chapters 1 and 2, and to Ruth Faden for her reading of Chapters 5 and 6. We are also grateful to John Hasnas and Madison Powers for their criticisms of the new section on casuistry.

Several articles critical of aspects of our book have appeared in the literature of biomedical ethics in recent years. Although we do not always concur with our critics, we are especially grateful to our friends John Arras, Dan Clouser, Bernie Gert, and Ron Green for some very probing and often penetrating suggestions.

Special acknowledgment is due to a talented research staff that has assisted us in the collecting of materials. Catherine Marshall, Brian Tauscher, Liz Emmett, and Felicia Cohn provided invaluable assistance and advice in this process, as well as in the revision of drafts of chapters. They repeatedly forced us to make our sections more pertinent and readable. Emily Wilson, Andrew Dodge, and Brian Marshall helped with page proofs and the index. In addition, our university offices provided superb assistance by faithfully preparing draft after draft. We are especially indebted for this assistance to Moheba Hanif and Diana McKenzie.

Some parts of chapters were presented at the seminars of the Kennedy Institute of Ethics. Many arguments were changed as a result of the comments and responses of our critics on these occasions. We also acknowledge with due appreciation the support provided by the Kennedy Institute's library and information retrieval systems, which kept us in touch with new literature and reduced the burdens of library research. In particular, we thank Mary Coutts for her faithful and precise searching of data bases.

Washington, D.C.   T.L.B.
Charlottesville, Virginia   J.F.C.
November 1993

Contents

Principles of Biomedical Ethics

1

Morality and Moral Justification

Medical ethics enjoyed a remarkable degree of continuity from the days of Hippocrates until its long-standing traditions began to be supplanted, or at least supplemented, around the middle of the twentieth century. Scientific, technological, and social developments during that time produced rapid changes in the biological sciences and in health care. These developments challenged many prevalent conceptions of the moral obligations of health professionals and society in meeting the needs of the sick and injured. The objective of this book is to provide a framework for moral judgment and decisionmaking in the wake of these developments.

Although major writings in ancient, medieval, and modern health care contain a rich storehouse of reflection on the relationship between the professional and the patient, this history is often disappointing from the perspective of contemporary biomedical ethics. It shows how inadequately, and with what measure of insularity, problems of truthfulness, privacy, justice, communal responsibility, and the like were framed in past centuries. To avoid a similar inadequacy, we begin with a study of ethics that may appear to be distant from both history and contemporary problems in the biological sciences, medicine, nursing, and other modes of health care. Our objective is to show how ethical theory can illuminate problems in health care and can help overcome some limitations of past formulations of ethical responsibility. However, it is unreasonable to expect any theory to overcome all the limitations of time and place and reach a universally acceptable perspective.

Morality and Ethical Theory

Ethics is a generic term for various ways of understanding and examining the moral life. Some approaches to ethics are normative (that is, they present standards of right or good action), others are descriptive (that is, they report what people believe and how they act), and still others analyze the concepts and methods of ethics.

Approaches to Ethics

Normative ethics. Inquiry that attempts to answer the question "Which general norms for the guidance and evaluation of conduct are worthy of moral acceptance and for what reasons?" is *general normative ethics.* The study of these norms has typically occurred while developing an ethical theory, although the concept of "normative ethics" is a distinctly twentieth-century notion not invoked in pre-twentieth-century theories. Ideally, such a theory satisfies a set of criteria for theories that is developed in Chapter 2, thereby making it a comprehensive inquiry into moral concepts, principles, reasoning, and the like. However, numerous practical questions would remain unanswered even if a fully satisfactory general ethical theory were available, for reasons explained at the end of this chapter.

The attempt to work out the implications of general theories for specific forms of conduct and moral judgment will be called *practical ethics* here, although it is often misleadingly called *applied ethics.* The term *practical* refers to the use of ethical theory and methods of analysis to examine moral problems, practices, and policies in several areas, including the professions and public policy. Often no straightforward movement from theory or principles to particular judgments is possible in these contexts, although general reasons, principles, and even ideals can play some role in evaluating conduct and establishing policies. Theory and principles are typically invoked only to help develop action-guides, which are also further shaped by paradigm cases of appropriate behavior, empirical data, and the like, together with reflection on how to put these influential sources into the most coherent whole.

Although general normative ethics is distinguished from practical ethics by being more general and by a weaker connection to concerns about practical affairs, no sharp distinction should be drawn between the two. In this book we are mainly concerned with interpreting principles and developing general moral action-guides for use in the biomedical fields, but we will also examine moral motives and character. (*Biomedicine* is a shorthand expression for the biological sciences, medicine, and health care.)

Nonnormative ethics. In addition to normative ethics, there are two broad types of nonnormative ethics. First, *descriptive ethics* is the factual investigation of moral behavior and beliefs. It uses standard scientific techniques to study how people reason and act. For example, anthropologists, sociologists, psychologists, and historians determine which moral norms and attitudes are expressed in professional practice, in codes, and in public policies. They study different beliefs and practices regarding surrogate decisionmaking, treatment of the dying, the nature of consent obtained from patients, and the like.

Second, *metaethics* involves analysis of the language, concepts, and methods of reasoning in ethics. For example, it addresses the meanings of such ethical terms as *right, obligation, virtue, principle, justification, sympathy, morality,* and *responsibility.* It also includes study of moral epistemology (the theory of moral knowledge) and the logic and patterns of moral reasoning and justification. Metaethical questions for analysis include whether social morality is objective or subjective, relative or nonrelative, and rational or emotive.

Descriptive ethics and metaethics are grouped together as nonnormative because their objective is to establish what factually or conceptually is the case, not what ethically ought to be the case. Often in this book we cite descriptive ethics—for example, by presenting what professional codes require. However, the underlying question is usually whether the described prescriptions of such codes are defensible, which is a normative issue. We also frequently engage in metaethics. Chapter 1 is largely an exercise in metaethics, whereas Chapter 2 is devoted to general normative ethics. However, such distinctions should be used with caution.[1] Metaethics frequently takes a sharp turn toward the normative, as our discussion of the justification of moral standards later in this chapter indicates. Likewise, normative ethics relies heavily on metaethics. Just as no sharp distinction should be drawn between practical ethics and normative ethics, so no clear line should be drawn to distinguish normative ethics and metaethics.

The Common Morality

In addressing the question "What is morality?" we may be tempted to answer that morality is a theory about right and wrong. However, the words *ethics* and *morality* should not be confined to theoretical contexts. *Ethical theory* and *moral philosophy* are the appropriate terms to refer to philosophical reflection on morality's nature and function. The purpose of theory is to enhance clarity, systematic order, and precision of argument in our thinking about morality. The term *morality* refers to social conventions about right and wrong human conduct that are so widely shared that they form a stable (although usually incomplete) communal consensus, whereas *ethics* is a general term referring to both morality and ethical theory. (The terms *ethical* and *moral* are here construed as identical in meaning.) *Ethical theory, moral philosophy,* and *philosophical ethics,* then, are reserved for philosophical theories, including reflection on the common morality. Similarly, *moral theology, theological ethics,* and *religious ethics* are reserved for reflection on morality in light of theological convictions in particular religious traditions.

In its broadest and most familiar sense, the *common morality* comprises socially approved norms of human conduct. For example, it recognizes many legitimate and illegitimate forms of conduct that we capture by using the language of "human rights." The common morality is a social institution with a code of learnable norms. Like languages and political constitutions, the common morality exists before we are instructed in its relevant rules and regulations. As we develop beyond infancy, we learn moral rules along with other social rules, such as laws. Later in life, we learn to distinguish general social rules held in common by members of society from particular social rules fashioned for and binding on the members of special groups, such as the members of a profession.

The common morality is not faultless or complete in its recommendations, but we will later argue that it forms the right starting point for ethical theory.

Codes of Professional Ethics

Influential reflection on problems of biomedical ethics within the health care professions has evolved through formal codes of medical and nursing ethics, codes of research ethics, and reports by government-sponsored commissions. *Particular* codes written for groups such as physicians, nurses, and psychologists are sometimes defended by appeal to general norms such as not harming others (nonmaleficence) and respecting autonomy and privacy, even if these were not explicitly considered in the drafting of the codes. Codes can be validly criticized or defended by appeal to general norms, as can many public policies and regulations that have been formulated to guide professionals' conduct.

Before we assess professional codes, the nature of professions needs brief discussion. According to Talcott Parsons, a profession is "a cluster of occupational roles, that is, roles in which the incumbents perform certain functions valued in the society in general, and by these activities, typically earn a living at a full-time job."[2] Under this definition circus performers, exterminators, and waitresses are professionals; prostitutes probably are not (because their function is not "valued in the society in general"), despite prostitution's reputation as "the world's oldest profession." However, it is not surprising to hear prostitution characterized as a profession, inasmuch as the word *profession* has come, in common use, to mean almost any occupation in which a person earns a living.

We need a more restricted meaning for the term *profession,* as used in *professional ethics.* Professionals are usually identified by their commitment to provide important services to clients or consumers and by their specialized

training. Professions maintain self-regulating organizations that control entry
into occupational roles by formally certifying that candidates have acquired the
necessary knowledge and skills. The concept of a medical professional is
closely tied to a background of distinctive education and skills that patients
typically lack and that morally must be used to benefit patients. In learned
professions such as medicine the background knowledge of the professional
derives from closely supervised training, and the professional is one who provides a service to others. However, not all professions are either learned or
service-oriented.

Health care professions typically specify and enforce obligations, thereby
seeking to ensure that persons who enter into relationships with their members
will find them competent and trustworthy. The obligations that professions attempt to enforce are role obligations that are correlative to the rights of other
persons. Problems of professional ethics usually arise from conflicts of values,
sometimes conflicts within the profession and sometimes conflicts of professional commitments with commitments of persons outside the profession. A
professional code represents an articulated statement of the role morality of the
members of the profession, and in this way professional standards are distinguished from standards imposed by external bodies such as governments (although their norms sometimes overlap and agree).

Codes also often specify rules of etiquette and responsibilities to other members of the profession. For example, one historically significant code of the
American Medical Association instructed physicians not to criticize a fellow
physician previously in charge of a case and urged all physicians to offer professional courtesy.[3] These codes tend to foster and reinforce member-
identification with and institutional conformity to the prevailing values of the
profession. These professional codes are beneficial if they effectively incorporate defensible moral norms. Unfortunately, some professional codes oversim-
plify moral requirements or claim more completeness and authority than they
are entitled to claim. As a consequence, professionals may mistakenly suppose
that they satisfy all moral requirements if they obediently follow the rules of
the code, just as many people believe that they discharge their moral obligations when they meet all relevant legal requirements.

A pertinent question concerns whether the codes specific to areas of science,
medicine, and health care are comprehensive, coherent, and plausible in their
moral norms. Many medical codes develop the implications of some general
principles, such as "Do no harm," and of some rules, such as rules of medical
confidentiality. But only a few have anything to say about the implications of
other principles and rules, such as veracity, respect for autonomy, and justice,
which have been the subjects of intense contemporary discussion. Some of
these neglected principles and rules have recently been incorporated into statements of patients' rights that invoke, for example, the principle of respect for

autonomy and rules of veracity.[4] These statements of proper professional conduct do not derive from professional codes and differ from many codes by focusing on the *rights* of those receiving health services rather than on the *obligations* of health professionals. Unfortunately, such statements are also usually incomplete and lack an argued defense.

Reasons other than incompleteness and lack of stated justification also support skepticism about the adequacy of professional codes in health care. From the time of Hippocrates, physicians have generated codes without scrutiny or acceptance by patients and the public. These codes have rarely appealed to more general ethical standards or to a source of moral authority beyond the traditions and judgments of physicians. In some cases, the special rules in codes for professionals seem to conflict with and even override more general moral norms. The pursuit of professional norms in these circumstances may do more to protect the profession's interests than to introduce an impartial and comprehensive moral viewpoint. Other rules have traditionally been expressed in abstract formulations that dispense vague moral advice open to competing interpretations.

Related reservations about codes of medical ethics were poignantly expressed in 1972 by psychiatrist Jay Katz. Originally inspired by his outrage over the fate of Holocaust victims, Katz became convinced that only a persistent educational effort beyond traditional codes could provide meaningful guidance in research involving human subjects:

As I became increasingly involved in the world of law, I learned much that was new to me from my colleagues and students about such complex issues as the right to self-determination and privacy and the extent of the authority of governmental, professional, and other institutions to intrude into private life. . . . These issues . . . had rarely been discussed in my medical education. Instead it had been all too uncritically assumed that they could be resolved by fidelity to such undefined principles as *primum non nocere* or to visionary codes of ethics.[5]

Government Guidelines and Public Policy

Additional moral direction for health professionals and scientists is sometimes provided through the public policy process, which includes specific regulations and guidelines promulgated by government agencies. Public policies, such as those that fund health care for the indigent and those that protect subjects of biomedical research, usually incorporate moral considerations. Moral analysis is part of good policy formation, not merely a method for evaluating already formed policy.

Rights of patients and research subjects provide instructive examples. The U.S. government has promulgated several legally binding regulations intended to provide morally adequate protections for research subjects. In 1974, Congress created a national commission to recommend research guidelines to the secretary of the Department of Health, Education and Welfare (now the Department of Health and Human Services) that would become federal regulations unless the secretary publicly justified not implementing them. In 1980, a president's commission was assembled to further examine these issues in research and other issues, such as access to health care and decisionmaking in clinical-patient relations.[6] Finally, in December 1991, the Patient Self-Determination Act (PSDA) went into effect.[7] Congress passed this law as the first federal legislation to ensure that health care institutions inform patients about their rights under state law and about institutional policies to accept or refuse medical treatment and to formulate advance directives.

Several U.S. federal agencies and courts regularly use ethical premises in the development of their health policies, rules, decisions, or analyses. These agencies include the Centers for Disease Control (CDC), the National Institutes of Health (NIH), the Office of Technology Assessment (OTA), and the U.S. Supreme Court. On the state level, formal ethical analysis also often plays a prominent role in policy formation in bioethics. Examples include the widely examined work of the New York Task Force on Life and the Law and of the New Jersey Bioethics Commission. Such commission reports and government acts, along with other government policies pertaining to biomedicine, raise vital questions explored later in this book about the proper relation between government and professional groups in formulating standards of practice.

These questions are also raised by the prominent role of the courts in the United States in developing case law that sets standards for science, medicine, and health care. These legal decisions have been significant resources for ethical reflection about moral responsibilities and public policy. Examples include decisions about informed consent (see Chapter 3) and terminating life-sustaining treatment (see Chapter 4). In the latter, the line of court decisions since the Karen Ann Quinlan case in the mid-1970s constitutes a nascent moral tradition of reflection that has been influenced by extralegal writings on topics such as whether artificial nutrition and hydration should be viewed as a medical treatment subject to the same standards of decisionmaking as other forms of treatment.

The term *public policy* is used in this text to refer to a set of normative, enforceable guidelines that have been accepted by an official public body, such as an agency of government or a legislature, to govern a particular area of conduct. The policies of corporations, hospitals, trade groups, and professional societies sometimes have a deep impact on public policy; but these policies are private rather than public (although these bodies are frequently regulated by public policies). A far closer connection exists between law and public policy, inasmuch as all laws constitute public policies; but not all public policies are, in the conventional sense, laws. In contrast to laws, public policies need not be explicitly formulated or codified. For example, an official who decides not to fund a program that has no prior history of funding formulates a public policy. Decisions not to act as well as decisions to act can constitute public policies.

Policy formation and criticism involve more complex forms of judgment than merely invoking ethical principles and rules.[8] The ethics of public policy must proceed from impure and unsettled cases, in which there are profound social disagreements, uncertainties, different interpretations of history, and imperfect procedures to resolve the disagreements. Obviously, no body of abstract principles and rules can dictate policy, because it cannot contain enough specific information or provide direct and discerning guidance. The specification and implementation of moral principles and rules must take account of problems of feasibility, efficiency, cultural pluralism, political procedures, uncertainty about risk, noncompliance by patients, and the like. Principles and rules provide background moral considerations for policy evaluation, but a policy must also be shaped by empirical data and by special information available in relevant fields of medicine, economics, law, psychology, and so on. In this process, moral principles and various uses of empirical data are often closely connected. For example, techniques such as risk–benefit analysis are not purely empirical and value-free, because they involve moral evaluation and need constraint by principles of justice.

Finally, when using moral principles or rules to formulate or criticize public policies, we cannot move with assurance from a judgment that *act x* is morally right (or wrong) to a judgment that a *law* or *policy y* is morally right (or wrong) because it mandates or encourages (or prohibits) act *x*. The judgment that an act is morally wrong, then, does not necessarily lead to the judgment that the government should prohibit it or refuse to allocate funds to support it. For example, one can consistently argue that sterilization or abortion is morally wrong without holding that the law should prohibit it or deny public funds to those who otherwise could not afford the procedure.

Similarly, the judgment that an act is morally acceptable does not imply that the law should permit it. For example, the thesis that active euthanasia is morally justified if patients face uncontrollable pain and suffering and request death is consistent with the thesis that the government should legally prohibit active euthanasia because it would not be possible to control abuses if it were legalized. We are not here defending particular moral judgments about the justifiability of such acts. We are maintaining only that the connections between moral action-guides and judgments about policy or law or legal enforcement are complicated and that a judgment about the morality of acts does not entail a particular judgment about law and policy. Factors such as the symbolic value of law, the costs of a program and its enforcement, and the demands of competing programs must also be considered.

Moral Dilemmas

Facing and reasoning through dilemmas to conclusions and choices is a familiar feature of the human condition. Consider a particular case (Case 1 in the appendix). Some years ago the judges on the California Supreme Court had to reach a decision about a possible violation of medical confidentiality. A man killed a woman after confiding to a therapist his intention to commit the act. The therapist attempted unsuccessfully to have the man committed but, in accordance with his duty of medical confidentiality to the patient, did not communicate the threat to the woman when the commitment attempt failed. The majority opinion of the court held that "When a therapist determines, or pursuant to the standards of his profession should determine, that his patient presents a serious danger of violence to another, he incurs an obligation to use reasonable care to protect the intended victim against such danger." Accordingly, this obligation extends to notifying the police and directly warning the intended victim. The justices in the majority opinion argue that therapists generally ought to observe the rule of medical confidentiality but that this rule must yield in this case to the "public interest in safety from violent assault." Although they recognize that rules of professional ethics have substantial public value, they hold that matters of greater importance, such as protecting others against violent assault, can override the rules.

In a minority opinion, a justice disagrees with this analysis and argues that doctors violate patients' rights if they fail to observe standard rules of confidentiality. If it were common practice to break these rules, he reasons, the fiduciary nature of the relationship between physicians and patients would begin to erode. The mentally ill would refrain from seeking aid or divulging critical information, because of the loss of trust that is essential for effective treatment. As a result, violent assaults would more than likely increase. This case presents a straightforward moral dilemma (as well as a legal dilemma), because both judges cite good and relevant reasons to support their conflicting judgments.

Moral dilemmas occur in at least two forms.[9] (1) Some evidence indicates that act x is morally right, and some evidence indicates that act x is morally wrong, but the evidence on both sides is inconclusive. Abortion, for example, is sometimes said to be a terrible dilemma for women who see the evidence in this way. (2) An agent believes that, on moral grounds, he or she both ought and ought not to perform act x. In a moral dilemma with this form, an agent is obligated by one or more moral norms to do x and obligated by one or more moral norms to do y, but the agent is precluded in the circumstances from doing both. The reasons behind alternatives x and y are good and weighty, and neither set of reasons is obviously dominant. If one acts on either set of reasons, one's actions will be morally acceptable in some respects but morally unacceptable in others. Some have viewed the intentional cessation of lifesaving therapies in the case of persistent vegetative state patients, such as Karen Ann Quinlan and Nancy Cruzan, as dilemmatic in this second way.

Dilemmas can be created by conflicting moral principles and rules, as popular literature, novels, and films about difficult choices often illustrate. For example, an impoverished person steals to save a family from starvation, a mother kills one of her children to save a second child, or a person lies to protect a family secret. The only way to comply with one obligation in such situations is by contravening another obligation. No matter which course is elected, some obligation must be set aside. However, it is both awkward and misleading to say that we are, in the circumstances, obligated to perform both actions. We should discharge the obligation that in the circumstances overrides what we would have been firmly obligated to perform were it not for the conflict.

Conflicts between moral requirements and self-interest sometimes produce a *practical* dilemma that is not a *moral* dilemma. If moral reasons compete with nonmoral reasons, difficult questions about priority can still be posed even though moral dilemmas are not present. Numerous examples appear in the work of anthropologist William R. Bascom, who collected hundreds of "African Dilemma Tales" transmitted for decades or centuries in African tribal societies. One traditional dilemma posed by the Hausa tribe of Nigeria is called *cure for impotence:*

A friend gave a man a magical armlet that cured his impotence. Later he saw his mother, who had been lost in a slave raid, in a gang of prisoners. He begged his friend to use his magic to release her. The friend agreed on one condition—that the armlet be returned. What shall his choice be?[10]

Hard choice? Perhaps, but not a hard *moral* choice. The obligation to the mother is moral in character, whereas retaining the armlet is a matter of self-interest. (We are assuming that no moral obligation exists to a sexual partner; in some circumstances such an obligation could produce a moral dilemma.)

Some moral philosophers and theologians have argued that many types of *practical* dilemmas exist, but never genuine *moral* dilemmas. They do not deny that agents experience moral perplexity, moral conflict, and moral disagreement in difficult cases, but they insist that if there were moral dilemmas two moral *oughts* would conflict, so that one could not perform an action that one ought to perform without forgoing another action one also ought to perform. The belief that one *cannot* do what one *ought* to do seems to these writers a confusion about the nature of moral language and obligation. Some major figures in the history of ethics have defended this conclusion, both because they accept one supreme moral value as overriding all other conflicting values (moral and nonmoral) and because they regard it as incoherent to allow contradictory oughts. The only *ought,* they maintain, is the *ought* generated by the supreme value.[11]

By contrast, we will maintain that various moral principles can and do conflict in the moral life. On some occasions the conflict produces a moral dilemma with no supreme principle to determine an overriding *ought*. Nonetheless, there are ways of reasoning about what should be done. In some cases the dilemma can be resolved, but in other cases the dilemma only becomes more difficult and remains unresolved after careful reflection.

Method, Justification, and Truth

A person of good will typically has no difficulty in making moral judgments about telling the truth and avoiding untenable conflicts of interest. Our routine moral judgments are reached through a mix of appeals to guidelines, models, parables, and the like. These moral beacons usually suffice, because we are not asked to deliberate about or justify either our judgments or the standards that underlie them. However, when we experience moral perplexity or uncertainty, we are led to moral reasoning about what morality recommends or requires of us and to deliberation about what we should do. From there we often find a need for moral justification.

Deliberation is primarily problem solving in which individuals or groups struggle to develop and assess their beliefs in order to reach a decision. As John Dewey once observed, deliberation begins with "an imaginative rehearsal of various courses of action." [12] As we deliberate, we usually consider which among the possible courses of action is morally justified, i.e. which has the strongest moral reasons behind it. The reasons we finally accept express the conditions under which we believe some course of action is morally justified.

But what, more precisely, is justification in ethics, and by what method of reasoning do we achieve it? *Justification* has several meanings in English, some specific to disciplines such as theology and law. In its customary sense, to justify is to show to be right, to vindicate, to furnish adequate grounds for, to warrant, and the like. In some theological traditions, justification is the condition under which a person is freed from sin and made righteous. In law, justification is a showing in court that one has a sufficient reason for one's claim or for what one has been called to answer. In ethical discourse, the legal sense provides the closest analogue. The objective is to establish one's case by presenting sufficient grounds for belief and action. To demonstrate that one is justified in a moral belief requires that one make explicit one's underlying warrants for the belief. A mere listing of beliefs will not suffice, because an *alleged* reason often provides no support for an intended conclusion. Not all reasons are good reasons, and not all good reasons are sufficient for justification. There is, then, a need to distinguish a reason's *relevance* to a moral judgment from its final *adequacy* for that judgment, and also to distinguish an *attempted* justification from a *successful* justification.

For example, the presence of dangerous toxic chemicals in a work environment was widely offered by chemical companies in the United States as a legally and morally sound reason to exclude women of childbearing age from a hazardous workplace, but in 1991 the United States Supreme Court overturned these policies as discriminatory.[13] The dangers to health and life presented by hazardous chemicals constitute a *good* reason for removing employees from the workplace, but this reason may not be a *sufficient* reason for a ban exclusively directed at women. No matter which position is defended, we expect proponents to give us a further account of why their reasons amount to both good and sufficient reasons.

Three Models of Justification

Several models of justification are operative in ethical theory. We will evaluate three that are both instructive and influential. The first approaches justification from a top-down perspective that emphasizes general norms and ethical theory as the proper basis for reaching correct moral judgments. The second approaches justification from a bottom-up perspective that emphasizes moral tradition, experience, and judgment as the bases of both general norms and theory. The third refuses to assign priority to either a top-down or a bottom-up strategy. We will discuss each approach and then defend a version of the third that incorporates important parts of the other two.

Deductivism: the covering-precept model. The covering-precept model—or, as it is now widely called, *deductivism*—holds that justified moral judgments are deduced from a preexisting theoretical structure of normative precepts that cover the judgment. This model is inspired by justification in disciplines such as mathematics, in which a claim is shown to follow logically (deductively) from a credible set of premises. This mode of argument is occasionally used in ethics, and deductivists promote it as the best model of justification. The idea is that justification occurs if and only if general principles and rules, together with the relevant facts of a situation, support an inference to the correct or justified judgment(s). This model is simple and conforms to the way virtually all persons first learn to think morally: Moral judgment is the application of a rule (principle, ideal, right, etc.) to a clear case falling under the rule. The deductive form is therefore sometimes said to be a top-down "application" of general precepts—a conception that motivated use of the term "applied ethics." The deductive form in the application of a rule is the following (here using what is *obligatory,* rather than what is *permitted* or *prohibited,* although the deductive model is the same for all three):

1. Every act of description *A* is obligatory.
2. Act *b* is of description *A*.

Therefore,

3. Act *b* is obligatory.

Using this schematic model, consider the following example:

1x. Every act in a patient's overall best interest is obligatory for the patient's doctor.[14]

2x. Act of resuscitation *b* is in this patient's overall best interest.

Therefore,

3x. Act of resuscitation *b* is obligatory for this patient's doctor.

Covering precepts, as in 1 and 1x, occur at various levels of generality. A particular judgment, belief, or hypothesis may be justified by bringing it under one or more moral rules, or the rules may be justified by bringing them under principles, or both rules and principles may be defended by a full ethical theory. As an example, consider a nurse who refuses to assist in an abortion procedure. The nurse might attempt to justify the act of refusal by the rule that it is wrong to kill an innocent human being intentionally. If pressed for further justification, the nurse may justify this moral rule by reference to a principle of the sanctity of human life. Finally, the particular judgment, the rule, and the principle might all be justified by an ethical theory that is only implicit and inchoate in the nurse's original judgment. From a pure deductivist perspective, the primary problem of practical ethics is the choice of an ethical theory to apply. Presumably each competitive theory commits a proponent to different norms and different solutions of problems.

This model, then, directs attention from the level of particular judgments to a covering level of generality (rules and principles that cover and justify particular judgments), and then on to the level of ethical theory (which covers and warrants rules and principles). This account can be diagrammed as follows (where each arrow describes a direction of justification, indicating that the less general assertion is justified by appeal to a covering, more general norm):

4. Ethical Theory

↑

3. Principles

↑

2. Rules

↑

1. Particular Judgments

This model functions smoothly whenever a judgment can be brought directly under a rule or a principle without intervening complexities such as appeals to several principles.

This model of justification does not capture how moral reasoning and justification proceed in complicated cases. Oversimplification appears in its linear conception, in which particular judgments and rules are derivative in direct descent from more general principles. Consider the apparently deductivist justification, "You must tell Mr. Sanford that he has cancer and will probably die soon, because rules of truthfulness are essential in order to properly respect the autonomy of patients." The above model suggests that "You should not lie to Mr. Sanford" descends in its moral content directly from the covering principle "You should respect autonomy" and the covering rule "You shouldn't lie to patients." While much in the moral life does conform loosely to this linear-dependence conception, much also does not. For several reasons, actual moral reasoning and justification exhibit greater complexity.

First, general action-guides are reciprocally related to particular elements in experience. The relationship between general norms and the particulars of experience is bilateral, not unilateral; and, as Jerome Schneewind has argued, there is no "context-free order of dependence among moral propositions."[15] Whether a moral proposition is known by inference or is known independent of inference cannot be decided by either the content of the proposition or its degree of generality. Whether a general action-guide depends on particular experiences, or the converse, is a matter of what is known and inferred in specific contexts (so-called inferential support as a matter of epistemic context). Moral beliefs arise both by generalization from the particulars of experience and by making judgments in particular circumstances by appeal to general precepts. No essential order of inference or dependence fixes how we come to have moral knowledge.

Particular moral judgments also often involve specifying and balancing norms for concrete situations, not merely bringing a particular judgment under a covering rule or principle. The abstract rules and principles in moral theories are extensively indeterminate; that is, the act descriptions used to point to obligations lack sufficient determinative content for many practical judgments. In the process of specifying and balancing norms and in making particular judgments, we often must consider factual beliefs about the world, cultural expectations, judgments of likely outcome, precedents previously encountered, and the like to help fill out and give weight to rules, principles, and theories.

Moral judgments about the justifiability of abortion, for example, typically depend less on moral rules and principles than on beliefs about the nature and development of the fetus. Disputants agree on the general rule that it is wrong to kill innocent persons directly, but traditional customs, scientific theories, metaphysical convictions, conceptual accounts, and religious beliefs often underlie interpretations of situations. As a result, moral debate sometimes stems more from disagreement about the correct scientific, metaphysical, or religious description of the situation or from different conceptual accounts than from disagreement about the relevant moral action-guides.

The facts of a situation are often such that no general norm (principle or rule) clearly applies, even if we do not disagree about the rules or principles of morality. For example, destroying a nonviable human fetus is not a clear violation of rules against killing or murder, and the rule that one has a right to protect one's bodily integrity and property similarly does not clearly apply to the problem of abortion. Typically, the facts are complex, and several different moral norms can be brought to bear on the facts, but with inconclusive and even contradictory results. In the case of abortion, even if we have our facts straight, the choice of facts and the choice of rules will generate a judgment that is incompatible with another choice of facts and rules. Obtaining the right set of facts and bringing the right set of rules to bear on these facts are not reducible to either a deductive form of judgment or to the resources of a general ethical theory.

A further problem is that deductivism creates a potentially infinite regress of justification—a never-ending demand for final justification—because each level of appeal to a covering precept requires some further level to justify it. This problem can perhaps be handled by presenting a principle that is self-justifying or one that it is irrational not to hold. But if a deductivist demand for justification were to entail that every standard used to justify another standard is itself unjustified until brought under a different covering precept, then there cannot in principle be an adequate foundation for moral judgments or for the institution of morality.

Finally, the appeal to a level of theory in the covering-precept model suggests that only one correct normative theory exists, yet many distinct theories have been developed and ably defended, without a substantial consensus as to which system best meets the tests for a theory. To the surprise of many philosophers in the last twenty years, often little is lost in practical moral decisionmaking by dispensing with general moral theories. The rules and principles shared across these theories typically serve practical judgment more adequately (as starting points) than the theories. This paradox provides one major reason why covering-precept theories have recently diminished in influence. However, the model of covering precepts applied in moral judgments can be retained as long as it is complemented by other models that capture the greater complexity of moral reasoning and justification.

Inductivism: the individual-case model. Many people now believe, and we agree, that moral justification proceeds inductively (bottom-up) no less than deductively (top-down). Inductivism maintains that we must use existing social agreements and practices as a starting point from which to generalize to norms such as principles and rules, and inductivists emphasize the role of particular and contextual judgments as a part of our evolving moral life. A society's moral views are not justified by an ahistorical examination of the logic of moral discourse or by some theory of rationality, but rather by an embedded moral tradition and a set of procedures that permit new developments. A static or morally conservative conception of morality does not follow from this account as long as the tradition presents methods and procedures for reflection on and development of the tradition. New experiences and innovations in the patterns of collective life lead to modifications in beliefs, and the institution of morality cannot be separated from a cultural matrix of beliefs that has grown up and been tested over time.

Inductivists argue that induction (reasoning from particular instances to general statements about the instances), including analogy (a species of induction in which similarities between acts or events support a hypothesis that the acts or events are similar in other respects as well), is central to deliberation and justification. They propose that certain kinds of cases and particular judgments about those cases can be relied upon as warrants for the acceptance of moral conclusions independently of either general norms or a historical tradition. As our experience and thinking develop, we then generalize beyond such judgments to create rules and principles that carry over to analogous contexts, but the inductivist believes that these rules and principles are *derivative* in the order of knowledge, not primary. New and revealing cases lead us to progressive refinements of our judgments and generalizations. Moral rules, then, are provisionally secure points in a cultural matrix of guidelines.

Consider an example from the explosion of interest since 1976 in surrogate decision making. A series of cases beginning with the aforementioned Quinlan case challenged medical ethics and the courts to develop virtually an entire new framework of substantive rules for responsible surrogate decisionmaking about life-sustaining treatments, as well as authority rules regarding who should make those decisions. This framework was created by working through cases analogically, and testing hypotheses against preexisting norms. In both ethics and law, a string of cases with some similar (and some dissimilar) features set the terms of the ethics of surrogate decisionmaking. Even when a principle or rule was not entirely novel in a proposed framework, its content was shaped by problems needing resolution in the cases. Gradually a loose consensus emerged in the courts and in ethics about a framework for such decisionmaking. It would falsify history to say that this framework was already available and was simply applied to new cases.

Some inductivists incorporate features of deductivism, understood as the claim that preexisting norms inform the process of analogy. This breadth makes inductivism more attractive, but not beyond criticism. There remains a certain haziness about the role of particular experience and individual judgment. If the judgments of individuals are basic, do general norms have any critical power to correct biased judgments or biases that might be built into the norms generalized from particular experiences? What could give general rules authority over particular judgments?

During a discussion of this problem, Henry Sidgwick argues that if "the particular case can be satisfactorily settled by conscience [i.e., practical judgment] without reference to general rules," then "we shall have no *practical* need of any such general rules." And if we were able to "form general propositions by induction from these particular conscientious judgments, and arrange them systematically . . . any interest which such a system may have will be *purely speculative*," not practical.[16] Sidgwick's insight cuts deeply against pure inductivism, and he builds on the point by arguing that we use general norms to constrain and evaluate particular moral judgments. Theoretical interest in the general, then, is not entirely for the sake of a speculative typology of what we already know from particular cases. We are interested in general standards because we are interested in knowing what we ought to do.

A familiar problem haunts pure inductivism. We frequently criticize inadequate judgments or traditions by appeal to general standards such as human rights. What justification could inductivism provide for our use of these general standards if they stand outside the framework of experience and judgment being criticized? Inductivism also has little to say about the common circumstance in which conflicting judgments are reached in particular cases by equally well-informed and dispassionate moral agents. Inductivist theory, then, needs to be buttressed by an account of the proper role of rules and principles in adjudicating disputes and constraining particular judgments.

Before we look at the third of our three approaches to see if it can meet this condition, we need to summarize how far we have come. We have discussed two broad approaches to method and justification. When the limits of these approaches are acknowledged, we see no inconsistency between them and no reason to reject them outright. Inductivism rightly emphasizes that history and philosophy do not produce static systems of moral norms. We constantly engage in reasoned decisionmaking, moving from new experiences and problems to new or more refined action-guides. Deductivism rightly notes that once we have a fairly settled (although not necessarily final) body of general guidelines, moral judgments are often warranted by direct appeal to those general guidelines.

A confusing feature of contemporary moral theory is that false rivalries and misleading statements of method often result from pigeonholing theories too readily, and assuming that the proponents of one method exclude the other methods in their moral thinking. Here are two examples involving writers in biomedical ethics to whom we return later (see pp. 94–96 and 106–107). First,

Bernard Gert and Danner Clouser express their method as follows: "In formulating theory we start with particular moral judgments about which we are certain, and we abstract and formulate the relevant features of those cases to help us in turn to decide the unclear cases." [17] This statement is arresting because Gert and Clouser have gained a reputation (whether deserved or not) as full-fledged deductivists. Yet this statement of method looks more like inductivism.

Second, Albert R. Jonsen and Stephen Toulmin have gained a reputation (whether deserved or not) as leading proponents of an inductivism that emphasizes analogical reasoning, case-by-case, from already well–navigated moral territory—a method they call *casuistry*. Yet they describe "good casuistry" as an account that "applies general rules to particular cases with discernment." [18] Jonsen forthrightly supports a strategy that delineates general principles that are powerful enough to provide direction in new territory in which analogies seem insufficient or perilous. For example, he maintains that our cumulative experience and case reports are often insufficient to provide answers to emerging moral problems presented in new areas such as reproductive technologies and genome mapping.[19] Toulmin similarly acknowledges that principles have a central role to play in contexts in which the actors are strangers rather than intimates, as occurs increasingly in health care institutions.[20] In these reflections, their methodology looks more deductivist than inductivist, although final assessment depends on whether they view principles as entailing or directly supporting particular moral judgments.

An important lesson can be learned about the use of these labels. It is easy to mislabel and stereotype philosophical methods. Once the label is attached, the theory can be altogether dismissed through objections such as those we have offered. We again emphasize that we find much more that is acceptable than unacceptable in the work of authors who are committed to these broad approaches to justification, and we will draw from both. At the same time, we do not regard even both approaches together as adequate. We will spend the remainder of this chapter depicting the third, and our favored, account of justification.

Coherentism. "Coherentism," as the third approach may be called, is neither top-down nor bottom-up; it moves in both directions. John Rawls has used the term *reflective equilibrium* to refer to the goal of this form of justification, and we will adopt some central features in his analysis. Rawls views the acceptance of theory in ethics as properly beginning with our "considered judgments," the moral convictions in which we have the highest confidence and believe to have the lowest level of bias. Rawls's term *considered judgments* refers to "judgments in which our moral capacities are most likely to be displayed without distortion." Examples are judgments about the wrongness of racial discrimination, religious intolerance, and political representation. These considered judgments occur at all levels of generality in our moral thinking, "from those about particular situations and institutions through broad standards and first principles to formal and abstract conditions on moral conceptions." [21]

A considered judgment of long-standing prominence in medicine is the rule, "A physician must not exploit patients for the physician's own gain because the patient's interests come first." This rule implies that it is inappropriate to permit certain physician interests to coexist with a fundamental commitment to the patient. For example, entrepreneurial physicians with ownership or investment interests in laboratories and for-profit medical centers have an unwarranted conflict of interest if they create self-referral arrangements with centers in which they have a financial interest. This conduct in medicine is unprofessional, although it is acceptable practice in many areas of business. Businesspersons are not always constrained by a rule such as "the client's and customer's interest comes first." One difference between many medical and business codes of ethics springs from the above rule, a considered judgment, about the patient–physician relationship.

However, even the considered judgments that we accept "provisionally as fixed points" are, Rawls argues, "liable to revision." The goal of reflective equilibrium is to match, prune, and adjust considered judgments so that they coincide and are rendered coherent with the premises of theory.[22] That is, we start with paradigm judgments of moral rightness and wrongness, and then construct a more general theory that is consistent with these paradigm judgments (so that they are as coherent as possible); any loopholes are closed, as are all forms of incoherence that are detected. The resultant action-guides are then tested to see if they too yield incoherent results. If so, they are readjusted or given up, and the process is renewed, because we can never assume a completely stable equilibrium. The pruning and adjusting occur by reflection and dialectical adjustment, in view of the perpetual goal of reflective equilibrium. To refer again to the rule about putting the patient's interest first, we would seek in biomedical ethics to make this rule as coherent as possible with other considered judgments about clinical teaching responsibilities, responsibilities in the conduct of research involving human subjects, and responsibilities to patients' families.

As we argue in Chapter 7, it is difficult to bring these diverse commitments into coherence along with other moral rules of impartiality and fairness. The rule about putting the patient's interest first is an acceptable starting premise, but it is not categorical for all possible cases. We are left with a range of options about how we should and should not specify and balance the rule. As long as contingent conflicts occur under the recognized and legitimate principles and rules of a moral system or theory, some measure of incoherence is present. For example, to take a relatively uncomplicated example in the ethics of organ transplantation, imagine that we are attracted to each of the following two moral considerations: (1) Distribute organs by expected number of years of survival, and (2) Distribute organs by time on the waiting list in order to give every candidate an equal opportunity. As they stand, these two distributive principles are not coherent, because use of either will undercut or eliminate the other. We can retain both (1) and (2) in a defensible theory of fair distribution, but to do so we will have to introduce limits on these principles as well as accounts of how to balance them. These limits and accounts will, in turn, have to be made coherent with other principles and rules, such as norms regarding discrimination against the elderly and the role of ability to pay in the allocation of expensive medical procedures.

This analysis suggests—rightly, we believe—that all moral systems present some level of indeterminateness and incoherence, revealing that they do not have the power to eliminate various contingent conflicts among principles and rules. So understood, coherence and reflective equilibrium are not achieved merely by an absence of inconsistencies in a system. Coherence is a matter of the further development and mutual support of norms.

So-called wide reflective equilibrium occurs when we evaluate the strengths and weaknesses of all plausible moral judgments, principles, and relevant background theories. That is, we incorporate as wide a variety of kinds of legitimate moral beliefs as possible, including hard test cases in experience.[23] We emphasize again the ideal (although not utopian) character of this procedure: No matter how wide the pool of beliefs, there is no reason to anticipate that the process of pruning, adjusting, and rendering coherent will either come to an end or be perfected. Virtually any set of theoretical generalizations achieved by reflective equilibrium will fall short of full coherence with considered judgments, and the only relevant model for moral theory is the *best approximation to full coherence*. We should assume that we are confronted with a never-ending search for defects of coherence, for counterexamples to our beliefs, and for novel situations.[24]

Ethical theories presumably can be made to cohere with considered judgments through this process of reflective equilibrium without incorporating controversial theoretical commitments about what is rational and irrational to accept. That is, many strands in the moral life can be reflectively considered, and brought into equilibrium, without introducing views about the rationality or irrationality of theories that deeply divide contemporary philosophers and theologians. From this perspective, moral thinking is analogous to hypotheses in science that are tested, modified, or rejected through experience and experimental thinking. Justification is neither purely deductivist (giving general action-guides preeminent status), nor purely inductivist (giving experience and analogy preeminent status). Many different considerations provide reciprocal support in the attempt to fit moral beliefs into a coherent unit. This is how we test, revise, and further specify moral beliefs. This outlook is very different from deductivism, because it holds that ethical theories are never sufficiently complete and applicable to moral problems; instead, theory itself must be tested for adequacy by its practical implications. But the goal of reflective equilibrium protects against the the risk of prejudice and merely intuitive moral judgments, because theory and practice have a relation of reciprocity that is mutually constraining.

To conclude, we have agreed with Rawls that justification is "a matter of the mutual support of many considerations, of everything fitting together into one coherent whole."[25] We will now pursue this thesis by developing our own coherence-based account of justification.

A Coherence Theory of Justification

In the late 1970s, when the first edition of this book was published, we sketched an account of justification for practical ethics in response to a crisis then bedeviling the underdeveloped field of biomedical ethics. At that time there was no sustained theory of biomedical ethics and no systematic account of its principles and normative rules. As our editions have evolved, many readers have requested that we state our views on method and justification in greater depth. We do so in this section.

Following Joel Feinberg and certain traditions in Greek philosophy, we initially described the relation between moral experience and moral theories as *dialectical*. We develop theories to illuminate experience and to determine what we ought to do, but we also use experience to test, corroborate, and revise theories.[26] If a theory yields conclusions at odds with our considered judgments—for example, if it allows children but not adults to be used without consent as subjects of biomedical research—we have reason to be suspicious of the theory and to modify it or seek an alternative theory. We regard this dialectical strategy as a way to work toward coherence between particular and general judgments.[27] As Feinberg notes, this procedure is similar to the reasoning that occurs in courts of law. On the one hand, if a principle commits one to an antecedently unacceptable judgment in a particular case, then one should modify or supplement the principle so as to render it coherent with one's particular and general beliefs taken as a whole. On the other hand, when a well-founded principle indicates the need to change a particular judgment, the overriding claims of coherence require that the judgment be adjusted.[28] It seems mistaken, then, to say that principles are not *drawn from* cases but only *applied to* cases. Furthermore, both general and particular considered judgments provide data for theory and are theory's testing ground. They lead us to modify and refine embryonic theoretical claims, especially by pointing to inadequacies in or limitations of theories.[29]

Although justification is a matter of coherence, bare coherence has seemed to many philosophers an insufficient basis for justification, because the substantive body of judgments and principles that cohere could themselves be morally unsatisfactory. There also could be a series of alternative coherent systems, each with a claim as valid as the next if coherence alone is the judge of theories. Moral justification and knowledge could never be achieved unless some criterion independent of coherence were added to the account. An example of this problem appears in the so-called Pirates' Creed of Ethics or Custom of the Brothers of the Coast.[30] Formed under a democratic confraternity of marauders circa 1640, this creed for pirates is a coherent, carefully delineated set of rules governing mutual assistance in emergencies, penalties for prohibited acts, the distribution of spoils, modes of communication, compensation for injury, and "courts of honour" that resolve disputes. This substantive body of rules and principles, although coherent, is morally unsatisfactory. Its appeal to "spoils," its awarding of slaves as compensation for injury, and the like involve immoral activities. But what justifies us in saying this coherent code is not an acceptable code of ethics?

This question points to the importance of starting with considered judgments that are settled moral convictions in a broad expanse of ethics, and then casting the net more broadly in specifying, testing, and revising those convictions. Coherentism is not exhausted by a relentless reduction of any set of beliefs to coherence. We start in ethics, as elsewhere, with a particular set of beliefs— the set of considered judgments (also called self-evident norms and plausible intuitions) that are acceptable initially without argumentative support. We cannot justify every moral judgment in terms of another moral judgment without generating an infinite regress or vicious circle of justification in which no judgment is justified. The only avenue of escape is to accept some judgments as justified without recourse to other judgments; and these judgments form our starting point.

These considered judgments typically have a history rich in moral experience that underlies our sense that they are credible and trustworthy; considered judgments are therefore not merely a matter of individual intuition. Any moral certitude associated with these norms is likely to derive from beliefs that are acquired, tested, and modified over time in light of the purposes served by the norms. Coherence among these initial norms is essential to their acceptability, and incoherence is a sound reason for rejecting one or more such "foundational" but fallible propositions. The Pirates' Creed, while coherent and acceptable among pirates, fails the test of initial moral acceptability.

Although we start with initially credible premises, the persons, codes, institutions, or cultures from which the premises descend need not themselves be in every case highly reliable or comprehensive in their reports and documents.

For example, the Hippocratic tradition—the starting point in medical ethics for centuries—has turned out to be a limited and generally unreliable basis for medical ethics. This problem can be overcome in a coherence theory by calling on a wider body of experience to collect points of convergence. To use an analogy to eye-witnesses in a courtroom, if a sufficient number of entirely independent witnesses converge to agreement in recounting the facts of a story, the story gains credibility beyond the credibility of the individuals who tell it. At the same time, we can eliminate the witnesses' stories that do not converge and cannot be made consistent with the main lines of convergence. The greater the coherence in a broadly based account that descends from initially credible premises, the more likely we are to believe it. The same point holds in moral theory: As we increase the number of accounts, establish convergence, and increase coherence, the best explanation is that the beliefs are justified and should be accepted. When we find wider and wider confirmation of hypotheses, the best explanation is that these hypotheses are the right ones. Such confirmation is the proper goal of moral theory, however difficult it is to accomplish.

Does it follow that there are *degrees* of justification and knowledge? Often we can achieve only a weak coherence, using more or less reliable reports. The extent to which we can speak of beliefs as justified is comparative, contingent upon evidence and degree of coherence. Justification in areas such as abortion and animal rights is notoriously difficult and resistant to solution by the ideal of reflective equilibrium. We will hereafter assume, without further argument, that this degrees-of-justification thesis is correct. We will also assume that coherence is the central condition in moral justification, but not that it is the sole condition.

In addition, several safeguards should be recognized in attempts to reconstruct moral concepts and norms on the model of coherence. These safeguards function to protect against faulty coherence construction. One safeguard can be called *the resemblance condition*. It requires that a moral account remain faithful to (resemble) the principles and concepts that provided the starting point for that account. In selecting data and constructing a theory, the final product should resemble the principles and concepts that it explicates. For example, suppose we are attempting to develop a coherent account of medical confidentiality that will remove several serious problems in our current system of confidentiality in health care; and suppose we rely so heavily in our account on rights of privacy that we completely lose sight of medical confidentiality and supply only a list of rights of privacy that hospitals should acknowledge. If confidentiality has been lost in the process, we have failed to do what we set out to do, even if the product exhibits a high degree of coherence. Although room exists for disagreement over the proper departure point for such an analysis (and therefore over what the final product must resemble), resemblance is an important constraint on theory construction. At the same time, resemblance must not be construed to preclude the possibility of radical shifts in normative perspective. The resemblance condition does not allow one principle or concept to be turned into another, but it also does not preclude our coming to the view that our initial judgment or position was flatly wrong.

Second, *universalizability* is a widely accepted condition that serves a safeguarding function. This condition does not imply that a society's distinct norms (those that differ from another society's) logically could not constitute a moral code or that all moral judgments and standards are identical for all persons— leaving no room for individual or group differences, for diverse moral traditions, for special relationships, and for autonomous judgments and moral disagreements. Rather, the condition of universalizability requires that any person who judges that action x is morally required (or morally worthy, morally virtuous, etc.) in circumstance C_1 is thereby committed to the premise that x is morally required (or morally worthy, morally virtuous, etc.) in circumstance C_2 if C_1 and C_2 are not different in any morally relevant respect. One therefore can universalize by advocating that all persons act in a certain way in a type of circumstance; but equally informed, rational, and impartial persons can advocate different actions in that type of circumstance. Universalizability is not a moral norm parallel to a material principle of justice or a demand for equal treatment; it is a formal condition rather than a substantive principle.

This condition implies that basic moral principles must be formulated in terms of universal rather than particular properties. Morality does not, for example, recognize a relevant difference between *I* and *he* or *she* in formulating norms of right or wrong.[31] This is one way in which morality protects against bias, prejudice, and idiosyncratic preference—at the same time recognizing that relevant differences exist between persons such as being a parent, being a supervisor, being experienced in a job, and the like. Universalizability, then, demands consistency of commitment within a moral system of judgments, rules, and principles, but it leaves open for discussion exactly what will count as morally relevant similarities and differences and whether unanimity is reachable over principles and rules.

Other safeguards also deserve mention. The comparative endurance, resilience, and output power of a principle or theory are clearly points in its favor. That a principle or theory *endures* through competitive encounters, is *adaptive to novelty,* and meets new problems with *creative and practical solutions* are all criteria of acceptability that promote reflective equilibrium. In Chapter 2 we develop a framework for theory construction that further supports the thesis that degrees of adequacy in theory are to be expected. In defending a coherence theory of justification, then, we do not mean to suggest that the criterion of coherence alone determines the merit of a theory.

Coherence and Noncoherence Accounts of Truth

It is customary in moral theory, epistemology, and philosophy of science to distinguish truth and justification. Problems such as the one encountered in our discussion of the Pirates' Creed suggest to some people that a moral theory must be *true,* not merely coherent. Others urge that a coherence theory of justification can double as a theory of truth. The idea is that convergence toward truth, not simply justification, is achieved by coherence (using an ideal such as reflective equilibrium). Still others deny this claim, saying that coherence is not constitutive of truth. They ask whether if several inconsistent theories generated from plausible initial premises can each claim a strong measure of internal coherence and consistency, we must then say that several true theories exist—for example, several true theories of justice.

This question leads us to ask whether a better criterion exists of the truth of a moral system than coherence among its norms. The problem with this proposal is that if a coherence theory is the right account of justification and no alternative route exists to the justification of a moral claim, there is no alternative way to check up on the results of a coherence account except coherence together with careful inspection of initial premises and of the safeguarding conditions mentioned above. To demonstrate the falsity of a belief, one would have to present a reasoned challenge to the results in the coherence account. But how would this challenge be mounted, except by casting more broadly the net of beliefs brought into coherence, which is part of the method of coherence?

The best explanation in the face of unshakable coherence is that the system has captured what is right, virtuous, and the like. If this result is what moral truth consists in, then the net of coherence has captured the truth. We would likely make such a claim in parallel cases of scientific knowledge: If a stable coherence is achieved after repeated testing, the best explanation is that the system of scientific beliefs so achieved either expresses or approximates the truth. If this is a sound account of scientific truth, is it not likewise a sound account of moral truth?

Yet it is far from settled that this treatment of moral truth is adequate. It is doubtful that a successful body of coherent beliefs, no matter how stable, yields truth. For one reason, it is doubtful that moral statements have truth values and that truth is a category that should appear in moral theory. For another reason, we would need a theory of *truth,* itself a complicated and controversial subject. We are content to conclude here that justification successfully occurs in ethics and that the right approach to justification is the coherence account we have outlined above and will augment in Chapter 2. If, in addition, some want to say that *justified* beliefs are *true* beliefs, we have no objection to this language, but we make no such extended claim for the conclusions expressed in this volume, and we believe that such a claim is likely to produce more misunderstanding than illumination.

Specifying and Balancing Principles

We are now in a position to develop the methods of specification and balancing mentioned previously. These methods fill out the coherence model and provide strategies for the resolution of moral problems and the avoidance of intractable conflict.

Specification

Philosopher G. W. F. Hegel fittingly criticized Immanuel Kant for developing an "empty formalism" that preached obligation for obligation's sake, without any power to develop an "immanent doctrine of duties." Hegel thought all "content and specification" in a living code of ethics had been replaced by abstractness in Kant's account.[32] Ethical theory that features *principles* has been similarly accused.[33] These criticisms point to an important problem. Every general norm, indeed morality itself, contains regions of indeterminacy that need reduction through further development and enrichment. If the principles discussed in this book are to have sufficient content, we must be able to specify the content in a way that surpasses ethereal abstractness, while also indicating the cases that properly fall under the principles.[34] If a principle lacks adequate specificity, it is empty and ineffectual.

Consider a simple example of this problem. Nonmaleficence is the principle that we ought not to inflict evil or harm on others. This principle provides only a rough starting point for guidance about the conditions under which harmful actions are prohibited. Normally we regard causing someone's death as a harm, but are assisted suicide and voluntary active euthanasia *harmful* actions that are absolutely proscribed by the principle of nonmaleficence? Are acts of mercy killing themselves sometimes acts of nonmaleficence, or even beneficence? If we question whether a physician who helps a patient commit suicide thereby harms or benefits the patient, no guidance is forthcoming from an unspecified principle of nonmaleficence. Without further specification, nonmaleficence is a bare starting point for resolving such problems as assisted suicide and euthanasia.

Abstract principles, then, often must be developed conceptually and shaped normatively to connect with concrete action-guides and practical judgments. In tightening our principles, we must take into account various factors such as efficiency, institutional rules, law, and clientele acceptance. Eventually we need to provide a practical strategy for real-world problems involving the demands of political procedures, legal constraints, uncertainty about risk, and the like. In light of the indeterminacy inherent in general norms, we accept Henry Richardson's argument that the specification of our principles is essential to determining what counts as an instance of that principle and to overcome some moral conflicts. Richardson notes that we sometimes *apply* norms directly to cases and that we often try to *balance* conflicting norms. Both techniques work on some occasions. But in managing new, complex, or problematic cases, the first line of attack should be to specify our norms and thereby to specify unclarities and problems away. In difficult cases, direct application rarely works, whereas balancing often appears to be too subjective, and fails to reduce conflict or the potential for further conflict. Specification, then, is an attractive strategy for the hard cases as long as the specification can be justified.[35] Of course, many already specified rules will need further specification to handle new circumstances of conflict. Progressive specification often must take place to handle the variety of problems that arise, gradually reducing the dilemmas and circumstances of conflict that the abstract principle has insufficient content to resolve.

As a simple example of specification, consider again the rule "Doctors should put their patients' interests first." A fact of life in modern medicine in the United States is that patients sometimes can afford the best treatment strategy only if their physicians falsify information on insurance forms, or at least only thinly spread the truth. It does not follow from a proper understanding of the rule of patient-priority that a physician should act illegally by lying or distorting the description of a patient's problem on an insurance form. Our rules against deception and for patient-priority are not categorical demands, and they stand in need of specification to give fuller, more concrete moral advice to physicians who wonder whether they should deceive payers, and, if so, under which conditions.

Nonetheless, the specification of a physicians' commitment to patients and to nondeception faces many problems, as a recent survey of practicing physicians' attitudes toward deception illustrates. Dennis H. Novack and several colleagues used a questionnaire to obtain physicians' responses to four difficult ethical problems that potentially could be resolved by deception. In one scenario, a physician recommends an annual screening mammography for a 52-year-old woman who protests that last year her insurance company would not cover the test and she had to pay herself, although she could not afford it. A secretary suggests that the patient's insurance company would cover the costs of the mammography if the physician stated the reason as "rule out cancer" rather than "screening mammography," although the latter alone was the reason. Almost seventy percent of the physicians responding to this survey indicated that they would put "rule out cancer," and eighty-five percent of this group insisted that their act would not involve "deception."[36]

These physicians' decisions can be interpreted as crude attempts to specify rules against deception. Most physicians in the study apparently did not operate with the definition of deception favored by the researchers ("to deceive is to make another believe what is not true, to mislead"). Perhaps the physicians believed that deception involves withholding information from or misleading someone who has a *right* to that information, and also believed that an insurance company with unjust policies of coverage has no right to accurate information. Or perhaps they believed that "deception" occurs when one unjustifiably misleads another, and that it was justifiable to mislead the insurance company in these circumstances. Yet another possibility is that these physicians understood the rule against deception to prohibit only self-serving actions or actions that harm other individuals, or to permit deceptive actions on behalf of one's patients whose interests should come first.

These physicians would not agree on how to specify rules against deception as well as rules requiring that patients' interests be first. Each of the proposed specifications would resolve the conflict (or, perhaps better, would *dissolve* it), but there would be debate about the justifiability of each specification. This survey provides an example of eliminating an apparent dilemma without either "applying" or "balancing" norms, yet any *proposed* specification may fail to provide the most adequate or justified resolution. To say that a problem or conflict is "resolved" or "dissolved" is here only to say that norms have been made determinate in content so that, when cases fall under them, we can decide what ought to be done.

An adequate specification requires that one justify the claim that the proposed specification is coherent with other relevant moral norms. Specification is a way of resolving problems through deliberation, but no proposed specification is justified without a showing of coherence. All moral norms are, in principle, subject to such revision, specification, and justification. The reason for this constant need for further content, as Richardson puts it, is that "the complexity of the moral phenomena always outruns our ability to capture them in general norms."[37] These problems about specification do not undercut the practical point that we can sometimes satisfactorily resolve conflicts and dilemmas by adequate specification.

Whether our framework is a workable account for biomedical ethics depends in part on whether its principles and related rules can be specified and the specifications justified. The substantive rules, authority rules, and procedural rules discussed below (pp. 38–39) involve specifications of our framework principles, and much of the argument of Chapters 3–7 is intended to show this process in action.

However, we still need to note some limitations and weaknesses in the method of specification, to make clear that we do not view the method as a cure-all for our deepest dilemmas. First, opposition between the model of specification and the models of balancing and applying norms should not be overstated. Nothing in the model of specification indicates that there is a way around balancing in the very act of specifying principles and rules; and nothing in the model shows that straightforward application never works. In any given problematic or dilemmatic case, several competing specifications will typically constitute possible resolutions, thereby returning us to conflicts of the sort that drove us to specification in the first place. (We explicate the model of balancing below.) Second, if one believes, as we do, that some moral conflict is inevitable and cannot always be avoided or eliminated by even tightly knit specifications, then the method is suited only for contexts in which specification has a reasonable hope of acceptance. Third, making norms more specific does not itself preclude the use of dogmatic, biased, arbitrary, or irrational views to make one's favored conclusion correct by fiat. Even if a specification eliminates contingent conflict, the specification may be arbitrary, lack impartiality, or fail for other reasons. As Richardson forthrightly acknowledges, "once the operation of specification has been adequately understood, it may then be admitted that it should be supplemented by application and balancing in a more complex hybrid model."[38]

Specification as a method must be indissolubly connected with a larger model of coherence that appeals to considered judgments and to the overall coherence introduced by a proposed specification. This is a general model that we accept, as does Richardson (who holds that specification and the coherence ideal dovetail, but have distinctive roles). So understood, specification holds out the possibility of a continually expanding normative viewpoint that is faithful to initial beliefs (which are not renounced) and that tightens rather than weakens coherence among the full range of accepted norms.

What advantage, then, does specification have over other attempts to resolve problems? Richardson's response, like ours, is that this question should be "answered in terms of the overall coherence and mutual support of the whole set of moral norms. . . . A coherence standard for the rationality of specification . . . in effect carries the Rawlsian idea of 'wide reflective equilibrium' down to the level of concrete cases."[39] From this perspective, specification is one arm of a larger method of coherence—a view that reinforces our earlier arguments that the central condition of justification is coherence and that interpretation, construction, and reconstruction are essential in both ethical theory and practical ethics. A particular specification is justified only if it is more coherent with the whole set of relevant norms than any other available specification.

The upshot of our analysis of coherence and specification is the following: One goal of a moral theory, and central to its account of justification, is to move from general levels of theory to particular rules, judgments, and policies that are in close proximity to everyday decisions in the moral life. Like a tributary with many forks into different territories, the principles and rules in a theory can be made to fork outward through specification and feed different parts of the moral life. Appropriate specification conserves or elevates the coherence already present in the theory. When moral conflicts occur, specification supplies an *ideal* of repeated coherence testing and modification of a principle or rule until the conflict is specified away, but specification is also a useful tool for the development of *policies* in biomedical ethics.

To accept this ideal is not to assume that conflicts can always be specified away by developing rules or policies. The moral life will be plagued by contingent conflicts that cannot be eliminated. Our pragmatic goal should be a method of resolution that often helps, not a method that will invariably resolve our problems.

Balancing and Overriding

Principles, rules, and rights require *balancing* no less than *specification*. Principles (and the like) direct us to certain forms of conduct, but principles by themselves do not settle conflicts of principle. Whereas specification entails a substantive development of the meaning and scope of norms, balancing consists of deliberation and judgment about the relative weights of norms. Balancing sometimes occurs in specification, and specification also sometimes occurs in balancing. Specification and balancing can best be conceived as mutually facilitative approaches, methods, or strategies that fit coherently within the larger method of coherence outlined above. Balancing is especially useful for individual cases, whereas specification is especially useful for policy development.

Avoiding balancing through "absolute" norms. Throughout this book we view the norms to be balanced—principles, rules, rights, and the like—as *prima facie* (see below, pp. 33–37), and not as absolute, as rules of thumb, or as hierarchically (lexically or serially) ordered. However, some specified norms are virtually absolute, and therefore usually escape the need to balance. Examples include prohibitions of cruelty and torture, where these actions are defined as gratuitous infliction of pain and suffering. (Other prohibitions, such as rules against murder, are absolute only because of the meaning of their terms. For example, to say "murder is categorically wrong" is to say "unjustified killing is unjustified.")

Defensible substantive absolutes are thorough and decisive specifications of principles. They are rare and rarely play a role in moral controversy. More interesting are norms that are formulated with the goal of including all legitimate exceptions, but whose formulation remains controversial. An example is "Always obtain oral or written informed consent for medical interventions with competent patients, *except* in emergencies, in low-risk situations, or when pa-

tients have waived their right to adequate information." This norm clearly
needs interpretation and a specification of what constitutes an informed consent, an emergency, a waiver, and a low risk, but this rule would be absolute
if all legitimate exceptions were included in its formulation and specification.
Depending on how far specification goes and whether all exceptions are built
in and defended, a rule could turn out to be legitimately absolute and thereby
escape balancing because its potential for conflict with other principles and
rules would have been eliminated. However, if such rules exist, they are rare.
Moreover, in light of the enormous range of possibilities for contingent conflicts among rules, absolute rules are best construed as ideals rather than fin-
ished products.

Balancing prima facie norms. Drawing on W. D. Ross, we distinguish *prima
facie* obligations from *actual* obligations. *Prima facie obligation* indicates an
obligation that must be fulfilled unless it conflicts on a particular occasion with
an equal or stronger obligation. A prima facie obligation is binding unless overridden or outweighed by competing moral obligations. Acts often have several
morally relevant properties or consequences. For example, an act of lying may
also promote someone's welfare, and an act of killing may involve the relief
of pain and suffering as well as respect for a patient's autonomy through causing the patient's death at the patient's request. Such acts are at once prima
facie wrong and prima facie right, because two or more norms conflict in the
circumstances. The agent must then determine what he or she ought to do by
finding an actual or overriding (in contrast to prima facie) obligation; that is,
the agent must locate what Ross called "the greatest balance" of right over
wrong. An agent's actual obligation in the situation is determined by the balance of the respective weights of the competing prima facie obligations (the
relative weights of all competing prima facie norms such as beneficence, fidelity, and justice).[40] This metaphor of larger and smaller weights moving a scale
up and down graphically depicts the balancing process, but it may also obscure
what happens in the process of balancing by misleadingly suggesting an intuitive or subjective assessment. Justified acts of balancing entail that good reasons be provided for one's judgment.

For example, suppose a physician encounters an emergency case that would
require her to extend an already long day so that she would be unable to keep
a promise to take her son to the library. She will then engage in a process of
deliberation that leads her to consider how urgently her son needs the visit to
the library, whether they could go very late to the library, whether another
physician could handle the case, etc. If she determines to stay deep into the
night with the patient, this obligation will have become overriding because she
has a good and sufficient reason. A life hangs in the balance, and she alone
has the knowledge to deal adequately with the full array of the circumstances.

Her action of canceling her evening with her son, painful and distressing as it is, can be justified by this good and sufficient reason for doing what she does. Balancing, then, is a process of justification only if adequate reasons are presented.

One way of viewing this process brings it close to and perhaps merges it with specification. As David DeGrazia has pointed out to us, the good and sufficient reasons that one offers in *an act of balancing* can be viewed as a *specification of norms that incorporates one's reasons.* These reasons can be generalized for similar cases: "If a patient's life hangs in the balance and the attending physician alone has the knowledge to deal adequately with the full array of the circumstances, then the physician's conflicting domestic obligations must yield." This merging of specification and balancing has merits, but it may be too neat and too sweeping to handle all situations of balancing and specification. Balancing often eventuates in specification, but it need not; and specification often involves balancing, but it also might only add details. Accordingly, we do not propose to merge the two methods. The point is that balancing does not compete with specification, and they both coherently augment the model of coherence. We therefore propose that balancing and specification be seamlessly united with a general model of coherence that requires us to defend the reasons we give for actions and norms. As noted previously, balancing is particularly useful for case analysis, and specification for policy development.

Conditions that restrict balancing. As a response to criticisms that the model of balancing is too intuitive and open-ended, we can list a few minimal conditions that reduce the amount of intuition involved. These conditions add content to the requirement of giving good reasons for actions and norms. The following conditions must be met to justify infringing one prima facie norm in order to adhere to another (however, these conditions, being norms themselves, are also prima facie, not absolute):

1. Better reasons can be offered to act on the overriding norm than on the infringed norm (for example, typically if persons have a *right,* their interests deserve a special place when balancing those interests against the interests of persons who have no comparable right).
2. The moral objective justifying the infringement has a realistic prospect of achievement.
3. No morally preferable alternative actions can be substituted.
4. The form of infringement selected is the least possible, commensurate with achieving the primary goal of the action.
5. The agent seeks to minimize the negative effects of the infringement.

Although some of these conditions appear to be tautological, or at least entirely noncontroversial, in our experience they often are not observed in moral deliberation and would lead to different actions were they observed. For example, many proposals in biomedical ethics about the use of life-extending technologies seem to violate (2) by endorsing certain actions in which no realistic prospect exists of achieving the goals of a proposed medical intervention. Typically this occurs when the intervention is regarded by the health professionals as legally required, but in some cases the intervention occurs merely as a matter of routine practice. Even more commonly violated is condition (3). Actions are frequently performed without serious consideration being given to the range of preferable alternative actions that might be taken when one obligation is in conflict with another obligation. For example, in animal care and use committees, a common conflict involves the obligation to approve a good scientific protocol and the obligation to protect animals against unnecessary suffering. The protocol is typically approved if a standard form of anaesthesia is proposed in the protocol. But standard forms of anaesthesia are often not the best way to protect the animal, and further inquiry is needed to determine the best anaesthetic for the interventions proposed. In our schema of conditions, it is *unjustifiable* to approve the protocol or to conduct the experiment without this additional inquiry. Accordingly, we think the above conditions are morally demanding, not simply obvious or tautological. When conjoined with our requirements of coherence, these minimal conditions should help us achieve some measure of protection against arbitrary, purely intuitive judgments.

But even with these safeguards, controversy will arise regarding which norm should triumph in a particular conflict with another norm. We could try to introduce further criteria or safeguards, such as, "rights override non-rights" and "liberty principles override nonliberty principles," but these meta-rules are certain to fail in many circumstances in which rights claims and liberty interests are relatively minor. Honesty about the process of balancing and overriding compels us to return to our earlier discussion of dilemmas and to acknowledge that in some circumstances we will not be able to determine which moral norm is overriding. Balancing is further complicated by the wide range of relevant considerations. Sometimes we must consider matters such as whether a personal relationship with a long history gives special weight to one party's interests or claims, whether one party likely to suffer a loss can be compensated for the loss whereas another party cannot be compensated, and whether being responsible for causing a harm gives the party harmed a special claim that another party does not have. To illustrate the last circumstance, suppose X causes a harmful outcome to Y. We typically think Y has a greater claim for assistance or compensation from X than does Z who, like Y, has suffered a harmful outcome, but not one caused by X; Y's interests usually deserve more weight in X's balancing even if Z has suffered the greater harm.

In all of these cases some intuitive judgments and subjective weightings are unavoidable, just as they are everywhere in life when we must balance competing goods (for example, in the foods we eat, in the strategies we try in tennis, and in the way we allocate time in our daily schedules). But this fact does not reduce the process of balancing and overriding to arbitrary or merely subjective preferences. Consider a typical example. The principle of respect for autonomy and the principle of beneficence (which requires acts of preventing harm to others) sometimes conflict in the AIDS epidemic. Respect for autonomy sets a prima facie barrier to the mandatory testing of people who are at risk of HIV infection and whose actions may put others at risk, and yet society has a prima facie obligation to act to prevent harm to those at risk. The two prima facie principles conflict, but to justify overriding respect for autonomy, one must show that the mandatory testing of certain individuals is necessary to prevent harm and has a reasonable prospect of preventing harm. If it meets these conditions, mandatory testing will still need to pass the least-infringement test, and agents must seek to reduce the harmful effects (such as the negative consequences that individuals fear from testing). As we will see in Chapter 7, many (but not all) proposed forms of mandatory testing cannot be justified, because other available alternatives would have a higher probability of success without infringing personal autonomy.[41]

As with specification, the process of balancing cannot be rigidly dictated by some formulaic "method" in ethical theory. The model of balancing will satisfy neither those who seek clear-cut, specific guidance about what one ought to do in particular cases nor those who believe in a lexical or serial ranking of principles, with automatic overriding conditions. Some have therefore attempted to circumvent balancing judgments by delineating automatic-overriding features in their ethical theories. For example, some have spoken of rights as *trumps* (Ronald Dworkin) and as *side constraints* on permissible judgments (Robert Nozick). But these attempts have failed because the proposed trumps and side constraints themselves must be balanced in many circumstances (see Chapter 2, pp. 71–72).

Ross's distinction between prima facie and actual obligations, as well as his model of balancing, are also attractive in that they conform closely with our experience as moral agents. The lingering concern about the role of intuition and subjectivity, even in the context of giving good reasons, does not disqualify the model. We can reflect on troublesome moral problems even if plural and conflicting values make comparisons difficult. A plurality of values and judgments does not by itself stifle sound deliberation, balancing, justification, and decisionmaking. Almost daily we are confronted with situations in which we must make choices between plural and conflicting values in our personal lives, and we must balance several considerations. Some of these choices are moral, but many are nonmoral. For example, our budget may require that we make a choice between buying books or buying a train ticket to see our parents. Not having the books will be an inconvenience and a loss, and not visiting home will make our parents unhappy. The choice is not easy, perhaps, but usually we think through the alternatives, deliberate, balance, and reach a conclusion.

Our concern in this section has not been to produce a mechanistic method for balancing, any more than we produced a definitive method of specification in the preceding section. We have proposed that a model of balancing deserves the same serious consideration as the model of specification and that both are needed for an account of moral judgment. In reaching our conclusions about method and justification, we have yet to defend any normative premises or principles. In the remainder of this chapter, we will outline (but not yet defend) the structural features of the normative framework adopted in this book.

The Place of Principles

We defend what has sometimes been called the *four-principles approach* to biomedical ethics,[42] and also called, somewhat disparagingly, *principlism*.[43] These principles initially derive from considered judgments in the common morality and medical tradition that form our starting point in this volume. For example, the principle of beneficence derives, in part, from long-standing, professional role obligations in medicine to provide medical benefits to patients. Our goal is to specify and balance these principles by the methods of ethical theory previously discussed. Both the set of principles and the content ascribed to the principles are based on our attempts to put the common morality as a whole into a coherent package.

In this section we sketch our ethical framework by providing an analytical breakdown of its elements. We distinguish several types of normative action-guides as components in our framework, including principles, rules, rights, and virtues. Although rules, rights, and virtues are of the highest importance for health care ethics, principles provide the most abstract and comprehensive norms in the framework. These principles will be individually analyzed in later chapters. This chapter presents only the structural shell.

Four Clusters of Basic Principles

We begin with our assumptions. That four clusters of moral ''principles'' (in another framework they might be developed as ''rights,'' ''virtues,'' or ''values'') are central to biomedical ethics is a conclusion we have reached by the search for considered judgments and coherence, not a position that receives an argued defense. However, we will in later chapters defend the choice of each principle as well as the independent significance of each. We also operate with only a loose distinction between rules and principles. Both are normative generalizations that guide actions, but, as we analyze them, *rules* are more specific in content and more restricted in scope than principles. Principles do not function as precise action guides that inform us in each circumstance how to act in the way more detailed rules do. *Principles* are general guides that leave considerable room for judgment in specific cases and that provide substantive guidance for the development of more detailed rules and policies. This limitation is no defect in principles; rather, it is a part of the moral life in which we are expected to take responsibility for the way we bring principles to bear in our judgments about particular cases. We also need to distinguish both rules and principles from the coherent, systematic body of norms that comprise *theories*. Our discussion of the coherence theory has already given some insight into our views about the nature of theory and its construction, but we defer further discussion until Chapter 2.

The four clusters of principles are (1) respect for autonomy (a norm of respecting the decisionmaking capacities of autonomous persons), (2) nonmaleficence (a norm of avoiding the causation of harm), (3) beneficence (a group of norms for providing benefits and balancing benefits against risks and costs), and (4) justice (a group of norms for distributing benefits, risks, and costs fairly). Nonmaleficence and beneficence have played a central historical role in medical ethics, whereas respect for autonomy and justice were neglected in traditional medical ethics but have came into prominence because of recent developments.

To illustrate this point about historical significance and neglect, British physician Thomas Percival furnished our first well-formed doctrine of medical ethics in 1803. His work served as the prototype for the American Medical Association's (AMA) first code of ethics in 1847. Easily the dominant influence in both British and American medical ethics of the period, Percival argued (using somewhat different language) that nonmaleficence and beneficence fix the physician's primary obligations and triumph over the patient's preferences and rights in any circumstance of serious conflict.[44] Percival failed to foresee the power of principles of respect for autonomy and distributive justice, but in fairness to him, it should be acknowledged that considerations of respect for autonomy and distributive justice are now ubiquitous in discussions of biomedical ethics in a way they were not when he wrote in late eighteenth century Britain.

Types of Rules

In addition to the four clusters of principles, we defend several types of rules that specify principles and guide actions.

Substantive rules. Rules of truthtelling, confidentiality, privacy, fidelity, and various rules pertaining to the allocation and rationing of health care, omitting treatment, physician-assisted suicide, and informed consent need to be formulated as guides to action that are more specific than abstract principles. A typical example of a rule that specifies the principle of respect for autonomy by giving it more content is, "Follow a patient's advance directive whenever it is clear and relevant."

Authority rules. We also defend rules about decisional authority—that is, rules regarding *who* may and should perform actions. For example, *rules of surrogate authority* determine who should serve as surrogate agents in making decisions for incompetent persons, and *rules of professional authority* determine who, if anyone, should make decisions to override or to accept a patient's decisions if they are medically damaging and poorly considered. Another example is found in *rules of distributional authority* that determine who should make decisions about the allocation of scarce medical resources. These authority rules do not delineate substantive standards or criteria for making decisions. Substantive standards—such as *guidance rules* for surrogate decisionmaking (advance directives, substituted judgment, and best interests) and *rationing rules* for the allocation of scarce resources (such as constituency priority and medical utility)—are moral directives that belong in the first category of substantive rules. Although authority rules are distinct in type from substantive rules, they interact in both theory and practice. For instance, authority rules are justified in part by how well they express substantive rules and principles.

Procedural rules. We also defend rules that establish procedures to be followed. Procedures for determining eligibility for scarce medical resources and procedures for reporting grievances to higher authorities are typical examples. We often resort to procedural rules when we run out of substantive rules and when authority rules are incomplete or inconclusive. For example, if substantive or authority rules are inadequate to determine which patients should be given scarce medical resources, we resort to procedural rules such as first-come-first-served, queuing, and lottery. (See pp. 382–384 in Chapter 6.)

Rights, Virtues, Emotions, and Assorted Moral Considerations

Our framework of principles and rules, as expressed above, does not specifically incorporate the rights of persons, the character and virtues of the agents who perform actions, or the moral emotions. These moral considerations all merit attention in a comprehensive theory. Rights, virtues, and emotional responses are in some contexts of greater moral importance than principles and rules. For example, an ethics of virtue helps us see why good moral choices depend on more than principles, and it also allows us to assess a person's moral character in a richer way than an ethics of principles and rules does. At this point we note only two points about our basic framework. First, it does not exclude categories such as rights, emotions, and virtues; we will in due course incorporate these categories. Second, we believe that for biomedical ethics, which has concentrated on guidelines for action, principles and rules are both indispensable and central to the enterprise. However, we will qualify this conclusion in Chapters 2 and 8, in which we clarify the role of these various categories.

Conclusion

In this chapter we have explained why moral reasoning is more complicated than the outmoded label "applied ethics" suggests. We have also hinted at an interdisciplinary account of biomedical ethics. Any solidly grounded discipline of ethics involves obtaining relevant factual information, assessing its reliability, and mapping out alternative solutions to problems that have been identified. This mapping sometimes entails presenting and defending reasons in support of factual, conceptual, and moral claims, while at the same time analyzing and assessing basic assumptions and commitments. Ethical theory, then, is but one vital contributor among other disciplines, including medicine, nursing, public health, law, and the social sciences.

We limited our discussion of theory in this chapter primarily to questions of method, deliberation, justification, and truth. These problems belong to metaethics. Except for a brief sketch of our normative framework, we have avoided discussion of types of normative theory that stand to make a substantive contribution to biomedical ethics. That topic is the subject of our next chapter.

Notes

1. For discussion of whether a sharp distinction can be drawn between metaethics and normative ethics, see David O. Brink, *Moral Realism and the Foundations of Ethics* (Cambridge: Cambridge University Press, 1989).
2. Talcott Parsons, *Essays in Sociological Theory,* Rev. Ed. (Glencoe, IL: The Free Press, 1954), p. 372.
3. The American Medical Association Code of Ethics of 1847, largely adapted from Thomas Percival's *Medical Ethics; or a Code of Institutes and Precepts, Adapted to the Professional Conduct of Physicians and Surgeons* (Manchester: S. Russell, 1803), was a response to a crisis in public and professional confidence. See Donald E. Konold, *A History of American Medical Ethics 1847–1912* (Madison: State Historical Society of Wisconsin, 1962), ch. 1–3; and Chester Burns, "Reciprocity in the Development of Anglo-American Medical Ethics," in *Legacies in Medical Ethics,* ed. Chester Burns (New York: Science History Publications, 1977).

4. See Chapter 2 for a discussion of "The Patient's Bill of Rights." For its history, see Ruth R. Faden and Tom L. Beauchamp, *A History and Theory of Informed Consent* (New York: Oxford University Press, 1986), ch. 3.

5. Jay Katz, ed., *Experimentation with Human Beings* (New York: Russell Sage Foundation, 1972), pp. ix–x.

6. See the publications of the National Commission for the Protection of Human Subjects of Biomedical and Behavioral Research and of the President's Commission for the Study of Ethical Problems in Medicine and Biomedical and Behavioral Research, several of which are mentioned throughout this volume.

7. Omnibus Budget Reconciliation Act of 1990. Public Law 101–508 (Nov. 5, 1990), §§ 4206, 4751. See 42 USC, scattered sections.

8. See Dennis Thompson, "Philosophy and Policy," *Philosophy and Public Affairs* 14 (Spring 1985): 205–18; and a Symposium on "The Role of Philosophers in the Public Policy Process: A View from the President's Commission," with essays by Alan Weisbard and Dan Brock, in *Ethics* 97 (July 1987): 775–95.

9. See John Lemmon, "Moral Dilemmas," *Philosophical Review* 71 (1962): 139–58.

10. William R. Bascom, *African Dilemma Tales* (The Hague: Mouton, 1975), p. 145 (relying on anthropological research by Roland Fletcher).

11. See the essays in Christopher W. Gowans, ed., *Moral Dilemmas* (New York: Oxford University Press, 1987); see also Walter Sinnot-Armstrong, *Moral Dilemmas* (Oxford: Basil Blackwell, 1988) and Edmund N. Santurri, *Perplexity in the Moral Life: Philosophical and Theological Considerations* (Charlottesville: University Press of Virginia, 1987).

12. John Dewey, *Theory of the Moral Life* (New York: Holt, Rinehart and Winston, 1960), p. 135, and Dewey and James H. Tufts, *Ethics* (New York: Henry Holt and Co., 1908), p. 323.

13. *United Automobile Workers v. Johnson Controls, Inc.,* Slip opinion (Argued October 10, 1990—Decided March 20, 1991).

14. One who defends this proposition might wish to stipulate that it is possible for the doctor to perform the action, that the resources can be obtained, that no competing obligation is overriding in the circumstances, and so forth. However, the precise nature of a fully specified principle is independent of our present inquiry.

15. J. B. Schneewind, "Moral Knowledge and Moral Principles," in *Revisions: Changing Perspectives in Moral Philosophy,* ed. Stanley Hauerwas and Alasdair MacIntyre (Notre Dame, IN: University of Notre Dame Press, 1983), pp. 118–20.

16. Henry Sidgwick, *The Methods of Ethics* (Indianapolis, IN: Hackett Publishing Co., 1981), bk. I, ch. 8, § 2, p. 99.

17. K. Danner Clouser and Bernard Gert, "A Critique of Principlism," *The Journal of Medicine and Philosophy* 15 (April 1990): 232.

18. Albert R. Jonsen and Stephen Toulmin, *The Abuse of Casuistry* (Berkeley: University of California Press, 1988), p. 16.

19. Albert R. Jonsen, "Of Balloons and Bicycles or the Relationship between Ethical Theory and Practical Judgment," *Hastings Center Report* 21 (September–October 1991): 14–16.

20. Stephen Toulmin, "The Tyranny of Principles," *Hastings Center Report* 11 (December 1981): 31–39.

21. John Rawls, "The Independence of Moral Theory," *Proceedings and Addresses of the American Philosophical Association* 48 (1974–75): 8.

22. Rawls, *A Theory of Justice* (Cambridge, MA: Harvard University Press, 1971), pp. 20–21, 46–50, 579–80.

23. See Norman Daniels, "Wide Reflective Equilibrium and Theory Acceptance in Ethics," *Journal of Philosophy* 76 (May, 1979): 257ff. Henry Richardson has pointed out to us that Rawls does not make it a logically necessary condition of considered judgments that they be *shared* with others; nor does he make it a logically necessary condition of wide reflective equilibrium that it is shared. However, to make his enterprise of social justice work, the considered judgments he selects would have to be widely shared. The importance of shared agreement is brought out in Rawls's emphasis on his theory of justice as a liberal political theory. (Richardson also argues that Rawls's primary protection against local bias is in his account of the veil of ignorance rather than in wide reflective equilibrium. Of course one could argue that both serve this purpose.)

24. Compare Rawls, *A Theory of Justice*, pp. 195–201.

25. *A Theory of Justice*, pp. 21, 579.

26. *Principles of Biomedical Ethics*, 1st Ed. (1979), esp. pp. 13–14. Work in biomedical ethics in the 1970s consisted almost entirely of articles and essays. Various problem areas were treated, such as abortion, euthanasia, and the allocation of resources. The few systematic statements and their discussions were arranged in terms of these problem areas. Examples include Joseph Fletcher, *Morals and Medicine* (Princeton, NJ: Princeton University Press, 1954), Paul Ramsey, *The Patient as Person* (New Haven, CT: Yale University Press, 1970), and Howard Brody, *Ethical Decisions in Medicine* (Boston: Little, Brown and Company, 1976).

27. This perspective is suggested by Aristotle's discussion of dialectic as a means to first principles in the *Topics*; see *The Complete Works of Aristotle*, ed. Jonathan Barnes, vol. I (Princeton, NJ: Princeton University Press, 1984), 101a25–101b4.

28. Joel Feinberg, *Social Philosophy* (Englewood Cliffs, NJ: Prentice-Hall, 1973), pp. 34–35. Chaim Perelman's account also influenced us in our second edition (1983): "In morals absolute preeminence cannot be given either to principles—which would make morals a deductive discipline—or to particular cases—which would make it an inductive discipline. Instead, judgments regarding particulars are compared with principles and preference is given to one or the other according to a decision that is reached by resorting to the techniques of justification and argumentation." *The New Rhetoric and Humanities: Essays on Rhetoric and Its Applications* (Boston: D. Reidel, 1979), p. 33.

29. See Judith Jarvis Thomson, *Rights, Restitution, and Risk: Essays in Moral Theory* (Cambridge, MA: Harvard University Press, 1986), pp. 251–60.

30. Circa 1640. Published 1974 by Historical Documents Co.

31. See R. M. Hare, *Moral Thinking: Its Levels, Method and Point* (Oxford: Clarendon Press, 1981), p. 223. But see also proposed qualifications on this view introduced in our Chapter 2, especially in the discussion of the ethics of care.

32. G. W. F. Hegel, *Philosophy of Right*, T. M. Knox, trans. (Oxford: Clarendon Press, 1942), pp. 89–90, 106–7.

33. Clouser and Gert, "A Critique of Principlism," Ronald M. Green "Method in Bioethics: A Troubled Assessment," *The Journal of Medicine and Philosophy* 15 (1990): 179–97, and Stephen Toulmin, "The Tyranny of Principles."

34. As R. M. Hare notes, "any attempt to give content to a principle involves specifying the cases that are to fall under it. . . . Any principle, then, which has content goes some way down the path of specificity." *Essays in Ethical Theory* (Oxford: Clarendon Press, 1989), p. 54.

35. Henry S. Richardson, "Specifying Norms as a Way to Resolve Concrete Ethical Problems," *Philosophy and Public Affairs* 19 (Fall 1990): 279–310. See also David

DeGrazia's reflections on specification in "Moving Forward in Bioethical Theory: Theories, Cases, and Specified Principlism," *Journal of Medicine and Philosophy* 17 (1992): 511–39.

36. Dennis H. Novack, et al., "Physicians' Attitudes Toward Using Deception to Resolve Difficult Ethical Problems," *Journal of the American Medical Association* 261 (May 26, 1989): 2980–85.

37. Richardson, "Specifying Norms," p. 294. ("Always" in this formulation should perhaps be understood to mean "in principle always"; specification may, in some cases, reach a final form.) For an example of elementary specification (but not so called) using the four-principles approach, see Raanan Gillon, "Doctors and Patients," *British Medical Journal* 292 (1986): 466–69.

38. Richardson, "Specifying Norms," p. 280.

39. Ibid., pp. 299–300.

40. See W. D. Ross, *The Right and the Good* (Oxford: Clarendon Press, 1930), esp. pp. 19–36; and *The Foundations of Ethics* (Oxford: Clarendon Press, 1939).

41. See James F. Childress, "Mandatory Screening and Testing," in *AIDS and Ethics,* ed. Frederic G. Reamer (New York: Columbia University Press, 1991), pp. 50–76. For a sensitive attempt to balance the rights and interests of HIV infected surgeons and dentists against the rights and interests of their patients—an attempt that reaches conclusions similar to ours about balancing and overriding—see Norman Daniels, "HIV-infected Health Care Professionals: Public Threat or Public Sacrifice?," *The Milbank Quarterly* 70 (1992): 3–42, esp. 26–32.

42. See, for example, *Principles of Health Care Ethics,* ed. Raanan Gillon and Ann Lloyd (London: John Wiley & Sons, 1993).

43. Clouser and Gert, "A Critique of Principlism," pp. 219–36.

44. Thomas Percival, *Medical Ethics.* See note 4 above.

2

Types of Ethical Theory

A well-developed ethical theory provides a framework within which agents can reflect on the acceptability of actions and can evaluate moral judgments and moral character. This chapter concentrates on several types of ethical theory: utilitarianism, Kantianism, character ethics, liberal individualism, communitarianism, the ethics of care, casuistry, and common-morality accounts. Some knowledge of these theories is indispensable for reflective study in biomedical ethics because much of the field's literature draws on methods and conclusions found in these theories.

A conventional introduction to ethical theory explicates and then proceeds to criticize several leading ethical theories. Typically, the criticisms are so harsh that each theory seems demolished beyond repair. As a result, readers become skeptical about the value of ethical theory. This outcome is both unfortunate and unnecessary. Although defects and excesses appear in all theories, several contain insightful perspectives and compelling arguments. Only such theories are discussed in this chapter. Our goal is to eliminate what is unacceptable in these theories and to appropriate what is relevant and acceptable.

Occasionally we refer to our system and to arguments in this book as a *theory*. A word of caution is in order about this use of the word *theory*. This term is commonly used in ethics to refer to each of the following: (1) abstract reflection and argument, (2) systematic reflection and argument, and (3) an integrated body of principles that are coherent and well developed (in ways discussed in Chapter 1). We have attempted in this book to construct a coherent account adequate for the particular subject of biomedical ethics, but we do not claim to have developed or to presuppose any particular comprehensive ethical theory in ways suggested by (3). We engage *in theory* (for example, in evaluating other ethical theories), and so in abstract reflection and argument (1). We also present an organized system of principles, and so engage in systematic reflection and argument (2). But, at best, we present only some elements of a comprehensive *general* theory (3). Our relevant presuppositions and theses are presented in the section near the end of this chapter titled ''Principle-Based, Common-Morality Theories.''

Each section of this chapter, except the first and the last, is divided into subsections, as follows: (1) an overview of the characteristic features of the theory (introduced by examining how its proponents would approach a case); (2) a more detailed presentation of the salient features of the theory; (3) an examination of criticisms that point to the theory's limitations and problems; and (4) an indication of the theory's strengths. This structure suggests that we accept several moral theories. We are pluralists in that we accept as legitimate various *aspects* of several different theories advanced in the history of ethics.[1] However, we reject the view that all the leading principles in the major moral theories can be rendered coherent (they cannot), as well as the view that the major theories offer equally tenable moral systems (they do not).

Criteria for Theory Construction

We begin with eight conditions of adequacy for an ethical theory. These proposals for theory construction set forth exemplary conditions for theories, but not so exemplary that a theory could not satisfy them. That all available theories only partially satisfy the demands in these conditions is not of concern here. The objective is to provide a basis from which to assess the defects and the strengths of theories. Satisfaction of these conditions protects a theory from criticism as a mere list of disconnected norms generated from our pretheoretic beliefs.The same general criteria of success in a moral theory can be used for any type of theory (for example, a scientific theory or a political theory). The eight conditions that follow express these criteria.[2]

1. Clarity. First, a theory should be as clear as possible, as a whole and in its parts. Although we can expect only as much precision of language as is appropriate, more obscurity and vagueness exists in the literature of ethical theory and biomedical ethics than is necessary or justified by the subject matter.

2. Coherence. Second, an ethical theory should be internally coherent. There should be neither conceptual inconsistencies (for example, ''strong medical paternalism is justified only by consent of the patient'') nor contradictory statements (for example, ''to be virtuous is a moral obligation, but virtuous conduct is not obligatory''). Ralph Waldo Emerson dismissed a foolish consistency as "the hobgoblin of little minds, adored by little statesmen and philosophers and divines." However, consistency is not a *sufficient* condition of a good theory, only a *necessary* condition. If an account has implications that are incoherent with other established parts of the account, some aspect of the theory needs to be changed in a way that does not produce further incoherence. Following the analysis in Chapter 1, a major goal of a theory is to bring into coherence all its various normative elements (principles, rights, considered judgments, etc.).

3. Completeness and Comprehensiveness. A theory should be as complete and comprehensive as possible. A theory would be entirely comprehensive if it included all moral values. Any theory that includes fewer moral values will be somewhere on a continuum from partially complete to void of important values. Although the principles presented in this book under the headings of respect for autonomy, nonmaleficence, beneficence, and justice are far from a complete system for general normative ethics, they do, when specified, provide a sufficiently comprehensive general framework for *biomedical* ethics. We do not need additional principles such as promise keeping, avoiding killing, keeping contracts, and the like. However, we draw on our principles to help justify rules of promise keeping, truthfulness, privacy, and confidentiality, among others (see esp. Chapter 7), and these norms increase the system's comprehensiveness by specifying commitments in the fundamental principles, as *specification* is defined in Chapter 1.

4. Simplicity. If a theory with a few basic norms generates sufficient moral content, then that theory is preferable to a theory with more norms but no additional content. A theory should have no more norms than are necessary, and no more than people can use without confusion. However, morality is complicated, and any comprehensive moral theory will be immensely complex. We can demand only as much simplicity in a moral theory as its subject matter permits.

5. Explanatory Power. A theory has explanatory power when it provides enough insight to help us understand the moral life: its purpose, its objective or subjective status, how rights are related to obligations, and the like.

6. Justificatory Power. A theory should also give us grounds for *justified* belief, not a reformulation of beliefs we already possess. For example, the distinction between acts and omissions underlies many critical beliefs in biomedical ethics, such as the belief that killing is impermissible and allowing to die permissible. But a moral theory would be impoverished if it only expressed this distinction without determining whether the distinction justifiably grounds those beliefs. A good theory also should have the power to criticize defective beliefs, no matter how widely accepted those beliefs may be.

7. Output Power. A theory has output power when it produces judgments that were not in the original data base of particular and general considered judgments on which the theory was constructed. If a theory did no more than repeat the list of judgments thought to be sound prior to the construction of the theory, nothing would have been accomplished. For example, if the parts of a theory pertaining to obligations of beneficence do not yield new judgments about role obligations of care in medicine beyond those assumed in constructing the theory, this failure of output suggests that the theory is purely a classification scheme. A theory, then, must generate more than a list of the axioms present in pretheoretic belief.

8. *Practicability.* A proposed moral theory is unacceptable if its requirements are so demanding that they probably cannot be satisfied or could be satisfied by only a few extraordinary persons or communities. A moral theory that presents utopian ideals, paltry expectations, or unfeasible recommendations fails the criterion of practicability. For example, if a theory proposed such high requirements for personal autonomy (see Chapter 3) or such lofty standards of social justice (see Chapter 6) that, realistically, no person could be autonomous and no society could be just, the proposed theory would be deeply defective.

Other general criteria could be formulated, but the eight sketched above are the most important for our purposes. A theory can receive a high score on the basis of one criterion and a low score on the basis of another. For example, early in this chapter utilitarianism is depicted as an internally coherent, simple, and comprehensive theory with exceptional output power, yet it is not coherent with some of our vital considered judgments, especially with certain judgments about justice, human rights, and the importance of personal projects. By contrast, Kantian theories are consistent with many of our considered judgments, but their clarity, simplicity, and output power are limited.

A contested and appropriately criticized moral theory may nonetheless be defensible in light of the criteria we have proposed. Although we currently have no perfect or even best moral theory, several good theories are available.

Utilitarianism: Consequence-Based Theory

Consequentialism is a label affixed to theories holding that actions are right or wrong according to the balance of their good and bad consequences. The right act in any circumstance is the one that produces the best overall result, as determined from an impersonal perspective that gives equal weight to the interests of each affected party. The most prominent consequence-based theory, utilitarianism, accepts one and only one basic principle of ethics: the principle of utility. This principle asserts that we ought always to produce the maximal balance of positive value over disvalue (or the least possible disvalue, if only undesirable results can be achieved). The classical origins of this theory are found in the writings of Jeremy Bentham (1748–1832) and John Stuart Mill (1806–1873).

At first sight, utilitarianism seems entirely compelling. Who would deny that evil should be minimized and positive value increased? Moreover, utilitarians offer many examples from everyday life to show that the theory is practicable and that we all engage in a utilitarian method of calculating what should be done by balancing goals and resources and considering the needs of everyone affected. Examples include designing a family budget to meet the family's needs and creating a new public park in a wilderness region. Utilitarians maintain that their theory renders explicit and systematic what is already implicit in everyday deliberation and justification.

The Concept of Utility

Although utilitarians share the conviction that human actions should be morally assessed in terms of their production of maximal value, they disagree concerning which values are most important. Many utilitarians maintain that we ought to produce *agent-neutral or intrinsic* goods—that is, the goods every rational person values.[3] These goods are valuable in themselves, without reference to their further consequences or to the particular values held by individuals.

Bentham and Mill are *hedonistic* utilitarians because they conceive utility entirely in terms of happiness or pleasure, two broad terms they treat as synonymous.[4] They appreciate that many human actions are apparently not performed for the sake of happiness. For example, when highly motivated professionals, such as research scientists, work themselves to the point of exhaustion in search of new knowledge, they often do not appear to be seeking pleasure or personal happiness. Mill proposes that such persons are initially motivated by success or money, both of which promise happiness. Along the way, either the pursuit of knowledge provides pleasure, or such persons never stop associating their hard work with the success or money they hope to gain.

However, many recent utilitarian philosophers have argued that values other than happiness have intrinsic worth. Some list friendship, knowledge, health, and beauty among these intrinsic values, whereas others list personal autonomy, achievement and success, understanding, enjoyment, and deep personal relationships.[5] Even when their lists differ, these utilitarians concur that the greatest good should be assessed in terms of the total intrinsic value produced by an action. Still other utilitarians say that the concept of utility does not refer to intrinsic goods, but to an individual's preferences.

A Case of Risk and Truthfulness

To sketch the major themes of each theory, each section in this chapter devoted to a theory explicates how its proponents might approach the same case, which centers on a five-year-old girl who has progressive renal failure and is not doing well on chronic renal dialysis. The medical staff is considering a renal transplant, but its effectiveness is "questionable" in her case. Nevertheless, a "clear possibility" exists that the transplanted kidney will not be affected by the disease process. The parents concur with the plan to try a transplant, but an additional obstacle emerges: The tissue typing indicates that it would be difficult to find a match for the girl. The staff excludes her two siblings, ages two and four, as too young to be donors. The mother is not histocompatible, but the father is compatible and has "anatomically favorable circulation for transplantation."

Meeting alone with the father, the nephrologist gives him the results and indicates that the prognosis for his daughter is "quite uncertain." After reflection, the father decides that he does not wish to donate a kidney to his daughter. His several reasons include his fear of the surgery, his lack of courage, the uncertain prognosis even with a transplant, the slight prospect of a cadaver kidney, and the suffering his daughter has already sustained. The father then asks the physician "to tell everyone else in the family that he is not histocompatible." He is afraid that if family members know the truth, they will accuse him of intentionally allowing his daughter to die. He maintains that truth-telling would have the effect of "wrecking the family." The physician is uncomfortable with this request, but after further discussion he agrees to tell the man's wife that "for medical reasons the father should not donate a kidney."[6]

Utilitarians evaluate this case in terms of the consequences of the different courses of action open to the father and the physician. The goal is to find the single greatest good by balancing the interests of all affected persons. This evaluation depends on judgments about probable outcomes. Whether the father ought to donate his kidney depends on the probability of successful transplantation as well as the risks and other costs to him (and indirectly to other dependent members of the family). The probability of success is not high. The effectiveness is questionable and the prognosis uncertain, although a possibility exists that a transplanted kidney would not undergo the same disease process, and there is a slight possibility that a cadaver kidney could be obtained.

The girl will probably die without a transplant from either a cadaveric or a living source, but the transplant also offers only a chance of survival. The risk of death to the father from anesthesia in the kidney removal is 1 in 10,000–15,000; it is difficult to put an estimate on other possible long-term health effects. Nevertheless, with a sufficiently high probability of success and a sufficiently low probability of harm, many utilitarians would hold that the father or anyone else similarly situated is *obligated* to undertake what many would consider a heroic act that *surpasses* obligation. On a certain balance of probable benefits and risks, an uncompromising utilitarian would suggest tissue typing the patient's two siblings and then removing a kidney from one if there were a good match and parental approval. However, utilitarians differ among themselves in these various judgments because of different theories of value and different assessments of probable outcomes.

Probabilistic judgments would likewise play a role in the physician's utilitarian calculation of the right action in response to the father's request to camouflage why he will not donate a kidney. Primary questions include whether a full disclosure would actually wreck the family, whether lying to the family would have serious negative effects, and whether the father would subsequently experience serious guilt from his refusal to donate, thereby jeopardizing relations within the family. Studies indicate that families caring for chronically ill children break up at a higher rate than other families, and perhaps this family is already beyond repair. The utilitarian holds that the physician is obligated to consider the whole range of facts and possible consequences in light of the best available information about their probability and magnitude.

So far we have taken primarily the perspective of a utilitarian who focuses on *particular acts*. Other utilitarians focus on the relevant *principles and rules* of parental obligation and professional practice that, over time, maximize overall welfare. We turn now to this distinction between different types of utilitarian theory.

Act and Rule Utilitarianism

The principle of utility is the ultimate standard of rightness and wrongness for all utilitarians. Controversy has arisen, however, over whether this principle pertains to particular acts in particular circumstances or instead to general rules that determine which acts are right and wrong. Whereas the rule utilitarian considers the consequences of adopting rules, the act utilitarian skips the level of rules and justifies actions by appealing directly to the principle of utility, as the following chart indicates:

Rule Utilitarianism	*Act Utilitarianism*
Principle of Utility	Principle of Utility
↑	
Moral Rules	↑
↑	
Particular Judgments	Particular Judgments

The act utilitarian asks, "What good and bad consequences will result from this action in this circumstance?," not "What good and bad consequences will result from this sort of action in such circumstances?" The act utilitarian sees moral rules as somewhat useful in guiding human actions, but also as expendable if they do not promote utility in a particular context. For the rule utilitarian, by contrast, an act's conformity to a justified rule (that is, a rule justified by utility) makes the act right, and the rule is not expendable in a particular context, even if following the rule in that context does not maximize utility.

Physician Worthington Hooker, a prominent nineteenth-century figure in academic medicine and medical ethics, was a rule utilitarian who attended to rules of truth-telling in medicine as follows:

The good, which may be done by deception in a *few* cases, is almost as nothing, compared with the evil which it does in *many,* when the prospect of its doing good was just as promising as it was in those in which it succeeded. And when we add to this the evil which would result from a *general* adoption of a system of deception, the importance of a strict adherence to the truth in our intercourse with the sick, even on the ground of expediency, becomes incalculably great.

Hooker agreed that a patient's health is sometimes maximally advanced through deception, but he argued that a widespread use of deception in medicine will have an increasingly negative effect over time and will eventually cause more harm than good. He therefore defended the rule-utilitarian conclusion that deception should be prohibited in medicine.[7]

Act utilitarians, by contrast, argue that observing a rule such as truth-telling does not always maximize the general good, and that the rule is properly understood as a rough guideline. They regard rule utilitarians as unfaithful to the fundamental demand of the principle of utility: Maximize value. In some circumstances, they argue, abiding by a generally beneficial rule will not prove most beneficial to the persons affected by the action, even in the long run. Why, then, should a rule be obeyed if obedience will not maximize value? According to a contemporary act utilitarian, J. J. C. Smart, a third possibility exists between never adopting any rules and always obeying rules; namely, *sometimes* obeying rules.[8] From this perspective, physicians do not and should not always tell the truth to their patients or their families, just as the physician uses misleading language to protect the father in the above case. Sometimes physicians even must lie to give hope. They do so justifiably if it is better for the patients and for all concerned and if their acts do not undermine general conformity to moral rules. According to Smart, selective obedience does not erode either moral rules or general respect for morality. Rules, then, are stabilizing but nonbinding guides in the moral life.

Because of the benefits to society of the general observance of moral rules, the rule utilitarian does not abandon them even in difficult situations (although the rule utilitarian may accept rules only as statements of prima facie obligation). Abandonment threatens the integrity and existence of both the individual rules and the whole system of rules.[9] The act utilitarian's reply is that although promises usually should be kept in order to maintain trust, this consideration should be set aside in cases in which overall good would be produced by breaking the promise. The act utilitarian might also argue that making exceptions to accepted rules is consistent with ordinary moral beliefs, because we often make exceptions to rules without acting wrongly. The act utilitarian also contends in some cases when breaking rules clashes with our considered moral convictions, we need to revise our ordinary convictions rather than discard act utilitarianism.

An example of the act utilitarian's point appears in a comment by former Colorado governor Richard Lamm, who once observed that in light of increasing financial costs of medical care the terminally ill have "a duty to die and get out of the way with all of our machines and artificial hearts and everything else." This statement clearly conflicts with ordinary morality, and there was an outcry of indignation and shock that a public official would brush aside considered moral rules that protect our rights. Lamm chose an unfortunate word when he stated that the terminally ill have a "duty" to die. But in context he was giving an act-utilitarian answer to what he correctly referred to as an "ethical question." His point was that we cannot continue public funding for medical technology without assessing costs and trade-offs, even if we must subsequently revise our traditional views and let some people die because a technology is not funded. The act utilitarian believes that many other questions posed by technological developments likewise cannot be handled by traditional moral rules.

An Absolute Principle with Derivative Contingent Rules

From the utilitarian's perspective only the principle of utility is absolute. No derivative rule is absolute, and no rule is unrevisable. Even rules against killing in medicine may be overturned or substantially revised. For example, we will have occasion later to discuss current debates in biomedical ethics regarding whether seriously suffering patients should, at their request, be killed rather than "allowed to die," although such acts would revise traditional beliefs in medicine. The rule utilitarian argues that we should support rules permitting killing if and only if those rules would produce the most favorable consequences. Likewise, there should be rules against killing if and only if those rules would maximize good consequences. The utilitarian views euthanasia as a delicate matter of balancing risks and interests, whether in public policy or in particular judgments.

Imagine that a physician has a patient who requests to be killed, and the best utilitarian outcome would result from killing the patient. But suppose the physician cannot bring himself or herself to perform the act. Here the utilitarian will judge that the physician has not done the right thing, but may, in addition, note that good social consequences flow to society by having physicians who care so deeply about not causing harm to patients. Utilitarians often point out that we do not presently permit physicians to kill patients because of the adverse social consequences that we believe would be produced for those directly and indirectly affected. But if, under a different set of social conditions, legalization of mercy killing would maximize overall social welfare, the utilitarian sees no reason to prohibit such killing. Utilitarians for this reason regard their theory as responsive in constructive ways to changing social conditions.

A Critical Evaluation of Utilitarianism

Several problems suggest that utilitarianism is not a fully adequate moral theory.

Problems with immoral preferences and actions. Problems arise for utilitarians who appeal to preferences when individuals have what our considered judgments tell us are morally unacceptable preferences. For example, if a research investigator derived supreme satisfaction from inflicting pain on animals or on human subjects in experiments, we would condemn this preference and would seek to prevent it from being actualized. Utilitarianism based on subjective preferences is a defensible theory only if a range of acceptable preferences can be formulated, where ''acceptability'' is determined independently of the preferences of agents. This task seems inconsistent with a pure preference approach, but will utilitarianism be destroyed by a second level that delineates what counts as an acceptable preference?

There is an additional problem of immoral actions. Suppose the only way to achieve the maximal utilitarian outcome is to perform an immoral act (as judged by the standards of the common morality). For example, suppose a war can be ended only by using extremely painful methods of torturing captured children who were told by their soldier fathers not to reveal their location. Utilitarianism seems to say not only that you are permitted to torture the children, but that you are morally required to do so. Yet this requirement seems blatantly immoral. Thus, utilitarianism seems to permit apparently immoral actions without giving sufficient reasons for us to abandon our reigning views.

Does utilitarianism demand too much? Many forms of utilitarianism also seem to demand too much in the moral life, because the principle of utility is a *maximizing* principle. Utilitarians have a difficult time maintaining a crucial distinction between (1) *morally obligatory actions,* and (2) *supererogatory actions* (those above the call of moral obligation and performed for the sake of personal ideals). This objection has been registered by Alan Donagan, who describes situations in which utilitarians are committed by their theory to regard an action as obligatory against our firm moral conviction that the action is ideal and praiseworthy rather than obligatory.[10]

Donagan would regard suicides by the frail elderly and persons with severe disabilities who are no longer of use to society as examples of an act that could never rightly be considered obligatory, irrespective of its consequences. Heroic donation of bodily parts such as kidneys and even hearts to save another person's life is another example. If utilitarianism makes such actions obligatory, then it is a defective theory. Donagan argues, and we agree, that all utilitarians face these problems, because none can rule out the ever-present possibility that what is today praiseworthy (but optional) will, through altered social circumstances, become obligatory by utilitarian standards. At the same time, we should recognize that utilitarians are sometimes right in arguing that ordinary morality is too weak or vague in its demands and should be upgraded by more demanding requirements.[11] Furthermore, in a changing social situation, our considered judgments may themselves undergo alteration.

Bernard Williams and John Mackie offer extensions of the thesis that utilitarianism demands too much. Williams argues that utilitarianism abrades personal integrity by making persons as morally responsible for consequences that they fail to prevent as for those outcomes they directly cause, even when the consequences are not of their doing. Mackie similarly argues that a utilitarian "test of right actions" is so distant from our moral experience as to be "the ethics of fantasy," because it demands that people strip themselves of many goals and relationships they value in life in order to maximize outcomes for others. From this perspective, the utilitarian demands that we act like saints who are without personal interests and goals.[12] These criticisms suggest that utilitarianism fails the test of *practicability* presented at the beginning of this chapter.

Problems of unjust distribution. A third problem is that utilitarianism in principle permits the interests of the majority to override the rights of minorities, and cannot adequately disavow unjust social distributions. The charge is that utilitarians assign no independent weight to justice and are indifferent to unjust distributions, instead insisting that value be distributed by net aggregate satisfaction. If an already prosperous group of persons could have more value added to their lives than the value that could be added to the lives of the indigent in society, the utilitarian must recommend that the added value go to the prosperous group.

An example of problematic (although not necessarily unjust) distribution appears in the following case. Two researchers wanted to determine the most cost-effective way to control hypertension in the American population. As they developed their research, they discovered that it is more cost-effective to target patients already being treated for hypertension than to identify new cases of hypertension among persons without regular access to medical care: younger men, older women, and patients with exceptionally high blood pressure. And they concluded that "a community with limited resources would probably do better to concentrate its efforts on improving adherence of known hypertensives, even at a sacrifice in terms of the numbers screened." If accepted by the government, this recommendation would exclude the poorest sector, which has the most pressing need for medical attention, from the benefits of high blood pressure education and management.

The investigators were concerned because of the apparent injustice in excluding the poor and minorities by a public health endeavor aimed at the economically advantaged sector of society. Yet their statistics were compelling. No matter how carefully planned the efforts, nothing worked efficiently (that is, nothing produced utilitarian results) except programs directed at known hypertensives already in contact with physicians. The investigators therefore recommended what they explicitly referred to as a utilitarian allocation.[13]

A Constructive Evaluation of Utilitarianism

Despite these criticisms, utilitarianism has many strengths, two of which we appropriate in later chapters. The first is the acceptance of a role for the principle of utility in the formation of public policy. The utilitarian's requirements of an objective assessment of everyone's interests and of an impartial choice to maximize good outcomes for all affected parties are acceptable norms of public policy. Second, when we formulate principles of beneficence in Chapter 5, utility plays an important role. Although we have characterized utilitarianism as primarily a *consequence*-based theory, it is also *beneficence*-based. That is, the theory sees morality primarily in terms of the goal of promoting welfare.

A theory with a principle of beneficence balanced by other principles should eliminate all the problems with an unqualified use of the principle of utility that we encountered in the criticisms offered in the preceding section. This point holds even if beneficence is developed primarily in terms of producing good consequences. As political economist Amartya Sen notes, "Consequentialist reasoning may be fruitfully used even when consequentialism as such is not accepted. To ignore consequences is to leave an ethical story half told."[14]

A *strict* or *pure* utilitarianism also has strengths, as we can see by reconsidering the objection that utilitarianism is overdemanding. Utilitarianism often demands more than the rules of the common morality do, but this apparent weakness is also a hidden strength. For example, ordinary morality demands that we not override the rights of individuals to maximize social consequences. But if we can more widely and more effectively protect almost everyone's interests by overriding some property and autonomy rights, then it is far from clear that this course of action would be wrong merely because it contravenes ordinary morality and pursues the goal of social utility. In many circumstances the utilitarian makes a compelling case in advising us to rely less on everyday convictions and more on judgments of overall benefit.

Kantianism: Obligation-Based Theory

A second type of theory denies much that utilitarian theories affirm. Often called *deontological* (i.e. a theory that some features of actions other than or in addition to consequences make actions right or wrong), this type is now increasingly called *Kantian,* because the ethical thought of Immanuel Kant (1724–1804), has shaped many of its formulations.

Consider how a Kantian might approach the above-mentioned case of the five-year-old in need of a kidney. A Kantian would first insist that we rest our moral judgments on reasons that can be generalized for others who are similarly situated. If the father has no generalizable moral obligation, no basis is available for moral criticism of him. The strict Kantian takes this point to be a rigid demand. If the father chooses to donate out of affection, compassion, or concern for his dying daughter, his act would actually lack moral worth, because it would not be based on a recognition of generalizable obligation. It would also not be legitimate to use one of the girl's younger siblings as a source of a kidney, because that recourse would involve using persons entirely as means to others' ends. This same principle would also exclude coercing the father to donate against his will.

Regarding the physician's options after the father requests deception of the family, a strict Kantian views lying as an act that cannot without contradiction be universalized as a norm of conduct. Thus, the physician should not lie to the man's wife or to other members of the family, even if the lie would function to salvage the family (a consequentialist appeal). Even if the physician's statement is not, strictly speaking, a lie, he intentionally used this formulation to conceal relevant facts from the wife, an act Kantians typically view as morally unacceptable.

A Kantian will also consider whether the rule of confidentiality has independent moral weight, whether the tests the father underwent with the nephrologist established a relationship of confidentiality, and whether the rule of confidentiality protects the information about the father's histocompatibility and his reasons for not donating. Even without considering possible effects on the family, the Kantian seems destined to face a difficult conflict of obligations: truthfulness in conflict with confidentiality. But before we can address a possible Kantian strategy for resolving this conflict, we need to understand more about Kantian theory.

Obligation from Categorical Rules

In an attempt to combat skeptical challenges to ethics, Kant argued that morality is grounded in pure reason, not in tradition, intuition, conscience, emotion, or attitudes such as sympathy. Kant saw human beings as creatures with rational powers to resist desire, the freedom to do so, and the capacity to act by rational considerations. He held that the moral worth of an individual's action depends exclusively on the moral acceptability of the rule (or "maxim") on which the person acts. As Kant puts it, moral obligation depends on the rule that determines the individual's will. An action possesses moral worth only if performed by an agent with a good will, which entails that a morally valid reason justify the action.[15]

For Kant, one must act not only *in accordance with* but *for the sake of* obligation. That is, to have moral worth, a person's motive for acting must come from a recognition that he or she intends what is morally required. For example, if an employer discloses a health hazard to an employee only because the employer fears a lawsuit, and not because of the importance of truth-telling or concern about the employee's health, then the employer has done the right thing but deserves no moral credit for the action. If agents do what is morally right simply because they are scared, because they derive pleasure from doing that kind of act, or because they are selfish, they lack the requisite good will that derives from acting for the sake of obligation.

Imagine a man who desperately needs money and knows that he will not be able to borrow it unless he promises repayment in a definite time, but who also knows that he will not be able to repay it within this period. He decides to make a promise that he knows he will break. Kant asks us to examine the man's reason, what Kant calls the maxim of the action: "When I think myself in want of money, I will borrow money and promise to pay it back, although I know that I cannot do so." This maxim, Kant says, cannot pass a test that he calls the *categorical imperative*. This imperative tells us what must be done irrespective of our desires. It requires unconditional conformity by all rational beings. In its major formulation, Kant states the categorical imperative as follows: "I ought never to act except in such a way that I can also will that my maxim become a universal law." Kant says that all particular imperatives of obligation (all "ought" statements that morally obligate) are justified by this one principle.

The categorical imperative, then, is a canon of the acceptability of moral rules—that is, a criterion for judging the acceptability of the maxims that direct actions.[16] This imperative adds nothing to a maxim's content. Rather, it determines which maxims are objective and valid. The categorical imperative functions by testing what Kant calls the consistency of maxims: A maxim must be capable of being conceived and willed without contradiction. When we examine the maxim of the person who deceitfully promises, we discover, according to Kant, that this maxim is incapable of being conceived and willed without contradiction. It is inconsistent with what it presupposes. The maxim would make the purpose of promising impossible, because no one would believe promises. Many examples from everyday life illustrate this thesis. For instance, maxims of lying are inconsistent with the practices of truth-telling they presuppose, and maxims permitting cheating on tests are inconsistent with the practices of honesty they presuppose.

Kant appears to have more than one categorical imperative, because his several formulations are not equivalent. His second formulation is at least as influential as the first: "One must act to treat every person as an end and never as a means only." [17] It has often been said that this principle categorically requires that we should never treat another as a means to our ends, but this interpretation misrepresents his views. He argues only that we must not treat another *exclusively* as a means to our ends. When secretaries type manuscripts and human research subjects volunteer to test new drugs, they are treated as a means to others' ends, but they have a choice in the matter and retain control over their lives. Kant does not prohibit such uses of consenting persons. He insists only that they be treated with the respect and moral dignity to which every person is entitled.

Autonomy and Heteronomy

In contemporary biomedical ethics the word *autonomy* typically refers to what makes a life one's own; viz. that it is shaped by personal preferences and choices. This conception of autonomy is emphatically not Kant's. A person has "autonomy of the will" for Kant if and only if the person knowingly acts in accordance with the universally valid moral principles that pass the requirements of the categorical imperative. He contrasts this *moral* autonomy with "heteronomy," which is any controlling influence over the will other than motivation by moral principles.[18] If, for example, a person acts from passion, ambition, or self-interest, the person acts heteronomously, not from a rational will that chooses autonomously. Kant thus regards acting from desire, fear, impulse, personal projects, and habit as no less heteronomous than actions manipulated or coerced by others.

To say that an individual must "accept" a moral principle in order to be autonomous does not mean that the principle is subjective or that each individual must create (author or originate) his or her moral principles. Kant only requires that each individual *will the acceptance* of moral principles. By contrast, Kant's theory is exclusively one of the moral self-legislation of objective rules. If a person freely accepts objective moral principles, that person is a law-giver unto himself or herself. The importance of this account for Kant also extends beyond the *nature* of autonomy to its *value*. "The principle of autonomy," he holds, is "the sole principle of morals," and autonomy alone gives people respect, value, and proper motivation. A person's dignity—indeed, "sublimity"—comes from being morally autonomous.[19]

Contemporary Kantian Ethics

Several writers in contemporary ethical theory have accepted and developed a
Kantian account, broadly construed. A straightforward example is *The Theory
of Morality* by Alan Donagan. He seeks the "philosophical core" of the morality expressed in the Hebrew-Christian tradition, now interpreted in secular
rather than religious terms. Donagan's philosophical elaboration of this point
of view relies heavily on Kant's theory of persons as ends in themselves, especially the imperative that one must treat humanity as an end and never as a
means only. Donagan expresses the fundamental principle of the Hebrew-
Christian tradition as a Kantian principle grounded in rationality: "It is impermissible not to respect every human being, oneself or any other, as a rational
creature." [20] Donagan believes that all other moral rules rely upon this fundamental principle and that Kant's theory captures the rational basis of these
rules.

A second theory has encouraged the use of Kantian insights in contemporary
ethics. John Rawls, whose theory of reflective equilibrium was examined in
Chapter 1, challenges utilitarian theories while attempting to develop Kantian
themes of reason, autonomy, equality, and opposition to utilitarianism. For
example, Rawls argues that vital moral considerations, such as individual rights
and the just distribution of goods among individuals, depend less on social
factors, such as individual happiness and majority interests, than on Kantian
conceptions of individual worth, self-respect, and autonomy.[21]

For Rawls, a social arrangement is a communal effort to advance the good
of all. Inequalities of birth, natural endowment, and historical circumstance are
undeserved, and persons in a cooperative society should make more equal the
situation of persons disadvantaged through no fault of their own. Those who
are naturally endowed with more advantageous properties by luck of the draw
do not deserve their advantageous properties, and hence a just society would
seek in its scheme of justice to overcome advantages stemming from the accidents of biology and history. Rawls uses a hypothetical social contract, in
which valid principles are those to which we would all agree if we could freely
consider the social situation from a standpoint he calls the "original position,"
in which individuals are equally ignorant of the particular characteristics and
advantages they do or will possess. They know that they live together in a
cooperative venture, but they are blinded to their individual desires, interests,
and objectives. In Kant's terms, they are purely rational agents behind what
Rawls calls a "veil of ignorance." [22]

Rawls aligns his original position with the Kantian theory of autonomy. Individuals give themselves the law from the perspective of rationality alone. Autonomy is moral self-legislation through a structure of reason and will that is
common to all rational agents. Persons are autonomous in the original position

because they choose and give to themselves the moral law out of their nature as rational, independent, and mutually disinterested persons. While treating Kantian autonomy, Rawls considers Henry Sidgwick's objection to Kant, that the principles of the scoundrel and the principles of the saint could both be accepted autonomously.[23] Rawls appropriately argues that this objection springs from a misunderstanding of Kantian theory. Although a free self *could* choose as a scoundrel would, this choice would be inconsistent with the choices that rational beings expressing their nature as such would make. For Rawls, any philosophy in which the right to individual autonomy legitimately outweighs the dictates of objective moral principles is unacceptable. Even courageous and conscientious actions do not merit respect unless they accord with objective moral principles. If society restricts conscientious actions that violate valid public principles, "no violation of our [moral] autonomy" exists, because these acts are not morally autonomous—no matter how freely and conscientiously chosen.[24]

In his recent writings, Rawls has stressed that his work presents a political conception of justice, rather than a comprehensive moral theory. That is, his account is "a moral conception worked out for a specific subject, namely, the basic structure of a constitutional democratic regime." As such, it does not presuppose a comprehensive moral doctrine such as Kant's. Rawls maintains that his theory is Kantian by "analogy not identity." He points to several Kantian perspectives with which he identifies, including the priority of the right over the good and persons as free, equal, and capable of autonomy.[25] The upshot seems to be that Rawls is expressing Kantian themes without making a full commitment to a Kantian or deontological moral theory. The same can be said of many other contemporary Kantians.

A Critical Evaluation of Kantianism

Like utilitarianism, Kantian theory fails to provide a full and adequate theory of the moral life, for reasons we shall now discuss.

The problem of conflicting obligations. Kant has a problem with conflicting obligations. Suppose we have promised to take our children on a long-anticipated trip, but now find that if we do so, we cannot assist our sick mother in the hospital. This conflict is generated between a rule of promise-keeping and a rule of assistance, perhaps based on a debt of gratitude. The conflict sometimes arises from a single moral rule rather than from two different rules in conflict—as, for example, when one has made two promises that now come into conflict, although one could not have anticipated the conflict at the time one made the promises.

Because he makes all moral rules absolute, Kant often seems to say that we are obligated to do the impossible and perform both actions. We cannot at the same time both take our children on a trip and help our mother in the hospital; yet Kant seems to require both. Any ethical theory that leads to this conclusion is incoherent, yet no clear path exists out of Kant's absolutistic framework. If even as many as two absolute rules exist, they will conflict on some occasions. Either we must accept a system with only one absolute, or we must give up absolutes altogether unless their meaning and scope can be specified to avoid conflict. (Our solution to this problem is found on pp. 104–106 below.)

Overemphasizing law, underemphasizing relationships. Kant's arguments concentrate on lawful obligations, and recent Kantian theories, such as Rawls's, feature a contractual basis for obligations. But whether freedom, choice, equality, contract, law, and other staples of Kantianism deserve to occupy such a central position in a moral theory is questionable. (They are, we can agree, central ingredients in legal and political theories.) These visions of the moral life fail to capture much in personal relationships, which generate various responsibilities. Among friends and family we rarely think or act in terms of law, contract, or absolute rules. This suggests that Kant's theory (as with utilitarianism) is better suited for relationships among strangers than for relationships among friends or other intimates. Parents, for example, do not see responsibilities to their children in terms of contracts, but in terms of care, needs, sustenance, and loving attachment. Only if all forms of moral relationship—and our moral sentiments, motivations, and virtues—could be reduced to a law-governed exchange would Kantian theory be defensible.

The limitations of the categorical imperative. Many immoral actions cannot be pronounced "contradictory" as easily as Kant's tidy examples suggest, and Kant's categorical imperative is both obscure and difficult to render functional in the moral life. Few philosophers would now hold, as Kant appears to, that universalizability is sufficient to determine the moral acceptability of rules, although many concur with him that universalizability is a necessary condition of ethical judgments, rules, and principles. As long as these questions hang over Kant's central principles, questions will persist about the theory's output, explanatory, and justificatory power.

Many arguments Kant adduces to explain the categorical imperative carry little conviction beyond those already convinced. His arguments are sometimes so unconvincing that he himself draws on a source outside the categorical imperative. For example, to argue against the moral acceptability of suicide, he maintains that suicide violates an obligation to God, because the suicide "leaves the post assigned him" as a "sentinel on earth" and "violates a holy trust." He notes that "as soon as we examine suicide from the standpoint of religion we immediately see it in its true light. . . . God is our owner; we are

His property.''[26] Kant's moral arguments from the categorical imperative, then, are unconvincing because his position often appears to rely on an external source, such as theology.

Abstractness without content. In Chapter 1 we mentioned Hegel's criticism that Kant's theory lacks the power to develop an "immanent doctrine of obligations" and obliterates all "content and specification" in favor of abstractness.[27] We agree that concepts such as "rationality" and "humanity" are too thin a basis for a determinate set of moral norms. Kant's relatively empty formalisms have little power to identify or assign specific obligations in almost any context of everyday morality, thereby raising questions about the theory's practicability. Both their abstractness and this impracticability provide reasons why method in ethics should start with considered judgments and then to specify principles and test moral claims in light of coherence.

A Constructive Evaluation of Kantianism

Kant held that any person who judges that X is morally required in one circumstance is thereby committed to the view that X is morally required in any relevantly similar circumstance. To be consistently committed to a moral system of rules and principles is a moral requirement that Kant analyzed with profound insight. The basic idea is that when a moral judgment is supported by good reasons, those reasons are good for any relevantly similar circumstance. As a point of consistency, this claim is undeniable, and it is far-reaching. Persons cannot act morally and make themselves privileged or exempt. Relevant differences exist across persons and groups, and there are valid exceptions to all general rules; but when persons are situated in relevantly similar ways, consistency requires that they use the same justifying reasons and treat persons in the same ways. If Kant had done nothing else than establish this point, he would have made a significant contribution to ethical theory.

Character Ethics: Virtue-Based Theory

Utilitarian and some Kantian theories attempt to shape various moral phenomena into integrated frameworks structured by a single dominant principle. Despite the attractiveness of their formulations, recent ethical theory has attended to some neglected moral phenomena, including character and virtue.[28] Whereas utilitarian and Kantian theories are principally expressed in the language of obligations and rights, with a focus on situations of choice, *character ethics* or *virtue ethics* emphasizes the agents who perform actions and make choices. Following the tradition of Plato and Aristotle, character ethics assigns virtuous character a preeminent position.

From this standpoint, the father's confession of a lack of courage in the case previously considered is relevant to an evaluation of him and his refusal to donate. But he has other reasons as well, some possibly involving self-deception. He points to his daughter's "degree of suffering," which suggests that he believes she might be better off without a transplant. From this viewpoint, his motives are partially altruistic, not purely self-centered. However, this judgment of altruism seems feeble in light of his comment about failed courage and may not be sustainable because of the delicate balance of benefits and risks, burdens, and costs that the family and the daughter face. A defender of character ethics would still wonder whether the father was sufficiently compassionate and caring about her welfare. Failed courage seems to have overwhelmed compassion and fidelity in the father.

Several other judgments of virtue and character are possible in this case. We lack a full description of his wife, but the father apparently worried that she would be vindictive and unforgiving in accusing him of "allowing his daughter to die." This belief underlies his request that the physician lie. The physician, we saw, focused on how the act of deception might compromise his integrity. Apparently he thought he could sidestep this problem, at least avoiding a severe compromise of integrity, by saying "for medical reasons" the father should not donate a kidney. However, the fact that he "felt very uncomfortable" about the man's request to conceal information indicates an ongoing concern about both truthfulness and moral integrity, two central virtues. Questions can also be raised about whether the physician deceived himself when he recognized and acted on a perilous distinction between a direct lie (for instance, "he cannot donate because he is not histocompatible") and deliberate, effective deception ("for medical reasons he should not donate").

The Concept of Virtue

A *virtue* is a trait of character that is socially valued,[29] and a *moral virtue* is a trait that is morally valued. The fact that courage, for example, is a socially valued trait does not necessarily make courage a moral virtue. Moral courage occurs only if the context is a moral one, and it is not sufficient that social groups approve of a trait and regard it as moral. Moral reasons must support a claim or perception of moral virtue. Persons are sometimes disvalued in a community when they act virtuously, and robbers and pirates are sometimes admired in their communities for their meanness and churlishness. It is a mistake, then, to reduce moral virtue to whatever is socially approved.

Some have defined moral virtue as a disposition to act or a habit of acting in accordance with moral principles, obligations, or ideals.[30] The moral virtue of nonmalevolence, for example, is understood as the trait a person has of abstaining from causing harm to others when it would be wrong to harm them.

However, this definition unjustifiably makes virtues wholly derivative from principles and fails to capture the importance of motives. Virtue is intimately connected to characteristic motives. We care morally about how persons are motivated, and we care especially about their *characteristic* forms of motivation. Persons who are motivated by sympathy and personal affection, for example, meet our approval when others who act the same way but from different motives would not meet our approval. Properly motivated persons often do not merely follow rules; they also have a morally appropriate desire to act as they do.

Imagine that a person discharges an obligation *because* it is an obligation, but intensely dislikes being placed in a position in which the interests of others are overriding. This person does not love, feel friendly toward, or cherish others and respects their wishes only because obligation requires it. This person can nonetheless perform a morally right action and have a disposition to perform that action. All he or she needs is a disposition to follow rules and perform obligation. But if the motive is improper, a vital moral ingredient is missing; and if a person *characteristically* lacks this motivational structure, a necessary condition of virtuous character is absent. The act may be right and the actor without blame, but neither the person nor the act is virtuous. In short, it is possible to be disposed to do what is right, to intend to do it, and to do it, while also yearning to avoid doing it. Persons who characteristically perform *morally right actions* from such a motivational structure are not *morally virtuous* even if they always perform the morally right action.

Aristotle expressed an important (although underdeveloped) distinction between right action and proper motive, which he also analyzed in terms of the distinction between external performance and internal state. An action can be right without being virtuous, he said, but an action can be virtuous only if performed from the right state of mind of the person. Both right action and right motive should be present in a virtuous action: "The agent must . . . be in the right state when he does [the actions]. First, he must know [that he is doing virtuous actions]; second, he must decide on them, and decide on them for themselves; and third, he must also do them from a firm and unchanging state," including the right state of emotions and desires. "The just and temperate person is not the one who [merely] does these actions, but the one who also does them in the way in which just or temperate people do them."[31]

Our analysis of the virtues in terms of motivational structure needs supplementation in the light of Aristotle's observations. First, in addition to being properly *motivated* to action, a virtuous person often must experience appropriate *feelings*, such as sympathy and regret—even when the feelings are not motives and no action can result from the feelings. Second, many virtues have no clear link to either motives or feelings. Moral discernment and moral integrity—two of the primary virtues treated in Chapter 8 (where we return to these problems)—are typical examples. Here behavior and psychological properties other than motives and feelings are paramount.

A Special Place for the Virtues

Some writers in character ethics maintain that the language of obligation is *derivative* from moral circumstances in which persons display a lack of virtue in not performing certain actions. Accordingly, one who is disposed by character to have the right motives and desires is the basic model of the moral person.[32] This model is more important, they claim, than a model of action-from-obligation, because right motives and character tell us more about moral worth than do right actions.

This position is attractive, because we are often more concerned about the character and motives of persons than about the conformity of their acts to rules. When a friend performs an act of "friendship," we expect it not to be motivated entirely from a sense of obligation to us, but rather because the person has a desire to be friendly, feels friendly, wants to keep friends in good cheer, and values friendship. The friend who acts only from obligation lacks the virtue of friendliness, which is vital. Absent this virtue, the relationship lacks moral merit.[33]

Some writers in biomedical ethics have also argued that the attempt in obligation-oriented theories to replace the virtuous judgments of health care professionals with rules, codes, or procedures will not result in better decisions and actions. For example, rather than using rules and government regulations to protect subjects in research, some claim that the most reliable protection is the presence of an "informed conscientious, compassionate, responsible researcher."[34] The underlying view is that character is more important than conformity to rules and that virtues should be inculcated and cultivated over time through educational interactions, role models, and the like.

Gregory Pence contends that moral issues in medicine and health care should be discussed in the framework of virtues, because almost any health professional can successfully evade a system of rules. We should, he says, create a climate in which health professionals "desire not to abuse their subjects—a point harking back to our definition of the good person as one who has the right kind of desires."[35] This argument provides a significant reason for incorporating the virtues into biomedical ethics and in medical and nursing education, but it needs elaboration.

A morally good person with the right configuration of desires and motives is more likely than others to understand what should be done, more likely to attentively perform the acts that are required, and even more likely to form and act on moral ideals. A person we trust is one who has an ingrained motivation and desire to perform right actions. Not the rule follower, then, but the person disposed by character to be generous, caring, compassionate, sympathetic, fair, and the like, is the one we will recommend, admire, praise, and hold up as a moral model.

If a virtuous person makes a mistake in judgment, thereby performing a morally wrong act, he or she would be less blameworthy than an habitual offender who performed the same act. The person's character informs our judgment of the individual and how we assess his or her actions. In his chronicle of life under the Nazi SS in the Jewish ghetto in Cracow, Poland, Thomas Keneally describes a physician faced with a grave dilemma: either inject cyanide into four immobile patients or abandon them to the SS, who were at that moment emptying the ghetto and had already proved that they would brutally kill all captives and patients. This physician, Keneally reports, "suffered painfully from a set of ethics as intimate to him as the organs of his own body."[36] Here is a person of the highest moral character and virtue, motivated to act rightly and even heroically, yet who at first had no idea what was the morally right action.

Ultimately, with uncertainty and reluctance, the physician elected active euthanasia without the consent or knowledge of the four doomed patients (using forty drops of hydrocyanic acid)—an act almost universally denounced by the canons of professional medical ethics. Even if one thinks that the physician's act was wrong and blameworthy, a judgment we reject, no one could reasonably make a judgment of blame or demerit directed at the physician's motives or character. Having already risked death by choosing to remain at his patients' beds in the hospital rather than take a prepared escape route, this physician is a moral hero who has displayed an extraordinary moral character.

Judgments of an agent's merit and praiseworthiness or demerit and blameworthiness are tied to the person's motives, not merely to the person's actions. To speak of a good, praiseworthy, or virtuous action is elliptical for our evaluation of the motive underlying the action—for example, the motive of benefiting another person.[37] However, in contrast to some radical forms of character ethics, the merit in an action is not in motive or character alone. The action must be appropriately gauged to bring about the desired result and must be morally justified in conformity with relevant principles and rules. For example, the physician who is appropriately motivated to help a patient but who acts inappropriately to bring about the desired result does not act in a praiseworthy manner.

The Compatibility of Virtues and Principles

Although the virtues do have a special place in the moral life, this fact is not sufficient evidence for an exclusive primary role, as if a virtue-based theory could replace or take precedence over obligation-based theories. The two kinds of theory have different emphases, but they are compatible and mutually reinforcing. As the case of the Cracow physician shows, persons of good moral character sometimes have trouble discerning what is right and may be the first to recognize that they need principles, rules, and ideals to determine right or good acts.

In circumstances of conflicting motivation from different virtues, we also need to ask questions about which action is right, best, or obligatory. One often cannot act virtuously unless one makes judgments about the best ways to manifest sympathy, desire, and the like.[38] Consider what a generous and tolerant person would do in a circumstance in which outrage or punishment is an appropriate response to someone's wrongdoing. It would be improper behavior to be generous or tolerant toward the wrongdoer. To see that normally appropriate responses are here wrong requires a balancing of conflicting values. Such judgments are based on general norms, not on the virtues alone. This suggests that the virtues need principles and rules to regulate and supplement them. As Aristotle suggests, ethics involves judgments like those in medicine: Principles guide us to actions, but we still need to assess a situation and formulate an appropriate response, and this assessment and response flow from character and training as much as from principles.

To defend the compatibility of virtues and principles is not to argue for a perfect correspondence. That is, one need not argue that every moral virtue has a corresponding moral principle of obligation. The proposal that there might be such a correspondence is displayed in schematic form in the following diagram (in which "exceptional standards" are moral ideals, as discussed in Chapter 8).[39]

	Action Guides [correspond to]	*Virtue Standards*
Ordinary Standards	Principles or Rules of Obligation	Virtue Standards
Exceptional Standards	Ideals of Action	Ideals of Virtue

The following list illustrates the correspondence between some specific action guides and virtues.

Principles	*Corresponding Virtues*
Respect for Autonomy	Respectfulness
Nonmaleficence	Nonmalevolence
Beneficence	Benevolence
Justice	Justice or Fairness

Rules	*Corresponding Virtues*
Veracity	Truthfulness
Confidentiality	Confidentialness

Privacy	Respect for Privacy
Fidelity	Faithfulness
Ideals of Action	*Ideals of Virtue*
Exceptional Forgiveness	Exceptional Forgiveness
Exceptional Generosity	Exceptional Generosity
Exceptional Compassion	Exceptional Compassion
Exceptional Kindness	Exceptional Kindness

This list could be expanded to include many additional action-guides and virtues, but a systematic program of correspondence likely cannot be developed from this programatic idea. Many virtue-standards do not directly correspond to action-guides. No one-to-one correspondence exists, even if there is some form of relationship. For example, concern, compassion, caring, sympathy, courage, modesty, and patience do not correspond to norms of obligation. This problem is broader than an absence of one-to-one relationships. Many virtues seem to have no direct connection to norms of obligation, although they contribute to or even improve actions done from obligation. Typical examples are cautiousness, integrity (in the sense of consistently upholding and standing firm in one's values), cheerfulness, unpretentiousness, sincerity, appreciativeness, cooperativeness, and commitment.

A Critical Evaluation of Character Ethics

We can now investigate some limitations of virtue theories.

Morality in relations between strangers. Not all areas of the moral life can be forced into the language and the framework of virtue theory without a loss of vital moral protections. Character judgments will often play a less significant role than rights and procedures (such as committee review), especially when strangers meet. For example, when a patient first encounters a physician, the physician's conformity to rules or principles (and even explicit contracts backed by sanctions) may be essential for their subsequent relationship. This reliance on principles and rules does not presuppose an unacceptable form of distrust. A presumption of trust can be combined with a recognition that people who are typically trustworthy at least occasionally need guidance from principles and rules.

Virtue is not enough. The first criticism leads to a second. It is doubtful that character ethics can adequately *explain* and *justify* assertions of the rightness or wrongness of specific actions. It is unacceptable to claim that if persons display a virtuous character, their acts are therefore morally acceptable. People of good character who act virtuously can perform wrong actions. They may have incorrect information about likely consequences, make incorrect judgments, or fail to grasp what should be done. Defenders of character ethics cannot plausibly maintain that just and unjust actions consist only in what just and unjust persons do. We sometimes cannot even evaluate a motive as being appropriate unless we know that certain forms of conduct are obligatory, prohibited, or permissible.

The defender of a pure character ethics must say that the virtues themselves, not principles or rules, guide action. The strength of this account is in the strength of character of the virtuous person. In a virtuous person who is decisive and resolute, this character should prove to be as functional in guiding action as rules and principles. When confronted with the question, which actions should be performed, a virtue theory can answer, "those actions that an exemplary moral agent would perform."[40] Although we deeply respect this point (and develop it further in Chapter 8), it needs qualification. In many circumstances, principles and rules are essential to guide conduct.

A Constructive Evaluation of Character Ethics

A proponent of character ethics need not claim that analysis of the virtues subverts or discredits ethical principles and rules. It is enough to argue that ethical theory is more complete if the virtues are included and that moral motives deserve to be at center stage in a way some leading traditional theories have inadequately appreciated. When the feelings, concerns, and attitudes of others are the morally relevant matters, rules and principles are not as likely as human warmth and sensitivity to lead us to notice what should be done. Even a seldom noticed virtue, such as cheerfulness or tactfulness, can be far more significant than standard rules in some contexts. Furthermore, forms of loyalty, reliability, and commitment to other persons can, across time, be more integral to an adequate or full moral life than following principles or rules.

To look at acts without also looking at the moral appropriateness and desirability of feelings, attitudes, forms of sympathy, and the like is to miss a large area of the moral picture. We do not merely expect persons to act in certain ways. We also expect them to have certain emotions, certain forms of responsiveness, and a trustworthy character. Character ethics helps us introduce this subtlety in moral theory, as we will see in later chapters.

Liberal Individualism: Rights-Based Theory

Thus far we have primarily been using terms such as the following from moral discourse: *obligation, permissible action, virtue,* and *justification.* It may seem odd that we have not often used the language of rights, given their historical importance and their recent role in ethics and foreign policy. Statements of rights provide vital protections of life, liberty, expression, and property. They protect against oppression, unequal treatment, intolerance, arbitrary invasion of privacy, and the like. Many philosophers and framers of political declarations therefore regard rights language as supplying the basic terminology for expressing the moral point of view.

An ethical analysis of the case of the five-year-old needing a transplant would, from this perspective, focus on the rights of all the parties, in an effort to determine the meaning and scope as well as the weight and strength of those rights. The father could be viewed as having rights of autonomy, privacy, and confidentiality that call for the protection of his bodily integrity and sphere of decisionmaking from interference by others. In addition, he has a right to information, which he apparently received, about the risks, benefits, and alternatives of living kidney donation.

The father's decision not to donate is within his rights, as long as it does not violate another's rights. No apparent grounds support a right to assistance that could permit anyone, including his daughter, to demand a kidney. However, there are some special rights to assistance, and it could be argued that the daughter has a right to receive a kidney from her father, on the basis of either parental obligations or medical need. But even if such a right exists, it would be sharply bounded. For example, it is implausible to suppose that such a right could be enforced against the girl's two siblings. Their right to noninterference, when the procedure is not for their direct benefit and carries risks, protects them against recruitment as sources for a kidney.

An analysis in terms of rights might also notice that the father exercises his rights of autonomy and privacy in allowing the physician to run some tests, and then seeks protection behind a right of confidentiality, which allows him to control further access to information generated in his relationship with the physician. The scope and limits of those rights and of competing rights need attention. For example, does the mother have a right to the information generated in the relationship between the father and the nephrologist, particularly information bearing on the fate of the daughter?

An analysis using rights would also consider whether the physician has a relevant right of conscience. For example, the physician might resist becoming an instrument of the father's desire to keep others from knowing why he is not donating a kidney. But even if the physician does have a right to protect his integrity, does this right outstrip or trump the rights of others? Can a physician justifiably say ''I have a right of conscience'' and use this trump to back out of a moral dilemma?

The Nature of Liberal Individualism

Rights theory will here be analyzed as liberal individualism, the conception that in a democratic society a certain space must be carved out within which the individual is protected and allowed to pursue personal projects. Liberal individualism has, in recent years, challenged the reigning utilitarian and Kantian models. H. L. A. Hart has described this challenge as a switch from an "old faith that some form of utilitarianism . . . *must* capture the essence of political morality" to a new faith in "a doctrine of basic human rights, protecting specific basic liberties and interests of individuals."[41]

There may be a new faith, but liberal individualism is not a new development in moral and political theory. At least since Thomas Hobbes, liberal individualists have employed the language of rights to buttress moral and political arguments, and the Anglo-American legal tradition has incorporated this language. The language of rights has served on occasion as a means to oppose the status quo, to assert claims that demand recognition and respect, and to promote social reforms that aim to secure legal protections for individuals. Historically this language was instrumental in securing certain freedoms from established orders of religion, society, and state, such as freedom of the press and freedom of religious expression.

The vital role of civil, political, and legal rights in protecting the individual from societal intrusions is now beyond serious dispute, but the idea that rights provide the fountainhead for ethical and political theory has been strongly resisted (for example, by many utilitarians and Marxists). Individual interests are often at odds with communal or institutional interests. In discussions of health care delivery, for example, proponents of a broad extension of medical services often appeal to the "right to health care," whereas opponents sometimes appeal to the "rights of the medical profession." Many participants in these moral, political, and legal debates seem to presuppose that arguments cannot be made persuasive unless they can be stated in the language of rights, although other participants prefer to avoid the confrontational connotation of rights language.

The Nature and Status of Rights

Rights are justified claims that individuals and groups can make upon others or upon society. To have a right is to be in a position to determine, by one's choices, what others are to do or need not do.[42] Rights give us a claim based on a system of rules that authorize us to affirm, demand, or insist upon what is due. If a person possesses a right, others are validly constrained from interfering with the exercise of that right. Claiming will hereafter be understood as a rule-governed activity. The rules may be legal rules, moral rules, institutional rules, or rules of games, but all rights exist or fail to exist because the relevant rules either allow or disallow the claim or entitlement in question. These rules distinguish valid claims from invalid claims. *Legal* rights are claims that are justified by legal principles and rules, and *moral* rights are claims that are justified by moral principles and rules. A right, then, is a justified claim or entitlement, validated by moral principles and rules.[43]

A rights holder need not assert his or her rights in order to have them. For example, small children, the comatose, and the mentally handicapped may not be able to claim their rights. Nonetheless, claims can be made for them by authorized representatives.

Absolute and Prima Facie Rights

Some rights may be absolute, such as the right to choose one's religion or to reject all religion, but typically rights are not absolute. Like principles of obligation, rights assert only prima facie claims (in the sense of "prima facie" introduced in Chapter 1). Some writers have asserted that rights are absolute, at least in restricted contexts. Ronald Dworkin is well known for his view that rights are individuals' "political trumps" and cannot be overridden to advance social interests. Although political decisions normally advance communal interests, he argues that the whole point of rights language is to constrain the community from acting at the expense of individuals. However, as Dworkin recognizes, if the claims of public utility are highly significant, it is not justifiable to allow the individual to play a trump card.[44] Dworkin, then, advances a sound theory about the *purpose* of having rights, rather than about their stringency or absoluteness.

Legitimate conflicting rights must be balanced or specified to reduce the conflict. Even the right to life is not absolute, irrespective of competing claims or social conditions, as evidenced by common moral judgments about killing in war and killing in self-defense. We have a right not to have our lives taken without justification, not an absolute right to life. Any right can be legitimately exercised and can create obligations on others only if the right overrides competing rights. Rights such as a right to give an informed consent or refusal, a right to die, and a right to lifesaving medical technology must compete with other rights, often producing a need to further specify the rights or to balance competing claims.[45]

In light of this need for balance, a *violation* of a right should be distinguished from an *infringement* of a right.[46] Violation refers to an unjustified action against a right, whereas infringement refers to a justified action overriding a right. When a right is justifiably overridden, it is infringed but not violated.

Positive Rights and Negative Rights

Whereas a positive right is a right to be provided with a particular good or service by others, a negative right is a right to be free from some action taken by others. A person's positive right entails another's obligation to do something for that person; a negative right entails another's obligation to refrain from doing something.[47] Examples of both sorts of rights are found in biomedical practice, research, and policy. If a right to health care exists, for example, it is a positive right to goods and services grounded in a claim of justice (see Chapter 6, pp. this 348–358). However, the right to forgo a recommended surgical procedure is a negative right grounded in the principle of respect for autonomy. The liberal individualist tradition has generally found it easier to justify negative rights, but the recognition of welfare rights in modern societies has extended the scope of rights to positive rights.

Confusion about public policies governing biomedicine can often be traced to a failure to distinguish positive and negative rights. One example involves the U.S. Supreme Court decisions on abortion. Those who contend that the various abortion decisions are inconsistent fail to see that the Court first recognized a negative right and later refused to recognize a positive right. The Court first ruled that a woman's right to privacy gives her a right to have an abortion prior to fetal viability (and after fetal viability if her life or health is threatened). The constitutionally protected right of privacy is here construed exclusively as a negative right that limits state interference. Many people thought that the Court had concomitantly recognized a positive right in its early decisions, namely a right to receive aid and assistance. They were surprised when the Court later ruled that the federal and state governments do not have obligations to provide funds for nontherapeutic abortions.[48] The Court's reasoning is consistent. It affirms a negative right and denies a positive right. (Our analysis is limited to this issue of consistency. We are not evaluating the substance of the court decisions.)

This controversy, and rights generally, should be analyzed by reference to the distinction between the statements (1) "X has a right to do Y" and (2) "X acts rightly in doing Y." The distinction is between rights (or a right) and right conduct, as well as between rights and their right exercise.[49] Sometimes when we say that a person "has a right to do X," we mean that he or she does not do wrong in performing X. But often our statement that someone "has a right to do X" implies nothing about the morality of the act, other than that others have no right to interfere with it. Thus, one can consistently affirm that a woman has a moral or a legal right to have an abortion and likewise affirm that she is not acting rightly in exercising her right.

The Correlativity of Rights and Obligations

How are rights connected to obligations? To answer this question, consider the meaning of "X has a right to do or have Y." X's right entails that some party has an obligation either not to interfere if X does Y or to provide X with Y. If a state has an obligation to provide goods such as food or health care to needy citizens, then any citizen who meets the relevant criteria of need can claim an entitlement to food or health care. This analysis suggests a firm but untidy *correlativity* between obligations and rights.[50]

Suppose a physician agrees to take John Doe as a patient and commences treatment. The physician incurs an obligation to Doe, and Doe gains correlative rights. There may be rights to a certain level of care and rights in care, such as the right to refuse treatment. This correlativity of rights and obligations is untidy because one use of the words *requirement, obligation,* and *duty* suggests that obligations do not always imply corresponding rights. For example, although we sometimes refer to requirements or obligations of charity, no person can claim another person's charity as a matter of right. If such norms express what we "ought to do," they do so not from obligation but from personal ideals that exceed obligation. These commitments are best construed as self-imposed "oughts" that are not required by morality and that do not generate rights-claims for other persons.

A traditional distinction between obligations of perfect obligation and obligations of imperfect obligation can help us analyze this problem. Justice exemplifies perfect obligation, which entails a correlative right; whereas kindness, generosity, and charity exemplify imperfect obligation, which entails no correlative right. Mill argued that "Justice implies something which is not only right to do, and wrong not to do, but which some individual person can claim from us as his moral right. No one has a moral right to our generosity or beneficence, because we are not morally bound to practice those virtues towards any given individual."[51] Mill rightly saw that obligations of justice have correlative rights and are perfect. But, as we explicate beneficence in Chapter 5, many obligations of beneficence are also perfect obligations. We therefore need to augment Mill's analysis (here using beneficence as an example): (1) Some obligations of beneficence are *perfect* (for example, the obligations of rescue discussed in Chapter 5 and parental obligations to protect children), and (2) some obligations of beneficence are *imperfect* (for example, kindness and generosity), just as Mill describes them. But (3) some so-called "obligations" of beneficence are *self-imposed* requirements that are neither perfect nor imperfect obligations (for example some forms of kindness and generosity). For type 1, perfect obligations, the correlativity thesis always holds; these obligations and rights are those we typically find proper for enforcement by moral and legal sanctions, because a violation of rights and a failure of obligation are involved. Self-imposed requirements of type 3, by contrast, are optional and never have correlative rights. Obligations of type 2 may or may not have correlative rights. (We examine these problems further in Chapters 5 and 8.)

It is sometimes unclear without additional specification which obligation is correlative to a right, although it is clear that *some* obligation is correlative. Consider again the right to life. "X has a right to life" means that the moral system (or the legal system) imposes an obligation on other persons not to deprive X of life. However, this right does not specifically entail that X cannot come to an agreement with another party to end X's life through an act of euthanasia. What X *wants* makes a difference to how we understand rights, waivers of rights, and the exercise of rights. We conclude that rights language is correlative to obligation language, but in an untidy way requiring careful attention to particular contexts and often further specification of both rights and their correlative obligations.

The Primacy of Rights

The correlativity thesis does not determine whether rights or obligations, if either, is the more fundamental or primary category. The proposal that ethical theory should be "rights-based" [52] springs from a conception of the function and justification of morality. If the function of morality is to protect individuals' interests (rather than communal interests), and if rights (rather than obligations) are our primary instruments to this end, then moral action-guides are rights-based. Rights thus precede obligations and any other forms of protection.

This proposal can be illustrated by a theory we encounter in Chapter 6: the libertarian theory of justice. One representative, Robert Nozick, maintains that "Individuals have rights, and there are things no person or group may do to them (without violating their rights)." [53] He takes the following rule to be basic in the moral life: All persons have a right to be left free to do as they choose. The obligation not to interfere with this right follows from the right itself. That it "follows" is an indication of the priority of a rule of right over a rule of obligation. That is, an obligation is derived from a right.

Another rights-based argument that uses *positive or benefit* rights has been advanced by Alan Gewirth:

Rights are to obligations as benefits are to burdens. For rights are justified claims to certain benefits, the support of certain interests of the subject or right-holder. Obligations, on the other hand, are justified burdens on the part of the respondent or duty-bearer; they restrict his freedom by requiring that he conduct himself in ways that directly benefit not himself but rather the right-holder. But burdens are for the sake of benefits, and not vice versa. Hence obligations, which are burdens, are for the sake of rights, whose objects are benefits.

Rights, then, are prior to obligations in the order of justifying purpose . . . in that respondents have correlative obligations *because* subjects have certain rights. [54]

These rights-based accounts do not reject the correlativity thesis. Rather, they accept a priority thesis holding that obligations follow from rights, not the converse. Rights form the justificatory basis of obligations because they best capture the purpose of morality, which is to secure liberties or other benefits for a rights-holder.

A Critical Evaluation of Liberal Individualism

Problems with rights-based theories. One problem with basing ethics in rights is that rights are only a piece of a more general account that stakes out what makes a claim valid. Justification of the system of rules within which valid claiming occurs is not itself rights-based. Pure rights-based accounts also run the risk of truncating or impoverishing our understanding of morality, because rights cannot account for the moral significance of motives, supererogatory actions, virtues, and the like. Such a limited theory would fare poorly under criteria of comprehensiveness and explanatory and justificatory power. Accordingly, rights-based accounts should not be understood as a comprehensive or complete moral theory, but rather as an account of the minimal and enforceable rules that communities and individuals must observe in their treatment of all persons.

Normative questions about the exercise of rights. Often the question is not whether someone has a right, but whether the right possessed should or should not be exercised. If a person says, "I know you have the right to do x, but you should not do it," this moral claim cannot be reduced to a statement of a right. One's obligation or character, not one's right, is in question. Even if we had a full and complete theory of rights, we would still need a theory of obligation, at least about the appropriate exercise of rights, and it does not appear possible to develop a satisfactory account by attention only to rights and their limits.

The neglect of communal goods. Liberal individualists sometimes write as if the major concern of social morality is the protection of individual interests against government intrusion. This vision is too limited, because it excludes not only bona fide communal demands and group interests, but also communal goods and forms of life such as public health, biomedical research, and the protection of animals. The better perspective is that social ideals and principles of obligation are as critical to social morality as rights, and that neither is dispensable. Rights can sometimes be overridden by momentous communal interests.

The adversarial character of rights. Finally, the language of *claims* and *entitlements* is often unnecessarily adversarial. For example, the current interest in children's rights gives children many vital protections against abuse (for instance, when parents refuse to authorize lifesaving therapies for children for inappropriate reasons), but the notion that children have claims against their parents is an inadequate framework to express the moral character of the parent–child relationship. The attempt to understand this relationship and others such as health care relationships strictly in terms of rights neglects and may even undermine the affection, sympathy, and trust at the core of the relationship. This is not to suggest that rights are inherently adversarial or that they are dispensable, but rather to note that rights theory is a partial framework.

A Constructive Evaluation of Liberal Individualism

In recent ethical theory some writers have sought to replace the language of rights altogether. The thought is either that rights language can be replaced by another vocabulary (obligations, virtues, etc.) or that the assertion of valid individual claims against society has risky implications. We reject such views, and we accept both the correlativity thesis and the moral and social purposes served by traditional interpretations of basic human rights.

We suspect that no part of the moral vocabulary has done more to protect the legitimate interests of citizens in political states than the language of rights. Predictably, injustice and inhumane treatment occur most frequently in states that fail to recognize human rights in their political rhetoric and documents. As much as any part of moral discourse, rights language crosses international boundaries and enters into treaties, international law, and statements by international agencies and associations. Rights thereby become acknowledged as international standards for the treatment of persons and the evaluation of communal action.

Being a rights-bearer in a society that enforces rights is both a source of personal protection and a source of dignity and self-respect. By contrast, to maintain that someone has an *obligation* to protect another's interest may leave the recipient in a passive position, dependent upon the other's good will in fulfilling the obligation. When persons possess enforceable rights correlative to obligations, they are enabled to be active, independent agents pursuing their projects and making claims. What we often cherish most is not that someone is obligated to us, but that we have a right that secures for us the opportunity to pursue and claim as ours the benefit or liberty that we value.

Communitarianism: Community-Based Theory

Communitarian theories view everything fundamental in ethics as deriving from communal values, the common good, social goals, traditional practices, and the cooperative virtues. Conventions, traditions, and social solidarity play a far more prominent role in communitarian theories than in the types of theory discussed to this point.

How might communitarians approach the case of potential kidney transplantation discussed previously in this chapter? Their first inquiry would not be which rights are at stake, but which communal values and relationships are

present or absent. They would focus on the family as a small community inter-
mediate between the individual and the state. They would likely ask which
acts, rules, and policies of living organ donation, privacy, and confidentiality
best reinforce and promote communal values, including family values.

Communitarian critics of the father's behavior, which reduces his daughter's
chances of survival, would charge that he is insufficiently committed to the
goods of the family and presupposes the values of liberal individualism in
standing on his rights, without adequately attending to his responsibilities. Critics would likely see the father as a twisted product of a society that focuses too
much on protecting rights such as autonomy and privacy, and they may view
the physician in the same light. The physician would certainly be expected to
consider whether his actions conform to traditions of medicine, with its communal goods, codes, and virtues. In this tradition, deception has often been
justified in the treatment of the patient, but the father requests that others be
deceived, a relatively rare request and one with less clear historical precedent
in medical practice. By contrast, nondisclosure to others because of confidentiality does have clear historical precedent in medicine, but these rules are not
absolute and have often been overridden by a larger social interest.

The communitarian will support actions that express communal values as
well as actions having a positive impact on a community. The father contends
that if the physician tells other members of the family the true reasons for his
decision not to donate, it would wreck the family. The father's prediction about
this negative impact may or may not be correct, but what his actions express
about his own lack of commitment to the family's welfare is notable. From the
communitarian's perspective, the father embodies the vices of liberal individualism rather than the cooperative virtues.

The Repudiation of Liberalism

Contemporary communitarians repudiate central tenets in what is often called
liberalism, a term that is defined through cardinal premises in the types of
theory we have discussed in three previous sections: utilitarian, Kantian, and
liberal individualist theories. What makes them jointly "liberal" is their commitment to what Mill defended as *individuality*, what Kant called *autonomy,*
and what liberal individualists protect as *rights of the person.* Each type of
theory protects the individual against the state, and—on the communitarian
interpretation—each also asserts that the state should neither reward nor penal-
ize different conceptions of the good life held by individuals. Postulates of
individual autonomy, rights against the state, and community neutrality toward
conflicting values, then, are the central elements of liberalism to which communitarians object.

In reacting critically to liberalism, contemporary communitarians repudiate the *theory* as well as *current societies* established on the premises of liberal theory, including many contemporary Western political states.[55] According to communitarians, these societies lack a commitment to the general welfare, to common purposes, and to education in citizenship, while expecting and even encouraging social and geographic mobility, distanced personal relations, welfare dependence, breakdowns in family life and marital fidelity, political fragmentation, and the like. The number of abandoned children and elderly parents, social and familial fragmentation, the disappearance of meaningful democracy, and the lack of effective communal programs are, according to communitarians, the disastrous products of liberalism.

The meaning of *community* and its synonyms varies. Some communitarians refer almost exclusively to the political state as the community, whereas others refer to smaller communities and institutions with defined goals and role obligations. Some include the family as a basic communal unit, within which being a parent and being a child involve specific roles and responsibilities. Much of what one ought to do in communitarian theories is determined by the social roles assigned to or acquired by a person as a member of the community. Understanding a particular system of moral rules, then, requires an understanding of the community's history, sense of cooperative life, and conception of social welfare.

With regard to theory, communitarian criticisms have often been directed at Mill and Kant, but recently they have been aimed at Rawls, whose liberal principle that the rights of individuals cannot legitimately be sacrificed for the good of the community has been a particular target of communitarian censure.[56] These communitarian criticisms of liberal theories seem to amount to the following: Liberalism (1) fails to appreciate the constructive role of the cooperative virtues and the political state in promoting values and creating the conditions of the good life, (2) fails to acknowledge shared goals and obligations that come not from freely made contracts among individuals, but from communal ideals and responsibilities, and (3) fails to understand the human person as historically constituted by and embedded in communal life and social roles.

Michael Sandel describes the positive aspect of communal life that is allegedly missed by liberal theory:

> In so far as our constitutive self-understandings comprehend a wider subject than the individual alone, whether a family or tribe or city or class or nation or people, to this extent they define a community in the constitutive sense. And what marks such a community is not merely a spirit of benevolence, or the prevalence of communitarian values, or even certain "shared final ends" alone, but a common vocabulary of discourse and a background of implicit practices and understandings.[57]

Communitarians thus revitalize Hegel's criticism of Kant that was mentioned in Chapter 1 (namely, Kant presents an "empty formalism" without an "immanent doctrine of duties") and apply it to liberals: They miss the essence of morality by emphasizing abstract principles and abstract agents, while failing to see that both principles and agents are social products of communal life. Communitarians also propose that we give up the principles, politics, and language of rights in favor of the principles, politics, and language of the common good and the community's way of life.[58]

Militant and Moderate Forms of Communitarianism

Communitarianism can be distinguished into *militant* and *moderate* forms. Militants firmly support community control and reject liberal theories. This approach has been supported by influential contemporary moral, social, and political thinkers, including Alasdair MacIntyre, Charles Taylor, and Michael Sandel. By contrast, moderates emphasize the importance of various forms of community—including the family and the political state—while attempting to accommodate rather than reject strands in liberal theories. This sense of communitarianism includes figures as diverse as Aristotle, Hugo Grotius, David Hume, G. W. F. Hegel, John Mackie, and Michael Walzer. For them social order and morality rest on historically developed norms, and moral rules derive their acceptability and correctness from these shared conventions. Although *communitarianism* is a recently coined term typically used for the militant form, we will use it for both forms. We will criticize militant theories, while relying on the moderate theories for our constructive evaluation.

Militant communitarianism is hostile to rights, sees liberalism as "born of antagonism to all tradition," and aims to perpetuate and even impose on individuals conceptions of virtue and the good life that limit the rights conferred by liberal societies. These communitarians see persons as intrinsically *constituted* by communal values and as best suited to achieve personal goods through communal life.[59] In addition, MacIntyre argues that we have inherited many incoherent fragments of once coherent schemes of thought and action, and only if we understand our peculiar historical and cultural situation can we recognize the problematic dimensions of the enterprise of moral evaluation and moral theory.[60]

The moderate communitarian takes a stance far less opposed to autonomy and individual rights. A typical example is J. L. Mackie's appeal to "intersubjective standards," meaning that community-wide agreements form the basis of acceptable moral rules and that these intersubjective agreements cannot be further validated or invalidated by appeal to rationality. Mackie understands morality entirely in terms of social practices that express what is demanded, allowed, enforced, and condemned in the community. Nonetheless, he insists that moral judgments need not be viewed as unchanging conventional rules beyond the possibility of reform: "Of course there have been and are moral heretics and moral reformers. . . . But this can usually be understood as the extension, in ways which, though new and unconventional, seemed to them to be required for consistency of rules to which they already adhered as arising out of an existing way of life."[61]

The Primacy of Social Practices

Alasdair MacIntyre and other communitarians have traced to Aristotle the thesis that local community practices and their corresponding virtues should have priority over ethical theory in normative decisionmaking. MacIntyre uses "practice" to designate a cooperative arrangement in pursuit of goods that are internal to a structured communal life. Social roles of parenting, teaching, governing, healing, and the like involve practices. "Goods internal to a practice" are achievable, according to MacIntyre, only by engaging in the practice and conforming to its constraints and standards of excellence. In the practice of medicine, for example, goods internal to the profession exist, and these determine what it is to be a good physician. The virtues of physicians flow from communal and institutional practices of care, practical wisdom, and teaching. Medicine, like other professions and political institutions, has a history that sustains a tradition requiring participants in the practice to cultivate certain virtues.[62]

The importance of traditional practices and the need for communal intervention to correct socially disruptive outcomes are standard themes in communitarian thought. For example, Sandel proposes that we disallow plant closings that devastate local communities and that we ban pornography when it deeply offends a community's way of life.[63] As an example of communitarians' promotion of the common good in biomedical ethics, consider their debate with liberal individualists over policies of obtaining cadaveric organs for transplantation. Based on principles of liberal individualism, but with an interest in obtaining cadaveric organs to save lives, all states in the United States adopted the Uniform Anatomical Gift Act in the late 1960s and early 1970s. This act gives individuals the right to make decisions about the donation of their organs through a donor card. If the individual has not made a decision prior to death, the law authorizes the family to decide whether to donate the decedent's organs. On the basis of opinion polls, it was expected that individuals would sign donor cards and provide a sufficient supply of organs, thereby avoiding the need to search for living donors of kidneys.

In practice, however, few individuals sign donor cards, the cards are rarely available at the time of death, and procurement teams virtually always check with the family even if the decedent left a valid donor card. As a result, a communitarian focus has emerged. The family has become the primary donor (that is, the decisionmaker about donation) rather than the individual, and because the supply of organs has remained limited, various policies have been considered and some adopted that aim to promote the common good more vigorously. Even approaches that protect individual rights attempt to educate people about the need for organs, and some propose *requiring* people to make a decision about donation, for instance, when obtaining a driver's license. Laws and regulations have also been implemented to require hospitals to ask families whether they know the wishes of the decedent and want to donate the decedent's organs.

Some communitarians now recommend still stronger laws to make organ procurement a well-defined community project rather than a matter of individual or even family decisions. They defend *presumed consent* laws, which would parallel laws in several states for corneas and laws in several countries for solid organs. These laws presume that individuals or families have decided to donate unless they have registered a dissent. A more stringent proposal is the routine salvaging of organs unless objections are registered. Here communitarians defend a policy of organ retrieval on grounds that members of a community should be willing to provide others objects of lifesaving value when no cost to themselves is required.[64] A few commentators even recommend harsher policies of conscription of cadaveric organs to reflect community ownership of cadaveric body parts. The latter approach conflicts so deeply with liberal individualistic values that it has not received serious consideration. Nevertheless, an extreme alternative approach based on liberal individualism, a market in organs, has been declared illegal in the United States because of concern about exploitation and coercion. Proponents of a market in organs typically view their communitarian opponents as zealous and inconsistent, because they allow and encourage individual or family *gifts* to benefit others but rule out *sales* that would provide the same benefit and perhaps even increase the supply of organs for transplantation.[65]

An emphasis on the community and the common good also appears in debates about the allocation of health care. In Daniel Callahan's communitarian account, we should enact public policy from a shared consensus about the good society, not on the basis of individual rights. Liberal assumptions about state neutrality should be scrapped, and society should be free to implement a substantive concept of the good. According to Callahan, biomedical ethics should use communitarian values to implement or revise social laws and regulations governing the promotion of health, the use of genetic knowledge, the use of advances in medical technology, responsibilities to future generations, and the limits of health care for the elderly. In each case, the question to be asked is, "What is most conducive to a good society?," not "Is it harmful or does it violate autonomy?"[66] Here we see a close similarity to utilitarian proposals. However, communitarians typically reject the principle of utility on grounds that it is remote from actual communal decisionmaking and, in any event, is individualistic in its effort to sum up individual benefits and costs for public policy.

Although many communitarians critique and propose specific acts, practices, and policies, such as procuring organs or allocating health care, few systematic communitarian proposals have emerged for biomedical ethics as a whole. One exception is Ezekiel Emanuel's vision of medical ethics, which rests on the following claims: The ends of medicine, as affirmed by the profession, have been shaped by public laws and public values. These ends are understood through a framework of shared political convictions, conceptions of justice, and ideas of the good life. In place of the liberalism that has typically undergirded medical ethics, Emanuel proposes a moderate communitarianism closely connected to political theory. This communitarianism is moderate by virtue of its acceptance of pluralistic conceptions of the good life and its recognition of some individual rights. Yet it remains communitarian because democratic initiatives will be needed to fashion a community's conceptions of the good life into policies and laws. Emanuel envisions thousands of community health plans in which citizen-members deliberate about conceptions of the good life and debate policies such as those for termination of life-sustaining treatment for incompetent patients and the allocation of medical resources.[67]

A Critical Evaluation of Communitarian Ethics

Several claims by militant communitarians rely on questionable accusations and arguments. We will concentrate on these problems in our criticisms. However, many themes in moderate communitarianism are unproblematic and even acceptable to many advocates of liberal theories. We focus on these unproblematic positions in our constructive section below.

An unfair account of liberal theories. Militant communitarians suggest that liberal theorists defend atomic, isolated individuals and have a corrupting skepticism about communal goods.[68] This characterization is inaccurate and unfair. Mill and Rawls, the figures most frequently attacked by communitarians, never depict either individuals or the communal good in these terms, and both philosophers develop a theory of the common good, as well as an account of social traditions and political community.[69] Mill thought he had captured how historical traditions converge to the principle of utility, which he construed as a principle of communal welfare. Even in *On Liberty,* Mill argued that a community should take steps to ensure adequate public discussion of what constitutes the good of the community. Liberty functions in his arguments to protect individuals against mistakes in planning communal pursuits of the good, and he defends individuality *because* it conduces to a constantly readjusted and improved social unit. Rawls defends rights and the value of liberty in society, in part, because social ends can be corrected better in an open society than in a society controlled by tradition.[70]

A false dichotomy: community or autonomy. Communitarians present us with two false dichotomies: (1) either liberal accounts of rights and justice have priority or the communal good has priority,[71] and (2) either radical autonomy in decisionmaking is protected or communal determination of social goals is protected against the individual. A more accurate picture is that we inherit various social roles and goals from traditions. We then critique, adjust, and attempt to improve our beliefs over time through free discussion and collective arrangements. Individuals and groups alike progressively interpret, revise, and sometimes even replace traditions with new conceptions that adjust and foster community values. This outlook of liberalism is, as Joel Feinberg notes, entirely compatible with communal interests: "It is impossible to think of human beings except as part of ongoing communities, defined by reciprocal bonds of obligation, common traditions, and institutions. . . . The ideal [in liberals' accounts] of the autonomous person is that of an authentic individual whose self-determination is as complete as is consistent with the requirement that he is, of course, a member of a community."[72]

A failed challenge to rights. Communitarians sometimes argue against rights (especially natural rights) on grounds that they do not exist.[73] At other times they argue against rights on grounds that rights stall communal organization and dull our sense of social union. Both claims miss the valuable consequences that rights have for communities. We value rights because, when enforced, they provide protections against unscrupulous behavior, promote orderly change and cohesiveness in communities, and allow diverse communities to coexist peacefully within a single political state.[74] As Judith Jarvis Thomson notes,

How much more satisfying the life in an 'organic community' than the life of alienation in a modern state! The ideal of the hive is seductive and fuels all communitarian ideologies. But the bee-like creatures of our hive-like world are not in fact kind to each other; each is indifferent to the others except insofar as the others are parts of the whole. . . . The ideal of the state as hive cannot be made real: it is amazing that communitarians have expected otherwise.[75]

Even if we grant communitarian arguments that the best life is communal life, it would not follow that communities should determine the individual's goals or truncate individual rights. The major reason for the prominence of rights in moral and political theory is that they stand as a shield against communal intrusion by governments. This and similar criticisms raise profound questions about how well communitarianism fares on several of the criteria for theory construction presented in the beginning of this chapter, especially output, explanatory, and justificatory power.

A Constructive Evaluation of Communitarianism

By emphasizing historical traditions and institutional practices, communitarian theories have made a substantial contribution to the redirection of ethical theory in recent years, and have also helped us rediscover the importance of community even if we accept liberal values. Communitarians rightly emphasize the need to foster neighborhood associations, create communal ties, promote public health, and develop national goals. Also to be welcomed is the return in some communitarian theories to such landmarks in ethical theory as the writings of Aristotle, Hume, and Hegel. These more community-minded philosophers deserve status as great classical theorists, alongside Mill and Kant.

Ethics of Care: Relationship-Based Accounts

Another family of moral reflections is widely referred to as the *ethics of care*. It shares some premises with communitarian ethics, including some objections to central features of liberalism and an emphasis on traits valued in intimate personal relationships, such as sympathy, compassion, fidelity, discernment, and love. *Caring* in these accounts refers to care for, emotional commitment to, and willingness to act on behalf of persons with whom one has a significant relationship. Noticeably downplayed are Kantian universal rules, impartial utilitarian calculations, and individual rights.

Proponents of an ethics of care would approach the case we have been examining by focusing on relationships involving care, responsibility, trust, fidelity, and sensitivity. The father who elects not to donate a kidney expresses some concern about his daughter's suffering, but his response is arguably grounded mainly in concern about himself. He does not think he can justify his behavior to his wife, who will, he believes, distrust him and "accuse him of allowing his daughter to die." Even if we give the father the benefit of the doubt about motives and trustworthiness, whether his care is responsibly expressed in donation or nondonation will depend in part on the balance of risks and benefits and his courage in confronting the risks.

The physician in this case faced several conflicts within relationships of care—to the dying daughter, her siblings, the reluctant father, the mother, and the family as a unit. Just as many moral theories face conflicts of principles and rights, the ethic of care faces conflicts among responsibilities in such situations. Traditional moral theory has typically concentrated on answers to questions about whether to lie or break confidentiality. The ethic of care, by contrast, emphasizes that it is not only important what the physician does—for example, breaks or maintains confidentiality—but also how actions are performed, which motives underlie them and whether positive relationships are promoted or thwarted. The trustworthiness of the physician and the quality of his care and sensitivity in the face of the father's unusual request for deception are all integral moral elements from the perspective of the ethics of care.

Two Speakers in a Different Voice

The origin of the ethic of care was predominantly in feminist writings. The themes included how women display an ethic of care, by contrast to men, who predominantly exhibit an ethic of rights and obligations. We begin with two figures who have played prominent roles in this recent history, psychologist Carol Gilligan and philosopher Annette Baier.

Gilligan's psychological account. The hypothesis that "women speak in a different voice"—a voice that traditional ethical theory has drowned out—arose in Gilligan's book, *In a Different Voice.* She maintained that women's moral development is typically distinct from men's, a fact she thought disregarded by influential psychological studies of moral development whose conceptions were based on studies of males only. She claimed to discover "the voice of care" through empirical research involving interviews with girls and women. This voice, she said, stresses empathic association with others, not based on "the primacy and universality of individual rights, but rather on . . . a very strong sense of being responsible." In her studies, female subjects typically view morality in terms of responsibilities of care deriving from attachments to others, whereas male subjects typically see morality in terms of rights and justice. Men look to and are formed by freely accepted relationships and agreements; women look to and are formed by contextually given relationships such as those of the family.[76]

Gilligan, then, identified two modes of relationship and two modes of moral thinking: an ethic of care in contrast to an ethic of rights and justice. She does not claim that these two modes of thinking are strictly correlated with gender or that all women or all men speak in the same moral voice.[77] Rather, she believes that men *tend* to embrace an ethic of rights using quasi-legal terminology and impartial principles, accompanied by dispassionate balancing and conflict resolution, whereas women *tend* to affirm an ethic of care that centers on responsiveness in an interconnected network of needs, care, and prevention of harm. Taking care of others is the core notion, and it is modelled on relationships such as those between parent and child.[78]

Baier's philosophical account. Gilligan's interpretation of empirical data has parallels in philosophical ethics. In Annette Baier's account, the reasoning and methods of women who write in ethical theory is noticeably different from traditional theories. She claims to hear in contemporary female philosophers, despite their diversity, the same different voice that Gilligan heard in her studies, but one made "reflective and philosophical."[79] She deplores the near-exclusive emphasis in modern moral philosophy on universal rules and principles, and she sternly rejects Kantian contractarian models with their emphasis on justice, rights, law, and particularly autonomous choice among free and equal agents. The conditions of social cooperation, especially in families and in communal decisionmaking, are, Baier observes, typically unchosen and intimate, and they involve unequals in a relational network. Her thesis is not that traditional ethical theories are false or even outmoded, but that they capture only a piece of the larger moral world.[80]

Baier envisions not a grand system of ethics that holds together all the diverse strands, but smaller scale systems that pull together a few strands. In casting about for a connecting bridge to span an ethic of love with an ethic of obligation, she proposes "appropriate trust" as a bridging concept. She does not recommend that we discard categories of obligation, but that we make room for an ethic of love and trust, including an account of human bonding and friendship. Traditional models of ethical theory often fail to acknowledge how parents and health care professionals, for example, see responsibilities to their children and patients in terms of care, loving attachment, meeting needs, and providing sustenance.[81]

Criticisms of Traditional Liberal Theories

Proponents of the care perspective offer a direct challenge to liberal values. Two criticisms of liberalism deserve special mention.[82]

Challenging impartiality. According to the care perspective, liberalism has lost sight of the full sweep of morality by taking a standpoint of detached fairness. This orientation is suitable for some moral relationships, especially those in which persons interact as equals in a public context of impersonal justice and institutional constraints. But lost in this *detachment* is an *attachment* to that which we care about most and which is closest to us—for example, our loyalty to groups. In the absence of public and institutional constraints, partiality toward others is not only morally permissible but is the expected norm of interaction and is an ineliminable feature of the human condition. Without exhibiting partiality we stand to sever important relationships and to alienate others. In seeking a blinded impartiality, liberalism risks making us blind and indifferent to the special needs of and relationships with others. Although impartiality is a moral virtue in some contexts, it is a moral vice in others. This two-sidedness is overlooked in traditional liberal theory, which simply aligns good and mature moral judgment with moral distance.[83] The care perspective is especially meaningful for roles such as parent, friend, physician, and nurse, in which contextual response, attentiveness to subtle clues, and the deepening of special relationships are likely to be more momentous morally than impartial treatment.

Challenging universal principles. An aversion to abstract principles, the instruments of impartiality, is also characteristic of the ethics of care. As long as principles allow room for discretionary and contextual judgment, the ethics of care need not dispense with principles. However, like many proponents of virtue theory, defenders of the ethics of care find principles often irrelevant, unproductive, ineffectual, or constrictive in the moral life. A defender of principles could say that *principles* of care, compassion, and kindness tutor our responses in caring, compassionate, and kind ways. But this claim seems hollow. Our moral experience suggests that our responses rely on our emotions, our capacity for sympathy, our sense of friendship, and our knowledge of how caring people behave.

Consider, as an example, the following report by physician Timothy Quill and nurse Penelope Townsend of a discussion with a young woman who has just been told that she is HIV infected:[84]

PATIENT: Oh God. Oh Lord have mercy. . . . Please don't do it again. Please don't tell me that. Oh my God. Oh my children. Oh Lord have mercy. Oh God, why did He do this to me? . . .

DR QUILL: First thing we have to do is learn as much as we can about it, because right now you are okay.

PATIENT: I don't even have a future. Everything I know is that you gonna die anytime. What is there to do? What if I'm a walking time bomb? People will be scared to even touch me or say anything to me.

DR QUILL: No, that's not so.

PATIENT: Yes they will, 'cause I feel that way . . .

DR QUILL: There is a future for you . . .

PATIENT: Okay, alright. I'm so scared. I don't want to die. I don't want to die, Dr Quill, not yet. I know I got to die, but I don't want to die.

DR QUILL: We've got to think about a couple of things. . . .

Quill and Townsend have moral responsibilities to their patient, but it is difficult to capture their responsibilities through principles and rules. We can produce rough generalizations about how caring physicians and nurses respond to patients, for example, but these generalizations will not be subtle enough to give helpful guidance for the next patient. Each situation calls for a set of responses exceeding what the generalization captures, and behavior that in one context is caring seems to intrude on privacy or to be offensive in another setting.

Relationship and Emotion

Two constructive themes are central to the ethics of care: mutual interdependence and emotional response.

Mutual interdependence in relationships. The ethics of care maintains that many human relationships—for example, in health care and research—involve persons who are vulnerable, dependent, ill, and frail and that the desirable moral response is attached attentiveness to needs, not detached respect for rights. Feeling for and being immersed in the other person establish vital facets of the moral relationship. Accordingly, this approach features responsibilities that a rights-based account may ignore in the attempt to protect persons from invasion by others.[85]

A role for the emotions. Ethical theory since the late eighteenth century has exhibited a cognitivist proclivity; that is, it has regarded theory and moral judgment as the affairs of reason, rather than of emotion or passion. Kant joined many other writers in the history of ethics, such as Plato, in depicting the emotions, feelings, passions, and inclinations as distracting impediments to moral judgment. These philosophers call for a struggle against desire, impulse, and inclination, in order that a more rational course of action will ensue. Actions done from desire, impulse, or inclination may be good in these theories, but not *morally* good, because they are not done from an appropriate cognitive framework.

The ethics of care corrects this cognitivist bias by giving the emotions a moral role. Having a certain emotional attitude and expressing the appropriate emotion in acting are morally relevant factors, just as having the appropriate motive for an action is morally relevant. The person who acts from rule-governed obligations without appropriately aligned feelings such as worry when a friend suffers seems to have a moral deficiency. In addition to expressing their feelings in their responses, agents also need to attend to the feelings of persons toward whom they act in moral relationships. Insight into the needs of others and considerate alertness to their circumstances often come from the emotions more than reason.[86] In the history of human experimentation, for example, those who first recognized that some subjects of research were being brutalized, subjected to misery, or placed at unjustifiable risk were persons who were able to feel compassion, disgust, and outrage through insight into the situation of these research subjects. They exhibited emotional discernment of and sensitivity to the feelings of subjects, where others lacked comparable responses.

This emphasis on the emotional dimension of the moral life does not reduce moral response to emotional response. Caring clearly has a cognitive dimension as well, because it involves an insight into and understanding of another's circumstance, needs, and feelings. As Hume pointed out, emotions motivate us and tell us much about a person's character, but it is the understanding that directs us in choosing a path of action.

A Critical Evaluation of the Care Ethic

The ethics of care emphasizes engaged, contextual, and even passionate moral thinking. As long as both passion and dispassion are acknowledged, few if any crippling criticisms can be brought against the ethics of care. Nonetheless, some problems need attention.

Underdeveloped theory. If one takes seriously the eight criteria for theory construction developed at the beginning of this chapter, then the ethics of care seems to fall short on criteria such as completeness, comprehensiveness, and explanatory and justificatory power. Of course, there may be a bias in the criteria: Because this list grows out of *traditional* accounts of theory that are often opposed by proponents of the ethics of care, it might be expected to reach a negative judgment on the ethics of care, which explicitly departs from traditional theory. But the heart of the problem is the lack of a developed and integrated body of reflections to supply the concepts and connections needed to satisfy these criteria. As Baier has pointed out, the ethics of care needs one or more central concepts and a set of bridging concepts to link it to the legitimate concerns of traditional theory. The ethic of care, then, is an underdeveloped theory, but not necessarily an incorrect one.

Should impartiality be rejected? In deemphasizing justice, impartiality, rights, and obligations, the ethics of care must confront situations in which bona fide requirements of impartiality conflict with acting partially from care. Acting partially clearly must sometimes yield to acting impartially. On at least some occasions we need an impartial judgment to arbitrate between conflicting moral judgments or feelings.[87] It is doubtful that many who endorse the ethics of care want their theory to be interpreted so narrowly as to exclude all impartial judgments and considerations of justice and the public good. But a problem remains about whether the theory can successfully incorporate these moral notions without losing much of its critical thrust and uniqueness. The ethic of care, as Gilligan and others have defended it, recognizes that two perspectives exist, but can they can be made *coherent?* Alternatively, one might argue (as Nel

Noddings does) that the ethics of care is the fundamental form of morality and that it is internally coherent. The latter, we suggest, simply gives up too much in the moral life.[88]

Too contextual and hostile to principles. One proponent of the ethics of care argues that in a defensible ethical theory, action should be "sometimes principle-guided, rather than always principle-derived."[89] This statement is a move in the right direction of coherence. However, if principles are accommodated by an ethics of care, does this inclusion undercut the grounds for antipathy to principles? The question is again one of coherence. Can the theory coherently trade on a rejection of some principles (Kantian principles, say), and at the same time accept a vital role for other principles (prima facie principles, say)?

We think principles will reappear in a more comprehensive theory and will enhance rather than weaken the ethics of care. If we agree that certain forms of sympathy and emotion are appropriate bases of motivation, we should be prepared for situations in which our actions are too partial and in need of correction by impartial principles. We are likely to judge more favorably persons who are close to us in intimate relationships, and yet on some occasions those who are distant from us deserve to be judged more favorably.

Feminist reservations about an ethics of care. Although initiated by feminist writers, the ethics of care has been sharply criticized by some feminists who worry that it attends to women's experiences as givers of care in traditional roles of self-sacrifice, but often neglects feminist insights into problems of oppression and dominance. Susan Sherwin argues that feminists should "be cautious about the place of caring in their approach to ethics; it is necessary to be wary of the implications of gender traits within a sexist culture. Because gender differences are central to the structures that support dominance relations, it is likely that women's proficiency at caring is somehow related to women's subordinate status."[90] She sees a need to examine the social context of care as well as to establish limits to the ethics of care. Both enterprises involve appeals to justice.

Without a broader framework, the ethics of care is too confined to the *private* sphere of intimate relationships and may serve to reinforce an uncritical adherence to traditional social patterns of assigning caretaker roles to women. Among health professionals, the ethic of care has been most widely appropriated by nurses. Without further explication, there is a danger that the ethics of care will be primarily located in nursing and primary care specialties in medicine to which many women are attracted, without having a major impact on health care as a whole.[91]

A Constructive Evaluation of the Care Ethic

The care ethic provides a needed corrective to two centuries of system-building in ethical theory and to the tendency to neglect themes such as sympathy, the moral emotions, and women's experiences. A morality centered on care and concern can potentially serve health care ethics in a constructive and balanced fashion, because it is close to the processes of reason and feeling exhibited in clinical contexts. We have seen that sympathy, friendliness, compassion, and trust cannot easily be brought under rules of behavior or even under a principle such as beneficence. Physician and nursing ethics have recently been presented in codes that express obligations and rights, but the ethics of care can retrieve basic commitments of caring and caretaking and help free health professionals from a narrow conception of their role responsibilities. Caring involves an open-minded responsiveness to another's needs as the other sees those needs, and therefore runs counter to the assumption that an established medical good will best meet those needs.

Disclosures, discussions, and decisionmaking in health care typically become a family affair, with support from a health care team. The ethics of care fits this context of relationships, whereas rights theory, for example, seems poorly equipped for it. Finally, correcting an undue obsession with impartiality requirements in traditional theories promises to have positive consequences because many aspects of character, forms of sensitivity, and modes of practical judgment exceed appeals to impartial principles. We return to these moral qualities in Chapter 8.

Casuistry: Case-Based Reasoning

Recently ethical theory has seen a revival of an approach with impressive influence in medieval and early modern philosophy. *Casuistry,* as it is called, focuses on practical decisionmaking in particular cases.[92] Casuists are skeptical of rules, rights, and theories divorced from history, precedent, and circumstance. Appropriate moral judgments occur, casuists say, through an intimate understanding of particular situations and the historical record of similar cases.[93]

Consider first how the casuist might approach the case of the father's refusal to become a donor. The casuist would begin by identifying particular features in the case rather than appealing to universal principles, utilitarian calculations, or rights. The casuist would then attempt to identify the relevant precedents and prior experiences with other cases, attempting to determine how similar and different this case is from experiences with other cases. In assessing what the father should do, the casuist would determine whether we typically insist, in relevantly similar cases, that parents bear comparable inconvenience and risk to offer their children some chance of survival. In determining what the physician should do, analogous cases would be considered in which breaches of confidentiality are justified or unjustified. The objective is to act in light of any strong social consensus found in precedent cases in medicine and law. Such cases would indicate, for example, that physicians have a right and sometimes an obligation to breach confidentiality in order to prevent harm to others. Examples of these cases include reporting gunshot wounds and venereal diseases and in some contexts warning intended victims of a patient's threatened violence.

The casuist might also ask whether the father's refusal to donate would cause a *harm* to his daughter or would only *fail to benefit* her and whether a threatened or actual breach of confidentiality might be justified in an effort to force him to donate. Similarly, the casuist would ask whether a lie ("the father is not histocompatible") or a milder form of deception ("for medical reason the father should not donate") could be justified to prevent wrecking the family. The casuist would attempt to answer these questions by appeal to maxims grounded in experience and tradition, as well as by reasoning from analogous cases.

The Recent Recovery of Casuistry

The recent rise of casuistry has surprised many, because in the last three hundred years casuistry had fallen into a disrepute rivaling astrology.[94] To illustrate its former low repute, when *An Encyclopedia of Religion* was published in 1945, then-prominent philosopher Edgar Sheffield Brightman wrote the entry on "casuistry," which read (in full):[95]

1) The application of ethical principles to specific cases. 2) Quibbling, rationalization, sophistry or an attempt to justify what does not merit justification; this meaning is often associated with methods used by Jesuits. See equivocation.

This definition is still typical of entries in reference works. But contemporary casuists would argue that Brightman and mainstream critics have matters upside-down. Casuists claim that their approach is not an application of principles to cases—quite the reverse, it moves up from cases to principles—and is a system of justification that tries to surmount the sophistry of "applying" principles.

A Repudiation of the Mainstream in Modern Ethics

As with communitarian theories and the ethics of care, the casuist is motivated in part by a dissatisfaction with the dominant ethical theories, including Kantianism, utilitarianism, and rights theory. In particular, casuists dispute the use of the model of scientific theory for ethical theory, the accompanying account of moral judgments, and the insistence on firm, universal principles.

Repudiating the model of a philosophical moral science. Some nineteenth- and twentieth-century philosophers seem to presuppose a model of a tidy, unified theory containing general and universal principles—in effect, a philosophical moral science.[96] Casuists reject this model, sometimes under the influence of Aristotle's conceptions of science and ethics. Aristotle noted the idea of a "first principle" that is certain and inherently justified belongs to science conceived on an axiomatic model,[97] but he held that principles in ethics are deeply embedded in the concrete world of human social conduct. Philosophers must obtain first principles by abstracting them from the mass of human actions and social practices.[98]

Casuists agree. Although there conceivably could be a first foundational principle for ethics that has absolute priority (not one from which all other moral content would follow), they maintain that moral beliefs and reasoning in fact do not follow this pattern. Ethics is not a demonstrative science, but a set of practices and types of judgment rooted in experience, wisdom, and prudence.

Repudiating moral judgment based on principles. Casuists interpret many moral philosophers to hold that cases are devoid of material that informs moral judgment, and thereby are powerless to determine obligation, blameworthiness, or praiseworthiness. Cases *illustrate* principles, *exemplify* dilemmas, *motivate* people to right actions, and the like; but cases are otherwise irrelevant to moral judgment. By contrast, casuists maintain that some forms of moral reasoning and judgment make no appeal to principles, rules, rights, or virtues. These forms include appeals to narratives, paradigm cases, analogies, models, classification schemes, and even immediate intuition and discerning insight.[99]

Rules and principles need not be excluded from moral thinking, but the casuist insists that moral judgments can be and often are made when no appeal to principles is possible. For example, we make moral judgments when principles, rules, or rights conflict and no further recourse to a higher principle, rule, or right is available. When principles are interpreted inflexibly irrespective of the nuances of the case, some casuists see a "tyranny of principles."[100] As a result, attempts at the resolution of moral problems suffer from a gridlock of conflicting principles, and moral debate becomes intemperate and interminable. This impasse can often be avoided, Albert Jonsen and Stephen Toulmin argue, by focusing on points of shared agreement about cases rather than on principles. The following is their prime example, drawn from their personal experiences during four years of work with the National Commission for the Protection of Human Subjects of Biomedical and Behavioral Research:

The one thing [*individual* commissioners] could not agree on was *why* they agreed. . . . Instead of securely established universal principles, . . . giving them intellectual grounding for particular judgments about specific kinds of cases, it was the other way around.

The *locus of certitude* in the commissioners' discussions . . . lay in a shared perception of what was specifically at stake in particular kinds of human situations. . . . That could never have been derived from the supposed theoretical certainty of the principles to which individual commissioners appealed in their personal accounts.[101]

In this account, casuistical reasoning rather than universal principles forged agreement. The commission functioned successfully by appeal to paradigms, particular cases, and families of cases, despite the various principles and inchoate moral theories individual commissioners held. Consensus about policies was reached by agreement on cases, when agreement would have been impossible to achieve on principles or theory. Although commissioners cited moral principles to justify their collective conclusions, Jonsen and Toulmin argue that these principles were less certain and central for commissioners in their deliberations than their particular judgments about cases.[102]

We agree that evidence supporting this interpretation exists in the work of the commission, but equally weighty evidence supports a justificatory role for principles in its deliberations, as we will see below.

Case-Based Reasoning and Judgment

Casuists typically hold that moral belief and knowledge evolve incrementally through reflection on cases, without essential recourse to a top-down theory. To support this thesis, casuists sometimes ask us to consider an analogy to case law. When the decision of a majority of judges becomes authoritative in a case, their judgments are positioned to become authoritative for other courts hearing cases with *similar* facts. This is the doctrine of precedent. Casuists see moral authority similarly: Social ethics develops from a social consensus formed around cases. This consensus is then extended to new cases by analogy to the past cases around which the consensus was formed. The underlying consensus and the paradigm cases become enduring and authoritative sources of appeal. For example, in the current literature of biomedical ethics, cases such as the Quinlan case, the Tuskegee Syphilis experiments, and the Quill case are constantly invoked not only to illustrate claims, but as sources of authority for new judgments.

As a history of similar cases and similar judgments mounts, we become more confident in our judgments. A "locus of moral certitude" is found in the judgments, and the stable elements crystallize in the form of tentative principles. As confidence in these generalizations increases, they are accepted less tentatively and moral knowledge develops. Just as case law (legal rules) develops incrementally from legal decisions in cases, so the moral law (moral rules) develops incrementally.[103]

Casuists find "the essence of the casuistic mode of thinking" in a gradual movement from clear and resolvable cases to more complex and difficult cases. There is an "ordering of cases under a principle by paradigm and analogy." The process is similar to that of a physician in clinical diagnosis and recommendations. Paradigms of accurate diagnosis and proper treatment function as sources of comparison when new problem cases arise. Recommendations are made by analogy to the paradigm. If the analogy is proper, a resolution of the problem and a recommendation will be achieved, but if no close analogy is available, uncertainty will remain.[104]

Consider the following example (ours, not that of any casuist known to us): If a particular act of suicide is paradigmatically wrong, then it will have certain relevant similarities with other wrong actions of suicide. Again, if a particular act of suicide is justifiable, then it will share relevant features with other acts of suicide that are morally acceptable. When confronted with a case of *assisted* suicide by a physician, these analogous, settled cases will constitute primary (but not exhaustive) resources for reasoning about the new moral problem of assisted suicide. No principle about suicide or killing need be invoked in this process if the paradigms are sufficiently powerful.

What Role for Theory?

Casuists disagree among themselves about the value and limitations of theory in practical ethics. While some casuists are sharply critical of theory, others encourage theory construction as well as generalization from cases. Baruch Brody, for example, insists that ethical theory is both possible and desirable. Case-based judgment that rests on plausible intuition "is only the *first* stage in the process of coming to have moral knowledge. The *next* stage is that of theory formation. . . . The goal is to find a theory that systematizes these intuitions, explains them, and provides help in dealing with cases about which we have no intuitions. In the course of this systematization, it may be necessary to reject some of the initial intuitions on the grounds that they cannot be systematized into the theory."[105] This theory-accessible casuistry is more appealing than a casuistry that denounces or evades theory.[106]

A Critical Evaluation of Casuistry

Casuists have sometimes overstated the promise and output power of their account, while understating the value of competing accounts. These problems need to be corrected.

Problems of case interpretation and conflicting judgments. Casuists often write as if cases speak for themselves or inform moral judgment by their facts alone. Clearly they do not. *Interpretation* of cases is essential for moral judgment, and principles and theory typically play a legitimate role in the interpretation. For the casuist to move constructively from case to case, some recognized rule of moral relevance must connect the cases. The rule will not be a part of the case, but a way of interpreting and linking cases. Jonsen treats this problem by distinguishing descriptive elements in a case from moral maxims that inform judgment about the case: "These maxims provide the 'morals' of the story. For most cases of interest, there are several morals, because several maxims seem to conflict. The work of casuistry is to determine *which maxim* should *rule the case* and to what extent." [107] So understood, casuistry presupposes rather than defeats the claim that principles (or maxims or rules) are essential moral elements. The principles are held prior to the decision, and then are selected and weighed in the circumstances.

Further, just as Kant and many other philosophers have a problem with conflicting principles, so casuists have a problem with conflicting analogies and judgments. Cases that are amenable to many competing judgments, including the choice of analogies, are common in ethics. In a given sequence of events, discussants sometimes even see different *cases*. It is not enough to be told that cases point beyond themselves and evolve into generalizations. Perhaps cases will evolve in the wrong way because they were wrongly treated from the outset. Casuists have no clear methodological resource to prevent a biased development of cases and a neglect of relevant features of cases.

This problem leads to questions regarding the justificatory power of casuistry. How does *justification* occur? The casuists' answer rests on social convention and the patterns of judgment traced through their methods. But given the many different types of appeal that might be made (analogies, generalizations, character judgments, etc.), there apparently can be many different "right" answers on a single occasion. Without some stable framework of general norms, there is no control on judgment and no way to prevent prejudiced or poorly formulated social conventions.

Do case judgments have epistemic priority? Jonsen and Toulmin argue for the priority of cases and case judgments in moral knowledge, as does Brody for moral intuition and intuitive perceptiveness. Such claims are sometimes followed in casuistic arguments by a qualifying statement to the effect that particular moral judgments amend and augment general norms, but do not displace them. This qualification, however, seems to undermine rather than to qualify the priority thesis, and in any event is not the best model. If, as we argued in Chapter 1, a relationship of mutual adjustment exists between general norms and particular circumstances, neither the general nor the particular should be granted an *order of priority*. The justification of beliefs moves from generalizations to cases *and* from cases to generalizations.

An overreaction to principles. An ambivalence about principles in the casuistry of Jonsen and Toulmin has never been consistently handled, raising questions about both the clarity and the coherence of the approach. On the one hand, they suggest a limited, conditional role for principles, and Jonsen explicitly says, "This casuistic analysis does not deny the relevance of principle and theory." [108] On the other hand, they eschew the use of principles such as those in this book, denounce firm and firmly held principles as tyrannical, and call the use of principles a "moralistic" use that is "not a serious ethical analysis." [109] This ambivalence mars their analysis and promotes an unnecessary rejection of principles.

Consider again Jonsen and Toulmin's example of the National Commission for the Protection of Human Subjects. Their constructive account of the commission's method of deliberation is unobjectionable. Commissioners reported that they were impressed by a history in medicine of cases of diagnostic, therapeutic, and preventive measures that formed a basis for their conclusions. However, the commissioners also reported a locus of certitude in moral principles. The transcripts of the commission's deliberations show a constant back-and-forth movement from principle to case, and from case to principle. Cases or examples favorable to one point of view were brought forward, and counterexamples to those cases were then advanced by a second commissioner against the examples and claims of the first. Principles were invoked to justify the choice and use of both examples and counterexamples. On many occasions a suggestion was made that a principle needed modification in light of a case, or an argument was offered that a case judgment was irrelevant or immoral in light of the commitments of a principle.[110] The commission's deliberations and conclusions are best understood, then, as examples of dialectical reasoning in which principles become interpreted, modified, and specified in context by the force of examples and counterexamples drawn from real-life cases.[111]

Jonsen and Toulmin appear to confuse the lack of a practical need for *theory* with the lack of a practical need for *principles,* as well as certitude about principles with certitude about theory. We believe the commission, the general public, and the mainstream of moral philosophy find a locus of certitude in the principles we present in this book, which do not sharply differ from the principles accepted by the commissioners. We agree that in practical deliberation we often do have more certitude about particular cases and conclusions (as well as maxims) than we do about various moral *theories*. But Jonsen and Toulmin suggest a lack of certitude surrounding *principles* (part of the common moralpity), when they should be pointing to the lack of certitude surrounding theories (which are not part of the common morality). Moreover, only deductivist theories seem damaged by their critical arguments. Theories with principles of prima facie obligation do not seem similarly damaged.

Mill argued that utilitarianism and other general theories can successfully face casuistical reservations about theory and general standards:

There is no ethical creed which does not temper the rigidity of its laws, by giving a certain latitude, under the moral responsibility of the agent, for accommodation to peculiarities of circumstances; and under every creed, at the opening thus made, self-deception and dishonest casuistry get in. There exists no moral system under which there do not arise unequivocal cases of conflicting obligation. . . . They are overcome practically with greater or with less success according to the intellect and virtue of the individual; but it can hardly be pretended that any one will be the less qualified for dealing with them, from possessing an ultimate [general] standard to which conflicting rights and obligations can be referred.[112]

Mill rightly believes that the person skilled in case judgments will be aided by, not hindered by, general moral standards. We agree that every significant normative ethical theory must face the limits of its principles and rules, the necessity of moral judgment, the role of interpretation in particular cases, and the importance of circumstances. But, if so, what does casuistry add to our understanding of decisionmaking that these theories fail to provide? Does casuistry deserve to score higher on the criterion of *practicability* than the other theories we have studied? If not, the failure would be particularly devastating, because the major goal of recent casuistry has been to reach a practicable method.

A Constructive Evaluation of Casuistry

Today's casuists have resourcefully reminded us of the importance of analogical reasoning, paradigm cases, and practical judgment. Biomedical ethics, like ethical theory, has unduly minimized this avenue to moral knowledge. Casuists also have rightly pointed out that generalizations are often best learned, accommodated, and implemented by using cases, case discussion, and case methods. These insights can be utilized by connecting them to an appropriate set of concepts, principles, and theories that control the selection and analysis of cases. Biomedical ethics has long been driven by two kinds of analysis: case study and ethical theory. Cases such as *Quinlan, Bouvia,* and *Tarasoff* are discussed across the literature of the field, form a shared resource, and become integral to the way we think and draw conclusions. They profoundly influence our standards of fairness, negligence, paternalism, and the like.

Finally, a proper account of moral judgment is critical for biomedical ethics, which cannot flourish without a link between theory, principles, and decisionmaking. Sensitivity to context and individual differences is essential for a discerning use of principles. Casuistry would be notable if for no other reason than its long history of attempting to deal with this problem.

Principle-Based, Common-Morality Theories[113]

We will now turn attention to theories that both find their source in the common morality and use principles as their structural basis. A common-morality theory takes its basic premises directly from the morality shared in common by the members of a society—that is, unphilosophical common sense and tradition. Such a theory need not be principle-based, but we treat these two types of theories together in order to develop the tradition of ethics in which our account should be situated. This section, then, is best understood overall as a statement of the type of ethical theory that we accept and utilize in subsequent chapters.

Principle-based theories share with utilitarian and Kantian theories an emphasis on principles of *obligation,* but these theories share little else. Two main differences distinguish them. First, utilitarianism and Kantianism are *monistic* theories. One supreme, absolute principle supports all other action-guides in the system. Common-morality theories, as we here stipulatively define them, are *pluralistic.*[114] Two or more nonabsolute (prima facie) principles form the general level of normative statement. Second, common-morality ethics relies heavily on ordinary shared moral beliefs for its content, rather than relying on pure reason, natural law, a special moral sense, and the like. The principles embedded in these shared moral beliefs are also usually accepted by rival ethical theories. Although not the most general principles in many normative theories, the principles are nonetheless accepted in most types of ethical theory. The four principles developed in Chapters 3–6 should be understood as principles of this description.

Any theory that eventuates in moral judgments that cannot be brought into reflective equilibrium with pretheoretical commonsense judgments will be considered seriously flawed. However, this is not to maintain *either* that (for reasons discussed in Chapter 1) a common-morality theory is merely a systematizing of commonsense judgments *or* that all *customary moralities* qualify as part of the *common morality.* An important function of the standards in the common morality (from which the principles we defend and their correlative rights are developed) is to provide a basis for the evaluation and criticism of actions in countries and communities whose customary moral viewpoints fail to acknowledge basic principles. A customary morality, then, is not synonymous with the common morality. The latter is a pretheoretic moral point of view that transcends merely local customs and attitudes. Analogous to beliefs in the universality of basic human rights, the principles of the common morality are universal standards.

Our method in this book is to unite principle-based, common-morality ethics with the coherence model of justification delineated in Chapter 1. This strategy allows us to rely on the authority of the indispensable principles in the common morality, while incorporating tools to refine and correct its weaknesses and unclarities and to allow for additional specification. Because our strategy accepts the goal of reflective equilibrium and, in part, *constructs* principles and rules from considered judgments in the common morality, while also *specifying* principles and rules, we will not end with the identical content with which we began.

We can again illustrate this type of theory by reference to the case of the daughter who needs a kidney transplant. Unlike utilitarian and Kantian strategies, common-morality theories have no overarching principle to justify obligations or to adjudicate conflicts. Judgment requires interpreting as well as weighing and balancing moral norms to determine whether to respect the father's refusal to donate or to prod him into donating, whether to protect confidentiality or to lie, and whether to involve or to exclude the girl's siblings. When the father refuses to donate his kidney, the principle of respect for autonomy and related rules of privacy and liberty require that his choice not be forcibly overridden. These principles and rules are not absolute, but they do have sufficient weight in these circumstances to preclude forcible or coercive intervention to try to save the daughter. However, the physician has the right and perhaps even the responsibility to try to persuade the father to donate, at least by explaining and balancing probable benefits to the daughter and risks to the father. With a sufficiently high probability of successful transplantation and a sufficiently low risk to himself, the father may well have an obligation to donate, based on parental responsibilities. At some level of probable benefits and risks, the father's decision not to donate falls short of the ideal of parental love, and is therefore morally deficient, although no moral grounds warrant compelling him to donate.

Regarding the father's request to the physician to tell the family that he is not histocompatible, his predicted outcome of wrecking the family is a morally relevant consideration. But theories based on the common morality (like many other theories) would inquire whether alternatives short of lying or nondisclosure, such as counseling, could also prevent this outcome. A conflict is also present in this case between rules of truth-telling and confidentiality. Although direct lying is not always wrong from the perspective of prima facie principles, it requires principled justification. For example, lying is sometimes justified to shield a vulnerable teenager who does not want to donate a kidney to a sibling. The nature and defense of such judgments require us to examine further how principles function in common-morality theories.

The Common Morality as Primary Source

As a rough generalization, what Henry Sidgwick called the commonsense morality (morality's core principles and assorted rules of veracity, fidelity, and the like) is the source of the initial moral content for this type of theory. Ethical theory augments this spare content by a method (1) to clarify and interpret the content, (2) to make the various strands coherent, and (3) to further specify and balance the requirements of norms (as discussed in Chapter 1).

Consider why the common morality should play an essential role in ethical theory. If we could be confident that some abstract moral theory was a better source for codes and policies than the common morality, we could work constructively on practical and policy questions by progressive specification of the norms in that theory. But fully analyzed norms in ethical theories are invariably more contestable than the norms in the common morality. We cannot reasonably expect that a contested moral theory will be better for practical decisionmaking and policy development than the morality that serves as our common denominator. Far more social consensus exists about principles and rules drawn from the common morality (for example, our four principles) than about theories. This is not surprising, given the central social role of the common morality and the fact that its principles are, at least in schematic form, usually embraced in some form by all major theories. Theories are rivals over matters of justification, rationality, and method, but they often converge on mid-level principles (see pp. 109–111 below).

Common-morality ethics does not preclude the possibility of reform, which often occurs through interpretation, specification, and balancing. We earlier noted John Mackie's observation that interpretation and innovation are almost always carried out by appeal to justifications *within* rather than *beyond* norms already shared in the community. For example, if our policies on AIDS are so uncompassionate that we need to alter our conception of how therapeutic drugs are brought to the market, purchased, and distributed, this reevaluation will invoke available conceptions of compassion, fair funding, and distribution, rather than totally new principles of justice. Moreover, social agreements, traditions, and norms are inherently indeterminate, thereby failing to adequately anticipate the full range of moral problems and solutions. Interpretation and specification of norms, reconstruction of traditional beliefs, balancing different values, and negotiation are essential. This approach to construction in theory invites evolutionary change while insisting that the common morality provides the starting point and the constraining framework.

Two Examples of Principle-Based Theories

Commonsense convictions played only a minor role in ethical theory prior to the eighteenth century, when philosophers such as Francis Hutcheson, Jean-

Jacques Rousseau, and Joseph Butler argued that a native moral sense or an intuitive conscience possessed by all persons is far more important in the moral life than the more complicated systems of philosophers. Their moral psychology did not survive, but their commonsense emphasis did, and Hume, Kant, Hegel, and other leading moral theorists were deeply affected by it. Two twentieth-century writers in ethical theory will serve here to illustrate how a principle-based, common-morality theory is still alive and well.

Frankena's theory. An elegant and simple example of a common-morality theory that resembles ours is William Frankena's version of Hume's postulate that the two major "principles of morals" are beneficence and justice. Frankena appeals to what Bishop Butler called "the moral institution of life," together with what Frankena calls "the moral point of view," meaning a dispassionate attitude of sympathy in which moral decisions are reached by appeal to principled good reasons. For Frankena, the principle of beneficence (presented below on pp. 190–192, 260ff) resembles, but is not identical to, the utilitarian demand that we maximize good over evil, whereas the principle of justice (primarily an egalitarian principle) guides "our distribution of good and evil" independently of judgments about maximizing and balancing good outcomes. Frankena's theory comprises these two general principles, together with an argument that they capture the essence of the moral point of view.[115]

Ross's theory. A second example is the ethics of W. D. Ross, who has had a particularly imposing influence on twentieth-century ethical theory, and more influence on the present authors than any recent writer in ethical theory. He is best known for his intuitionism and his scholarship on Aristotle, but we will largely ignore these dimensions of his work. Ross's starting point is Aristotelian. The moral convictions of thoughtful persons are "the data of ethics just as sense-perceptions are the data of a natural science. Just as some of the latter have to be rejected as illusory, so have some of the former."[116] The "plain" person is, for Ross, the beginning rather than the end of the matter. Using this data base of ordinary standards, Ross thinks *acts* are properly categorized as right and wrong, whereas *motivation* and character are good and bad. This allows him to say that a right act can be done from a bad motive and that a good motive may eventuate in a wrong act.

Ross defends several basic and irreducible moral principles that express prima facie obligations. For example, promises create obligations of fidelity, wrongful actions and debts create obligations of reparation, and the generous services or gifts of others create obligations of gratitude. In addition to fidelity, reparation, and gratitude, Ross lists obligations of self-improvement, justice, beneficence, and nonmaleficence.[117] He holds that the principle of nonmaleficence (noninfliction of harm) takes precedence over the principle of beneficence (production of benefit) when the two come into conflict, but he assigns no priorities among the other principles. This list of obligations is not grounded in any overarching principle.

In a noteworthy methodological statement, Ross maintains that principles are "recognized by intuitive induction as being implied in the judgments already passed on particular acts."[118] His studies of Greek philosophy also led him to distinguish knowledge from opinion. We know principles in the same way the plain person knows the main lines of moral obligation. Here we have *knowledge,* not *opinion.* However, when two or more obligations conflict and balancing, overriding, and judgment are necessary, Ross says we must examine the situation carefully until we form a "considered opinion (it is never more)" that one obligation is more incumbent in the circumstances than any other.[119] These judgments are about the *weight* of principles. They are not judgments that straightforwardly *apply* principles.

The Centrality of Principles and Rules

We can now develop the perspectives and assumptions in this book that make it a form of common-morality ethics.

The source of the principles. To say that principles have their origins in the common morality is not to suggest that the final form in which they greet a reader of this book is identical to their appearance in the common morality. Conceptual clarification and methods to introduce coherence are needed to give shape and substance to our moral commitments, much as grammarians, lexicographers, and stylists investigate the nature of our commitments in using words, punctuation, forms of citation, and the like. If unacceptable content is discovered in formulations of principles (for example, if a vigorous strong paternalism in clinical medicine is uncovered) or if incoherence is located, an attempt is made to find acceptable content and achieve coherence. This is work *in* ethical theory, even if its product should not be spoken of as *an* ethical theory. The objective is to give each principle a precise, plausible, thorough, and independent statement, without presupposing that our familiar ways of formulating principles are necessarily the best or the most coherent ways. After the principles are so formulated, they will still have to be further interpreted, specified, and balanced to produce an ethics for biomedicine. This is the heart of our strategy.

The prima facie and specifiable nature of the principles. Like Ross, we construe principles as prima facie binding. Some theories recognize rules, but treat them as expendable rules of thumb that summarize past experience by expressing better and worse ways to handle recurrent problems. Other theories contain absolute principles. Still other theories give a hierarchical (or lexical) ordering to moral norms. We reject all three interpretations as inadequate to capture the nature of moral norms and moral reasoning. Rules of thumb permit too much discretion, as if principles or rules were not binding; absolute principles and rules disallow all discretion for moral agents and also encounter unresolvable moral conflicts; and a hierarchy of rules and principles suffers from damaging counterexamples whose force depends on our reservoir of considered judgments. (Unlike Ross, we assign no form of priority weighing or hierarchical ranking to our principles.)

By contrast, we treat principles as both prima facie binding and subject to revision. So understood, a prima facie principle is a normative guideline stating conditions of the permissibility, obligatoriness, rightness, or wrongness of actions that fall within the scope of the principle. The latitude to balance principles in cases of conflict leaves room for compromise, mediation, and negotiation. The account is thereby rescued from the charge that principles cannot be compromised and so become tyrannical. In stubborn cases of conflict there may be no single right action, because two or more morally acceptable actions are unavoidably in conflict and yet have equal weight in the circumstances. Here we can give good but not decisive reasons for more than one action.

For instance, although murder is absolutely prohibited because of the normative content in the word *murder,* it is not plausible to hold that killing is absolutely prohibited. Killing persons is *prima facie* wrong, but killing to prevent a person's further extreme pain or suffering is not wrong in every circumstance. Killing may be the only way to meet some obligations, even though it is prima facie wrong (see Chapter 4, pp. 219–241.) However, when a prima facie obligation is outweighed or overridden, it does not simply disappear or evaporate. It leaves what Nozick calls "moral traces,"[120] which should be reflected in the agent's attitudes and actions.

A disadvantage of this account, some say, is that it moves relentlessly to the paradoxical conclusion that, as Hume put it, "the principles upon which men reason in morals are always the same; though the conclusions which they draw are often very different."[121] True, a relativity of judgment is inevitable, but a relativity of the principles embedded in the common morality is not. When people reach different conclusions, their moral judgments are still subject to justification by good reasons. They are not purely arbitrary or subjective judgments. A judgment can be proposed for consideration on any basis a person chooses—random selection, emotional reaction, mystical intuition, etc.—but to propose is not to justify, and one part of justification is to test judgments and norms by their coherence with the other norms in the moral life.

We conclude that although flexibility and diversity in judgment are ineliminable, judgment generally should be constrained by the demands of moral justification, which typically involves appeal to principles. Our presentation of the principles—together with arguments to show the coherence of these principles with other aspects of the moral life, such as the moral emotions, virtues, and rights—*constitutes* the theory in the present volume. This web of norms and arguments *is* the theory. There is no single unifying principle or concept, no description of the highest good, and the like.

A Reply to Some Criticisms

Some commentators have criticized our account as a mere "mantra of principles," meaning that the principles often function like a ritual incantation of norms repeated with little reflection. H. Danner Clouser and Bernard Gert have so argued in an attack on "principlism," a term they use to designate all theories composed of a plural body of potentially conflicting prima facie principles—principally our account and Frankena's. They accuse us of the following defects in theory: [122] (1) The "principles" are little more than names, checklists, or headings for values worth remembering, leaving principles without deep moral substance or capacity to guide action. (2) Principle-analyses fail to provide a unified theory of justification or a general theory that ties the principles together as a systematic, coherent, and comprehensive body of guidelines, with the consequence that the alleged action-guides are ad hoc constructions lacking systematic order. (3) The prima facie principles (and other action guides in the framework) often conflict, and the underlying account is too indeterminate to provide a decision procedure to adjudicate those conflicts.

We do not deny that these problems are worthy of sustained reflection. We reject, however, certain assumptions that Clouser and Gert make, especially their requirement that there be "a single clear, coherent, and comprehensive decision procedure for arriving at answers." [123] We are skeptical of this enterprise, even as a model for ethical theory, for reasons presented in Chapter 1 (see pp. 13–37). Regarding their *first* criticism, that our principles are checklists or headings without deep moral substance, we agree that principles order, classify, and group moral norms that need additional content and specificity. Until the principles are *interpreted and analyzed* (as they are in every first section of Chapters 3–6) and *specified and connected to other norms* (as they are in later sections of these chapters), it is unreasonable to expect much more than a classification scheme that organizes the normative content. [124]

Regarding the *second* criticism, [125] that our principle-analysis fails to provide a systematic theory, we see the point but view it as irrelevant. We have not attempted a general ethical theory and do not claim that our principles mimic, are analogous to, or substitute for the foundational principles in leading classical theories such as utilitarianism (with its principle of utility) and Kantianism (with its categorical imperative). We have expressed a constrained skepticism about this foundationalism and are doubtful that such a unified foundation for ethics is discoverable. As we have acknowledged, even the core principles in our account are so scant that they cannot provide an adequate basis for deducing most of what we can justifiably claim to know in the moral life.

Regarding the *third* criticism, that principles compete in ways our account cannot resolve, we acknowledge that conflicts among principles cannot be resolved a priori. No system of guidelines could reasonably anticipate the full range of conflicts, and the point of our discussion of dilemmas was to indicate circumstances in which principles (and other commitments) pull us in different directions. No one escapes this problem in living the moral life. It does not follow that these principles are inconsistent or that we encounter incompatible moral commitments by accepting these principles. It is a virtue of our theory that it requires specification, and a defect in Clouser and Gert's account that it purports through its rules to escape the need for specification. Only a theory that could put enough content in its norms to escape conflicts and dilemmas in all contexts could live up to the Clouser-Gert demand, and no theory has come close to doing so. It is therefore essential to leave room for interpretation, specification, and balancing of principles and rules in the face of recurrent and recalcitrant conflicts.

Here experience and sound judgment are indispensable allies. It is insupportably optimistic, for several reasons, to suppose we have attained or will attain a fully specified system of norms for health care ethics. Thomas Nagel has forcefully argued that an unconnected heap of obligations and values is an ineradicable feature of morality, and Ross rightly argued that his Kantian and utilitarian critics forced an "architectonic" of "hastily reached simplicity" on ethics. Whereas critics of Ross's account (and ours) rely on an ideal of systematic unity, we see disunity, conflict, and moral ambiguity as pervasive aspects of the moral life. Untidiness, complexity, and conflict are unfortunate features of communal living, but a theory of morality cannot be faulted for a realistic appraisal of them.

Persons typically lack a complete understanding of the full range of commitments they make in accepting a principle, because of its indeterminateness and our inability to specify it all the way down to the concrete cases. We come to understand principles, and what they exclude and include, by making judgments in particular circumstances. For example, many of us likely have a poor idea of the demands of the principle of respect for autonomy in an institution serving persons with serious mental disabilities. But if we were in that environment on a daily basis, we probably would develop a better set of ideas. The judgments that we make achieve an increased specificity, which then loops back and in some cases forces a revised gloss on the norms in our moral framework.

This growth of moral understanding is to be encouraged. Only a faulty conception of the nature and interpretation of principles would lead to the conclusion that principles have no integral role in moral reasoning in concrete circumstances. The more accurate estimate is that principles point us in the right direction, but we then typically encounter a host of other considerations that must be accommodated, such as institutional practices, limited resources, judgments about acceptable risk, religious beliefs, and personal projects and aspirations.

Critical Evaluation

Although we accept a version of principle-based, common-morality ethics, we acknowledge that this approach has unresolved problems. Three are of interest for the present chapter on types of theory.

Specification and judgment. Do principles, when specified for behavior, enable us to reach practical judgments, or are they either too indeterminate or too determinate to eventuate in judgments? Again we confront a problem of practicability. We must be careful both to specify in order to escape abstractness and not to *overspecify* a principle or rule, because it then becomes too rigid and insensitive to circumstances. We have argued that the best course of action is to accept both abstract principles and a method for specifying those principles, in order that they can be appropriately implemented for specific circumstances. But can this goal be achieved in practice? For example, if in specifying the principle of respect for autonomy and rules of truth-telling in medicine, the resultant rules require too little education of and conversation with patients in some cases and too much in other cases (where the health care system will not bear the time and cost of the requirements), then the specification is inadequate. Many specified principles and rules will encounter this problem of too-little and too-much for some contexts, which is one reason why balancing and judgment are as consequential as specification. But without tighter controls on permissible balancing than common-morality theories propose, critics charge that too much room is left for judgments that are unprincipled and yet sanctioned or permitted by the theory. Can the conditions on balancing presented in Chapter 1 reduce intuition to an acceptable level? Can the constraints of coherence be tightened to adequately respond to these concerns? In Chapter 8, we will argue that these problems are actually more complicated, requiring acceptance of important parts of character ethics and a distinction between principles of obligation and the judgments that are guided by those principles.

Can the common morality be rendered coherent? We have linked a coherence theory of justification to a common-morality theory, but can the common morality be made coherent? If one argues (as we did above, citing Nagel) that an unconnected heap of obligations and values comprises the common morality, is there any hope of rendering the heap coherent, short of so radically reconstructing the norms that they become only a distant cousin of the common morality? Is the goal of coherence more an article of faith than a demonstrable achievement?

Consider, for example, the use of animals as research subjects. Across society we disagree regarding the "considered judgments" that might form our starting place, and it is doubtful that the common morality can be tapped to find shared considered judgments. On the one hand, one might argue that we need to search for a wider body of beliefs that can be brought into reflective equilibrium. On the other hand, we might simply specify our personal considered judgments. Either way, no clear starting point and body of beliefs exist to be rendered coherent, mainly because of a lack of agreement about the status of animals and our obligations, if any, to them. Many other controversies similarly invite disagreement over appropriate *initial* beliefs.

Is there a theory to be constructed? These problems of coherence lead straight to some connected problems about theory. The language of a "common-morality *theory*" suggests either that a theory underlies the common morality or that a theory can be philosophically constructed from it. Is there good reason to believe that a theory (not merely an unconnected group of coherent principles and rules) is possible? Perhaps mid-level principles, polished analyses of the moral virtues, and coherent statements of transnational human rights are all that should be attempted, rather than a theory that conforms to the criteria delineated at the beginning of this chapter. Perhaps "moral theory" has been so diluted in meaning in "common-morality theories" that the goal of a theory should be abandoned altogether, in favor of a more modest goal, such as "moral reflection and construction." A related problem is that attempts to bring the common morality into greater coherence risk decreasing rather than increasing moral agreement in society. That is, a theory can introduce claims that generate disagreements not found in the initial considered judgments; or, as we have often seen in the history of ethics, the theory may turn out to be less clear and reliable for practical decisionmaking than the common morality.

In part these problems turn on one's expectations for a "theory." Clouser and Gert expect a strong measure of unity and systematic connection among rules, a clear pattern of justification, and a practical decision procedure that flows from a theory, whereas Annette Baier is skeptical of each of these conditions, and even of the language of "theory."[126] We need not here debate the theory of theories, but we do need to return to the theme of convergence among ethical theories.

Convergence Across Theories

Whenever several competing theories or systems of belief are available, we seek out the best and affiliate with it, while rejecting the others. However, affiliation with one type of theory is not always the best strategy in either general ethics or biomedical ethics. If the two authors of this book were forced to rank the types of theory examined in this chapter other than common-morality theory, we would differ. We have reached different estimates after testing available theories under the criteria established early in this chapter. But for both of us, the most satisfactory theory—if we could find *one* to substitute for a common-morality theory—would be only slightly preferable, and no theory would fully satisfy all the criteria.

Differences between types of theory are exaggerated if they are presented as warring armies locked in combat. Many different theories lead to similar action-guides and to similar estimates of the role of character in ethics. It is possible from several of these standpoints to defend roughly the same principles, obligations, rights, responsibilities, and virtues. For example, although utilitarianism is often depicted both as starkly different from and as hostile to the other theories, when utilitarian Richard Brandt states his view, it is strikingly reminiscent at the level of principle and obligation to Ross's estimate, which we have seen to be sharply critical of utilitarianism:

> [The best code] would contain rules giving directions for recurrent situations which involve conflicts of human interests. Presumably, then, it would contain rules rather similar to W. D. Ross's list of prima facie obligations: rules about the keeping of promises and contracts, rules about debts of gratitude such as we may owe to our parents, and, of course, rules about not injuring other persons and about promoting the welfare of others where this does not work a comparable hardship on us.[127]

That Brandt appeals to utility and Ross to intuitive induction to justify similar sets of rules is a significant difference at the level of moral justification, and the two authors might interpret and specify their rules differently. Yet, they exhibit only trivial differences in their lists of primary obligations. This convergence is not restricted to Brandt and Ross. It is common in normative theories that provide frameworks of principles and rules. Such agreement springs in part from an initial shared data base, namely, the norms of the common morality.

This convergence offers encouragement to practical ethics, although in itself it does not resolve either theoretical differences or practical problems. Convergence as well as consensus about principles among a group of persons is common in assessing *cases* and framing *policies,* even when deep theoretical differences divide the group. Agreement may similarly be reached regarding precedent cases. This is not to deny that theoretical differences do sometimes eventuate in practical disagreements, in different policies, and in unresolvable dilemmas. For example, utilitarians tend to support various types of research involving human subjects because of the potential benefits the research offers for future patients. Many nonutilitarians tend to be skeptical of some of this research on grounds of its actual or potential violation of individual rights. But utilitarians and their theoretical opponents also often cross over these lines of demarcation and agree that any adequate ethical approach to research involving human subjects must include some of the constraints and considerations that have been highlighted by proponents of both types of theory (and that are now embedded in the major codes and regulations of research involving human subjects).

Reasons exist, then, for holding that distinctions between types of theory are not as significant for *practical* ethics as has sometimes been proclaimed. It is a mistake to suppose that a series of continental divides separates moral theorists into distinct and hostile groups who reach different practical conclusions and fail to converge on principles. We should not overlook the fact that some theories are closer in substantive principles and rules to supposedly rival theories than they are even to some theories of their own "type."

Conclusion

Contemporary biomedical ethics incorporates theoretical conflicts of considerable complexity, and the diverse theories explored in this chapter help us see why. Competition exists among the various normative theories, and in addition we find a body of competing conceptions as to how such theories should be related to biomedical practice. Thus, persons who agree on a particular type of ethical theory may still find themselves in sharp disagreement regarding how to relate their theory to the treatment of particular moral problems.

Nonetheless, we stand to learn from all of these theories. Where one theory is weak in accounting for some part of the moral life, another is often strong. Although each type of theory clashes at some point with deep moral convictions, each also articulates norms that we are reluctant to relinquish. Each of the theories discussed in this chapter has led to the development and rejection of prominent hypotheses in moral theory. Although we have described our approach as principle-based, we reject the assumption that one must defend a single type of theory that is solely principle-based, virtue-based, rights-based, case-based, and so forth. In moral reasoning we often blend appeals to principles, rules, rights, virtues, passions, analogies, paradigms, parables, and interpretations. To assign priority to one of these factors as the key ingredient is a dubious project, as is the attempt to dispense with ethical theory altogether. The more general (principles, rules, theories, etc.) and the more particular (feelings, perceptions, case judgments, practices, parables, etc.) should be linked together in our moral thinking. We will have more to say about how these strands are mutually supportive in Chapters 7 and 8, after we develop our framework of principles in Chapters 3–6.

Notes

1. See Baruch Brody's definition of "pluralism" in *Life and Death Decision Making* (New York: Oxford University Press, 1988), p. 9. Our views on pluralism are

influenced by Thomas Nagel, "The Fragmentation of Value," in *Mortal Questions* (Cambridge: Cambridge University Press, 1979), pp. 128–37.

2. Our discussion in this edition has profited from Shelly Kagan, *The Limits of Morality* (Oxford: Clarendon Press, 1989), esp. pp. 11–15, and from criticisms by David DeGrazia.

3. For recent analysis of this utilitarian thesis, see Samuel Scheffler, *Consequentialism and its Critics* (Oxford: Clarendon Press, 1988).

4. Jeremy Bentham, *An Introduction to the Principles of Morals and Legislation,* ed. Burns & Hart (Oxford: Clarendon Press, 1970), pp. 11–14, 31, 34. John Stuart Mill, *Utilitarianism,* in vol. 10 of the *Collected Works of John Stuart Mill* (Toronto: University of Toronto Press, 1969), ch. 1, p. 207; ch. 2, pp. 210, 214; ch. 4, pp. 234–35.

5. A representative of the first list is G. E. Moore, *Principia Ethica* (Cambridge: Cambridge University Press, 1903), pp. 90ff; a representative of the latter list is James Griffin, *Well-Being: Its Meaning, Measurement and Moral Importance* (Oxford: Clarendon Press, 1986), p. 67.

6. This case is based on Melvin D. Levine, Lee Scott, and William J. Curran, "Ethics Rounds in a Children's Medical Center: Evaluation of a Hospital-Based Program for Continuing Education in Medical Ethics," *Pediatrics* 60 (August 1977): 205.

7. Worthington Hooker, *Physician and Patient* (New York: Baker and Scribner, 1849), pp. 357ff, 375–81.

8. J. J. C. Smart, *An Outline of a System of Utilitarian Ethics* (Melbourne: University Press, 1961); and "Extreme and Restricted Utilitarianism," in *Contemporary Utilitarianism,* ed. Michael Bayles (Garden City, NY: Doubleday and Co., 1968), esp. pp. 104–7, 113–15.

9. Richard B. Brandt, "Toward a Credible Form of Utilitarianism," in *Contemporary Utilitarianism,* pp. 143–86, and in Brandt's *Morality, Utilitarianism, and Rights* (Cambridge: Cambridge University Press, 1992).

10. Alan Donagan, "Is There a Credible Form of Utilitarianism?" in *Contemporary Utilitarianism,* pp. 187–202.

11. A subtle argument to this conclusion is found in Kagan, *The Limits of Morality, passim.*

12. Williams, "A Critique of Utilitarianism," in J. J. C. Smart and Bernard Williams, *Utilitarianism: For and Against* (Cambridge: Cambridge University Press, 1973), pp. 116–17, and J. L. Mackie, *Ethics: Inventing Right and Wrong* (New York: Penguin Books, 1977), pp. 129, 133.

13. Milton Weinstein and William B. Stason, *Hypertension* (Cambridge, MA: Harvard University Press, 1977), and their articles in *New England Journal of Medicine* 296 (1977): 716–21, and *Hastings Center Report* 7 (October 1977): 24–29.

14. Amartya Sen, *On Ethics and Economics* (Oxford: Basil Blackwell, 1987), p. 75.

15. Kant sought to show that reason unaided can be and should be a proper motive to action. What we should do morally is determined by what we would do "if reason completely determined the will." *The Critique of Practical Reason,* trans. Lewis White Beck (New York: Macmillan, 1985), pp. 18–19. Ak. 20. "Ak." designates the page-reference system of the 22-volume Preussische Akademie edition conventionally cited in Kant scholarship.

16. Kant, *Foundations of the Metaphysics of Morals,* trans. Lewis White Beck (Indianapolis, IN: Bobbs-Merrill Company, 1959), pp. 37–42; Ak. 421–24.

17. *Foundations,* p. 47; Ak. 429.

18. *Foundations,* pp. 51, 58–63; Ak. 432, 439–44.

19. *Foundations*, pp. 58; Ak. 439–40; and *Critique of Practical Reason*, p. 33; Ak. 33.

20. Alan Donagan, *The Theory of Morality* (Chicago: University of Chicago Press, 1977), pp. 63–66.

21. See *A Theory of Justice* (Cambridge, MA: Harvard University Press, 1971), pp. 3–4, 26–31. For Rawls's more technical interests in and development of Kant, see his "Themes in Kant's Moral Philosophy," in *Kant's Transcendental Deductions*, ed. Eckart Förster (Stanford, CA: Stanford University Press, 1989), pp. 81–113.

22. *A Theory of Justice*, pp. 102, 137, 252–55. In § 40 of *A Theory of Justice*, Rawls presents his "Kantian Interpretation of Justice as Fairness," as "based upon Kant's notion of autonomy."

23. Sidgwick, *The Methods of Ethics*, 7th Ed. (Indianapolis, IN: Hackett Publishing Co., 1981), p. 516.

24. Rawls, *A Theory of Justice*, pp. 252, 256, 515–19. See also, "A Kantian Conception of Equality," *Cambridge Review* (February 1975): 97ff.

25. Rawls, "The Priority of Right and Ideas of the Good," *Philosophy & Public Affairs* 17 (1988): 252, and "Justice as Fairness: Political not Metaphysical," *Philosophy & Public Affairs* 14 (1985): 223–51, esp. 224–25.

26. "The Doctrine of Virtue," Part II of *The Metaphysic of Morals*, trans. Mary J. Gregor (Philadelphia: University of Pennsylvania Press, 1964), p. 85, Ak, 421–22; See also *Lectures on Ethics*, ed. Louis Infield (New York: Harper and Row, 1963), pp. 150–54.

27. G. W. F. Hegel, *Philosophy of Right*, trans. T. M. Knox (Oxford: Clarendon Press, 1942), pp. 89–90, 106–7.

28. For two influential anthologies of recent work, see *Midwest Studies in Philosophy Volume XIII—Ethical Theory: Character and Virtue*, ed. Peter A. French, Theodore E. Uehling, Jr., and Howard K. Wettstein (Notre Dame, IN: University of Notre Dame Press, 1988); and *Identity, Character, and Morality*, ed. Owen Flanagan and Amélie Oksenberg Rorty (Cambridge, MA: MIT Press, 1990). For two very different treatments of the Aristotelian perspective, see Nancy Sherman, *The Fabric of Character: Aristotle's Theory of Virtue* (Oxford: Clarendon Press, 1989); Alasdair MacIntyre, *After Virtue*, 2d Ed. (Notre Dame, IN: University of Notre Dame Press, 1984).

29. This is not the broadest sense, inasmuch as machines, tools, horses, and the like are often said to have virtues. Some writers more tightly restrict the meaning of *virtue* than we do. For example, Aristotle required that virtue involve habituation rather than a natural character trait. *Nicomachean Ethics*, trans. Terence Irwin (Indianapolis, IN: Hackett Publishing Co., 1985), 1103a18–19. Thomas Aquinas (relying on a formulation by Peter Lombard) additionally held that virtue is a good quality of mind by which we live rightly and therefore *cannot be put to bad use*. *Treatise on the Virtues* (from *Summa Theologiae*, I–II), Question 55, Arts. 3–4, pp. 54–55.

30. This definition is the primary use reported in the *O.E.D.* It is defended by Alan Gewirth, "Rights and Virtues," *Review of Metaphysics* 38 (1985): 751, and R. B. Brandt, "The Structure of Virtue," in *Midwest Studies in Philosophy* 13 (1988): 76. Edmund Pincoffs presents a definition of virtue in terms of desirable dispositional qualities of persons, in *Quandaries and Virtues: Against Reductivism in Ethics* (Lawrence: University Press of Kansas, 1986), pp. 9, 73–100. We accepted a definition similar to these in the first two editions of this book, for which we were criticized by John Waide, "Virtues and Principles," *Philosophy and Phenomenological Research* 48 (1988): 455–72.

31. *Nicomachean Ethics,* bk. II, 1105^{a}17–33, 1106^{b}21–23; cf. bk. VI, 1144^{a}14–20 (trans. Irwin).
32. See Philippa Foot, *Virtues and Vices* (Oxford: Basil Blackwell, 1978), Rodger Beehler, *Moral Life* (Oxford: Basil Blackwell, 1978), Gregory Trianosky, "Supererogation, Wrongdoing, and Vice," *Journal of Philosophy* 83 (1986): 26–40.
33. See Michael Stocker, "The Schizophrenia of Modern Ethical Theories," *Journal of Philosophy* 73 (1976): 453–66. One might try to amend Kant to overcome this objection. See Kurt Baier, "Radical Virtue Ethics," *Midwest Studies in Philosophy* 13 (1988): 130–31.
34. H. K. Beecher, "Ethics and Clinical Research," *New England Journal of Medicine* 274 (1966): 1354–60.
35. G. Pence, *Ethical Options in Medicine* (Oradell, NJ: Medical Economics Co., 1980), p. 177.
36. Thomas Keneally, *Schindler's List* (New York: Penguin Books, 1983), pp. 176–80.
37. This formulation is indebted to David Hume, *A Treatise of Human Nature,* 2d Ed., ed. L. A. Selby-Bigge and P. H. Nidditch (Oxford: Clarendon Press, 1978), p. 478.
38. See William K. Frankena, *Ethics,* 2d Ed. (Englewood Cliffs, NJ: Prentice-Hall, 1973), p. 65; and Kurt Baier, "Radical Virtue Ethics," pp. 133–34.
39. This schema has been adapted, with modifications, from Tom L. Beauchamp, *Philosophical Ethics,* 2d Ed. (New York: McGraw-Hill, 1991), ch. 6.
40. See David Solomon, "Internal Objections to Virtue Ethics," *Midwest Studies in Philosophy* 13 (1988): 439.
41. Hart, "Between Utility and Rights," in *Jurisprudence and Philosophy* (Oxford: Clarendon Press, 1983), p. 198. For debates about liberalism, see Nancy L. Rosenblum, ed. *Liberalism and the Moral Life* (Cambridge, MA: Harvard University Press, 1989).
42. Compare H. L. A. Hart, "Bentham on Legal Rights," in *Oxford Essays in Jurisprudence,* 2nd series. ed. A. W. B. Simpson (Oxford: Oxford University Press, 1973), pp. 171–98.
43. See Joel Feinberg, *Social Philosophy* (Englewood Cliffs, NJ: Prentice-Hall, 1973), p. 67.
44. Dworkin, *Taking Rights Seriously* (Cambridge, MA: Harvard University Press, 1977), pp. xi, 92, 191, and "Is there a Right to Pornography?" *Oxford Journal of Legal Studies* 1 (1981): 177–212.
45. See James Griffin, "Towards a Substantive Theory of Rights," in *Utility and Rights,* ed. R. G. Frey (Minneapolis: University of Minnesota Press, 1984), pp. 155–58.
46. See Judith Jarvis Thomson, *The Realm of Rights* (Cambridge, MA: Harvard University Press, 1990), pp. 122ff.
47. See Feinberg, *Social Philosophy,* p. 59; and Eric Mack, ed., *Positive and Negative Duties* (New Orleans: Tulane University Press, 1985).
48. The first decade of decisions began with *Roe v. Wade* 410 U.S. 113 (1973) and ran through *City of Akron v. Akron Center for Reproductive Health* (June 1983). Decisions of major importance pertaining to indigency and funding were *Maher v. Roe,* 432 U.S. 464 (1977) and *Harris v. McRae,* 448 U.S. 297 (1980). In *Planned Parenthood v. Casey* (June 28, 1992), the U.S. Supreme Court further upheld the pregnant woman's right to terminate her pregnancy within limits, while abolishing the trimester framework. It recognized the state's interest in fetal life

from the beginning of the pregnancy and allowed states to institute requirements that do not impose an undue burden on the pregnant woman's decisions and
actions.

49. See A. I. Melden, *Rights and Right Conduct* (Oxford: Basil Blackwell, 1959).

50. See David Braybrooke, "The Firm but Untidy Correlativity of Rights and Obligations," *Canadian Journal of Philosophy* 1 (1972): 351–63.

51. Mill, *Utilitarianism*, in *Collected Works*, p. 247.

52. Ronald Dworkin argues that political morality is rights-based in *Taking Rights Seriously*, pp. 169–77, esp. 171. John Mackie has applied this thesis to morality generally in "Can There Be a Right-Based Moral Theory?" *Midwest Studies in Philosophy* 3 (1978), esp. p. 350.

53. Robert Nozick, *Anarchy, State, and Utopia* (New York: Basic Books, 1974), pp.
ix, 149–82.

54. Gewirth, "Why Rights are Indispensable," *Mind* 95 (1986): 333.

55. See Michael Sandel, "The Political Theory of the Procedural Republic," *Revue
de métaphysique et de morale* 93 (1988): 57–68, esp. 64–67; Sandel, "Democrats
and Community," *The New Republic*, February 22, 1988: 20–23; Alasdair
MacIntyre, *After Virtue*, pp. 235–37; Michael Walzer, "The Communitarian Critique of Liberalism," *Political Theory* 18 (1990): 6–23. See also Shlomo Avineri
and Avner de-Shalit, eds., *Communitarianism and Individualism* (Oxford: Oxford University Press, 1992); David Rasmussen, ed., *Universalism vs. Communitarianism: Contemporary Debates in Ethics* (Cambridge, MA: MIT Press,
1990); and Donald L. Gelpi, ed., *Beyond Individualism: Toward a Retrieval of
Moral Discourse in America* (Notre Dame, IN: University of Notre Dame Press,
1989).

56. See Sandel, *Liberalism and the Limits of Justice* (Cambridge: Cambridge University
Press, 1982), pp. 15–17.

57. Ibid., p. 172; cf. p. 179. See similar statements in MacIntyre, *After Virtue*, pp.
203–6.

58. Sandel, "Introduction," in *Liberalism and Its Critics*, ed. Sandel (New York: New
York University Press, 1984), p. 6, and "Morality and the Liberal Ideal," *The
New Republic* (May 7, 1984), pp. 15–17; MacIntyre, *After Virtue*, ch. 1.

59. Sandel, *Liberalism and the Limits of Justice*, 15–23, 84–87, 92–94, 139–51;
MacIntyre, *Whose Justice? Which Rationality?* (Notre Dame, IN: University of
Notre Dame Press, 1988), p. 10, and *After Virtue*, p. 206.

60. *After Virtue*, p. 53.

61. Mackie, *Ethics*, pp. 30, 36–37; see also 106–10, 120–24.

62. Alasdair MacIntyre, *After Virtue*, pp. 17, 187, 190–94.

63. "Morality and the Liberal Ideal," p. 17.

64. See James L. Nelson, "The Rights and Responsibilities of Potential Organ Donors:
A Communitarian Approach," *Communitarian Position Paper* (Washington, DC:
The Communitarian Network, 1992); James Muyskens, "Procurement and Alloca-
tion Policies," *The Mount Sinai Journal of Medicine* 56 (1989): 202–6.

65. For the wide range of issues in organ procurement, see James F. Childress, "Ethical Criteria for Procuring and Distributing Organs for Transplantation," *Journal of
Health Politics, Policy and Law* 14 (1989): 87–113.

66. Callahan, *What Kind of Life* (New York: Simon and Schuster, 1990), ch. 4, esp.
pp. 105–13, and *Setting Limits* (New York: Simon and Schuster, 1987), esp. pp.
106–14.

67. Ezekiel J. Emanuel, *The Ends of Human Life: Medical Ethics in a Liberal Polity* (Cambridge, MA: Harvard University Press, 1991). See also Troyen Brennan, *Just Doctoring: Medical Ethics in the Liberal State* (Berkeley: University of California Press, 1991).

68. See esp. Charles Taylor, *Philosophy and the Human Sciences,* Philosophical Papers, vol. 2 (Cambridge: Cambridge University Press, 1985), ch. 7, "Atomism."

69. See arguments to this conclusion in Will Kymlicka, "Liberalism and Communitarianism," *Canadian Journal of Philosophy* 18 (June 1988): 181–204, and "Liberal Individualism and Liberal Neutrality," *Ethics* 99 (July 1989): 883–905. Even in John Locke and Thomas Hobbes—the communitarians' arch-enemies (see MacIntyre, *After Virtue,* pp. 233–34)—there is a considerable emphasis on promoting the commonweal. Locke gives an elegant statement in *Two Treatises of Civil Government, Works* (London: C. and J. Rivington, 1824), 12th Ed., bk. 2, note 8, p. 357.

70. See Amy Gutmann, "Communitarian Critics of Liberalism," *Philosophy and Public Affairs* 14 (Summer 1985): 308–22.

71. Sandel interprets Rawls as creating this dilemma by his account of the priority of the right over the good. *Liberalism and the Limits of Justice,* pp. 1–10, 17–24, 168–72, and "Morality and the Liberal Ideal," pp. 16–17.

72. Joel Feinberg, *Harm to Self,* vol. 3 in *The Moral Limits of the Criminal Law* (New York: Oxford University Press, 1986), p. 47.

73. See MacIntyre, *Against Virtue,* pp. 67–68.

74. See Allen Buchanan, "Assessing the Communitarian Critique of Liberalism," *Ethics* 99 (July 1989): 852–82, esp. 862–65, and William A. Galston, *Liberal Purposes* (Cambridge: Cambridge University Press, 1991).

75. Thomson, *The Realm of Rights,* p. 223.

76. Carol Gilligan, *In a Different Voice* (Cambridge, MA: Harvard University Press, 1982), esp. p. 21. For these themes in her later work, see her "Mapping the Moral Domain: New Images of Self in Relationship," *Cross Currents* 39 (Spring 1989): 50–63.

77. Gilligan and many others deny that the two distinct voices correlate strictly with gender. See Gilligan and Susan Pollak, "The Vulnerable and Invulnerable Physician," in *Mapping the Moral Domain,* ed. C. Gilligan, J. Ward, and J. Taylor (Cambridge, MA: Harvard University Press, 1988), pp. 245–62.

78. See Gilligan and G. Wiggins, "The Origins of Morality in Early Childhood Relationships," in *The Emergence of Morality in Young Children,* ed. J. Kagan and S. Lamm (Chicago: University of Chicago Press, 1988). See also Sara Ruddick, *Maternal Thinking: Toward a Politics of Peace* (Boston: Beacon Press, 1989).

79. Baier, "What Do Women Want in a Moral Theory?" *Nous* 19 (March 1985): 53.

80. Ibid., pp. 53–56.

81. Cf. Baier, *Postures of the Mind* (Minneapolis: University of Minnesota Press, 1985), pp. 210–19.

82. Our formulation of these criticisms of liberalism is influenced by Alisa L. Carse, "The 'Voice of Care': Implications for Bioethical Education," *The Journal of Medicine and Philosophy* 16 (1991): 5–28, esp. 8–17.

83. Baier, "Trust and Antitrust," *Ethics* 96 (1986): 248.

84. Quill and Townsend, "Bad News: Delivery, Dialogue, and Dilemmas," *Archives of Internal Medicine* 151 (March 1991): 463–64.

85. See Nel Noddings, *Caring: A Feminine Approach to Ethics and Moral Education* (Berkeley: University of California Press, 1984).

86. See Nancy Sherman, *The Fabric of Character* (Oxford: Oxford University Press, 1989), pp. 13–55, and Martha Nussbaum, *Love's Knowledge* (Oxford: Oxford University Press, 1990).

87. See the Kantian arguments in Barbara Herman, "Integrity and Impartiality," *Monist* 66 (April 1983): 233–50, and Marcia Baron, "The Alleged Repugnance of Acting from Duty," *Journal of Philosophy* 81 (April 1984): 197–220.

88. For a recent attempt to incorporate caring into a framework that retains impartiality, see Jeffrey Blustein, *Care and Commitment: Taking the Personal Point of View* (New York: Oxford University Press, 1991).

89. Carse, "The 'Voice of Care,' " p. 17.

90. Susan Sherwin, *No Longer Patient: Feminist Ethics and Health Care* (Philadelphia: Temple University Press, 1992), pp. 49–50. See also Laura Purdy, "A Call to Heal Ethics," in Helen Bequaert Holmes and Purdy, eds., *Feminist Perspectives in Medical Ethics* (Bloomington: Indiana University Press, 1992), p. 10.

91. See Hilde L. Nelson, "Against Caring," Nel Noddings, "In Defense of Caring," and Toni M. Vezeau, "Caring: From Philosophical Concerns to Practice," in *The Journal of Clinical Ethics* 3 (Spring 1992): 8–20. Two recent anthologies provide a good entry point for these debates: Claudia Card, ed., *Feminist Ethics* (Lawrence: University Press of Kansas, 1991), and Eve Browning Cole and Susan Coultrap-McQuin, eds., *Explorations in Feminist Ethics: Theory and Practice* (Bloomington: Indiana University Press, 1992). See also Christine Overall, *Ethics and Human Reproduction: A Feminist Analysis* (Boston: Allen and Unwin, 1987).

92. Casuists have had little to say about the nature of a case, but see the analysis in Albert R. Jonsen, "Casuistry as Methodology in Clinical Ethics," *Theoretical Medicine* 12 (December 1991): 298.

93. For leading expositions, see Albert R. Jonsen and Stephen Toulmin, *The Abuse of Casuistry: A History of Moral Reasoning* (Berkeley: University of California Press, 1988) and Brody, *Life and Death Decision Making.*

94. The casuistical tradition was prominent in the seventeenth century when it came under a severe and enduring attack by Blaise Pascal in his *Provincial Letters* (18 letters published in 1656–57, under the pseudonym Louis de Montalte). Jonsen and Toulmin assess the relevance and fairness of Pascal's attack in *Abuse of Casuistry,* ch. 12, esp. pp. 243–49.

95. *An Encyclopedia of Religion,* ed. V. Ferm (New York: The Philosophical Library, 1945), p. 124.

96. Here are two candidates. Jeremy Bentham: "From utility then we may denominate a principle, that may serve to preside over and govern . . . several institutions or combinations of institutions that compose the matter of this science." *A Fragment on Government,* ed. Burns and Hart (Oxford: Clarendon Press, 1977), Preface, p. 416. Henry Sidgwick: "Utilitarianism may be presented as [a] scientifically complete and systematically reflective form of th[e] regulation of conduct." *Methods of Ethics,* bk. 4, ch. 3, § 1, p. 425.

97. Aristotle, *Posterior Analytics* (Cambridge, MA: Harvard University Press, Loeb Library, 1960), $71^{b}18$–23, $72^{a}15$–23, $73^{a}23$–26. There is scholarly controversy about this reading of Aristotle in light of his discussion in the *Topics* of the use of dialectic as a method of reaching first principles.

98. Aristotle, *Nicomachean Ethics,* $1095^{b}1$ff.

99. Jonsen and Toulmin, *Abuse of Casuistry,* pp. 11–19, 251–54, 296–99; Jonsen, "Casuistry as Methodology in Clinical Ethics," pp. 299–302; Brody, *Life and Death Decision Making,* pp. 12–13, 15n.

100. Toulmin, "The Tyranny of Principles," *Hastings Center Report* 11 (December 1981): 31–39.

101. Jonsen and Toulmin, *Abuse of Casuistry*, pp. 16–19.

102. Ibid., and see Toulmin, "The National Commission on Human Experimentation: Procedures and Outcomes," in *Scientific Controversies: Case Studies in the Resolution and Closure of Disputes in Science and Technology*, ed. H. T. Engelhardt, Jr. and A. Caplan (New York: Cambridge University Press, 1987), pp. 599–613, and Jonsen, "American Moralism and the Origin of Bioethics in the United States," *Journal of Medicine and Philosophy* 16 (1991): 113–30.

103. See John D. Arras, "Getting Down to Cases: The Revival of Casuistry in Bioethics," *Journal of Medicine and Philosophy* 16 (1991): 31–33; Jonsen and Toulmin, *Abuse of Casuistry*, pp. 16–19, 66–67; Jonsen, "Casuistry and Clinical Ethics," *Theoretical Medicine* 7 (1986): 67, 71.

104. Jonsen and Toulmin, *Abuse of Casuistry*, pp. 252–62.

105. Brody, *Life and Death Decision Making*, p. 13

106. Jonsen and Toulmin sometimes seem to criticize all theory and at other times only abuse and overstatement in theory (especially as Sidgwick conceived it). We interpret them as hostile primarily to theory that is deductivist or composed of allegedly universal, eternal, and unchallengeable principles. Pragmatic and nondogmatic theories, such as those of Aristotle and William James, seem to be acceptable, even laudable. See *Abuse of Casuistry*, pp. 23–27, 279–303.

107. Jonsen, "Casuistry as Methodology in Clinical Ethics," p. 298.

108. Jonsen, "Case Analysis in Clinical Ethics," *The Journal of Clinical Ethics* 1 (1990): 65. See *Abuse of Casuistry*, p. 10.

109. Jonsen, "American Moralism and the Origin of Bioethics in the United States," esp. pp. 117, 125–28.

110. The pertinent data appear in National Commission for the Protection of Human Subjects of Biomedical and Behavioral Research, "Transcript of the Meeting Proceedings." February 11–13, 1977, pp. 11–155; July 8–9, 1977, pp. 104–17; April 14–15, 1978, pp. 155–62; and June 9–10, 1978, pp. 113–19. The Commission's general principles appear in *The Belmont Report: Ethical Guidelines for the Protection of Human Subjects* (Washington, DC: DHEW Publication (OS) 78-0012, 1978).

111. Cf. Jonsen and Toulmin, *Abuse of Casuistry*, pp. 11–16; Brody, *Life and Death Decision Making*, pp. 10–11.

112. *Utilitarianism*, ch. 2, p. 225.

113. Revisions in our theory in this edition have benefited from criticisms by David DeGrazia—see his "Moving Forward in Bioethical Theory: Theories, Cases, and Specified Principlism," *Journal of Medicine and Philosophy* 17 (October 1992): 511–39—and Ruth Faden.

114. H. A. Prichard presented powerful arguments in the common-morality tradition to show that all single or absolute-principle theories disintegrate in the face of the diversity in the considered judgments of pretheoretic commonsense morality. See his *Moral Obligation: Essays and Lectures*, ed. W. D. Ross (Oxford: Clarendon Press, 1949). However, Prichard rejected principle-based theories.

115. William K. Frankena, *Ethics*, pp. 4–9, 43–56, 113; *Thinking about Morality* (Ann Arbor: University of Michigan Press, 1980), pp. 26, 34. Frankena cites Butler on p. 6 of the first book.

116. Ross, *The Right and the Good* (Oxford: Clarendon Press, 1930), p. 41.

117. Ibid., pp. 21–22.

118. Ross, *The Foundations of Ethics* (Oxford: Clarendon Press, 1939), pp. 169–70.

119. Ross, *The Right and the Good*, p. 19.

120. See Robert Nozick, "Moral Complications and Moral Structures," *Natural Law Forum* 13 (1968): 1–50.

121. Hume, "A Dialogue," published with *An Enquiry Concerning the Principles of Morals*, pp. 335–36.

122. Clouser and Gert, "A Critique of Principlism," pp. 219–27.

123. "A Critique of Principlism," p. 233.

124. Gert's moral rules can be treated as rules falling under various principles. Gert has told us in private conversation that once principles are interpreted as headings under which rules fall, they become unobjectionable, but also expendable. For the general theory on which he and Clouser rely, see Gert, *Morality: A New Justification of the Moral Rules* (New York: Oxford University Press, 1988).

125. A variant of this criticism has also been leveled against us by Ronald Green, "Method in Bioethics: A Troubled Assessment," *The Journal of Medicine and Philosophy* 15 (April 1990): 188–89.

126. See *Postures of the Mind*, pp. 139–41, 206–17, 223–26, 232–37.

127. Brandt, "Toward a Credible Form of Utilitarianism," p. 166.

3

Respect for Autonomy

Respect for the autonomous choices of other persons runs as deep in common morality as any principle, but little agreement exists about its nature and strength or about specific rights of autonomy. Many philosophers have held that morality presupposes autonomous actors, but they have emphasized different themes associated with autonomy. These disagreements indicate a need for analysis of the concept of autonomy and for specification of the principle of respect for autonomy.

The concept of autonomy is used in this chapter primarily to examine decisionmaking in health care. Our account should be adequate to identify what is protected by rules of informed consent, informed refusal, truth-telling, and confidentiality. This account is essential to our objectives throughout subsequent chapters, which fill out and qualify the nature and importance of respect for autonomy.

The Concept of Autonomy

The word *autonomy,* derived from the Greek *autos* ("self") and *nomos* ("rule," "governance," or "law"), was first used to refer to the self-rule or self-governance of independent Hellenic city-states. *Autonomy* has since been extended to individuals and has acquired meanings as diverse as self-governance, liberty rights, privacy, individual choice, freedom of the will, causing one's behavior, and being one's own person. Thus, autonomy is not a univocal concept in either ordinary English or contemporary philosophy. Several ideas constitute the concept, creating a need to refine it in light of particular objectives. Like many philosophical concepts, "autonomy" acquires a more specific meaning in the context of a theory.

Toward this end, we start with what we take to be essential to personal autonomy, as distinguished from political self-rule: personal rule of the self that is free from both controlling interferences by others and from personal limitations that prevent meaningful choice, such as inadequate understanding.[1] The autonomous individual freely acts in accordance with a self-chosen plan, analogous to the way an independent government manages its territories and sets its policies. A person of diminished autonomy, by contrast, is in at least some respect controlled by others or incapable of deliberating or acting on the basis of his or her desires and plans. For example, institutionalized persons, such as prisoners and the mentally retarded, often have diminished autonomy. Mental incapacitation limits the autonomy of the retarded, and coercive institutionalization constrains the autonomy of prisoners.

Virtually all theories of autonomy agree that two conditions are essential: (1) *liberty* (independence from controlling influences) and (2) *agency* (capacity for intentional action). However, disagreement exists over the meaning of these two conditions and over whether some additional condition is needed. We will analyze autonomy in terms of three conditions in the next section.

Theories of Autonomy

Some theories of autonomy have featured the traits of the *autonomous person,* which include capacities of self-governance, such as understanding, reasoning, deliberating, and independent choice. However, our interest in decisionmaking leads us to focus on *autonomous choice,* which is actual governance rather than capacity for governance. Even autonomous persons with self-governing capacities sometimes fail to govern themselves in their choices because of temporary constraints imposed by illness or depression, or because of ignorance, coercion, or conditions that restrict options. An autonomous person who signs a consent form without reading or understanding the form is qualified to act autonomously by giving an informed consent, but has failed to do so. Similarly, some persons who are not generally autonomous can at times make autonomous choices. For example, some patients in mental institutions who are unable to care for themselves and have been declared legally incompetent may still be able to make autonomous choices such as stating preferences for meals, refusing some medications, and making telephone calls to acquaintances.

Some contemporary writers in ethical theory have maintained that autonomy is largely a matter of having the capacity to reflectively control and identify with one's basic (first-order) desires or preferences through higher-level (second-order) desires or preferences.[2] For example, an alcoholic may have a desire to drink, but also a higher-order desire to stop drinking that prevails over the lower-level desire. An autonomous person, in this account, is one who has the capacity to rationally accept, identify with, or repudiate a lower-order desire or preference in a manner that it is independent of the manipulation of desires. Such acceptance of or repudiation of first-order desires at the higher level (the capacity to change one's preference structure) constitutes autonomy.

However, serious problems confront this theory of autonomy. Acceptance or repudiation of a desire on one level can be motivated by an overriding desire that is simply *stronger,* not more *rational* or *autonomous.* Second-order desires can be caused by the potency of first-order desires or by the influence of a condition such as alcohol addiction that is antithetical to autonomy. (An addicted person, we sometimes say, is not his or her own person.) The background of alcohol consumption has created the overriding desire to continue consuming. The point can be generalized beyond circumstances of addiction: If second-order desires (decisions, volitions, etc.) are generated by prior desires or commitments, then the process of identification with one desire rather than another does not distinguish autonomy from nonautonomy. Very often a second-order identification with a first-order desire is assured by the strength of the first-order desire; such identification is simply an awareness of the already formed structure of one's preferences, not a new structuring of preferences or an exercise of autonomy. Such second-order desires are not significantly different from first-order desires, and the condition of higher-order desires is an unnecessary complication for a theory of autonomy.

It also appears that any act of identification with a desire that is genuinely autonomous necessarily requires an independent act of identification at a higher level. One would have to correct, identify with, or repudiate second-order desires by third-order desires, thereby generating an infinite regress of desires, and never arriving at autonomy. If the person's identification at any level is itself the result of a process of thoroughgoing conditioning, the identification is never sufficiently independent to qualify as autonomous. For example, the alcoholic who identifies with drinking is not autonomous if a second-level desire for alcohol derives from and then reinforces the first-level desire for alcohol. An alcoholic can reflect at ever-higher levels on lower-level desires without achieving autonomy. This theory therefore at least needs an account powerful enough to distinguish autonomy-robbing influences and desires from those that are consistent with autonomy.

But this theory also needs a more important condition: It needs a way of allowing ordinary persons to qualify as deserving respect for their autonomy even when they have *not* reflected on their preferences at a higher level, and this condition seems unlikely to be satisfied in this and various other theories of autonomy. Some theories of autonomy require that both persons and their actions meet still more rigorous standards than the standards in this theory to be autonomous. For example, some theories demand that the autonomous person be exceptionally authentic, self-possessed, consistent, independent, in command, resistant to control by authorities, and the original source of personal values, beliefs, and life plans.[3] Alternatively, some theories demand that an individual evaluate and accept each of the reasons on which the individual acts.[4] One problem with all such exacting requirements for autonomy, including second-order-desire theories, is that few choosers, and also few choices, would be autonomous if held to such standards, which in effect present an aspirational ideal of autonomy. No theory of autonomy is acceptable if it presents an ideal beyond the reach of normal choosers. Instead of depicting an ideal of this sort, our analysis will be closely tied to the assumptions of autonomy underlying moral requirements of "respect for autonomy."

We analyze autonomous action in terms of normal choosers who act (1) intentionally, (2) with understanding, and (3) without controlling influences that determine their action. The first of these three conditions of autonomy is not a matter of degree. Acts are either intentional or nonintentional. (See Chapter 4 for analysis of intention, pp. 208–210.) By contrast, the conditions of understanding and absence of controlling influences can both be satisfied to a greater or lesser extent. Actions therefore can be autonomous by degrees, as a function of satisfying these two conditions to different degrees. For both conditions, a broad continuum exists from fully present to wholly absent. Many children and many elderly patients, for example, exhibit various degrees of understanding and independence found on this continuum.[5]

For an action to be autonomous we should only require a substantial degree of understanding and freedom from constraint, not a full understanding or a complete absence of influence. To limit adequate decisionmaking by patients to the ideal of fully or completely autonomous decisionmaking strips these acts of any meaningful place in the practical world, where people's actions are rarely, if ever, fully autonomous. A person's appreciation of information and independence from controlling influences in the health care setting need not exceed, for example, a person's information and independence in making a financial investment, hiring a new employee, buying a new house, or selecting a university. Such consequential decisions are usually substantially autonomous, but far from fully autonomous.

The line between what is substantial and what is insubstantial often appears arbitrary, and therefore our analysis might seem imperiled. However, thresholds marking substantially autonomous decisions can be carefully fixed in light of specific objectives such as meaningful decisionmaking. Substantial autonomy is achievable in decisions about participation in research and acceptance

of proposed medical interventions, no less and no more than substantially autonomous choice is present elsewhere in life. Accordingly, appropriate criteria
of substantial autonomy are best addressed in a particular context, rather than
pinpointed through a general theory of a substantial amount.

Autonomy, Authority, and Community

Some people have argued that autonomous action is incompatible with the authority of church, state, or other communities that legislate persons' decisions.
They maintain that autonomous persons must act on their own reasons and can
never submit to an authority or choose to be ruled by others without losing their
autonomy. Because this conclusion might seem to follow from our analysis
of autonomous action, we need to consider whether autonomy is inconsistent
with authority.[6]

We believe no fundamental inconsistency exists, because individuals can exercise their autonomy in choosing to accept and submit to the authoritative
demands of an institution, tradition, or community that they view as a legitimate source of direction. Having welcomed the authority of his or her religious
institution, a Jehovah's Witness can refuse a recommended blood transfusion,
and a Roman Catholic can refuse to consider an abortion. Morality is not a set
of personal rules created by individuals isolated from society, and moral principles have authority over our lives by virtue of a social and cultural setting that
is independent of any single autonomous actor. That we share these principles
in no way prevents them from being an individual's own principles. Virtuous
conduct, role responsibilities, acceptable forms of loving, charitable behavior,
respect for autonomy, and many other moral notions are autonomously accepted by individuals but usually derive from cultural traditions. A principle
that is outside social arrangements would merely be one individual's belief or
policy. Rules or codes of professional ethics similarly are not an individual's
invention, yet they are compatible with autonomy.

This conclusion about the compatibility of autonomy, authority, and moral
tradition holds for medical as well as political and religious contexts. We encounter many problems of autonomy in medical contexts because of the patient's dependent condition and the medical professional's authoritative position. On some occasions authority and autonomy are incompatible, but not
because the two concepts are intrinsically incompatible. Conflict arises because
authority has not been properly delegated or accepted.

Some critics of the current emphasis on autonomy in ethical theory view it
as focused too narrowly on independence from others, while underestimating
the importance of intimate and dependent relationships. Religious traditions
are sometimes suspicious of appeals to autonomy that render the individual
independent of a transcendent power, and several philosophical traditions ques-

tion the model of an independent self, especially when presented as a rational will that is inattentive to communal life, reciprocity, and the development of persons over time. Some feminist critics view ethical theories that focus on autonomous individuals as unrealistic and even pernicious when a supreme and overriding value is placed on autonomy.[7] These criticisms typically apply to stark, individualistic conceptions of autonomy that more balanced theories avoid. Communal life and human relationships provide the matrix for the development of the self, and no defensible theory of autonomy denies this fact.

The Principle of Respect for Autonomy

Being autonomous is not the same as being respected as an autonomous agent. To respect an autonomous agent is, at a minimum, to acknowledge that person's right to hold views, to make choices, and to take actions based on personal values and beliefs. Such respect involves respectful *action,* not merely a respectful *attitude.* It also requires more than obligations of nonintervention in the affairs of persons, because it includes obligations to maintain capacities for autonomous choice in others while allaying fears and other conditions that destroy or disrupt their autonomous actions. Respect, on this account, involves treating persons to enable them to act autonomously, whereas disrespect for autonomy involves attitudes and actions that ignore, insult, or demean others' autonomy and thus deny a minimal equality to persons.

Why is such respect owed to persons? Two philosophers who have influenced contemporary interpretations of respect for autonomy were examined in Chapter 2: Immanuel Kant and John Stuart Mill. Kant argued that respect for autonomy flows from the recognition that all persons have unconditional worth, each having the capacity to determine his or her own destiny.[8] To violate a person's autonomy is to treat that person merely as a means, that is, in accordance with others' goals without regard to that person's own goals. Such treatment is a fundamental moral violation because autonomous persons are ends in themselves capable of determining their destinies. Mill was more concerned about the autonomy—or, as he preferred to say, the individuality—of persons in shaping their lives. He argued that citizens should be permitted to develop according to their personal convictions, as long as they do not interfere with a like expression of freedom by others; but he also insisted that we sometimes are obligated to seek to persuade others when they have false or ill-considered views.[9] Mill's position requires both noninterference with and an active strengthening of autonomous expression, whereas Kant's entails a moral imperative of respectful treatment of persons as ends rather than merely as means. In the final analysis, however, these two profoundly different philosophies both provide support for the principle of respect for autonomy.

The principle of respect for autonomy can be stated, in its negative form, as follows: *Autonomous actions should not be subjected to controlling constraints by others.* The principle asserts a broad, abstract obligation that is free of exceptive clauses such as "We must respect individuals' views and rights *so long as their thoughts and actions do not seriously harm other persons.*" Correlative to this obligation is the right to self-determination, which supports various autonomy rights, including those of confidentiality and privacy. This principle needs specification in particular contexts to become a practical guide to conduct, and appropriate specification will list the valid exceptions. Part of this process of specification will appear in rights and obligations of liberty, privacy, confidentiality, truthfulness, and consent (several of which receive sustained attention in Chapter 7). Wide disagreement exists in contemporary literature about the scope of these rights, but wide agreement exists that rights of autonomy are often legitimately constrained by the rights of others.

Respect for autonomy, then, has only prima facie standing and can be overridden by competing moral considerations. Typical examples are the following: If our choices endanger the public health, potentially harm innocent others, or require a scarce resource for which no funds are available, others can justifiably restrict our exercises of autonomy. The justification must, however, rest on some competing and overriding moral principles. The principle of respect for autonomy does not by itself determine what, on balance, a person ought to be free to know or do or what counts as a valid justification for constraining autonomy. For example, in Case 2 (see appendix) a patient with an inoperable, incurable carcinoma asks, "I don't have cancer, do I?" The physician lies, saying, "You're as good as you were ten years ago." This lie denies the patient information he may need to determine his future course of action, thereby infringing the principle of respect for autonomy. However, on balance the lie may be justified in this context by the principle of beneficence.

Many criticisms directed at current uses of the principle of respect for autonomy in biomedical ethics note that autonomy is not our only value and that respect for autonomy is not the only moral imperative.[10] These critics rightly point out that many decisions in health care depend less on respecting autonomy than on maintaining the capacity for autonomy and the conditions of meaningful life. Thus, respect for autonomy is often less prominent than expressions of beneficence and compassion. These criticisms, however, are effective only against ethical theories that recognize an unduly narrow principle of autonomy or that treat the principle as absolute or as lexically prior to all other principles. The principle of respect for autonomy should be viewed as establishing a stalwart right of authority to control one's personal destiny, but not as the only source of moral obligations and rights.

We can now consider the principle's affirmative demands, especially the *positive* obligation of respectful treatment in disclosing information and fostering autonomous decisionmaking. In some cases we are obligated to increase the options available to persons. Many autonomous actions could not occur without the material cooperation of others in making options available. Respect for autonomy obligates professionals to disclose information, to probe for and ensure understanding and voluntariness, and to foster adequate decisionmaking. As some contemporary Kantians declare, the demand that we treat others as ends requires that we assist persons in achieving their ends and foster their capacities as agents, not merely that we avoid treating them entirely as means to our ends.[11]

There is a temptation in medicine to use the authority of the physician's role to foster or perpetuate the dependency of patients, rather than to promote their autonomy. But discharging the obligation to respect patients' autonomy requires equipping them to overcome their sense of dependence and achieve as much control as possible or as they desire. These positive obligations of respect for autonomy derive in part from the special fiduciary relationships professionals have with their patients, including affirmative obligations of disclosure and conversation. In some cases the medical professional is obligated to restore ill patients to a condition in which meaningful autonomy is possible. From this perspective, respect for autonomy is not, as some critics allege,[12] a principle that brands medical professionals as agents of paternalism and counsels them to disregard difficult patients. To the contrary, the negative and positive sides of respect for autonomy jointly indicate that respecting another includes efforts to foster and effect that person's outlook on his or her interests.

Because of various ways in which these positive and negative principles function in the moral life, they are capable of supporting many more specific moral rules (although other principles, such as beneficence and nonmaleficence, also help justify some of these same rules). Typical examples include the following rules:
1. "Tell the truth."
2. "Respect the privacy of others."
3. "Protect confidential information."
4. "Obtain consent for interventions with patients."
5. "When asked, help others make important decisions."
Both the principle of respect for autonomy and its specifications in these moral rules are prima facie, not absolute.

Despite the breadth of our obligations to respect autonomy, the principle is not so broad that it covers nonautonomous persons. The principle should not be used for persons who cannot act in a sufficiently autonomous manner (and cannot be rendered autonomous) because they are immature, incapacitated, ignorant, coerced, or exploited. Infants, irrationally suicidal individuals, and drug-dependent patients are typical examples. Those who vigorously defend rights of autonomy in biomedical ethics, as do the present authors, have never denied that some forms of intervention are justified if persons are substantially nonautonomous and cannot be rendered autonomous for specific decisions. We will return to this problem of using respect for autonomy as a canopy to protect nonautonomous persons in this chapter's final section (and in Chapter 5 in a discussion of justifiable paternalistic interventions).

Interpreting Respect for Autonomy

The principle of respect for autonomy has been spiritedly attacked in biomedical ethics over the last several years. Many now believe that an emphasis on autonomy displaces or distorts other moral values, subverting the moral authority of medicine and leaving many patients isolated. One objective of this chapter is to interpret this complex principle so that such misconceptions and misguided criticisms are eliminated. We acknowledge, however, that many defenders of the principle have often encouraged critics because they have overextended or oversimplified it.

Varieties of "consent." The basic paradigm of autonomy in health care, politics, and other contexts is *express* and informed consent. Consent has long occupied a pivotal role in these settings because valid consent legitimates forms of authority and conduct that otherwise would not be legitimate and provides access that otherwise would be unobtainable. However, consent occurs under various conditions. It may be perfunctory or grudging, and it often occurs under intense pressures that may render it invalid. It also occurs in several forms. The paradigm of informed consent captures only one form of consent relevant to health care ethics. Another form is *tacit* consent, which is expressed passively by omissions. If residents of a long-term care facility are asked whether they object to having the time of dinner changed by one hour, a uniform lack of objection constitutes consent (assuming they understand the proposal and the need for consent). Similarly, *implicit* or *implied* consent is inferred from actions. For example, consent to one medical procedure is often implicit in a specific consent to another procedure. *Presumed* consent is still another variety, although if consent is presumed on the basis of what we know about a particular person, it closely resembles implied consent. By contrast, if it is presumed on the basis of a general theory of human goods or a theory of the rational will, the moral situation is both different and problematic. Consent should refer to an individual's own actions and inactions. Although we often legitimately make presumptions that a person's silence constitutes consent or that his or her consent is implicit in other statements or actions, these inferences can lack sufficient warrant.

Consider two situations in which non-express forms of consent—namely, implicit consent and presumed consent—are sometimes held to be morally relevant, even though their connection to autonomous choice is precarious. In current debates about organ procurement, concern exists that requirements of express consent by the decedent while alive or by the family after the relative's death impair rather than facilitate collection of needed organs. Several nations have adopted what is variously called *presumed, tacit,* or *implicit* consent for solid organs, and several states in the United States have done likewise for corneas. The moral rationale for the removal of corneas where the decedents have not registered their opposition is typically tacit consent. However, if no evidence of tacit consent exists—for example, if the decedents were unaware of the law—then the practice either falls under another form of consent or simply expropriates organs without regard to consent. It is difficult to see how consent to donation is implicit in the decedent's actions while alive, and presumed consent based on a theory of human goods is not bona fide consent. The principle of respect for autonomy, then, can be used unjustifiably through fictions of consent that are misleading and dangerous. (A related and also risky overextension is to refer to a cadaveric source of organs for transplantation as a "donor" when he or she never "donated," that is, never chose to donate.)

Another controversy about non-express forms of consent appears in the testing of hospital admittees for antibodies to the human immunodeficiency virus (HIV), which causes AIDS. Interest in testing hospitalized patients has emerged in part because treating HIV-infected patients creates risks for caregivers under some circumstances. If a newly admitted hospital patient gives express consent when asked for permission to perform an HIV-antibody test, the staff is authorized to proceed. If a patient is silent when told the test will be performed unless he or she objects, silence constitutes valid tacit consent as long as understanding and voluntariness are present. But if the question is not asked, the patient's failure to object to the test cannot be presumed to be a consent without some additional information, including the basis for presuming a general awareness of hospital testing policies.

Suppose, by contrast, that a patient has given consent for routine blood tests. Do health care professionals now have the patient's valid consent for an HIV test? Here the appeal might be to a specific consent implicit in the general consent to blood tests (or to admission to the hospital). There are reasons to be suspicious of this claim, because express consent is the only appropriate consent in these circumstances. Even if blood has already been drawn with consent, the test has psychological and social risks. For a seropositive individual, the psychological risks include anxiety and serious depression, and the social risks include stigma, discrimination, and breaches of confidentiality.[13] In general, hospitals are not justified in testing patients for HIV antibodies without specific consent.

A recent Virginia law (Virginia Code 32.1-45.1) invokes "deemed consent" in permitting a health care provider to test a patient's blood, without specific consent, following the provider's exposure to the patient's body fluids under circumstances that could spread HIV infection: "The patient whose body fluids were involved in the exposures shall be deemed to have consented to testing for infection with human immunodeficiency virus [and] to have consented to the release of such test results to the person who was exposed." The law assigns to health care providers the responsibility to inform patients of this rule of deemed consent prior to the provision of health care services, except in emergency circumstances. The patient's acceptance of health care following this disclosure counts under the statute as consent.

Although writers in biomedical ethics often resort to fictions such as deemed consent, it is more defensible to argue straightforwardly that a patient's autonomy, liberty, privacy, or confidentiality can be justifiably overridden to obtain information about an individual's HIV-antibody status in order to protect a health care provider who has been exposed to the risk of infection. A preferable approach is to obtain patients' advance express consent if accidental exposure occurs.

Consents and refusals over time. People's beliefs, choices, and consents emerge and are modified over time. Moral and interpretive problems emerge when a person's present choices contradict his or her prior choices, which may have been explicitly designed to prevent future changes of mind. In one case a twenty-eight-year-old man decided to terminate chronic renal dialysis because of his restricted lifestyle and the burdens on his family. He had diabetes, was legally blind, and could not walk because of progressive neuropathy. His wife and physician agreed to provide medication to relieve his pain and agreed not to put him back on dialysis even if he requested this action under the influence of pain or other bodily changes as he died. While dying in the hospital, the patient awoke complaining of pain and asked to be put back on dialysis. The patient's wife and physician decided to act on the patient's earlier request not to intervene, and he died four hours later.[14] In our judgment, the spouse and physician should have put the patient back on dialysis to determine if he had autonomously revoked his prior choice.

A key question in this and related cases is whether people have autonomously revoked their prior decisions. Whether actions are autonomous can turn in part on whether they are in character or out of character. For example, a sudden and unexpected decision to discontinue dialysis by a woman who has displayed considerable courage and zest for life despite years of disability is evidence (but not necessarily decisive evidence) that a decision may not be adequately autonomous. Actions are more likely to be substantially autonomous if they are in character (for example, when a committed Jehovah's Witness refuses a blood transfusion). However, acting in character is not a necessary condition of autonomy. At most, actions that are out of character can be caution flags that warn others to seek explanations and probe more deeply into whether the actions are autonomous.

Autonomous decisions that anticipate periods of incompetence. In recent years, advance directives have emerged as a way for people to control what happens to them in the event they become incompetent. Prospective decisions to forgo life-sustaining treatment in a period of incompetence provide one example, but advance directives can have a broader role in requests for treatment and donation of organs (see pp. 241–244). One issue concerns the extent to which a person's prior autonomously expressed wishes should be viewed as valid and binding after the person becomes incompetent or dies. Suppose that subsequent to an automobile accident, a Jehovah's Witness is taken to the hospital and, while competent in the emergency room, refuses medically essential blood transfusions and falls unconscious. Some contend that the patient's prior request should be honored because otherwise the physicians (1) would have to *harm* the patient by subsequently disclosing the fact of the transfusion, or (2) would have to *deceive* the patient by not telling him the truth if they provided the transfusion.[15] On the basis of respect for autonomy, a more direct and satisfactory conclusion is available. The transfusion of an incompetent patient who, while competent, refused a transfusion violates that person's autonomy, and is disrespectful and insulting to the person.

However, situations are often far more complicated. In some cases, courts have held that in serious life-threatening emergencies only a contemporaneous informed refusal of a blood transfusion must be respected, especially if a prior directive was given in contemplation of a routine procedure that usually does not involve life-threatening complications.[16] In one case, a twenty-two-year-old man hospitalized after an automobile accident was transferred after one week to another hospital where it was determined that his severe brain injury required immediate surgery. Although his parents consented to the surgery, they refused to consent to blood transfusions. The hospital twice sought and received authority from a court to administer blood transfusions. The Pennsylvania Supreme Court held that there was no error when a lower court failed to hear testimony by the patient's parents, fiancée, or minister regarding the patient's religious beliefs, because death would probably have occurred if the operation had not been performed immediately. The necessity to preserve life outweighed third-party judgments about what an unconscious patient would want. The court held that in emergency situations calling for immediate action, "nothing less than a fully conscious contemporaneous decision by the patient will be sufficient to overrule evidence of medical necessity." [17]

Problems about personal identity and continuity. Related issues arise about whether and to what extent the prior decisions and projects of those now dead should be honored. For example, concerns exist about proper respect for the dead in autopsy, transplantation, research, and medical education, including dissection, although the dead no longer have existing interests to be protected. Similar issues surround advance directives by patients who can be expected to survive, but never to regain competence. In Case 3 (see appendix) the staff debates whether to follow a man's request not to tell his father, who is in the early stages of Alzheimer's disease, the truth about his diagnosis. The nurse notes that the patient has a right to know and to make an advance directive prior to further deterioration, or at least to express his fears and feelings. The physician responds that the patient will lose his ability to change his mind once he loses his ability to make decisions. For the nurse, however, the patient's advance directive provides the best indication of what should later be done.

Interesting theoretical issues surrounding these controversies include personal identity and continuity of the self over time. Stated in an extreme form, the problem is that later selves can evolve to be so different from earlier selves that they are two different people. If so, it is not fair for self 1 to bind self 2 to a course of action through an advance directive—for example, when a severely demented condition causes radical changes.[18] Although this radical discontinuity thesis has some attractiveness, its plausibility and relevance in ethics are diminished when we try to envision ways to mark the point of discontinuity in order to draw the line between different selves and determine the inapplicability of advance directives. As with respect for prior wishes of the dead, we respect the previously expressed autonomous wishes of the now severely demented incompetent person because of our respect for the autonomy of the person who made the decision, as well as our own interest in securing control over our lives prior to becoming incompetent. Interventions against autonomous advance directives infringe the principle of respect for autonomy, although they can in some cases be justified.

Problems often exist in determining whether the chooser was competent when executing the advance directive, and in interpreting the directive. Similar problems about competence arise with contemporaneous choices, as we shall now see.

Competence and Autonomous Choice

Debates about competence focus on whether patients or subjects are capable, psychologically or legally, of adequate decisionmaking. Competence in decisionmaking is therefore closely connected to autonomous decisionmaking and to questions about the validity of consent.

The Gatekeeping Function

Competence judgments serve a gatekeeping role in health care by distinguishing persons whose decisions should be solicited or accepted from persons whose decisions need not or should not be solicited or accepted. Professional judgments of competence help determine whether a guardian should be appointed to look after a person's interests, whether involuntary institutionalization is appropriate, and the like. When legal incompetence has been established, a court appoints a surrogate decisionmaker who has either partial or plenary (full) authority over the incompetent individual.

In health care as well as other contexts, competence judgments distinguish the class of individuals whose autonomous decisions must be respected from those individuals whose decisions need to be checked and perhaps overridden by a surrogate.[19] No problem of competence exists if no problem exists of whether to respect a person's decisionmaking capacity. A competent decision is necessarily one for which a person can be held responsible, and a general presumption should exist that adults are competent to make decisions. Thus, the metaphor of gatekeeping is misleading if it suggests either that adults are presumed to be incompetent or that only professionals should determine whether their decisions be solicited and accepted. Moreover, if a health care professional has determined that a patient is not competent, the next step is to inquire whether capacity can be restored. When incompetence rests on a reversible cause, such as pain or overmedication, the immediate goal is to restore capacity prior to decisionmaking.

Competence judgments have a distinctive normative role of qualifying or disqualifying the person for certain decisions or actions. Even though such judgments of grading and sorting are normative, they are sometimes incorrectly presented as empirical findings. For example, a person who appears irrational or unreasonable to others might fail a psychiatric test, and so be declared incompetent. The test is an empirical measuring device, but normative judgments determine how the test will be used to sort persons into the two classes of competent and incompetent. They are normative judgments because they concern how persons ought to be or may permissibly be treated. These judgments are often justified, but they sometimes conceal an unduly narrow value perspective.

The Concept of Competence[20]

The special perspectives of medicine, psychiatry, law, philosophy, and other professions have led to competing accounts of the abilities persons must have to be competent. The word *competence* has thereby accumulated layers of meaning connected in diverse ways, but with different purposes and protective functions behind the various ideas. Consequently, some commentators believe there is no single acceptable *definition* of competence and no single acceptable *standard* of competence. They contend that no nonarbitrary line can be drawn between competent and incompetent persons. However, definitions, standards, tests, and boundary lines should be kept distinct. We confine attention for the moment to the problem of definition.

A single core meaning of the word *competence* is present in all the varied contexts in which it is properly used. That meaning is "the ability to perform a task."[21] By contrast to this core meaning, the criteria of particular competencies vary from context to context because the criteria are relative to specific tasks. The criteria for someone's competence to stand trial, to raise dachshunds, to write checks, or to lecture to medical students are radically different. The competence to decide is therefore relative to the particular decision to be made. Moreover, a person should rarely be judged incompetent with respect to every sphere of life. We usually need to consider only some type of competence, such as the competence to decide about treatment or about participation in research. These judgments of competence and incompetence affect only a limited range of decisionmaking. For example, a person who is incompetent to decide about financial affairs may be competent to decide to participate in medical research, or able to handle simple tasks easily while faltering before complex ones. Competence is therefore best understood as specific rather than global.

Many persons are incompetent to do something at one point in time and competent to perform the same task at another point in time. Judgments of competence about these persons can be complicated by the need to distinguish categories of illness that result in chronic changes of intellect, language, or memory from those characterized by rapid reversibility of these functions, as in the case of transient ischemic attack, transient global amnesia, and the like. In some of the latter cases competence varies from hour to hour.

Intermittent competence and specific competence are evident in the following case. A woman involuntarily hospitalized because of periods of confusion and loss of memory is competent most of the time to perform ordinary tasks. Health professionals and a court are called upon to determine whether this legally incompetent patient can be provided with an alternative medical therapy suitable to her situation.[22] In such legal cases, the concept of *specific incompetence* has been invoked to prevent vague generalizations about competence from excluding persons from all decisionmaking. When it proves too difficult at first to determine the level of competence, it is appropriate to evaluate the patient's understanding, deliberative capacity, and coherence over time, while supplying counseling and further support and information.

These conceptual points are of practical significance in several ways. The law has traditionally presumed that a person who is incompetent to manage his or her estate is also incompetent to vote, make medical decisions, get married, and the like. Such laws were usually aimed at the protection of property rather than persons and so were ill suited to medical decisionmaking. Their global sweep, based on a total judgment of the person, has at times been carried too far. To say that "person X is incompetent to do Y" does not necessarily imply that X is incompetent to do Z—that is, not competent to perform an action other than Y. In one classic case, a physician argued that a patient was incompetent to make decisions because of epilepsy.[23] Such judgments defy much that we now know about the etiology of various forms of incompetence, even in hard cases of mentally retarded individuals, psychotic patients, and patients with uncontrollably painful afflictions. Persons who are incompetent by virtue of dementia, alcoholism, immaturity, and mental retardation present radically different types and problems of incompetence.

Sometimes a competent person who is generally able to select means appropriate to reach chosen goals will act incompetently in a particular circumstance. Consider the following actual case of a patient hospitalized with an acute disc problem whose goal is to control back pain. The patient has decided to manage the problem by wearing a brace, a method she has used successfully in the past. She believes strongly that she should return to this treatment modality. This approach conflicts, however, with her physician's unwavering and insistent advocacy of surgery. When the physician—an eminent surgeon who alone in her city is suited to treat her—asks her to sign the surgical permit, she is psychologically unable to refuse. The patient's hopes are vested in this assertive and, in her view, powerful and authoritative physician. Her hopes and fears are exaggerated by her illness, and she has a passive personality. In the circumstance, it is psychologically too risky for her to act as she desires. She is competent to choose in general, but she is not competent to choose on this occasion because she lacks the needed capacity.

This analysis indicates that the concept of competence in decisionmaking has close ties to the concept of autonomy, as presented earlier. A patient or subject is competent to make a decision if he or she has the capacity to understand the material information, to make a judgment about the information in light of his or her values, to intend a certain outcome, and to freely communicate his or her wish to caregivers or investigators. Law, medicine, and to some extent philosophy presume a context in which the characteristics of the competent person are also the properties possessed by the autonomous person. Although *autonomy* and *competence* are different in meaning (*autonomy* meaning self-governance; *competence,* the ability to perform a task), the criteria of the autonomous person and of the competent person are strikingly similar. Two plausible hypotheses are that an autonomous person is (necessarily) a competent person (for making decisions), and that judgments of whether a person is competent to authorize or refuse an intervention should be based on whether the person is autonomous.

Persons are more and less able to perform a task to the extent that they possess a certain level or range of abilities, just as persons are more and less intelligent and athletic. For example, an experienced and knowledgeable patient is likely to be more qualified to consent to a procedure than a frightened, inexperienced patient in the emergency room. This ability continuum runs from full mastery through various levels of partial proficiency to complete ineptitude. However, it is confusing to think of this continuum as involving degrees of *competency*. For practical and policy reasons, we need threshold levels on this continuum below which a person with a certain level of abilities is incompetent.[24] Not all competent individuals are equally able and not all incompetent persons equally unable, but competence determinations sort persons into these two basic classes, and thus treat persons as either competent or incompetent. Where we draw the line will depend on the particular tasks involved.[25]

Although a continuum of abilities underlies the performance of tasks, the gatekeeping function of competence requires sorting persons into one of two classes: competent or incompetent. In this respect, competence is a threshold and not a continuum concept like autonomy. That is, its purpose is to divide persons into classes and not to place persons at various points on a continuum of abilities (as occurs in ratings for skating, gymnastics, and the like). Persons are not more or less competent, although they perform the tasks that determine competence more or less well. Above the threshold, persons are equally competent; below the threshold they are equally incompetent. Gatekeepers test to determine who is above and who is below this threshold.

Standards of Competence

Not surprisingly, a major question about competence in recent years has centered on standards for its determination—the conditions that must be satisfied to be judged to be competent. In law and medicine standards of competence tend to feature mental skills or capacities closely connected to the attributes of autonomous persons, such as cognitive skills and independence of judgment. In criminal law, civil law, and clinical medicine, standards for competence have clustered around various abilities to comprehend and process information and to reason about the consequences of one's actions. Although the properties most crucial to a determination of competence are controversial, in biomedical contexts a person has generally been viewed as competent if able to understand a therapy or research procedure, to deliberate regarding major risks and benefits, and to make a decision in light of this deliberation.

We agree that if a person lacks any of these capacities, competence to decide, consent, or refuse is doubtful. But there are many troublesome questions about how to classify persons who have diminished capacity to understand, deliberate, or decide. Some patients have a significant capacity to understand, deliberate, and reach conclusions without being competent. For example, some religious fanatics and many psychotic patients have fictitious and delusional beliefs that drive their actions. Nonetheless, they have considerable capacities to understand, deliberate, and decide. Patients with a low IQ as a result of meningitis at an early age can still have a significant capacity to refuse an intervention such as intubation or catheterization. So we need further qualifications and deeper insight than our rough-and-ready categories provide.

The following case illustrates some of the difficulties often encountered in attempting to judge competence. A man who generally exhibits normal behavior patterns is involuntarily committed to a mental institution as the result of bizarre self-destructive behavior (pulling out an eye and cutting off a hand), which is influenced by his unorthodox religious beliefs. He is judged incompetent, despite his generally competent behavior and despite the fact that his peculiar actions follow "reasonably" from his religious beliefs.[26] This troublesome case cannot be interpreted in terms of intermittent competence, but it might be argued that analysis in terms of limited competence is justified. However, such an analysis suggests that persons with unorthodox or bizarre religious beliefs are less than competent, even if they reason clearly in light of their beliefs. This criterion is morally perilous for policy purposes and difficult to accept as a guideline without specific and careful qualification.

Rival standards of incompetence. The following schema expresses the range of *in*abilities currently required by various competing standards of *in*competence.[27] These standards range progressively from the one requiring the least ability to the other end of the spectrum.

1. Inability to express or communicate a preference or choice
2. Inability to understand one's situation and its consequences
3. Inability to understand relevant information
4. Inability to give a reason
5. Inability to give a rational reason (although some supporting reasons may be given)
6. Inability to give risk/benefit-related reasons (although some rational supporting reasons may be given)
7. Inability to reach a reasonable decision (as judged, for example, by a reasonable person standard)

These standards cluster around three kinds of abilities or skills (each of which requires that a level of the ability be established at which the person satisfies the standard). Standard 1 looks for the simple ability to state a preference and is a weak standard. Standards 2 and 3 probe for abilities to understand information and to appreciate one's situation. Standards 4–7 look for the ability to reason through a consequential life decision, although only standard 7 restricts the range of acceptable outcomes of a reasoning process. These standards have been and still are used, either alone or in combination, in order to determine incompetence.

Operational tests for incompetence. A clinical need also exists to select, under one or more of these standards, an operational test of incompetence that establishes passing and failing grades. Dementia rating scales, mental status exams, and similar devices test for factors such as time-and-place orientation, perseveration, memory, understanding, and coherence. These tests are empirical, clinical assessments that are generally administered when incompetence is suspected. Although empirical, a normative judgment underlies the empirical test. Each of the following ingredients involves normative judgments.[28]

1. Establishing the relevant abilities for (in)competence
2. Fixing a threshold level of the abilities in item 1
3. Accepting an empirical test for item 2

For any test accepted under item 3, it is an empirical question whether someone possesses the requisite level of abilities, but this question can only be asked and answered if other criteria have already been fixed under items 1 and 2. These criteria are sometimes fixed by institutional rules or by tradition, but in other cases they are open to further modification. Generally, even established criteria could have been different and can shift over time.

The Sliding-Scale Strategy

Properties of autonomy and psychological capacity are not the only criteria used in fashioning competence *standards.* Many policies use pragmatic criteria of efficiency, feasibility, and social acceptability to determine whether a person is competent or has given a valid authorization. For example, age has conventionally been used as an operational criterion of valid authorization, with established thresholds of age varying in accordance with a community's standards, with the degree of risk involved, and with the importance of the prospective benefits. Criteria of this type are used to protect immature or mistake-prone persons against possible decisions that fail to promote their best interest. Many such persons are competent to perform the necessary tasks and yet are judged incompetent because they fail a pragmatic standard, such as age.

In medicine, the motive for determining incompetence is to protect patients against decisions they might make that are not in their interests. Many therefore believe that standards of competence should be closely connected to levels of experience, maturity, responsibility, and welfare. Some writers offer a sliding-scale strategy for how this goal might be accomplished. They argue that as an intervention in medicine increases the risks for patients, the level of ability required for a judgment of competence to elect or refuse the intervention should be increased. As the consequences for well-being become less substantial, the level of capacity required for competence should be decreased. The sliding-scale approach allows standards of competence in decisionmaking to shift with the risk attached to the decision. If a serious risk such as death is present, then a stringent standard of competence is needed; if a low or insignificant risk is present, then a relaxed standard of competence may be used. Thus, the same person might be competent to decide whether to take a tranquillizer but incompetent to decide whether to authorize an appendectomy.[29]

The sliding-scale strategy is attractive. A decision about which standard to use to determine competence for decisionmaking depends on several factors, and these factors are often risk-related. In health care institutions, the selection of abilities, thresholds, and standards will depend on moral and policy questions involving decisionmaking requirements. All methods for setting standards of incompetence encounter difficulties about whether to emphasize the patient's autonomy or to emphasize protecting the patient against harm, a moral rather than a medical choice. If one is especially concerned about preventing abuses of autonomy, one might accept standard 1 in the previous section as the only valid standard of incompetence, or perhaps one will accept only standards 1, 2, and 3. But if one's primary concern is that sick patients receive the best medical treatment possible, one might require patients to pass all the above standards, or at least standards 6 and 7. Those who accept a stringent standard of incompetence (such as 6 and 7) will place the welfare or medical interests and safety of patients above their autonomy interests.

The strength of the sliding-scale strategy is that our interests in ensuring good outcomes legitimately contribute to the way we inquire about and create standards for judging persons competent or incompetent. If the consequences for welfare are grave, our need to be able to certify that the patient possesses the requisite capacities increases, whereas if little in the way of welfare is at stake, the level of capacity required for decisionmaking might be reduced. For example, if enteral nutrition is needed to help a patient with a reversible dementia to recover, a powerful reason exists for protecting the patient against rash or imprudent decisionmaking by adopting a rigid standard of competence. But if the dementia is irreversible and the physician's primary purpose of enteral nutrition is simply to make the patient comfortable, the standard of competence might be relaxed.

The sliding-scale strategy is generally a sound protective device, but we risk confusion about the nature of both competence judgments and competence itself unless some conceptual and moral difficulties can be resolved. This position suggests that a person's *competence* to decide is contingent upon the decision's importance or upon some harm that might follow from the decision. But this position seems questionable. A person's competence to decide whether to participate in cancer research does not depend upon the decision's consequences. As risks increase or decrease, we can legitimately escalate or reduce the rules or measures we use to *ascertain* whether someone is competent; but in formulating what we are doing, we need to distinguish between our modes of ascertainment and the person's competence.

Two senses of *standard of competence* need to be distinguished. In one sense, *criteria* of competence are at stake—that is, the conditions under which a person is or is not competent. In a second sense, *standard of competence* refers to the *pragmatic guidelines* we use to determine competence. For example, a mature teenager could be competent to decide about a kidney transplant (satisfying criteria of competence) but could also be legally incompetent by virtue of age (failing pragmatic guidelines). In a more complicated case, a person with locked-in syndrome (involving total inabillity to communicate) is able to decide about medical care, satisfying criteria of competence, and yet fails to communicate adequately, thereby indicating through a test that the person is incompetent (failing pragmatic guidelines). To alleviate this problem of a dual meaning of *standard of competence* we will use the term *standard* only to mean a criterion for *determining* competence. Thus, a person could be correctly labeled incompetent in light of the best tests but nonetheless be competent.

Leading adherents of the sliding-scale strategy hold just the reverse— namely, that *competence* varies with risk. According to the most meticulous and convincing proponents of this strategy, Allen Buchanan and Dan Brock,

[J]ust because a patient is competent to consent to a treatment, it does *not* follow that the patient is competent to refuse it and vice versa. For example, consent to a low-risk life-saving procedure by an otherwise healthy individual should require only a minimal level of competence, but refusal of that same procedure by such an individual should require the highest level of competence.

Because the appropriate level of competence properly required for a particular decision must be adjusted to the consequences of acting on that decision, no single standard of decision-making competence is adequate. Instead, the level of competence appropriately required for decision making varies along a full range from low/minimum to high/ maximal. . . . The greater the risk relative to other alternatives . . . the greater the level of communication, understanding, and reasoning skills required for competence to make that decision. . . . [30]

The core thesis in this account seems both conceptually and morally perilous. A shift in risky consequences (from risk of a small scar, say, to risk of death) indicates that we should be cautious in permitting someone to assume the greater risk, and it is true that the level of competence to decide increases as the complexity or difficulty of a task increases (deciding about spinal fusion, say, as contrasted with deciding whether to take a minor tranquilizer). But the level of competence to decide does not increase as the risk of an outcome increases. It is confusing to blend the complexity or difficulty of a task with the risk of a decision. No basis exists for believing that risky decisions require more ability at decisionmaking than less risky decisions. To the contrary, a solid basis exists for believing that many non-risky decisions require more ability at decisionmaking than many risky decisions.

Furthermore, for any person whose competence is in question, it seems disrespectful of autonomy to say, in effect, "You are competent to decide what to do with your children, what to do with your financial affairs, and whether to be in this hospital, but you are not competent to refuse to be intubated or catheterized because of the increased risk." The sliding-scale strategy seems, then, to be incoherent. Inadequate distinctions lead to a conflation of riskiness and complexity as well as conflation of criteria for justified paternalism and standards of competence.[31] These problems can be avoided by holding that the level of evidence for determining competence should vary in accordance with risk, although competence itself varies only along a scale of difficulty in decisionmaking. Brock and Buchanan insist that the "required level of decisionmaking competence" should be placed on a sliding scale from low to high in accordance with risk, but we recommend that only the required standards of evidence for determining decisionmaking competence should be placed on a sliding scale (in accordance with risk).

It follows that judgments about whether to override patients' decisions should be distinguished from questions of whether the patients are competent. Paternalism has a valid place in medicine (see Chapter 5, pp. 278–287), but its place is not in fixing criteria of competence. The incompetent are usually those we treat paternalistically, but we may also have valid paternalistic grounds for overriding the decisions of competent persons. In any event, the issue of justified paternalism should be distinguished from criteria of competence, so as to avoid situations in which we decide that a patient's decision is too risky and that he or she is therefore incompetent.

In practice, challenges to a patient's competence rarely emerge unless a disagreement exists about values. As long as the patient concurs with the physician's recommendations, his or her competence to understand, to decide, and to consent to treatment is rarely examined. But conflict between the patient's wishes and the physician's judgment about that patient's best interests typically provokes an inquiry into the patient's competence.[32] This practice is not surprising. A general presumption exists that adults are competent to make their decisions, and when those decisions are unproblematic (in part because they concur with professional judgment), no motive exists to challenge competence.

In this section we have argued that competence is determined primarily by whether a person has the capacity to decide autonomously, and not by whether a person's best interests are protected. A different set of reasons will lead us (later in this chapter and the next two chapters) to take account of risks, benefits, and best interests. First, however, we need to examine the relationship between autonomy and informed consent.

The Meaning and Justification of Informed Consent

Since the Nuremberg trials, which presented horrifying accounts of medical experimentation in concentration camps, the issue of consent has been at the forefront of biomedical ethics. The term *informed consent* did not appear until a decade after these trials, and it did not receive detailed examination until around 1972. In recent years the focus has shifted from the physician's or researcher's obligation to *disclose* information to the quality of a patient's or subject's *understanding* and *consent*. The forces behind this shift of emphasis were autonomy-driven and were primarily external to codes of medical and research ethics. Throughout this section, we note how standards of informed consent have evolved through the regulation of research, case law governing medical practice, changes in the patient–physician relationship, and ethical analysis.

Functions and Justifications of Informed Consent Requirements

Virtually all prominent medical and research codes and institutional rules of ethics now hold that physicians and investigators must obtain the informed consent of patients and subjects prior to any substantial intervention. Procedures for consent have been designed to enable autonomous choice, but they serve other functions as well, including the protection of patients and subjects from harm and the encouragement of medical professionals to act responsibly in interactions with patients and subjects.

Two positions on the function and justification of informed consent requirements have dominated the literature. Throughout the early history of concern about research subjects, consent requirements were primarily viewed as a way to minimize the potential for harm. Risk reduction and avoidance of unfairness and exploitation still function as reasons for many professional, regulatory, and institutional controls. However, in recent years the primary justification advanced for requirements of informed consent has been protection of autonomous choice, a loosely defined goal that is often buried in vague discussions of protecting the welfare and rights of patients and research subjects. Historically, we can claim little beyond the indisputable fact that a general, inchoate societal demand has developed for the protection of patients' and subjects' rights, particularly their autonomy rights. Throughout this chapter we accept and attempt to give depth to the premise that the primary function and justification of informed consent is to enable and protect individual autonomous choice.

The Definition and Elements of Informed Consent

The concept of informed consent needs clarification before we can establish the conditions under which it is appropriate and mandatory to seek informed consent. Considerable vagueness surrounds the term, creating a need to sharpen the concept so that its meaning is stable and suitable.

Some commentators have attempted to reduce the idea of informed consent to shared decisionmaking between doctor and patient, so that *informed consent* and *mutual decisionmaking* are rendered synonymous.[33] Their thesis is not that *informed consent* has this meaning in ordinary language or law, but rather that it *should* have this meaning. This proposal is plausible when consent involves ongoing exchanges of information between patients and health care providers, rather than a single event of authorizing an intervention.[34] Informed consent is typically given over time and can be withdrawn over time. We agree that it is essential to understand informed consent in terms of a temporal process, and to avoid the common view that the signed consent form is the essence of informed consent.

However, informed consent cannot be reduced to shared decisionmaking. Informed consent is obtained and will continue to be obtained in many contexts of research and emergency medicine in which shared decisionmaking is a misleading model. Furthermore, in various clinical contexts the informational exchanges through which patients elect medical interventions should be distinguished from acts of approving and authorizing those interventions. Shared decisionmaking is a worthy ideal in medicine, but it neither defines nor displaces informed consent. By viewing informed consent as a temporal process, we can avoid the model of mutual decisionmaking and the model of a single event.

Two senses of "informed consent."[35] The question "What is informed consent?" should be addressed in relation to two different conceptions of informed consent that appear in current literature and practices. In the first sense, *informed consent* is analyzable through the account of autonomous choice presented earlier in this chapter: An informed consent is an *autonomous authorization* by individuals of a medical intervention or of involvement in research. In this first sense, a person must do more than express agreement or comply with a proposal. He or she must authorize through an act of informed and voluntary consent. In the classic case of *Mohr v. Williams,* a physician obtained Anna Mohr's consent to an operation on her right ear. While operating, the surgeon determined that the left ear instead needed surgery. A court found that the physician should have obtained the patient's consent to the surgery on the left ear: "If a physician advises a patient to submit to a particular operation, and the patient weighs the dangers and risks incident to its performance, and finally consents, the patient thereby, in effect, enters into a contract authorizing the physician to operate to the extent of the consent given, but no further."[36] An *informed consent* in the first sense occurs if and only if a patient or subject, with substantial understanding and in substantial absence of control by others, intentionally authorizes a professional to do something.

In the second sense, informed consent is analyzable in terms of *the social rules of consent* in institutions that must obtain legally valid consent from patients or subjects before proceeding with therapeutic procedures or research. Informed consents are not necessarily autonomous acts under these rules and sometimes are not even meaningful authorizations. *Informed consent* refers only to an institutionally or legally effective authorization, as determined by prevailing rules. A patient or subject can *autonomously* authorize an intervention, and so give an informed consent in the first sense, without *effectively* authorizing that intervention and thus without giving an informed consent in the second sense. For example, if a minor is not legally authorized to consent, he or she can autonomously authorize an intervention without thereby giving an effective consent under prevailing institutional rules (although some "mature minor" laws give minors the right to authorize medical treatments in a limited range of circumstances).

Institutional rules of informed consent have generally not been judged by the demanding standard of autonomous authorization. As a result, critics of health care institutions' rules argue that the courts impose on physicians and hospitals nothing more than an obligation to warn of risks of proposed interventions, and that consent under these circumstances is not bona fide informed consent.[37] Jay Katz, for example, maintains that a "judicially imposed obligation must be distinguished from the idea of informed consent, namely, that patients have a decisive role to play in the medical decision making process." Katz believes that courts as well as medical institutions have allowed "the idea of informed consent . . . to wither on the vine."[38] His criticisms can best be understood in terms of the gap between the two senses of informed consent: A physician who obtains a consent under institutional criteria can fail to meet the more rigorous standards of an autonomy-based model.

It is easy to criticize institutional rules as superficial, but health care professionals cannot always obtain a consent that satisfies the demands of rigorous autonomy-protecting rules. The rules may turn out to be excessively difficult or impossible to implement. Prevailing rules should be evaluated not only in terms of respect for autonomy but also in terms of the probable consequences of imposing burdensome requirements on institutions. Policies may legitimately take account of what is fair and reasonable to require of health care professionals and researchers, the effect of alternative consent requirements on efficiency and effectiveness in the delivery of health care and the advancement of science, and the effect of consent requirements on the welfare of patients. Nevertheless, we take it as axiomatic that the model of autonomous choice (the first sense) ought to serve as the benchmark for the moral adequacy of institutional rules.

The elements of informed consent. The received approach to the definition of *informed consent* has been to specify the elements of the concept, in particular by dividing the elements into an *information* component and a *consent* component. The information component refers to disclosure of information and comprehension of what is disclosed. The consent component refers to a voluntary decision and agreement to undergo a recommended procedure. Legal, regulatory, philosophical, medical, and psychological literatures tend to favor the following elements as the analytical components of informed consent:[39] (1) Competence, (2) Disclosure, (3) Understanding, (4) Voluntariness, and (5) Consent. These elements are then presented as the building blocks for a definition of *informed consent*. One gives an informed consent to an intervention if (and perhaps only if) one is competent to act, receives a thorough disclosure, comprehends the disclosure, acts voluntarily, and consents to the intervention.

This five-element definition is vastly superior to the one-element definition in terms of *disclosure* that courts and medical literature have often proposed,[40] but the definition is unduly influenced by medical convention and malpractice law. By making disclosure the key item, both approaches alike tend to warp informed consent. Any such definition incorporates dubious assumptions about medical authority, physician responsibility, and legal theories of liability, all of which delineate an *obligation to make disclosures* rather than a *meaning of informed consent*. The meaning of *informed consent,* as we saw above, is better analyzed in terms of autonomous authorization, which has nothing to do with disclosure specifically (even though disclosures must often be made for persons to gain an adequate understanding).

Disclosure of information is often less vital in clinical medicine than a health professional's recommendation of one or more actions. This is typically the case in direct exchanges between physicians and patients regarding surgery, medications, and the like; but it is also true, for example, of notifications to employees or pensioners by corporate medical divisions after routine surveillance or after a study of hazardous chemicals. Recommendations of treatments or of lifestyle changes such as smoking cessation are likely to be far more meaningful than information about the results of empirical studies or surveillance. Although recommendations are informational, they are also normative, and thus not appropriately described as disclosures, which are composed of descriptive statements.

Despite these reservations, we accept the premise that the above "elements" capture several basic notions about informed decision that need analysis. In this chapter each of the following seven elements is treated. (The importance of authorization in our analysis leads us to substitute elements 6 and 7 below for "Consent," which is listed above as element 5.)

I. Threshold Elements (Preconditions)
   1. Competence (to understand and decide)
   2. Voluntariness (in deciding)

II. Information Elements
    3. Disclosure (of material information)
    4. Recommendation (of a plan)
    5. Understanding (of 3. and 4.)
III. Consent Elements
    6. Decision (in favor of a plan)
    7. Authorization (of the chosen plan)

This list requires some qualifications. First, an *informed refusal* entails a modification of items under III by turning the categories into Refusal Elements—for example, 6. "Decision (against a plan)." Second, consent for research involving human subjects does not necessarily involve a recommendation. If a recommendation is made, it may be quite different from recommendations in clinical medicine. Third, competence is more a presupposition or condition of the practice of obtaining informed consent than an element.

Because this chapter is principally about autonomy rather than informed consent and refusal, our treatment of these elements will extend into several regions of autonomous choice. We will concentrate on the elements of general importance for the analysis of both informed consent and autonomy, beginning with disclosure.

Disclosure

We have just seen that the obligation to disclose information to patients has often been presented as a necessary, and sometimes as the sole, condition of valid informed consent. The legal doctrine of informed consent has been primarily a law of disclosure based on a general obligation to exercise reasonable care by giving information. Civil litigation has emerged over informed consent because of injury to one's person or property that is intentionally or negligently inflicted by a physician's failure to disclose, an injury measured in terms of monetary damages. This focus results from the legal system's need for a serviceable mechanism to assess injury and responsibility.

As litigation over legal requirements of consent to medical treatment evolved, a more complicated set of rules also evolved, especially regarding disclosure standards. The term *informed consent* was born in this legal context. However, from the moral viewpoint, informed consent has less to do with the liability of professionals as agents of disclosure and more to do with the autonomous choices of patients and subjects. Both health care professionals and patients need to ask and answer questions, and this process is less a matter of disclosing information than of discovering the relevant information and deciding how to frame and use it.

Nevertheless, disclosure is a pivotal topic. Without an adequate way to deliver information, many patients and subjects will have a substandard basis for decisionmaking. The professional's perspective, opinions, and recommendations are often essential for a sound decision. Professionals are obligated to disclose a core set of information, including (1) those facts or descriptions that patients or subjects usually consider material in deciding whether to refuse or consent to the proposed intervention or research, (2) information the professional believes to be material, (3) the professional's recommendation, (4) the purpose of seeking consent, and (5) the nature and limits of consent as an act of authorization.

Additional types of disclosure have also been proposed—for example, the names of persons in charge. Many controversies center on how much should be disclosed about a procedure's risks, as well as about its nature and its benefits, and any alternatives to the procedure, including new drugs, devices, and treatments.[41] If research is involved, disclosures should generally be made as to the aims, methods, anticipated benefits and risks of the research, any anticipated inconvenience or discomfort, and the subjects' right to withdraw from the research. Additional disclosures and special precautions to ensure that persons understand may also be necessary, including disclosure of the criteria used for the selection of subjects and an indication that the person has an opportunity to ask further questions. Such lists could be expanded almost indefinitely. For example, in one controversial decision, the California Supreme Court held that when seeking an informed consent "a physician must disclose personal interests unrelated to the patient's health, whether research or economic, that may affect the physician's professional judgment."[42] However, the central moral issues turn on the informational needs of particular patients and subjects, not on lists or categories of information.

Standards of Disclosure

The courts have struggled to determine which norms should govern the disclosure of information. Two competing standards of disclosure have emerged: the professional practice standard and the reasonable person standard. A third, the subjective standard, has also been proposed, but it has been implemented in the courts only as a causation standard—that is, as a way of determining whether a physician's failure to disclose caused injury to the patient—not as a disclosure standard. Discussion of these standards has set the terms for much of the current debate over informed consent requirements in medical ethics no less than in law.

The professional practice standard. The first standard holds that adequate disclosure is determined by a professional community's customary practices. This standard assumes that the doctor's proper role is to act in the patient's best medical interest. The custom in a profession establishes the amount and kinds of information to be disclosed. Disclosure, like treatment, is a task that belongs to physicians because of their professional expertise and commitment to the patient's welfare. As a result, only expert testimony from members of this profession could count as evidence that there has been a violation of a patient's right to information.[43]

Several difficulties affect this standard, which is sometimes called a *reasonable doctor standard*.[44] First, it is uncertain in many situations whether a customary standard exists for the communication of information in medicine. Second, if custom alone were conclusive, pervasive negligence could be perpetuated with impunity. The majority of professionals could offer the same inadequate level of information or be allowed total discretion to determine the scope of disclosure. The chief objection to the professional practice standard is that it subverts the right of autonomous choice. Professional standards in medicine are fashioned for medical judgments, but decisions for or against medical care, which are nonmedical, are rightly the province of the patient.

It is also questionable whether physicians have developed skills to determine the information that is in their patients' best interests. The assumption that they have such expertise is largely empirical, and yet no reliable data substantiate it.[45] The weighing of risks in the context of a person's subjective beliefs, fears, and hopes is not an expert skill, and information provided to patients and subjects sometimes needs to be freed from the entrenched values and goals of medical professionals.

The reasonable person standard. Although many legal jurisdictions retain the traditional professional practice standard, the reasonable person standard has gained some acceptance in over half of the states in the United States.[46] According to this standard, information to be disclosed is determined by reference to a hypothetical reasonable person. The pertinence of information is measured by the significance a reasonable person would attach to it in deciding whether to undergo a procedure. The authoritative determination of informational needs thus shifts from the physician to the patient, and physicians may be found guilty of negligent disclosures even if their behavior conforms to recognized professional practice. Proponents of the reasonable person standard believe that obligations to respect autonomy generally outweigh obligations of beneficence and that, on balance, the reasonable person standard better serves the autonomy of patients than does the professional practice standard.

Whatever its merits, this reasonable person standard is also plagued by conceptual, moral, and practical difficulties. First, "material information" and the central concept of the reasonable person have never been carefully defined. Second, questions exist about whether and how the reasonable person standard can be employed in practice. Its abstract and hypothetical character makes it difficult for physicians to use, because they have to project what a reasonable patient would need to know. A related problem has emerged from empirical studies examining whether patients use information disclosed to them in reaching their decisions. Data collected in one study indicate that although ninety-three percent of the patients surveyed believed they benefited from the information disclosed, only twelve percent used the information in their decisions to consent.[47] This study, involving family-planning patients, reaches conclusions similar to an earlier study of kidney donors.[48] In both studies the data indicate that patients generally make their decisions prior to and independent of the process of receiving information. Other studies indicate that patients often deferentially accept physicians' or parents' recommendations without carefully weighing risks and benefits,[49] and that many patients would agree to a procedure without any discussion of risks (eighty-six percent of upper gastrointestinal endoscopy patients in one study)[50] or during their first meeting with a physician (eighty-two percent of candidates for breast cancer adjuvant therapy in one study).[51]

These data do not always indicate that decisions by patients are uninformed or that disclosed information is irrelevant. The patients may have believed that additional information received from physicians did not alter their prior commitment to a course of action such as surgery. Nonetheless, these empirical findings raise questions about what should count as material information for the individual patient and whether this information is the same for the reasonable patient and the individual patient. This problem leads to the third standard of disclosure.

The subjective standard. In the subjective model, adequacy of information is judged by reference to the specific informational needs of the individual person, rather than the hypothetical "reasonable person." Individual needs can differ, because persons may have unconventional beliefs, unusual health problems, or unique family histories that require a different informational base than the reasonable person needs. For example, a person with a family history of reproductive problems might desire information that other persons would not want or need before becoming involved in research on sexual and familial relations or accepting employment in certain industries. If a physician knows or has reason to believe that a person wants such information, then withholding it may undermine autonomy.

At issue is the extent to which a standard should be tailored to the individual patient, that is, made subjective, so that a disclosure would have to include the factors particular to the patient's need for information that a physician could reasonably be expected to know. According to the subjective standard, the physician is obligated to disclose information a particular patient needs to know, so long as a reasonable connection exists between those needs and what the physician should know about the patient's position.[52]

Despite many problems that plague the subjective standard as a *legal* standard, it is a preferable *moral* standard of disclosure, because it alone acknowledges the independent informational needs of persons. Nevertheless, exclusive use of a subjective standard is insufficient for either law or ethics, because patients often do not know what information would be relevant for their deliberations, and a doctor cannot reasonably be expected to do an exhaustive background and character analysis of each patient to determine what information would be relevant. Again, the key question is not what quantum of information should be disclosed, but what professionals can do to facilitate informed decisionmaking.

The solution to the problem of disclosure should be found in active participation through mutual exchange of information. Neither the professional-practice standard nor the reasonable-person standard is a sufficient guide. What professionals customarily disclose and what an objective reasonable person needs often fail to contain some or all of the information material to the person making the decision. Legal and professional rules of disclosure should only serve, then, to initiate the communication process, and professionals and their institutions should not be satisfied with a signed consent form unless attention has also been paid to the process that led to it.

Intentional Nondisclosure

Several problems in biomedical ethics center on deliberate nondisclosure. Some types of research are incompatible with complete disclosure, and in certain clinical interventions physicians often claim that nondisclosures benefit the patient. Are such intentional nondisclosures justifiable?

The therapeutic privilege. Legal exceptions to the rule of informed consent allow the health professional to proceed without consent in cases of emergency, incompetency, waiver, and the like. A controversial exception is the therapeutic privilege, according to which a physician may legitimately withhold information, based on a sound medical judgment that to divulge the information would be potentially harmful to a depressed, emotionally drained, or unstable patient. Several harmful outcomes have been cited, including endangering life, causing irrational decisions, and producing anxiety or stress.[53] Despite the protected status this doctrine has traditionally enjoyed, in 1986 U. S. Supreme Court Justice Byron White vigorously attacked the idea that concerns about increasing a person's anxiety about a procedure provide grounds for an exception to rules of informed consent: "It is the very nature of informed consent provisions that they may produce some anxiety in the patient and influence her in her choice. This is in fact their reason for existence, and . . . it is an entirely salutary reason."[54] White suggested that the legal status of the doctrine of therapeutic privilege is no longer as secure as it once was.

The precise formulation of this therapeutic privilege varies across legal jurisdictions. Some formulations permit physicians to withhold information if disclosure would cause *any* countertherapeutic deterioration in the patient's condition. Other formulations permit the physician to withhold information if and only if the patient's knowledge of the information would have serious health-related consequences—for example, by jeopardizing the treatment's success or by critically impairing relevant decisionmaking processes. The narrowest formulation is analogous to a circumstance of incompetence: The therapeutic privilege can be validly invoked only if the physician has reason to believe that disclosure would render the patient incompetent to consent to or refuse the treatment. To invoke the therapeutic privilege under this condition does not in principle conflict with respect for autonomy, because the patient would not be capable of an autonomous decision at the point it would be needed.

It is doubtful, however, that a general criterion of physician discretion in disclosing information can be made coherent with the extensive disclosure of facts now demanded by many courts. Courts rarely mention valid exceptions to the legal rights they proclaim, and they also leave unclear whether remote risks—often the most anxiety-inducing—must be discussed. The moral issues are as tangled as the legal issues, as we can see in a case in which a woman had a fatal reaction during urography. The radiologist had intentionally not disclosed the chance of death (roughly one in ten thousand) because it might have upset the patient. The radiologist justified his nondisclosure on grounds that the disclosure would be "dangerous" and "not in the best interest of the patient."[55] Such nondisclosure may be warranted with exceptionally fragile patients, but the cases will be rare. Empirical evidence indicates more often than not that physician-hypothesized negative effects such as anxiety and reduced compliance do not materialize.[56] A more acceptable approach is found in the following recommendation by a group of anesthesiologists: "Tell all patients that there are serious, although remote, risks of anesthesia, but . . . allow the individual patient to decide how much additional information he or she wishes to obtain about these risks."[57]

Therapeutic use of placebos. The therapeutic use of placebos also involves intentional deception or incomplete disclosure. A placebo is a substance or intervention that the health care professional believes to be pharmacologically or biomedically inert for the condition being treated. Studies indicate that placebos relieve some symptoms in approximately thirty-five percent of patients who suffer from conditions such as angina pectoris, cough, anxiety, depression, hypertension, headache, and the common cold.[58]

One incautious, beneficence-based defense of placebos is that "deception is completely moral when it is used for the welfare of the patient."[59] This defense endangers autonomy and may founder on its assumptions. Some evidence suggests that the placebo effect—an improvement in the patient after use of a placebo—can sometimes be produced without nondisclosure, incomplete disclosure, or deception. For example, the placebo effect sometimes occurs even if patients have been informed that a substance is pharmacologically inert and have consented to its use.[60] In many cases placebos appear to work because of the "healing context," involving the professional's care, compassion, and skill in fostering hope and trust.[61] Thus, the placebo effect is sometimes produced without administering placebos.

Nevertheless, a placebo is less likely to be effective if used with the patient's knowledge. In one case, professionals thought that an undisclosed placebo offered the only hope of effective pain treatment. Mr. X had undergone several abdominal operations for gallstones, postoperative adhesions, and bowel obstructions, and subsequently experienced chronic pain. He became somewhat depressed, lost weight, had poor personal hygiene, was unkempt, and withdrew socially. After using the addictive drug Talwin six times a day for more than two years to control pain, he had trouble finding injection sites for the Talwin. He sought help "to get more out of life in spite of pain" and voluntarily entered a psychiatric ward that used relaxation techniques and other behavioral procedures.

In the ward he successfully reduced his Talwin usage to four times daily, but insisted that this level was necessary to control his pain. His therapists decided to withdraw the Talwin over time without his knowledge by diluting it with increasing proportions of normal saline. He experienced withdrawal symptoms of nausea, diarrhea, and cramps, which he thought were the result of the Elavil, which the therapists had introduced to relieve the withdrawal symptoms, again without informing him of the purpose. The physicians gradually increased the intervals between injections of the saline. X was aware of these changes, but did not know that the injections contained only saline. After three weeks, his therapist informed him of the placebo substitution. After his initial incredulity and anger subsided, the patient asked that the saline be discontinued and self-control techniques continued. When discharged three weeks later, he could control his abdominal pain more effectively with the self-control techniques than he had been able to with Talwin. Six months later he was still using self-control techniques and had resumed social activities.

The therapists defended their deception on the grounds that they "felt ethically obliged to use a treatment that had a high probability of success." Yet, the therapists continue, "We saw no option without ethical problems. Although it is precarious to justify the means by the end, we felt most obliged to use a procedure designed to help the patient achieve a personally and medically desirable goal." They argued, in effect, that the principle of beneficence overrode respect for autonomy in this case. They also hinted that their actions did not infringe X's autonomy because his autonomy was already compromised by his addiction. They further suggested that they did not violate X's rights, and even acted in accord with his autonomous choices by taking account of his own therapeutic goals.[62]

One defense of this claim appeals to X's alleged implicit consent when he admitted himself to a ward where adjustment in medication was a clear expectation. He accepted the therapy, "to get more out of life." However, what X implicitly consented to when he entered the psychiatric ward is unclear, because we do not know what he understood, and no appeal to implicit consent can be accepted for all maneuvers, because he expressly refused to allow further reduction in his Talwin dosage. A related justification for the undisclosed placebo is that X ratified the therapists' decision to use the placebo when he decided to continue the self-control techniques, rather than returning to Talwin. However, predicted future "consent" is only an expected future approval, not a *consent,* and at best rests on evidence about the patient's beliefs or goals. But even with such evidence, a predicted future ratification does not transform the current intervention into respect for the patient's autonomy.

The therapists note that they saw "no option without ethical problems," but they had not exhausted all moral options. One possibility was to obtain the patient's general consent to the administration of several drugs and placebos, as part of the effort to wean him from Talwin and to enable him to develop adequate self-control techniques to manage his pain. Such consent, obtained at the outset, would have obviated the need for specific consent to the placebo substitution. The staff's commitment to behavioral therapy may have blinded them to some aspects of the problem, leading them to focus on correctable behaviors, with less attention to the person behind the behaviors.[63] If the therapists had conceived X's problem in terms of the importance of autonomous choice, they might have discovered alternative procedures with fewer or no ethical problems. We conclude that the staff's justification is deficient in its appeals to implicit consent and future consent. However, we leave open the possibility that a paternalistic use of placebos of the sort found in this case may be justifiable on other grounds (see Chapter 5).

Withholding Information from Research Subjects. Problems of intentional nondisclosure in clinical practice have parallels in research, where investigators sometimes need to avoid sharing available information with subjects. Occasionally good arguments can be provided for such nondisclosure. Vital research in fields such as epidemiology could not be conducted if consent from subjects were required to obtain access to medical records, and their use without consent is sometimes ethically justified, for example, to establish the prevalence of a particular disease. Some research of this description is only the first phase of an investigation intended to determine whether a need exists to trace and contact particular individuals who are at risk of disease and obtain their permission for further participation in a study. There should be careful protection of confidential information used, but informed consent requirements are sometimes overly burdensome. Occasionally research subjects need not be contacted at all, for example, when hospital records are studied by epidemiologists without knowing the names of the patients. And in other circumstances persons need only to be *notified* in advance of how data being gathered will be used and given the opportunity to refuse participation in the research. That is, disclosures, warnings, and opportunities to decline involvement are sometimes legitimately substituted for obtaining an informed consent.

However, data collection and its analysis grow in unanticipated ways over time, and results occasionally appear late in the course of research that could not be anticipated at the beginning. A conscientious investigator will periodically consider whether informed consent is needed, and submit these judgments to a review committee. Such review may discover a need for informed consent where none previously existed or find a need to communicate study results to those whose records have been examined.

Many forms of intentional nondisclosure in research are difficult to justify. For instance, debate has emerged about a recent study, designed and conducted by two physicians at the Emory University School of Medicine to determine the prevalence of cocaine use and the reliability of self-reports by patients. Controversy centered on the questions that would be most likely to elicit accurate answers from a group of men in an Atlanta walk-in, inner-city hospital clinic that serves low-income, predominantly black residents. In this study, which was approved by the institutional human investigations committee, weekday outpatients at Grady Memorial Hospital were "asked to participate in a study about asymptomatic carriage of STDs," for which they would receive ten dollars. Study participants had to be between 18 and 39 years old and had to be sexually active within the previous six months. Eighty-two percent of those asked agreed to participate. The average age of the participants was 29.5 years; 91.6% were black, and 89% were uninsured.

The participants provided informed consent for the sexually transmitted disease study, but not for the unmentioned piggy-back study of recent cocaine use and reliability of self-reports of such use. Patients were informed that their urine would be tested for STDs, but they were not informed that it would be analyzed for cocaine metabolites. Of the 415 eligible men who agreed to participate, thirty-nine percent tested positive for a major cocaine metabolite, although seventy-two percent of those with positive urinary assays denied any illicit drug use in the three days prior to sampling. (The metabolite is cleared from the body within three days following single-dose cocaine injection.) In answering questions, subjects with positive urine assays were more likely to admit to "any illegal drug" use (87.5 percent) than admit to the more specific "any form of cocaine" use (60.6 percent) over the prior year. Overall, "42.4 percent of the 415 participants admitted to use of cocaine within one year." Researchers concluded:

Our findings underscore the magnitude of the cocaine abuse problem for young men seeking care in inner-city, walk-in clinics. Health care providers need to be aware of the unreliability of patient self-reports of illicit drug use. In this high-risk population, any admission of illicit drug use within the prior year, despite denial of ongoing abuse, should lead physicians to suspect recent use.[64]

The researchers deceived the subjects about some aims and purposes of the research (to study the prevalence of recent cocaine use and the reliability of patient self-reports) and did not disclose the means that would be used (testing their urine for recent cocaine use). Investigators faced a dilemma. On the one hand, accurate information was needed about illicit drug use for health care and public policy. On the other hand, obtaining adequate informed consent was difficult. If informed about the aims of the study, many potential subjects would either refuse to participate or would offer false information to researchers. These problems are increased in research that uses subjects' body fluids as a way to test the reliability of subjects' self-reports about illegal activities.

Requirements of informed consent should not be so easily set aside. These rules protect subjects from manipulation and abuse during the research process. For example, reports of this cocaine study stand to increase suspicion of medical institutions and professionals and could also function to make patients' self-reports of illegal activities even less reliable.[65] We have conceded that informed consent is sometimes unnecessary, but this study of cocaine use is not a legitimate example. Investigators would have been better advised to resolve their dilemma by developing alternative research designs, including sophisticated methods of using questions that can either reduce or eliminate response errors without abridging informed consent. (Another example of problematic partial nondisclosure appears in some clinical trials involving randomization, placebos, blind experiments, and the like; see Chapter 7, pp. 442–447).

As substantial deception or substantial risk is added in a research project, justifying the research becomes progressively more difficult. In Stanley Milgram's well-known experiments on obedience, recruits come to what appears to be a psychology laboratory to participate in what has been advertised as a study of memory and learning. One is designated a "teacher," the other a "learner." The investigator explains that the study will focus on how punishment affects learning. The learner is then seated, his or her arms are strapped to prevent excessive movement, and an electrode is attached to his or her wrist. The learner is told that he or she is to attempt to learn a list of word pairs. Whenever an error is made, electric shocks of increasing intensity will be administered by the other subject, the teacher. The subject assigned the role of teacher is deliberately deceived by the investigator. The learner is actually part of the research team, and the machine does not deliver shocks to the learner. The point of the experiment, as Milgram describes it, "is to see how far a person will proceed in a concrete and measurable situation in which he is ordered to inflict increasing pain on a protesting subject."[66]

In contrast to what consultants had predicted, Milgram reported that as many as 62.5 percent of the subjects continued to obey the investigator's order to inflict shock up to the maximum of 450 volts, labeled on the machine "Danger—Severe Shock." Through debriefing and friendly reconciliation with the "victim," Milgram tried to minimize any harms that the subjects might experience through stress, anxiety, guilt, and shame about their actions in the experiment. His primary defense of his methods is that the subsequent responses of the participants justify the research: "To my mind, the central moral justification for allowing my experiment is that it was judged acceptable by those who took part in it."[67] Eighty-four percent said they were glad to have been in it, fifteen percent were neutral, and one percent expressed negative opinions. These subsequent responses could be construed as indicating that the harms were minimal (and justified by the benefits) and as providing a form of retroactive approval and consent.

The extensive ethical debate over this research during the last thirty years has centered on the imposition of risks of harm to subjects without their informed consent.[68] Milgram contends that criticisms of his methods are unfair if the research is described as involving "deception." He proposes "morally neutral terms" such as "masking," "staging," and "technical illusions." However, these terms frustrate the debate by obscuring the fact that deception without the subjects' specific consent was essential for the research. The experiment may have eventuated in subsequent approval by subjects in their efforts to come to grips with their actions, but retroactive approval is not a substitute for informed consent or refusal. A more promising approach, as Milgram recognizes, is obtaining subjects' prior general consent to participate in research involving deception or nondisclosure.[69]

We believe that research cannot be justified if (1) significant risk is involved, and (2) subjects are not informed that they are being placed at risk. Again, the central question is whether subjects can voluntarily accept the risk with an adequate understanding of the deceptive practices. It is, in our judgment, an indefensible violation to deceive subjects while placing them at substantial risk, regardless of the research's importance. This conclusion does not imply that research involving deception can *never* justifiably be undertaken. Relatively risk-free research that requires deception or incomplete disclosure is often warranted in fields such as behavioral and physiological psychology, as well as the biomedical sciences. Simple examples include studies of visual and other perceptual responses, as well as some behavioral observation studies. Generally, however, deception should be permitted in research only if it is essential to obtain vital information, no substantial risk is involved, subjects are informed that deception is part of the study, and subjects consent to participate under these conditions. We return in Chapter 7 to some needed qualifications to this conclusion, especially in the context of randomized clinical trials.

Understanding

Traditional problems of disclosure need to be reconceived in terms of what professionals can do to facilitate good decisions based on substantial understanding. Asking questions, eliciting the concerns and interests of the patient or subject, and establishing a climate that encourages questions often do more to foster understanding than disclosed information does. However, clinical experience and empirical data indicate that patients and subjects exhibit wide variation in their understanding of information about diagnoses, procedures, risks, and prognoses. Some patients and subjects are calm, attentive, and eager for dialogue, whereas others are nervous or distracted in ways that impair or block understanding. Many conditions limit their understanding, including illness, irrationality, and immaturity.

The Nature of Understanding

No consensus exists about the nature of understanding, but an analysis sufficient for our purposes is that one understands if one has acquired pertinent information and justified, relevant beliefs about the nature and consequences of one's action. Such understanding need not be complete, because a substantial grasp of central facts and other descriptions is generally sufficient. Some facts are irrelevant or trivial; others are vital, perhaps decisive. In some cases, a person's lack of awareness of even a single risk, limitation, or missing fact can deprive him or her of adequate understanding. Consider, for example, the case of *Bang v. Miller Hospital,* in which patient Bang did not intend to consent to a sterilization entailed in prostate surgery.[70] Bang did, in fact, give a formal consent to prostate surgery, but without being told that sterilization was an inevitable outcome. (Sterilization is not necessarily an outcome of all prostate surgery, but it is inevitable in the specific procedure selected in this case.) Bang's failure to understand this one surgical consequence substantially compromised what was otherwise an adequate understanding and invalidated what otherwise would have been a valid consent.

Patients and subjects usually should understand at least what a health care professional believes a patient or subject needs to understand and should regard as material in order to authorize an intervention. Typically, diagnoses, prognoses, the nature and purpose of the intervention, alternatives, risks and benefits, and recommendations are essential. But patients or subjects also need to share an understanding with professionals about the terms of the authorization before proceeding. As in all contractual circumstances, unless agreement exists about the essential features of what is authorized, there can be no assurance that a patient or subject has made an autonomous decision. Even if both physician and patient use a word such as *stroke* or *hernia,* their interpretations will be vastly different if standard medical definitions and conceptions have no meaning or significance for the patient.

It is sometimes argued that many patients and subjects cannot comprehend enough information or appreciate its relevance sufficiently to make decisions about medical care or participation in research. Franz Ingelfinger maintains, for example, that "the chances are remote that the subject really understands what he has consented to."[71] Such statements are overgeneralizations based partially on unwarranted standards of full disclosure and full understanding. The ideal of complete disclosure of all possibly relevant knowledge promotes these claims about the limited capacity of subjects to comprehend. If this ideal standard is replaced by a more acceptable account of understanding relevant information, such skepticism can be put to rest. From the fact that actions are never *fully* informed, voluntary, or autonomous, it does not follow that they are never *adequately* informed, voluntary, or autonomous.

Some patients, however, have such limited knowledge bases that communication about alien or novel situations is exceedingly difficult, especially if new concepts and cognitive constructs are required. Studies indicate that their understanding of scientific goals and procedures is likely to be both impoverished and distorted.[72] But even under such difficult situations, enhanced understanding and adequate decisions are often possible. Successful communication of novel and specialized information to laypersons can often be accomplished by drawing analogies between this information and more ordinary events familiar to the patient or subject. Similarly, professionals can express risks in both numeric and nonnumeric probabilities, while helping the patient or subject to assign meanings to the probabilities through comparison with more familiar risks and prior experiences, such as risks involved in driving automobiles or using power tools.

However, to enable a patient not only to comprehend but also to appreciate risks and benefits can be a formidable task. For example, many patients confronted with coronary artery bypass, orthopedic operations, and many other forms of surgery understand that as a consequence of their consent to the surgery they will suffer postoperative pain. Nevertheless, their projected expectations of the pain are often altogether inadequate. Patients often cannot, in advance, adequately appreciate the nature of the pain, and many ill patients reach a point at which they can no longer balance with clear judgment the threat of pain against the risks of surgery. At this point the benefits of surgery are overwhelmingly attractive, and the risks are devalued. In one respect these patients correctly understand basic facts about procedures that involve pain, but in other respects their understanding is less than adequate.

Many situations in medicine require physicians to confront this problem. For example, in Case 4 (see appendix), a fourteen-year-old girl consents to donate a kidney to her mother. Although she has exhibited a perceptive and relatively unemotional grasp of the situation, many doubt that a fourteen-year-old child can in these circumstances either adequately appreciate the significance of future risks or carefully balance risks and benefits.

Problems of Information Processing

With the exception of a few limited studies of comprehension, studies of decisionmaking by patients typically pay little attention to information processing, which raises substantial issues about understanding. For example, information overload is sometimes an obstacle to adequate understanding and is as likely as underdisclosure to produce uninformed decisions. Information overload is exacerbated if unfamiliar terms are used or if information cannot be meaningfully organized, yet practical constraints generally require that disclosures occur in a compact presentation. Patients and potential subjects are likely to rely on some modes of selective perception, and it is often difficult to determine when words have special meaning for them, when preconceptions distort their processing of the information, and when other biases intrude.

Some valuable studies have uncovered difficulties in processing information about risks, indicating that risk disclosures often lead subjects to distort information and promote inferential errors and disproportionate fears of risks.[73] Some ways of framing information are so misleading that both health professionals and their patients regularly distort the content. For example, choices between risky alternatives can be heavily influenced by whether the same risk information is presented as providing a gain or an opportunity for a patient, or as constituting a loss or a reduction of opportunity.[74] One study asked radiologists, outpatients with chronic medical problems, and graduate business students to make a hypothetical choice between two alternative therapies for lung cancer: surgery and radiation therapy.[75] The preferences of all three groups were affected by whether the information about outcomes was framed in terms of survival or death. When faced with outcomes framed in terms of probability of *survival*, twenty-five percent chose radiation over surgery. However, when the identical outcomes were presented in terms of probability of *death*, forty-two percent preferred radiation. The mode of presenting the risk of immediate death from surgical complications, which has no counterpart in radiation therapy, appears to have made the decisive difference.

These framing effects reduce understanding of material information, with direct implications for autonomous choice. If a misperception prevents a person from adequately understanding the risk of death and this risk is material to the person's decision, then the person's choice of surgery is based on less than a substantial understanding and would not qualify as an autonomous authorization. The lesson to be learned is not skepticism about information processing, but rather the need for better understanding of techniques that will enable professionals to communicate the positive and the negative sides of information— for example, both the mortality and the survival information.[76]

Problems of Nonacceptance and False Belief

A person's ability to make decisions can be compromised by a breakdown in the ability to *accept* information as true or untainted, even if the person adequately *comprehends* the information. The distinction between comprehension of information and acceptance of information has often been obscured in the relevant literature by excessive reliance on recall tests. At best, "correct" answers on these tests provide evidence of a person's memory of what the physician or investigator has disclosed, not whether the subject interpreted correctly or believed what was disclosed.

However, a false belief can invalidate a decision by a patient or subject in the presence of suitable disclosure and comprehension. Here are three examples: (1) A person might falsely and irrationally believe that a doctor will not fill out insurance forms unless the patient consents to a procedure the doctor has suggested. (2) A sufficiently informed psychiatric patient capable of consent might agree to participate in nontherapeutic research under the false belief that it is therapeutic. (3) A seriously ill patient asked to make a treatment decision might refuse under the false belief that he or she is not ill. Even if the physician recognizes the person's false belief and adduces conclusive evidence to prove to the person that the belief is mistaken, and the person comprehends the information provided, the person may go on believing that what has been (truthfully) reported is false.

Inconclusive evidence and failure to achieve agreement about the truth or falsity of beliefs, sometimes after considerable discussion, further complicate these problems. Many beliefs that are central for a patient's decision are regarded by others, including health care professionals seeking consent, as highly questionable, poorly reasoned, or perhaps absurd. Sometimes overwhelming medical evidence indicates that a patient's belief is unjustified, but in other circumstances the patient's beliefs will be contestable without being refutable by hard counterevidence.

The probabilities and uncertainties that surround many beliefs suggest that truth claims should be judged by the available evidence, which is often subject to different interpretations. More than one standard of evidence may exist, and all evidence must be collected within some framework that determines what qualifies as evidence. No evidence is independent of the framework that it presupposes, yet two or more frameworks sometimes advance competing standards of evidence. If disagreement persists on the criteria for determining the justifiability of beliefs, there will be no adequate basis for determining whether a given belief compromises understanding or simply involves an essentially contestable proposition. This conclusion is not meant as a skeptical denial of the possibility of knowledge, but only as a warning that the evidence for thinking that a belief is false may be rationally contestable.

When beliefs are demonstrably false, the question arises whether patients and subjects should be forced to abandon their false beliefs to enable them to reach an informed decision. Some have argued that if autonomous subjects decline further information, it should not be imposed.[77] This proposal is attractive, but it also seems wrong to say that we should never pressure protesting patients or subjects to change their beliefs or to process information differently. If choice is limited by ignorance, as in the case of a demonstrably false belief, it may be permissible or possibly obligatory to promote autonomy by attempting to impose unwelcome information.

Consider the following case in which a false belief played a major role in a patient's refusal of treatment:[78]

A 57-year-old woman was admitted to the hospital because of a fractured hip. . . . During the course of the hospitalization, a Papanicolaou test and biopsy revealed stage 1A carcinoma of the cervix. . . . Surgery was strongly recommended, since the cancer was almost certainly curable by a hysterectomy. . . . The patient refused the procedure.

The patient's treating physicians at this point felt that she was mentally incompetent. Psychiatric and neurological consultations were requested to determine the possibility of dementia and/or mental incompetency. The psychiatric consultant felt that the patient was demented and not mentally competent to make decisions regarding her own care. This determination was based in large measure on the patient's steadfast "unreasonable" refusal to undergo surgery. The neurologist disagreed, finding no evidence of dementia. On questioning, the patient stated that she was refusing the hysterectomy because she *did not believe* she had cancer. "Anyone knows," she said, "that people with cancer are sick, feel bad and lose weight," while she felt quite well. The patient continued to hold this view despite the results of the biopsy and her physicians' persistent arguments to the contrary.

The physician seriously considered overriding the patient's refusal, because sound medical evidence demonstrated that she was unjustified in believing she did not have cancer. As long as this patient continues to hold such a false belief and it is material to her decision, her refusal cannot correctly be said to be an informed refusal. Several complexities inherent in achieving effective communication are illustrated by this case: The patient was a poor white woman from Appalachia with a third-grade education. The fact that her treating physician was black turned out to be the major reason for her false belief that she had no cancer. She would not believe what a black physician told her. However, intense discussions with a white physician and with her daughter eventually resulted in a change in her belief and a consent to a successful hysterectomy.

The Problem of Waivers

A further problem about understanding is presented by waivers of informed consent. In the exercise of a waiver, a patient voluntarily relinquishes the right to an informed consent and relieves the physician from the obligation to obtain informed consent. The patient delegates decisionmaking authority to the physician or asks not to be informed. In effect, the patient makes a decision not to make an informed decision.

Some courts have held that "a medical doctor need not make disclosures of risks when the patient requests that he not be so informed,"[79] and some prominent writers in biomedical ethics hold that "rights are always waivable,"[80] including the right to an informed consent. Various studies indicate that perhaps sixty percent of patients want to know virtually nothing about certain procedures or the risks of those procedures, that a high percentage would consent without knowledge of risk, and that only a small percentage use the information provided in reaching their decisions.[81] Some physicians claim that more uninformed patients defer to physicians' recommendations than seek pertinent information, although one study also indicates that physicians tend to underestimate patient preferences for information.[82]

There are two primary ways to manage the problem of waivers. The contemplated medical procedure might be withheld until sufficient understanding is present, notwithstanding the patient's autonomously expressed desire not to be informed. Persons would then not be coerced or manipulated into receiving undesired information. Alternatively, if a patient or subject adequately understands his or her situation and then waives the right to relevant information about proposed medical interventions, the professional might proceed without insisting on any understanding beyond the person's understanding that he or she is waiving a right. In this second approach, the waiver constitutes a valid consent to therapy or research, even if it is not an informed consent.

It is usually appropriate to recognize waivers of rights because we have discretion over rights, and because waivers do seem justified in many contexts of consent. For example, if a committed Jehovah's Witness were to inform a doctor that he wished to have everything possible done for him, but did not want to know if transfusions or similar procedures would be employed, it is difficult to construct a moral argument (although legal reasons might exist) to support the conclusion that he must give a specific informed consent to the transfusions. Nevertheless, a general practice of allowing waivers is dangerous. Many patients have an inordinate trust in physicians, and the general acceptance of waivers of consent in research and therapeutic settings could make patients more vulnerable to those who would abbreviate or omit consent procedures for convenience, already a serious problem in health care. Accordingly, the danger of abuse of the waiver in busy medical settings, together with problems of how to determine the conditions under which a patient can make a voluntary and informed decision to waive the right to relevant information, demand caution in implementing waiver policies.

No general solution to these problems about waivers is likely to emerge. Each case or situation of waiver needs to be considered separately. There may, however, be appropriate procedural responses. For example, rules could be developed that disallow waivers except when they have been approved by deliberative bodies, such as institutional review committees and hospital ethics committees. If a committee determined that the person's interest was best protected in a particular case by recognizing a proposed waiver, it could be sustained. This procedural solution is not simply an evasion of the problem. It would be easy to violate autonomy and to fail to discharge our responsibilities by inflexible rules that either permit or prohibit waivers in institutional settings. Close monitoring by review could provide the necessary level of protection for patients, as well as a flexible arrangement for deliberation and decision.

Voluntariness

Autonomous persons typically consider the freedom to act as no less important than adequate understanding. Under the category *voluntariness,* we will concentrate on a person's independence from others' manipulative and coercive influences. As the law has long recognized, a consent or refusal coerced by threats or manipulated by misrepresentation is invalid.

Our use of the term *voluntariness* is intentionally narrow to distinguish it from broader uses that make it synonymous with autonomy. Some have analyzed voluntariness in terms of the presence of adequate knowledge, the absence of psychological compulsion, and the absence of external constraints.[83] If we adopted this broad meaning, the voluntariness condition would be the necessary and sufficient condition of autonomous action. However, we hold only that a person acts voluntarily to the degree he or she wills the action without being under the control of another influence. We consider here only control by other individuals. However, voluntariness can also be diminished or voided by conditions such as debilitating disease, psychiatric disorders, and drug addiction.

Control over another person is necessarily an influence, but not all influences are controlling. If a physician orders a reluctant patient to undergo cardiac catheterization and coerces the patient into compliance through a threat of abandonment, then the patient is influenced by the physician's control. If, by contrast, a physician persuades the patient to undergo the procedure when the patient is at first reluctant to do so, then the patient is influenced by, but not controlled by the physician's actions. Many influences are resistible, and some are welcomed rather than resisted. The broad category of influence includes acts of love, threats, education, lies, manipulative suggestions, and emotional appeals, all of which can vary dramatically in their impact on persons.

Forms of Influence

Three primary categories of influence are present in our analysis: coercion, persuasion, and manipulation. Coercion, as we define it, occurs if and only if one person intentionally uses a credible and severe threat of harm or force to control another.[84] The threat of force or punishment used by some police, courts, and hospitals in acts of involuntary commitment for psychiatric treatment is a typical form of coercion. Society's use of compulsory vaccination laws is another. For a threat to be credible, both parties must believe that the person making the threat can effect it, or the one making the threat must successfully deceive the person threatened into so believing. A physician in a prison who tells an inmate he *must* submit to sedation will need an accompanying prison guard for the threat to be credible; only then will coercion occur.

Some threats will coerce virtually all persons (for example, a credible threat to kill the coerced person), whereas others will coerce only a few persons (for example, a threat presented by an employee to an employer of quitting a job unless a raise is offered). Whether coercion occurs depends on the subjective responses of the intended target of the coercion. However, a subjective response in which persons comply because they *feel* threatened does not qualify as coercion, because coercion requires that a real, credible, and intended threat be brought on a person so that his or her self-directedness is displaced. Coercion, so understood, voids an act of autonomy (that is, coercion renders even intentional and well-informed behavior nonautonomous), and so should be placed at one end of a continuum of types of influence.

In *persuasion,* as we use the term, a person must be convinced to believe in something through the merit of reasons advanced by another person. Accordingly, we do not recognize as a form of persuasion what Paul Appelbaum and Loren Roth label "forceful persuasion," which involves persistent forcefulness and sometimes misleading language. They cite a case of an intern who did not accept a patient's refusal of an X-ray. The intern insisted that he "absolutely must have the film and that he could not refuse it." The patient then reluctantly agreed.[85] In our usage, neither nonrational nor forceful "persuasion" qualifies as a form of persuasion, because both are forms of manipulation.

The word *manipulation* is a generic label for several forms of influence that are neither persuasive nor coercive. The essence of manipulation is swaying people to do what the manipulator wants by means other than coercion or persuasion. For purposes of decisionmaking in health care, the key form of manipulation is informational manipulation, a deliberate act of managing information that nonpersuasively alters the person's understanding of a situation and thereby motivates him or her to do what the agent of influence intends. Many forms of informational manipulation are incompatible with autonomous decisionmaking. For example, deception that involves such strategies as lying, withholding information, and misleading exaggeration to cause persons to believe what is false are all inconsistent with autonomous choice. In Milgram's obedience experiments, he deceived subjects about virtually every aspect of the research to which they consented. By our criteria, these consents were manipulated and, therefore, did not qualify as autonomous choices.

Several problems encountered previously in discussing understanding reappear as issues of informational manipulation. An underdiscussed problem in health care is the amount of routine care and testing ordered in health care facilities without an explanation to the patient, thereby denying the patient a choice among alternatives (if any exist) and a right to refuse. Far more often mentioned is clinicians' uses of the therapeutic privilege to withhold information to manipulate patients into consenting to a medically desirable procedure.[86] The manner in which information is presented by tone of voice, by forceful gesture, and by framing information positively ("we succeed most of the time with this therapy") rather than negatively ("we fail with this therapy in thirty-five percent of the cases") can easily manipulate a patient's perception and response, and thereby affect understanding. The major concern about manipulation in medicine has been expressed by Eliot Freidson:

It is my impression that clients are more often bullied than informed into consent, their resistance weakened in part by their desire for the general service if not the specific procedure, in part by the oppressive setting they find themselves in, and in part by the calculated intimidation, restriction of information, and covert threats of rejection by the professional staff itself.[87]

Nevertheless, one can easily inflate the threat of control by manipulation beyond its significance in health care. We typically make decisions in a context of competing influences, such as personal desires, familial constraints, legal obligations, and institutional pressures. Although significant, these influences need not be controlling to a substantial degree. From the perspective of decisionmaking by patients and subjects, we need only establish general criteria for the point at which autonomous choice is imperiled, while recognizing that no sharp boundary can be drawn in many cases between controlling and noncontrolling influences. Also, in each case the powers of an individual patient or subject must be assessed, and the health professional will need to consider the particular patient's subjective resistibility to influence, not the (so-called objective) reasonable person's ability to resist.

The Obligation to Abstain from Controlling Influence

Thus far we have attempted primarily to distinguish influences that are compatible with substantial autonomy from influences that are not compatible. Now we can examine the justifiability of exerting these forms of influence.

Many influences are welcomed by patients and subjects, and even unwelcome influences are sometimes compatible with autonomous decisionmaking. In some cases professionals are morally blameworthy if they do *not* attempt to persuade resistant patients to pursue treatments that are medically essential, and such persuasion need not violate respect for autonomy. Reasoned argument in defense of an option is a form of providing information and is often vital to ensuring understanding. It is never an unjustified form of influence, although in some cases it can be unduly intrusive and therefore unjustifiable.

We are assuming that influence by appeal to reason—persuasion—is in theory and practice distinguishable from influence by appeal to emotion. As applied to health care professionals, the problem is to distinguish emotional responses from cognitive responses and to determine which are likely to be evoked. The goal is to avoid overwhelming the person with frightening information, particularly if the person is in a psychologically vulnerable or compromised state. Disclosures or approaches that might rationally persuade one patient might overwhelm another patient whose fear or panic would short-circuit reason.

Coercion and controlling manipulation are occasionally justified, although these occasions are infrequent in medicine (by contrast to police work, where such techniques are more common and also more commonly justified). If a physician responsible for a disruptive and childishly noncompliant patient threatens to discontinue treatment unless the patient alters certain behaviors, the physician's mandate may be justified even though coercive. The most difficult problems about manipulation concern not punishment and threat, which are almost always unjustified in health care and research, but rather the effect of rewards, offers, and encouragement. An egregious example of an unjustified offer occurred during the aforementioned Tuskegee Syphilis experiments. Various offers were used to stimulate and sustain the interest of subjects in continued participation. Subjects were offered free burial assistance and insurance, free transportation to and from the examinations, and a free stop in town on the return trip. They were rewarded with free medicines and free hot meals on the days of the examination. The socioeconomic deprivation of these subjects made them vulnerable to these overt and unjustifiable forms of manipulation.[88] Problematic techniques in clinical practice are usually far more subtle and difficult to locate and analyze, but they can have the identical effect.

When an offer is made in a setting in which it is abnormally attractive—for example, an offer of large sums of money or freedom for destitute prisoners—it may be manipulative, but it is never coercive. To maintain that irresistibly attractive offers such as free medical care or freedom from involuntary commitment coerce patients or subjects deeply distorts the concept of coercion (unless the "offer" is in truth a disguised threat), because then anyone who intentionally and successfully influenced another by presenting an offer so attractive that the person was unable to resist it—for example, a large salary at a wonderful job—would have coerced the person. An offer of something irresistible is not coercive, although it does under some conditions manipulatively take advantage of a person's vulnerabilities.

The conditions under which an influence is controlling and morally unjustified may be clear in theory, but they are often unclear in concrete situations, and many borderline cases remain. Some difficult cases in health care consist of manipulation-like situations in which patients or subjects are in desperate need. To say that a person desperately needs something, such as a medication or a source of income, means that without it a high probability exists that the person (or some loved one) will be seriously harmed. Attractive offers such as free medication or extra money can leave persons without any meaningful choice besides accepting the offer. Such a person is constrained in a desperate situation, but not controlled by another person's intentional manipulation.

Some seem to believe that an offer of this magnitude to a person in desperate need is inherently exploitative. In some circumstances the offer is likely to appear to the beneficiary as a threat—for example, if an experimental therapy is the sole therapy and can be obtained only if a person becomes a research subject. However, such an offer is sometimes perceived differently. In 1722, Newgate Prison officials offered several inmates their freedom, as an alternative to hanging, if they volunteered to be subjects in an experiment on smallpox inoculation.[89] It might at first seem that they were coerced, because the offer appears to be a disguised threat on the order of "We will hang you unless you become an experimental subject." More plausibly, though, this manipulation-like circumstance involves a welcome offer made to persons in desperate need, who without the offer would be hanged anyway. The prisoners certainly considered the offer to be fortuitous, as these condemned men all survived and were released.

In contrast, influences that ordinarily are resistible can become controlling for abnormally weak, dependent, and surrender-prone patients, and compliance may be induced in these patients by contributing to or playing on their desperation, anxiety, boredom, or other emotions. The hope of more attention and better care can be a significant factor for a bedridden person. What a health professional intends as an attempt at rational persuasion can irrationally influence the patient by attacking his or her vulnerabilities. We are not implying that health professionals do routinely manipulate or exploit patient vulnerabilities, but only that many patients are susceptible to this kind of influence and need protection against it.[90]

It is especially vital to ensure that conditions permitting resistance to control are preserved in total institutions, whose populations are admitted involuntarily. The threat of exploitation is substantial in these institutions, yet neither coercive institutionalization nor coercive institutions entail that each decision made by a person in the institution is coerced. There is no reason why prisoners, for example, cannot validly consent to some research if coercive tactics are not involved in enlisting them as subjects and if there are no manipulative offers, such as unduly large payments for excessive risk taking.[91]

These problems are often more subtle and difficult in institutions to which persons are admitted voluntarily but in which rules, policies, and practices can work nonetheless to compromise autonomous choice. Perhaps nowhere is this compromise more evident than in long-term care. For example, the elderly in nursing homes frequently experience a constriction of their choices, particularly in routine or everyday matters. Many people in nursing homes have already suffered a decline in their ability to carry out personal choices because of physical impairments. This decline in *executional* autonomy need not be accompanied by a decline in *decisional* autonomy, and yet their autonomous choices and decisions are often neglected or overridden by the nursing home.[92]

These everyday matters often range over food (when, what kind, how prepared, and how much), roommates (who selects them and how to resolve conflicts), possessions (which to keep and how to protect them), exercise (when, what kind, and with what supervision), sleep (when and how much), clothes (what to wear and when to wash), as well as baths, medications, and restraints. The liberty of competent residents to live their lives in accord with their preferences and life plans must often be balanced against protecting their health, protecting the interests of others, promoting safety and efficiency in the facility, and allocating limited financial and other resources. Although respect for autonomy suggests individualized care in the nursing home setting, such care can rarely be individualized in the ways we expect outside such institutions.

Consider the following example from a facility named Mansion Manor. Mrs. Hollinger, who is seventy-six years old, has encountered difficulty with the nurses's aides about the facility's requirement that residents rise in time for breakfast, which is served at 7:30. She has never liked breakfast and she moves slowly after a second stroke. She finds the effort to make it to breakfast almost intolerable. She has been late each morning for two weeks, and the aides say that her late arrival disrupts the feeding of other residents and that she fails to finish her breakfast when she is late because she is a slow eater. The floor nurse warns her, in a manner she finds threatening, that if her tardiness for breakfast continues, she will be put with those who cannot feed themselves in a separate dining room. Her worries about being late for breakfast have begun to cause her trouble in sleeping and have increased her tiredness. The staff has had several earlier battles with Mrs. Hollinger, particularly ones centered on her charges that the staff "poked around" in her room and removed some of her belongings that were deemed to be unsafe to others who might wander into her room. The staff's animosity makes it difficult to determine whether Mrs. Hollinger's late arrival at breakfast in fact infringes on the rights of others and disrupts institutional order.

The staff's efforts at persuasion are justifiable, but their coercive threat to put her in the separate dining room is not justified unless her actions genuinely pose problems for others or for the institution. The aides could respond that they are not overriding Mrs. Hollinger's autonomy, only respecting it, because she accepted the rules and regulations that restrict liberty when she voluntarily entered the nursing home. Thus, the argument might go, she has an obligation of compliance, not only because of the need for institutional order but also because of her consent. However, before this claim can be sustained, we would need to know exactly what Mrs. Hollinger (and her son) were told at the outset about the rules and regulations. They might well have grounds to complain about initial disclosures or about the nursing home's narrowly legalistic interpretations of its rules and of governmental regulations.

The director of nursing explained that federal regulations require that the first meal of the day occur no more than 14 hours after a substantial evening meal the previous day, which for some residents is 4:30 p.m. This regulation is indispensable to protect nursing home residents from exploitation and harm. However, it could also be construed as establishing an option right, rather than a mandatory right, for residents. An option right can be waived, whereas a mandatory right such as the right to education cannot.[93] If an option right exists, autonomous residents would have the option to accept or refuse the meals. A strict interpretation of a mandatory right would require force-feeding of resistant autonomous residents, and the implausibility of such an interpretation provides a reason to suspect that the institution is displaying bad faith in its conflict with Mrs. Hollinger. Even if the principle of respect for autonomy can be justifiably overridden to protect others or to establish (legitimate) institutional order, the institution must choose the least restrictive alternative.[94]

Some contend that respect for autonomy, taken literally, demands too much of nursing homes and other long-term care facilities. They propose that this individualistic principle be replaced by a communitarian perspective in which informed consent is superseded by "negotiated consent" and individual rights are incorporated into a larger vision of community, with an emphasis on mutual responsibilities.[95] Although this alternative has attractive features, it is too obscure and risky without explicit protections against violations of autonomy. The presumption in favor of voluntariness and rights of autonomous choice should never be renounced. However, in some cases other persons—surrogate decisionmakers—should be granted some measure of decisional authority for residents, for reasons now to be discussed.

A Framework of Standards for Surrogate Decisionmaking

Surrogate decisionmakers reach decisions for doubtfully autonomous or nonautonomous patients. If a patient is not competent to choose or to refuse treatment, a hospital, a physician, or a family member may justifiably be placed in a decisionmaking role or go before a court or other authority to seek resolution of the issues before a decision is implemented. Courts and legislatures have been actively involved in this area since the Quinlan decision in 1976, and significant advances have been made in both law and ethics. However, much remains undecided, particularly with regard to patients who are incompetent and debilitated, yet conscious. Many judgments about terminating or continuing treatment are made daily for patients in this condition—for example, those suffering from stroke, Alzheimer's disease, Parkinson's disease, chronic depression affecting cognitive function, senility, and psychosis.

Celebrated legal cases have centered on formerly autonomous patients, including Karen Ann Quinlan, Earle Spring, Brother Fox, Claire Conroy, Paul Brophy, and Nancy Cruzan, as well as never-competent patients such as Joseph Saikewicz and John Storar. In such cases, courts have split over the use of two surrogate decisionmaking standards: best interests and substituted judgment. Neither has an entirely clear basis in autonomy, but appeals to autonomy are often used by defenders of these standards. Currently a received opinion operates in many courts about how treatment decisions should be reached for both formerly competent and never-competent patients. In this account, all patients have a right to decide, and their autonomous choices must be consulted whenever possible as the basis of any decision; an incompetent person is still a person with a right to choose. We will resist this framework, substituting a different account of decisionmaking standards and of the order of priority among them.

We will consider three general standards that surrogate decisionmakers might use: *substituted judgment,* which is often presented as an autonomy-based standard, *pure autonomy,* and the *patient's best interests.* Our objective is to structure and integrate this framework of standards for surrogate decisionmaking.

Although we assess these standards for law and policy, our underlying argument is independent of law and policy. The argument is a moral one that extends our earlier discussions of the value of protecting autonomy. Only in Chapter 4 will we consider *who* should be the surrogate decisionmaker.

The Substituted Judgment Standard

The standard of substituted judgment appears initially to be autonomy-based, and several influential judicial opinions have so viewed it. However, it is, at best, a weak autonomy standard. Substituted judgment begins with the premise that decisions about treatment properly belong to the incompetent or nonautonomous patient by virtue of rights of autonomy and privacy. The patient has the right to decide but is incompetent to exercise it. It would be unfair to deprive an incompetent patient of decisionmaking rights merely because he or she is no longer (or has never been) autonomous. Nonetheless, another decisionmaker should be substituted if the patient is currently unable to make autonomous decisions.

This standard requires the surrogate decisionmaker to "don the mental mantle of the incompetent," as the *Saikewicz* court put it—that is, to make the decision the incompetent would have made if competent. In *Saikewicz,* the court had to consider evidence that most reasonable persons with Joseph Saikewicz's illness choose treatment, but the court invoked the standard of substituted judgment to decide that Saikewicz, a never-competent patient, would not have chosen treatment had he been competent. The court defined its task as determining "how the right of an incompetent person to decline treatment might best be exercised so as to give the fullest possible expression to the character and circumstances of that individual." Asserting that what the majority of reasonable people would choose could differ from what a particular incompetent person would choose, the court proposed the following standard:

[T]he decision in many cases such as this should be that which would be made by the incompetent person, if that person were competent, but taking into account the present and future incompetency of the individual as one of the factors which would necessarily enter into the decision-making process of the competent person.[96]

Both the *Quinlan* and the *Saikewicz* courts used the substituted judgment standard, first attempting to determine the individual's subjective wants and needs and then attempting to decide how to proceed in light of the individual's value system. However, these two cases involve different interpretations and uses of the substituted judgment standard. In *Quinlan,* the court sought to protect an autonomy right for a person who could not assert the right because of her permanent vegetative state. The court authorized the patient's father to infer her wants and needs from her life as a competent person, despite the fact that his judgments involved several assumptions. The court did not frame the issue either in terms of parental rights over children or in terms of whether the father could decide in her best interests. Rather, the court attempted to protect her autonomy and privacy rights by asking the father to determine what she would have chosen if she had been able to choose. The court found that "Karen's right of privacy may be asserted on her behalf by her guardian whether she would exercise her right" to terminate care, "even if it meant the prospect of natural death."[97] This decision illustrates the scope courts often give to rights of privacy and autonomy.

In *Saikewicz*, the lack of evidence about the incompetent patient's likely choice forced the court to look to what is known about other people in his situation to help determine what a reasonable person in his circumstances, with his needs and desires (insofar as they are ascertainable), would decide. As understood in *Saikewicz*, and to some extent in *Quinlan*, the premise of the substituted judgment standard has a fictional component. An incompetent person cannot literally be said to have the right to make medical decisions if the right can only be exercised by competent persons. This fictional quality makes substituted judgment controversial. John Robertson has argued that it is desirable to treat incompetent persons as autonomous, despite the apparent absurdity of treating them in a way that diverges from their situation: "Eliminating this divergence would mean that we treat the incompetent in all respects as a nonthinking, nonchoosing, irrational being—in short, as a nonperson."[98]

Despite its established status, the standard of substituted judgment should be used for once-competent patients only if reason exists to believe that a decision can be made as the patient would have made it. In such cases, the surrogate's acquaintance with the patient should be sufficiently deep and relevant that a judgment will reflect the patient's goals and views. If the surrogate can reliably answer the question, "What would the patient want in this circumstance?," then substituted judgment is an appropriate standard. But if the surrogate can only answer the question, "What do you want for the patient?" then this standard is inappropriate, because all connection to the patient's former autonomy has vanished.

Similarly, the standard of substituted judgment should be rejected for never-competent patients, because their autonomy is not involved. No basis exists for a judgment of autonomous choice if a person has never had autonomy. The never-competent patient therefore should be considered relevantly different from those who can now make or who previously have made autonomous choices. Exponents of substituted judgment have failed to establish the relevance of the characteristic of autonomy for never-autonomous patients, leading one court to hold that trying to determine what a never-competent patient would have decided if competent is like asking, "If it snowed all summer, would it then be winter?"[99]

There are also problems with substituted judgment when used for incompetent but conscious patients such as Earle N. Spring, a senile man whose family and physicians considered his continuation on kidney dialysis to be of doubtful value (see Case 5 in the appendix). His wife and son petitioned a Massachusetts court for authorization to terminate dialysis. If a surrogate views such a patient in terms of what the patient might wish if competent, rather than in terms of his medical need, a danger arises of overlooking the person's stake in continued existence. Many debilitated incompetent patients, like Earle Spring, have their care terminated on the basis of highly tenuous judgments by financially strained relatives about what the person would have wanted if he or she could speak. In general, little is known at present about how accurately surrogate decisionmakers reflect the preferences of patients.[100] In the instance of *Spring,* the Massachusetts Supreme Court (unlike the original probate court) accepted the family's argument that Earle Spring had been an active, vigorous outdoorsman who hated confinement and killed suffering animals when he found them in the woods. Almost all senile individuals suffer a loss of activity, but this has never been considered a good or sufficient reason for terminating their lives.

Preservation of privacy and dignity are often given as reasons in such cases, even when for months little privacy or dignity has been available for such patients. A best interests test would lead to closer scrutiny of questions about the patient's welfare than does substituted judgment. This is a matter of practical importance, because many residents of nursing homes and state facilities routinely have such judgments made about their lives—especially regarding continuation of respirators, antibiotics, nutrition and hydration, and the like. We do not suggest that these judgments are poorly made, but we do hold that substituted judgment is a poor basis on which to make them. (There are parallel dangers with authorizing parental decisions for healthy minors—for example, when a parent makes a "substituted judgment" about whether a healthy minor child would want to give a kidney to a sibling.)

The rule of substituted judgment, then, helps us understand what should be done for once-competent patients whose relevant prior preferences can be discerned; but, so interpreted, it collapses into a pure autonomy standard that respects previous autonomous choices. We conclude that we should abandon substituted judgment insofar as possible in law and in ethics and substitute a pure autonomy standard in contexts in which explicit prior autonomous judgments are identifiable.

The Pure Autonomy Standard

The second standard, then, eliminates the ghost autonomy found in substituted judgment. It applies exclusively to formerly autonomous patients who expressed a relevant autonomous decision or preference. This standard makes

more specific the general commitments of the principle of respect for autonomy. One must respect past, self-regarding, autonomous decisions reached by
now-incompetent but previously competent persons. Whether or not there exists
a formal advance directive, prior autonomous judgments should be accepted.
(It is assumed that such judgments are known, not merely conjectured, and are
directly relevant to a contemplated action.) We find an instructive approach to
such formerly autonomous patients in the Claire Conroy case, in which the
New Jersey Supreme Court grappled with several standards of surrogate decisionmaking.[101]

Claire Conroy, an eighty-three-year-old nursing home resident, suffered from
irreversible physical and mental impairments, including organic brain syndrome, arteriosclerotic heart disease, hypertension, diabetes, necrotic ulcers on
her left foot, and a gangrenous left leg. She was awake enough to track persons
with her eyes, but was severely demented, lay in a fetal position, and was
unable to speak. She had no discernible cognitive or volitional functioning. She
could not swallow enough food and water to sustain herself, and she received
nutrition and hydration through a nasogastric tube. She could move a little, but
could not control her excretory functions. Certain stimuli resulted in an occa-
sional response. For example, she would sometimes smile when her hair was
combed or when she received a comforting rub, and she would occasionally
moan when moved or fed or when her bandages were changed.

Claire Conroy's nephew (Thomas Whittemore) was her guardian and only
surviving blood relative. He sought court permission to remove his aunt's nasogastric tube, which would result in her dehydration and death in about a
week. His petition was opposed by her physician, who viewed such an action
as a violation of medical ethics. The trial court decided to permit removal of
the feeding tube, although her dying might be painful, on grounds that her life
had become permanently burdensome. The court ordered removal, but a court-
appointed guardian ad litem appealed, and the order was stayed pending appeal. Conroy died during the appellate process, but two courts nevertheless
issued opinions.

A first appellate court reversed the trial court's judgment, on grounds that
removal of the feeding tube would cause her death and thus would constitute
an active and impermissible killing from dehydration and starvation. On further
appeal, the New Jersey Supreme Court held that any medical treatment, including artificial nutrition and hydration, may be withheld or withdrawn from an
incompetent patient under some circumstances. The court invoked the incompetent patient's autonomy right to accept or refuse medical treatment, even
though the right must be exercised by another decisionmaker. This court's language appears at first to be a mainline instance of the substituted judgment
standard. It asserts that "the goal of decision-making . . . should be to determine and effectuate . . . the decision that the patient would have made if com-

petent'' and that "the right of an adult who, like Claire Conroy, was once competent, to determine the course of her medical treatment remains intact even when she is no longer able to assert that right or to appreciate its effectuation.''

However, this court also makes direct appeals both to a pure autonomy standard and to a best interests standard. The court holds that life-sustaining treatment is legitimately withheld or withdrawn from an incompetent patient when it is clear from a "subjective test"—a demonstrable basis in former autonomous choices—that this particular patient, when autonomous, would have refused under the circumstances. If this subjective or autonomy test is not met, a best interests test then must be satisfied. The court here recognizes the patient's right of informed refusal as correlative to the right of informed consent.[102] The court reasons that the subjective or autonomy-based standard is in principle fulfilled by a written document (such as a living will); an oral directive to family member, friend, or health care provider; a durable power of attorney; the patient's convictions about medical treatment administered to others; religious beliefs and tenets; or the "patient's consistent pattern of conduct with respect to prior decisions about his own medical care.''

The court indicates that it had erred a decade earlier in *Quinlan* when it disregarded the evidence of "statements that Ms. Quinlan made to friends about the artificial prolongation of the lives of others who were terminally ill.'' Such evidence is "certainly relevant.'' But, the court notes, evidence has different degrees of probative value, "depending on the remoteness, consistency, and thoughtfulness of the prior statements or actions and the maturity of the person at the time of the statements or acts.'' For example, advance directives typically express a person's general standards, designate a decisionmaker, or combine the two. A living will that specifies personal standards for decisionmaking—for example, "I don't want to be kept alive by a respirator if I am permanently comatose''—can have high probative value, though it requires interpretation in particular situations. The court reasons that recognizing such advance directives respects incompetent patients' (previous) autonomy.

Ideally, a surrogate conveys rather than substitutes another's autonomous judgment. In many cases, however, questions exist about the reliability of evidence used to determine the patient's earlier preferences, such as whether he or she was sufficiently competent and clearly expressed relevant preferences. *Conroy* rightly notes that "in the absence of adequate proof of the patient's wishes, it is naive to pretend that the right to self-determination serves as the basis for substituted decision-making.'' (In the later, landmark *Cruzan* decision, the U.S. Supreme Court held that a state can legitimately require clear and convincing evidence of a patient's prior express wishes about forgoing or withdrawing life-sustaining treatment, rather than accepting a proxy's interpretation of those wishes.) Nevertheless, the *Conroy* court holds that an absence of adequate proof does not entail that life-sustaining treatment must be continued: "Life-sustaining treatment may also be withheld or withdrawn from a patient in Claire Conroy's situation if either of two types of 'best interest' test—a *limited-objective* or a *pure-objective* test—is satisfied."

In its reliance on "best interests," the court does not substantially deviate from considerations of autonomy in its "limited-objective test." Its test requires "some trustworthy evidence that the patient would have refused the treatment" along with the decisionmaker's conviction that "the burdens of the patient's continued life with the treatment outweigh the benefits of that life for him." If these conditions are satisfied, the treatment is deemed merely to prolong suffering. Any evidence mentioned under the subjective (pure autonomy) test could be sufficient in reaching judgments about the relevant burdens, although it might be "too vague, casual, or remote to constitute the clear proof of the patient's subjective intent that is necessary to satisfy the subjective test."

Even if no evidence exists about the patient's previous wishes, life-sustaining treatment is justifiably withheld or withdrawn if decisionmakers satisfy the pure-objective test, which is strictly a test of best interests: "The net burdens of the patient's life with the treatment should clearly and markedly outweigh the benefits that the patient derives from life" and "the recurring, unavoidable and severe pain of the patient's life with the treatment would be such that the effect of administering life-sustaining treatment would be inhumane." Although the New Jersey court limited its holding to previously competent patients in Claire Conroy's situation, its arguments about best interests extend to other classes of incompetent patients.[103] Paradoxically, the court determined that Claire Conroy herself did not satisfy any of the court's standards for withdrawing life-sustaining treatment, and, therefore, had she lived, the court would not have authorized removal of her feeding tube.

Although we also commend a pure autonomy standard, as appropriate, there are additional problems in *Conroy* and similar legal decisions regarding satisfactory evidence for acting under this standard. In the absence of explicit instructions, a surrogate decisionmaker might, for example, selectively choose from the patient's life history those values that accord with the proxy's own values, and then use only those selected values in reaching decisions. The proxy's findings might also be based on values of the patient that are only distantly relevant to the immediate decision—such as the patient's expressed dislike of hospitals. It is reasonable to ask what a decisionmaker can legitimately infer from Claire Conroy's prior conduct, especially her fear and avoidance of doctors and her earlier refusal to consent to amputation of a gangrenous leg.

A troublesome problem is that surrogates often assume an explicitness in a patient's directive about the future that does not, with sufficient directness, apply to the decision at hand. In *Evans v. Bellevue Hospital,* a formerly competent patient had executed a durable power of attorney authorizing another to make medical decisions in a circumstance of incompetence and had executed a second document refusing life-sustaining treatments if he suffered from "illness, disease or injury or experienced extreme mental deterioration, such that there is no reasonable expectation of recovering or regaining a meaningful quality of life." When the patient became incompetent and suffered from brain lesions due to toxoplasmosis, a form of infection, the designated surrogate refused treatment, allegedly following the executed document's declaration. Both physicians and a court rightly refused to recognize the proxy's decision, because the document did not clearly pertain to this condition, which was in principle treatable and had a chance of restoring the patient's capacity to communicate.[104] Such imprecise statements provide too little guidance and are sometimes dangerous. Often these cases need to be handled under the best interests standard rather than an autonomy standard, even when legally valid documents have been executed with the intent of exercising autonomous control.

There is also a procedural problem of ensuring that surrogates respect a patient's prior autonomous judgments or otherwise act responsibly as surrogates. It has become increasingly difficult to find suitable persons willing to assume the burdensome job of guardianship for institutionalized mentally disabled persons, and families sometimes make decisions that conflict with the apparent wishes of a now incompetent person. One study focused on decisions by surrogates (largely sons and daughters) for 168 elderly patients in nursing homes about whether to permit their participation as research subjects in a minimal risk study of morbidity associated with long-term urinary catheters. These surrogates tended to believe that research should not be conducted in nursing homes, that they themselves would not consent to participate, that the research would disturb the patient, and that the patient, if competent, would not consent. Nonetheless, fifty-four percent consented to the patient's participation in the study, and thirty-one percent of the surrogates who thought the patients would not consent if competent still consented for the patient. Because this discrepancy emerged only through interviews after completion of the project, the researchers did not confront the ethical dilemma of what to do when surrogates act against what they believe to be the patient's wishes.[105] The study's authors suggest that consent auditors are sometimes needed to ensure better decisions when the surrogate appears to act against the patient's preferences.

Another procedural problem has emerged from a recent study of gender bias in appellate judicial opinions regarding the termination of life-sustaining treatment for newly incompetent patients. The investigators concluded that "Judicial reasoning about profoundly ill, incompetent men accepts evidence of mens' treatment preferences to define the standing of personal autonomy in decisions about life-sustaining treatment. Judicial reasoning about women defines the role of caregivers in making treatment decisions after either rejecting or failing to consider evidence of women's preferences with regard to life-sustaining treatment.'' [106] For newly incompetent patients without a written advance directive, the appellate courts tended to adopt the male patient's preferences from reports of family and friends, whereas they rarely took this approach for newly incompetent female patients. The following tendencies were discovered in this study: A man's prior opinions are typically viewed as rational, whereas a woman's earlier comments are often viewed as unreflective, emotional, or immature. A woman's viewpoint, as reflected in prior statements, is sometimes neglected altogether. Statements about women's views and values are also subjected to a higher standard of clear and convincing evidence. Finally, the court opinions tend to depict men as subject to medical assault and women as vulnerable to medical neglect. Both men and women are placed at risk by such gender bias. Men are vulnerable to quick decisions about termination of life-sustaining treatment, whereas women are at risk of not having their autonomous decisions taken seriously.

In summary, we have argued that previously competent patients who autonomously expressed their preference in the form of an advance directive should be treated under the pure autonomy standard, and we have suggested an economy of standards. It is presently popular in biomedical ethics to hold that an ordered set of standards for surrogate decisionmaking runs from (1) autonomously executed advance directives to (2) substituted judgment to (3) best interests, with (1) having priority over (2) and (1) and (2) having priority over (3) in a circumstance of conflict. We have collapsed (1) and (2) as essentially identical. Their defense and only basis is in the principle of respect for autonomy, which applies if and only if a relevant autonomous judgment exists that constitutes an authorization. Where the previously competent person left no reliable traces of his or her wishes, surrogate decisionmakers should adhere only to (3). This conclusion takes us to an examination of the best interests standard.

The Best Interests Standard

Under the best interests standard a surrogate decisionmaker must determine the highest benefit among the available options, assigning different weights to interests the patient has in each option and discounting or subtracting inherent risks or costs. The term *best* is used because the obligation is to maximize benefit through a comparative assessment that locates the highest net benefit. The best interests standard protects another's well-being by assessing risks and benefits of various treatments and alternatives to treatment, by considering pain and suffering, and by evaluating restoration or loss of functioning. It is therefore inescapably a quality-of-life criterion.

Although a best interests judgment must evaluate risks and benefits for the person involved, such a judgment should not rest solely on known subjective preferences or other forms of personal value. It appeals indirectly to these autonomy considerations insofar as they provide a basis for understanding welfare and interpreting interests. Autonomous preferences should be considered under the best interests standard only as far as they affect interpretations of quality of life, direct benefit, and the like. They should be known preferences, not inferences about what the patient would think based on his or her broad expressed values.

The best interests standard has been widely used both in and beyond health care settings. Long before autonomy and privacy were pervasively applied through law to incompetents and minors, the responsibility of parents toward their children was legally defined as the responsibility to act in the best interests of those children. It was assumed in law that parents generally do act in their children's best interests and that the state should not interfere except in extreme circumstances in which the state and the parents disagree about some decision with potentially serious consequences for the child—for example, when Jehovah's Witness parents refuse lifesaving blood transfusions for their minor children. If a court rather than the family decides, the court has already made a judgment about the unjustifiability of the family's proposed course of action (or the family's incompetence to decide).

We believe there are circumstances in which the best interests standard, so understood, can validly be invoked to override advance directives executed by autonomous patients who have become incompetent, refusals by minors, and refusals by mental patients. This overriding can occur, for example, in a case in which a person has designated another by a durable power of attorney to make medical decisions on his or her behalf. If the designated surrogate makes a decision that is clearly against the patient's best interests, the decision should be overridden unless there is a clearly worded, second document executed by the patient that specifically supports the surrogate's decision. Overriding the surrogate's decision in such a case does not violate respect for autonomy or constitute a paternalistic intervention.

For previously competent patients whose prior preferences cannot be reliably traced and for never-competent patients, it is appropriate to rely on a best interests standard as more suitable than the pure autonomy standard and substituted judgment standards. Although it has been argued that substituted judgment is a standard that seeks "to implement the patient's best interests as that patient would have defined them" and, therefore, that "the substituted judgment approach is merely one way in which the best interests standard is given content," [107] this synthesis is too convenient and confusing. The best interests standard can in principle conflict with either an autonomy standard or a substituted judgment standard. As the authors of the above-mentioned study of surrogate decisions for the elderly note, these standards do in fact conflict in many cases. It is best to keep these standards as conceptually and normatively distinct as possible.

Courts, health care institutions, and religious traditions have too long been eager to assert that they do not make quality of life judgments, but only reach decisions in view of what the patient would have chosen. The substituted judgment standard has been popular, because it enables a decisionmaker to disclaim quality-of-life considerations altogether, while claiming to look exclusively at the individual's preferences. Courts have viewed quality-of-life judgments as comparative ways of expressing a person's social worth, and they have understandably wanted to avoid comparative ranking of the worth of individual lives. However, "quality-of-life judgments" are not about the social worth of individuals, but about the value of the life for the person who must live it. The value of a life is primarily (although not exclusively) the value it has for that person. Best interests judgments are one way to focus attention on this point, rather than on the value the person's life has for other persons. Accepting a best interests standard, properly so called, is tantamount to acknowledging that we have to decide in marginal cases what a patient's welfare interests are at the moment, not what they would have chosen in some imaginary possible world.

Unfortunately, the best interests standard has sometimes been interpreted as highly malleable, permitting values that are irrelevant to the patient's benefits or burdens and incorporating intangible factors of questionable value to the incompetent person. For example, when parents have sought court permission for a kidney transplant from an incompetent minor child to a competent sibling, parental judgments about the "donor's" best interests have on occasion taken into account projected psychological trauma from the death of the sibling and the psychological benefits of the unselfish act of "donation." [108] While we would not exclude such considerations altogether, they should be greeted with skepticism and with additional procedural protections, such as committee review. Best interests judgments should concentrate on tangible factors, such as physical suffering and medical diagnosis, and should be extended into other domains only with hesitation and great caution.

Under this formulation, questions arise about whether the burdens considered under the best interests standard should be limited to physical pain and suffering, as judicial language often suggests. If pain and suffering were the only relevant burdens, it would be difficult to justify withholding or withdrawing life-sustaining treatment for a permanently comatose patient. However, this range of concerns about the best interests standard cannot be examined until Chapters 4 and 5, where we discuss benefits and harms more comprehensively.

Conclusion

The intimate connection between autonomy and decisionmaking in health care unifies this chapter's several sections. Although we have justified the obligation to solicit decisions from patients by the principle of respect for autonomy, we have acknowledged that the principle's precise demands remain unsettled and open to interpretation and specification. For example, notable issues about the principle's connection to rules of truthfulness, confidentiality, and privacy are discussed in Chapter 7. We have thus far argued only that making respect for autonomy a trump moral principle, rather than one moral principle in a system of principles, gives it an excessive value. The human moral community, indeed morality itself, is rooted no less deeply in the three clusters of principles discussed in subsequent chapters. In many clinical circumstances the weight of respect for autonomy is minimal, and the weight of nonmaleficence or beneficence is maximal. Similarly in public policy, the demands of justice can easily outweigh the demands of respect for autonomy.

Several conclusions in this chapter could be viewed as one-sided in their deference to autonomy, on grounds that their implications for professional conduct exceed current legal and regulatory requirements. For example, our proposed shift from a focus on disclosure to a focus on understanding and effective communication entails a different and more burdensome way of structuring the consent-solicitation process. Nevertheless, we have not argued that our proposals should be transformed directly into enforceable legal requirements or into regulatory rules or hospital policies. It is not always justifiable to provide the resources needed to create a context in which professionals conduct themselves in accordance with the full set of strategies suggested in this chapter. This problem invites judgments about justice and resource allocation (see Chapter 6) that compete with the obligation to obtain informed consent.

Notes

1. The core idea of autonomy has been helpfully treated by Isaiah Berlin, "Two Concepts of Liberty," in *Four Essays on Liberty* (Oxford: Oxford University Press, 1969), pp. 118–72; Joel Feinberg, *Harm to Self,* vol. III in *The Moral Limits of Criminal Law* (New York: Oxford University Press, 1986), ch. 18 and 19; and Thomas E. Hill, Jr., *Autonomy and Self-Respect* (Cambridge: Cambridge University Press, 1991), ch. 1–4.
2. See Gerald Dworkin, *The Theory and Practice of Autonomy* (New York: Cambridge University Press, 1988), ch. 1–4; Harry G. Frankfurt, "Freedom of the Will and the Concept of a Person," *Journal of Philosophy* 68 (1971): 5–20.
3. See Stanley Benn, "Freedom, Autonomy and the Concept of a Person," *Proceed-*

ings of the Aristotelian Society 76 (1976): 123–30. In his earlier and later views, Benn notes that one can and should be a proper object of respect without satisfying the "exacting requirements of the ideal of autonomy." See *A Theory of Freedom* (Cambridge: Cambridge University Press, 1988), pp. 3–6, 155f, 175–83. For an emphasis on autonomy through authorship of one's life, see Joseph Raz, *The Morality of Freedom* (Oxford: Clarendon Press, 1986), pp. 145–62, 368–429, esp. 154–56, 368–72.

4. Dworkin, *The Theory and Practice of Autonomy,* pp. 15–20.

5. For practical implications and empirical studies, see Priscilla Alderson, "Consent to Children's Surgery and Intensive Medical Treatment," *Journal of Law and Society* 17 (1990): 52–65; and Barbara Stanley et al., "The Functional Competency of Elderly at Risk," *The Gerontologist* 28, Suppl. (1988): 53–58.

6. See Robert Paul Wolff, *In Defense of Anarchism* (New York: Harper and Row, 1970), pp. 4–6, 13f, and Arthur Kuflik, "The Inalienability of Autonomy," *Philosophy and Public Affairs* 13 (1984): 271–98. See also Joseph Raz, "Authority and Justification," *Philosophy and Public Affairs* 14 (1985): 3–29; and Christopher McMahon, "Autonomy and Authority," *Philosophy and Public Affairs* 16 (1987): 303–28.

7. Susan Sherwin, *No Longer Patient: Feminist Ethics and Health Care* (Philadelphia: Temple University Press, 1992), p. 138. However, she does not reject the relevance of moral considerations of autonomy. For a view that "feminists have reason to regard institutions and practices that undermine autonomy as especially detrimental to women," see Diana T. Meyers, *Self, Society, and Personal Choice* (New York: Columbia University Press, 1989).

8. Kant, *Foundations of the Metaphysics of Morals,* trans. Lewis White Beck (Indianapolis, IN: Bobbs-Merrill Company, 1959); *The Doctrine of Virtue,* part II of the "Metaphysics of Morals," trans. Mary Gregor (Philadelphia: University of Pennsylvania Press, 1964), esp. p. 127.

9. Mill, *On Liberty,* in *Collected Works of John Stuart Mill,* vol. 18 (Toronto: University of Toronto Press, 1977), ch. I, III.

10. See, for example, Daniel Callahan, "Autonomy: A Moral Good, Not a Moral Obsession," *Hastings Center Report* 14 (October 1984): 40–42; Robert M. Veatch, "Autonomy's Temporary Triumph," *Hastings Center Report* 14 (October 1984): 38–40; and James F. Childress, "The Place of Autonomy in Bioethics," *Hastings Center Report* 20 (January/February 1990): 12–16.

11. See Barbara Herman, "Mutual Aid and Respect for Persons," *Ethics* 94 (July 1984): 577–602, esp. 600–602; Onora O'Neill, "Universal Laws and Ends-in-Themselves," *Monist* 72 (1989): 341–61.

12. See Daniel Callahan, "Autonomy: A Moral Good, Not a Moral Obsession"; and Colleen D. Clements and Roger C. Sider, "Medical Ethics' Assault Upon Medical Values," *Journal of the American Medical Association* 250 (Oct. 21, 1983): 2011–15.

13. See Bernard Lo et al., "Voluntary Screening for Human Immunodeficiency Virus (HIV) Infection: Weighing the Benefits and Harms," *Annals of Internal Medicine* 110 (May 1989): 727–33; and Martha S. Swartz, "AIDS Testing and Informed Consent," *Journal of Health Politics, Policy, and Law* 13 (Winter 1988): 607–21.

14. Childress, *Who Should Decide?* (New York: Oxford University Press, 1982), pp. 224–25. This case was prepared by Gail Povar, M.D.

15. See Bernard Gert and Charles Culver, "The Justification of Paternalism," *Ethics* 89 (January 1979): 199–210.

16. *Werth v. Taylor,* 190 Mich App 141 (1991).

17. *In re Estate of Dorone,* 502 A.2d 1271 (Pa. Super. 1985)

18. See Rebecca Dresser and John Robertson, "Quality of Life and Non-Treatment Decisions for Incompetent Patients: A Critique of the Orthodox Approach," *Law, Medicine, and Health Care* 17 (1989): 234–44.

19. See Allen E. Buchanan and Dan W. Brock, *Deciding for Others: The Ethics of Surrogate Decision Making* (Cambridge: Cambridge University Press, 1989), pp. 26–27. This book helped us correct some parts of our argument as presented in our third edition.

20. The analysis in this section has profited from discussions with Ruth R. Faden, Nancy M. P. King, and Dan Brock.

21. See the analysis of the core meaning in Charles M. Culver and Bernard Gert, *Philosophy in Medicine* (New York: Oxford University Press, 1982), pp. 123–26.

22. See *Lake v. Cameron,* 267 F. Supp. 155 (D.D.C. 1967).

23. *Pratt v. Davis,* 118 Ill. App. 161 (1905), aff'd, 224 Ill. 300, 79 N.E. 562 (1906).

24. See Daniel Wikler, "Paternalism and the Mildly Retarded," *Philosophy and Public Affairs* 8 (Summer 1979): 377–92.

25. A number of subtleties and needed qualifications in this analysis are discussed in an important paper by Kenneth F. Schaffner, "Competency: A Triaxial Concept," in *Competency,* ed. M. A. G. Cutter and E. E. Shelp (Dordrecht, the Netherlands: Kluwer Academic Publisher, 1991), pp. 253–81.

26. This case was prepared by P. Browning Hoffman, M.D., for presentation in the series of "Medicine and Society" conferences at the University of Virginia.

27. This schema is indebted to Paul S. Appelbaum, Charles W. Lidz, and Alan Meisel, *Informed Consent: Legal Theory and Clinical Practice* (New York: Oxford University Press, 1987), ch. 5; Ruth Macklin, "Some Problems in Gaining Informed Consent from Psychiatric Patients," *Emory Law Journal* 31 (Spring 1982): 345–74; Paul S. Appelbaum and Thomas Grisso, "Assessing Patients' Capacities to Consent to Treatment," *New England Journal of Medicine* 319 (December 22, 1988): 1635–38.

28. For additional ways in which values are incorporated, see Loretta M. Kopelman, "On the Evaluative Nature of Competency and Capacity Judgments," *International Journal of Law and Psychiatry* 13 (1990): 309–29. For conceptual and epistemic problems in all available tests, see E. Haavi Morreim, "Competence: At the Intersection of Law, Medicine, and Philosophy," in *Competency,* pp. 93–125, esp. 105–8.

29. See Willard Gaylin, "The Competence of Children: No Longer All or None," *Hastings Center Report* 12 (April 1982): 33–38, esp. 35; Buchanan and Brock, *Deciding for Others,* pp. 51–70; and Dan Brock, "Children's Competence for Health Care Decisionmaking," in *Children and Health Care,* ed. Loretta Kopelman and John Moskop (Boston: Kluwer Academic Publishers, 1989), pp. 181–212.

30. Buchanan and Brock, *Deciding for Others,* pp. 52–55. For elaboration and defense, see Brock, "Decisionmaking Competence and Risk," *Bioethics* 5 (1991): 105–12.

31. Related problems in the Buchanan-Brock analysis are discussed in Mark R. Wicclair, "Patient Decision-Making Capacity and Risk," *Bioethics* 5 (1991): 91–104, esp. p. 98 (and see p. 120 for an additional "Response").

32. Wendy Carlton, *"In Our Professional Opinion . . ." The Primacy of Clinical Judgment over Moral Choice* (Notre Dame, IN: University of Notre Dame Press, 1978), pp. 5–6.

33. See Jay Katz, *The Silent World of Doctor and Patient* (New York: The Free Press, 1984), pp. 86–87; and President's Commission for the Study of Ethical Problems in Medicine and Biomedical and Behavioral Research, *Making Health Care Decisions* (Washington, DC: U.S. Government Printing Office, 1982), vol. I, p. 15. Alan Weisbard, a proponent of this approach, suggests abandoning "informed consent" in favor of a different term, in "Informed Consent: The Law's Uneasy Compromise with Ethical Theory," *Nebraska Law Review* 65 (1986): 767.

34. See Charles W. Lidz et al., "Two Models of Implementing Informed Consent," *Archives of Internal Medicine* 148 (June 1988): 1385–89.

35. The analysis in this subsection is based in part on Faden and Beauchamp, *A History and Theory of Informed Consent,* ch. 8.

36. *Mohr v. Williams,* 95 Minn. 261, 265; 104 N.W. 12, 15 (1905).

37. This conclusion is vigorously defended by Weisbard, "Informed Consent: The Law's Uneasy Compromise with Ethical Theory," pp. 749–67.

38. Jay Katz, "Disclosure and Consent," in *Genetics and the Law II,* ed. A. Milunsky and G. Annas (New York: Plenum Press, 1980), pp. 122, 128; for revisions and amplifications, see Katz, "Physician-Patient Encounters 'On a Darkling Plain,' " *Western New England Law Review* 9 (1987): 207–26, and Alan Meisel, "A 'Dignitary Tort' as a Bridge between the Idea of Informed Consent and the Law of Informed Consent," *Law, Medicine, and Health Care* 16 (1988): 210–18.

39. See, for example, Alan Meisel and Loren Roth, "What We Do and Do Not Know about Informed Consent," *Journal of the American Medical Association* 246 (1981): 2473–77; President's Commission, *Making Health Care Decisions,* vol. II, pp. 317–410, esp. p. 318, and vol. I, ch. 1, esp. pp. 38–39; National Commission for the Protection of Human Subjects of Biomedical and Behavioral Research, *The Belmont Report* (Washington, DC: DHEW Publication OS 78-0012, 1978), p. 10.

40. See, for example, *Planned Parenthood of Central Missouri v. Danforth,* 428 U.S. 52 at 67 n.8 (1976) (U.S. Supreme Court).

41. See the controversies catalogued in Hunter L. Prillaman, "A Physician's Duty to Inform of Newly Developed Therapy," *Journal of Contemporary Health Law and Policy* 6 (1990): 43–58.

42. *Moore v. Regents of the University of California,* 793 P.2d 479 (Cal. 1990) at 483.

43. See "Necessity and Sufficiency of Expert Evidence and Extent of Physician's Duty to Inform Patient of Risks of Proposed Treatment," *American Law Reports* 3d, 52 (1977): 1084; and "Physician's Duty to Inform of Risks," *American Law Reports* 3d, 88 (1986): 1010–25.

44. See *Largey v. Rothman,* 540 A.2d 504 (N.J. 1988), at 505.

45. See, for example, Charles Keown, Paul Slovic, and Sarah Lichtenstein, "Attitudes of Physicians, Pharmacists, and Laypersons Toward Seriousness and Need for Disclosure of Prescription Drug Side Effects," *Health Psychology* 3 (1984): 1–11, and Ruth R. Faden et al., "Disclosure of Information to Patients in Medical Care," *Medical Care* 19 (July 1981): 718–33.

46. See "Physician's Duty to Inform of Risks," pp. 1010–25 (and update, 50–60).

47. Ruth R. Faden and Tom L. Beauchamp, "Decision-Making and Informed Consent:

A Study of the Impact of Disclosed Information," *Social Indicators Research* 7 (1980): 313–36.

48. Carl H. Fellner and John R. Marshall, "Kidney Donors—The Myth of Informed Consent," *American Journal of Psychiatry* 126 (1970): 1245–50, and "Twelve Kidney Donors," *Journal of the American Medical Association* 206 (1968): 2703–7.

49. See L. A. Siminoff and J. H. Fetting, "Factors Affecting Treatment Decisions for a Life-Threatening Illness: The Case of Medical Treatment of Breast Cancer," *Social Science and Medicine* 32 (1991): 813–18; David G. Scherer and N. D. Reppucci, "Adolescents' Capacities to Provide Voluntary Informed Consent," *Law and Human Behavior* 12 (1988): 123–41.

50. Gerald T. Roling et al., "An Appraisal of Patients' Reactions to 'Informed Consent' for Peroral Endoscopy," *Gastrointestinal Endoscopy* 24 (November 1977): 69–70.

51. L. A. Siminoff, J. H. Fetting, and M. D. Abeloff, "Doctor-Patient Communication about Breast Cancer Adjuvant Therapy," *Journal of Clinical Oncology* 7 (1989): 1192–1200.

52. The Oklahoma Supreme Court has been particularly vigorous in asserting this conception of the need for information. See *Scott v. Bradford,* 606 P.2d 554 (Okla. 1979) at 559 (together with *Masquat v. Maguire,* 638 P.2d 1105, Okla. 1981).

53. *Canterbury v. Spence,* 464 F.2d 772 (1977), at 785–89. See also *Wilson v. Scott,* 412 S.W.2d 299, 301 (Tex. 1967), and F. F. W. van Oosten, "The So-Called 'Therapeutic Privilege' or 'Contra-Indication': Its Nature and Role in Non-Disclosure Cases," *Medicine and Law* 10 (1991): 31–41.

54. *Thornburgh v. American College of Obstetricians,* 106 S.Ct. 2169, at 2199–2200 (1986) (White, J., dissenting).

55. Robert W. Allen, "Informed Consent: A Medical Decision," *Radiology* 119 (April 1976): 233–34.

56. See Kimberly A. Quaid et al., "Informed Consent for a Prescription Drug: Impact of Disclosed Information on Patient Understanding and Medical Outcomes," *Patient Education and Counselling* 15 (1990): 249–59.

57. James W. Lankton, Barron M. Batehelder, and Alan J. Ominsky, "Emotional Responses to Detailed Risk Disclosure for Anesthesia: A Prospective, Randomized Study," *Anesthesiology* 46 (April 1977): 294–96.

58. See Howard Brody, *Placebos and the Philosophy of Medicine: Clinical, Conceptual, and Ethical Issues* (Chicago: University of Chicago Press, 1980), pp. 10–11; and Herbert Benson and Mark Epstein, "The Placebo Effect: A Neglected Aspect in the Care of Patients," *Journal of the American Medical Association* 232 (1975): 1225.

59. Alan Leslie, "Ethics and Practice of Placebo Therapy," in *Ethics in Medicine,* ed. S. Reiser, A. Dyck, and W. Curran (Cambridge, MA: MIT Press, 1977), p. 242.

60. See L. C. Park et al., "Effects of Informed Consent on Research Patients and Study Results," *Journal of Nervous and Mental Disease* 145 (1967): 349–57.

61. Brody, *Placebos and the Philosophy of Medicine,* pp. 110, 113, *et passim;* Katz, *The Silent World,* pp. 189–95. For a defense of placebos, see Howard Spiro, *Doctors, Patients, and Placebos* (New Haven: Yale University Press, 1986).

62. Philip Levendusky and Loren Pankratz, "Self-Control Techniques as an Alternative to Pain Medication," *Journal of Abnormal Psychology* 84, no. 2 (1975): 165–68.

63. See Herbert C. Kelman, ''Was Deception Justified—and Was It Necessary?'' *Journal of Abnormal Psychology* 84 (1975): 172–74.

64. Sally E. McNagy and Ruth M. Parker, ''High Prevalence of Recent Cocaine Use and the Unreliability of Patient Self-report in an Inner-city Walk-in Clinic,'' *Journal of the American Medical Association* 267 (February 26, 1992): 1106–8.

65. As Sissela Bok has argued in ''Informed Consent in Tests of Patient Reliability,'' *Journal of the American Medical Association* 267 (February 26, 1992): 1118–19.

66. Stanley Milgram, *Obedience to Authority: An Experimental View* (New York: Harper & Row, 1974), pp. 3–4. See also Milgram, ''Behavioral Study of Obedience,'' *Journal of Abnormal and Social Psychology* 67 (1963): 371–78; and ''Some Conditions of Obedience and Disobedience to Authority,'' *Human Relations* 18 (1965): 57–76.

67. Milgram, ''Subject Reaction: The Neglected Factor in the Ethics of Experimentation,'' *Hastings Center Report* 7 (October 1977): 19–21.

68. See Diana Baumrind, ''Some Thoughts on Ethics of Research: After Reading Milgram's 'Behavioral Study of Obedience,' '' *American Psychologist* 19 (1964): 421–23; Milgram, ''Issues in the Study of Obedience: A Reply to Baumrind,'' *American Psychologist* 19 (1964): 848–52; and Steven C. Patten, ''The Case That Milgram Makes,'' *Philosophical Review* 86 (July 1977): 350–64.

69. Milgram, ''Subject Reaction,'' p. 19.

70. *Bang v. Charles T. Miller Hospital*, 251 Minn. 427, 88 N.W. 2d 186 (1958).

71. Franz J. Ingelfinger, ''Informed (But Uneducated) Consent,'' *New England Journal of Medicine* 287 (August 31, 1972): 455–56. See also his ''Arrogance,'' *New England Journal of Medicine* 303 (December 25, 1980): 1507–11.

72. See Paul R. Benson et al., ''Information Disclosure, Subject Understanding, and Informed Consent in Psychiatric Research,'' *Law and Human Behavior* 12 (1988): 455–75.

73. The pioneering work was done by Amos Tversky and Daniel Kahneman. See ''Choices, Values and Frames,'' *American Psychologist* 39 (1984): 341–50; ''Judgment under Certainty: Heuristics and Biases,'' *Science* 185 (1974): 1124–31; ''The Framing of Decisions and the Psychology of Choice,'' *Science* 211 (1981): 453–58.

74. Kahneman and Tversky, ''Choices, Values and Frames,'' 344–46; and Tversky and Kahneman, ''The Framing of Decisions.''

75. S. E. Eraker and H. C. Sox, ''Assessment of Patients' Preferences for Therapeutic Outcome,'' *Medical Decision Making* 1 (1981): 29–39; Barbara McNeil et al., ''On the Elicitation of Preferences for Alternative Therapies,'' *New England Journal of Medicine* 306 (May 27, 1982): 1259–62.

76. See Jon F. Merz and Baruch Fischoff, ''Informed Consent Does Not Mean Rational Consent,'' *The Journal of Legal Medicine* 11 (1990): 321–50; Baruch Fischoff, Paul Slovic, and Sarah Lichtenstein, ''Knowing What You Want: Measuring Liable Values,'' in *Cognitive Processes in Choice and Decision Behavior*, ed. Thomas Wallsten (Hillsdale, NJ: Lawrence Erlbaum Associates, 1980), 117–41.

77. See Mark Siegler, ''Critical Illness: The Limits of Autonomy,'' *Hastings Center Report* 12 (October 1977): 12–15, and the reply to Siegler by Jay Katz, *The Silent World*, pp. 156–59.

78. Ruth Faden and Alan Faden, ''False Belief and the Refusal of Medical Treatment,'' *Journal of Medical Ethics* 3 (1977): 133–36.

79. *Cobbs v. Grant*, 502 P.2d 1, 12 (1972).

80. Baruch Brody, *Life and Death Decision Making* (New York: Oxford University Press, 1988), p. 22.
81. See Ralph J. Alfidi, "Controversy, Alternatives, and Decisions in Complying with the Legal Doctrine of Informed Consent," *Radiology* 114 (January 1975): 231–34.
82. William M. Strull, Bernard Lo, and Gerald Charles, "Do Patients Want to Participate in Medical Decisionmaking?" *Journal of the American Medical Association* 252 (1984): 2990–94.
83. See Joel Feinberg, *Social Philosophy* (Englewood Cliffs, NJ: Prentice-Hall, 1973), p. 48; *Harm to Self,* pp. 112–18.
84. Our formulation is indebted to Robert Nozick, "Coercion," in *Philosophy, Science and Method: Essays in Honor of Ernest Nagel,* ed. Sidney Morgenbesser, Patrick Suppes, and Morton White (New York: St. Martin's Press, 1969), pp. 440–72, and Bernard Gert, "Coercion and Freedom," in *Coercion: Nomos XIV,* ed. J. Roland Pennock and John W. Chapman (Chicago: Aldine, Atherton Inc. 1972), pp. 36–37.
85. Paul S. Appelbaum and Loren H. Roth, "Treatment Refusal in Medical Hospitals," in President's Commission, *Making Health Care Decisions,* vol. II, p. 443; see also pp. 452, 462, 466.
86. See Charles W. Lidz and Alan Meisel, "Informed Consent and the Structure of Medical Care," in President's Commission, *Making Health Care Decisions,* vol. II, pp. 317–410.
87. Eliot Freidson, *The Profession of Medicine* (New York: Dodd, Mead & Co., 1970), p. 376.
88. See James H. Jones, *Bad Blood* (New York: The Free Press, 1981); David J. Rothman, "Were Tuskegee & Willowbrook 'Studies in Nature'?" *Hastings Center Report* 12 (April 1982): 5–7.
89. Henry K. Beecher, *Research and the Individual: Human Studies* (Boston: Little, Brown, and Co., 1970), p. 6.
90. See Charles W. Lidz et al., *Informed Consent: A Study of Decisionmaking in Psychiatry* (New York: Guilford Press, 1984), ch. 7, esp. pp. 110–11, 117–23.
91. The problems mentioned in this paragraph were examined in *Kaimowitz v. Department of Mental Health,* Civil No. 73-19434-AW (Circuit Court, Wayne County, Mich., July 10, 1973), at 31–32.
92. For the distinction between decisional autonomy and executional autonomy, see Bart J. Collopy, "Autonomy in Long Term Care," *The Gerontologist* 28, Supplementary Issue (June 1988): 10–17.
93. For this distinction between option right and mandatory right, see Joel Feinberg, "Voluntary Euthanasia and the Inalienable Right to Life," *Philosophy and Public Affairs* 7 (1978): 93–123.
94. For this case, see "If You Let Them, They'd Stay in Bed All Morning: The Tyranny of Regulation in Nursing Home Life," in *Everyday Ethics: Resolving Dilemmas in Nursing Home Life,* ed. R. A. Kane and A. L. Caplan (New York: Springer Publishing Co., 1990), ch. 7. For autonomy in long-term care, see other chapters in *Everyday Ethics* and a special journal issue devoted to this subject: *The Gerontologist* 28 (June 1988).
95. For a defense of negotiated consent, see Harry R. Moody, *Ethics in an Aging Society* (Baltimore: The Johns Hopkins University Press, 1992), ch. 8.
96. *Superintendent of Belchertown State School v. Saikewicz,* Mass. 370 N.E. 2d 417 (1977). For developments in related court opinions, see Sean M. Dunphy and John

H. Cross, "Medical Decision Making for Incompetent Persons: The Massachusetts Substituted Judgment Model," *Western New England Law Review* 9 (1987): 153–67.

97. *In re Quinlan,* 70 N.J. 10, 355 A.2d 647 (1976), at 663–64.

98. John A. Robertson, "Organ Donations by Incompetents and the Substituted Judgment Doctrine," *Columbia Law Review* 76 (1976): 65.

99. See George Annas, "Help from the Dead: The Cases of Brother Fox and John Storar," *Hastings Center Report* 11 (June 1981): 19–20. For an extremely charitable defense of courts' ascriptions of rights of self-determination to incompetents, see Alan Strudler, "Self-Determination, Incompetence, and Medical Jurisprudence," *The Journal of Medicine and Philosophy* 13 (1988): 349–65.

100. See the empirical study and analysis in Allison B. Seckler et al., "Substituted Judgment: How Accurate are Proxy Predictions?," *Annals of Internal Medicine* 115 (1991): 92–98.

101. In re *Conroy,* 486 A.2d 1209 (N.J. 1985). All quotations below are taken from this source.

102. See the court's explicit recognition and development of this point in re *Jobes,* 108 NJ 394, 529 A.2d 434 (1987).

103. In a series of decisions in 1987, the New Jersey Supreme Court extended its analysis to other types of cases (In re *Farrell,* 529 A.2d 404, In re *Jobes,* 529 A.2d 434, In re *Peters,* 108 N.J. 865).

104. *In the Matter of the Application of John Evans against Bellevue Hospital,* Supreme Court of the State of New York, Index No. 16536/87 (1987).

105. John Warren et al., "Informed Consent by Proxy: An Issue in Research with Elderly Patients," *New England Journal of Medicine* 315 (October 30, 1986): 1124–28, esp. 1127–28.

106. Steven H. Miles and Alison August, "Courts, Gender and 'The Right to Die,' " *Law, Medicine and Health Care* 18 (Spring-Summer 1990): 85–95.

107. Appelbaum, Lidz, and Meisel, *Informed Consent: Legal Theory and Clinical Practice.*

108. The classic case is *Strunk v. Strunk,* 445 S.W.2d 145 (Ky 1969), which considered these benefits in terms of a standard of substituted judgment.

4

Nonmaleficence

The principle of nonmaleficence asserts an obligation not to inflict harm intentionally. It has been closely associated in medical ethics with the maxim *Primum non nocere:* "Above all [or first] do no harm." This maxim is frequently invoked by health care professionals, yet its origins are obscure and its implications unclear. Often proclaimed the fundamental principle in the Hippocratic tradition of medical ethics, it is not found in the Hippocratic corpus, and a venerable statement sometimes confused with it—"at least, do no harm"—is a strained translation of a single Hippocratic passage.[1] Nonetheless, an obligation of nonmaleficence and an obligation of beneficence are both expressed in the Hippocratic oath: "I will use treatment to help the sick according to my ability and judgment, but I will never use it to injure or wrong them."

In this chapter we examine the principle of nonmaleficence and various attempts to specify its implications for biomedical ethics. In particular, we critically examine distinctions between killing and letting die, intending and foreseeing harmful outcomes, withholding and withdrawing life-sustaining treatments, and extraordinary and ordinary treatments. Many controversies in biomedical ethics surround the terminally ill and the seriously ill and injured. A framework is therefore needed for decisionmaking about life-sustaining procedures and assistance in dying. We defend a framework that would considerably alter current medical practice and guidelines for both competent and incompetent patients. At the center of the framework is an interpretation of the principle of nonmaleficence that sanctions rather than suppresses quality-of-life judgments. This framework allows patients, guardians, and health care professionals under certain conditions to accept or refuse treatments after weighing the benefits and burdens of those treatments.

The Concept of Nonmaleficence

The Distinction between Nonmaleficence and Beneficence

A principle of nonmaleficence is recognized in many types of ethical theory, including utilitarian[2] and nonutilitarian writings.[3] Some philosophers join nonmaleficence and beneficence as a single principle. William Frankena, for example, treats the principle of beneficence as divisible into four general obligations, the first of which we will distinguish as the obligation of nonmaleficence and the other three of which we will refer to as obligations of beneficence:

1. One ought not to inflict evil or harm (what is bad).
2. One ought to prevent evil or harm.
3. One ought to remove evil or harm.
4. One ought to do or promote good.[4]

Frankena arranges these elements serially so that—other things being equal in a circumstance of conflict—the first takes moral precedence over the second, the second over the third, and the third over the fourth. Frankena acknowledges that the fourth element requires defense and qualification as a statement of *obligation,* for reasons we will address in Chapter 5.

If we try to encompass the ideas of benefiting others and not injuring them under a single principle, we will still be forced to distinguish, as Frankena does, among the various obligations embedded in this general principle. Although nonmaleficence and beneficence are similar and are often treated in moral philosophy as not sharply distinguishable, conflating them into one principle obscures relevant distinctions. Obligations not to harm others (for example, those prohibiting theft, disablement, and killing) are clearly distinct from obligations to help others (for example, by providing benefits, protecting interests, and promoting welfare). Obligations not to harm others are sometimes more stringent than obligations to help them, but obligations of beneficence are also sometimes more stringent than obligations of nonmaleficence. For example, the obligation not to injure others intuitively seems more stringent than the obligation to rescue them, but the obligation not to risk injury to research subjects through low-risk procedures is typically not as stringent as the obligation to rescue an injured research subject who underwent the procedures. If, in a particular case, the injury inflicted is very minor (swelling from a needlestick, say), but the benefit provided by rescue is major (a life-saving intervention, say), then the obligation of beneficence clearly takes priority over the obligation of nonmaleficence.

Many writers in ethics have maintained that one must accept substantial risks to one's safety in order not to cause harm to others, whereas acceptance of even moderate risks is not generally required to benefit others. But this claim too depends for its justification on particular situations, especially in professional ethics. For instance, public health officials in some countries cannot perform their jobs properly without undertaking at least moderate risks, such as exposing themselves to contagious diseases.

We might try to reformulate the idea of an increased stringency in nonmaleficence as follows: Generally, obligations of nonmaleficence are more stringent than obligations of beneficence; and, in some cases, nonmaleficence overrides beneficence when the best utilitarian outcome would be obtained by acting beneficently. For example, if a surgeon could save two innocent lives by killing a prisoner on death row to retrieve his heart and liver for transplantation, this outcome would have the highest net utility (in the circumstances), but it is not morally defensible. This formulation of the stringency of nonmaleficence has an initial ring of plausibility, especially if the act of benefiting involves committing a moral wrong. But again we should be cautious about axioms of priority. A utilitarian action does not necessarily take second place to an act of not causing harm. In cases of conflict, nonmaleficence is typically overriding, but the weights of these moral principles—like all moral principles—vary in different circumstances, and there thus can be no a priori rule that favors avoiding harm over providing benefit.

The claim that an order of priority exists among elements 1 through 4 in Frankena's scheme above is likewise difficult to sustain. Refraining from aiding another person (by not providing a good or by not preventing or removing harm) can be as morally wrong as inflicting a harm. Suppose the same harm occurs to X either by not assisting X, thereby permitting the harm to occur, or by inflicting the harm on X, and suppose the harm that is inflicted or allowed is equally intentional, equally sure to occur, and equally avoidable. Finally, suppose the actor is equally at negligible risk in the two scenarios. For example, the harm of death can be inflicted by killing a person with an injection or can be caused by failing to put a person on a respirator. The only difference in these cases is inflicting harm and refraining from assistance so as to allow harm, but this difference has no moral relevance. Thus, there is no moral difference between these two (or the above four) categories, and no order of priority among the categories.

It is preferable, we suggest, to distinguish the principles of nonmaleficence and beneficence conceptually in the following way, without proposing any normative ranking or hierarchical structure.

Nonmaleficence

1. One ought not to inflict evil or harm.

Beneficence

2. One ought to prevent evil or harm.
3. One ought to remove evil or harm.
4. One ought to do or promote good.

Each of these three forms of beneficence requires taking action by helping—preventing harm, removing harm, and promoting good—whereas nonmaleficence only requires intentionally refraining from actions that cause harm. Rules of nonmaleficence therefore take the form "Do not do X." Some philosophers accept only principles or rules that take a similarly proscriptive form. They interpret even rules of respect for autonomy as limited to rules of the form "Do not interfere with a person's autonomous choices." These philosophers reject all principles or rules that require helping, assisting, or rescuing other persons (although they recognize these norms as legitimate moral ideals). However, the mainstream of moral philosophy has not accepted such a *sharp* distinction between obligations of harming and helping—preferring instead to recognize and preserve the distinction in other ways. We will take this same path, and in Chapter 5 we will explain further the nature of the distinction and why conditions other than some form of *priority* for nonmaleficence can appropriately account for the distinction.

Legitimate disagreements have arisen about how to classify many actions under categories 1 through 4 as well as about the nature and stringency of the obligations that are involved in various circumstances. Consider, for example, the following case. Robert McFall was dying of aplastic anemia, and his physicians recommended a bone marrow transplant from a genetically compatible donor to increase his chances of living one additional year from twenty-five percent to a range of forty to sixty percent. The patient's cousin, David Shimp, agreed to undergo tests to determine his suitability to be a donor. After completing the test for tissue compatibility, he refused to undergo the test for genetic compatibility. He had changed his mind about donation. Robert McFall's lawyer asked a court to require that Mr. Shimp undergo the second test and donate his bone marrow if the test indicated a good match.[5]

Public discussion focused on whether David Shimp had an obligation of beneficence toward Robert McFall in the form of an obligation to prevent harm, to remove harm, or to promote McFall's welfare. McFall's lawyer contended (unsuccessfully) that even if Shimp did not have a legal obligation of beneficence to rescue his cousin, he had a legal obligation of nonmaleficence, which required that he not make McFall's situation worse. The lawyer argued that when Shimp agreed to undergo the first test and then backed out, he caused a "delay of critical proportions" and violated the obligation of nonmaleficence. However, the judge ruled that Shimp did not violate any legal obligations but held that his actions were "morally indefensible."[6] This case illustrates the difficulties of identifying specific obligations under the principles of beneficence and nonmaleficence.

The Concept of Harm

The concept of nonmaleficence is frequently explicated using the terms *harm* and *injury*. *Injury* refers to harm, on the one hand, and to injustice, violation, or wrong, on the other.[7] The term *harm* has a similar ambiguity. "X harmed Y" might mean that X wronged Y or treated Y unjustly, or only that X thwarted, defeated, or set back Y's interests. Wronging involves violating someone's rights, whereas harming need not involve a violation. People are harmed without being wronged by diseases, acts of God, and bad luck; and people are wronged without being harmed whenever a wrongful action such as withholding promised information accidentally redounds to their benefit.[8] To explicate the principle of nonmaleficence, we will construe harm only in the second and normatively neutral sense of thwarting, defeating, or setting back the interests of one party by causes that include self-harming conditions as well as the (intentional or unintentional) actions of another party. Therefore, a *harmful* invasion by one party of another's interests may not be *wrong or unjustified*, although it is prima facie wrong. Some harmful actions are justifiable setbacks to another's interests—as, for example, in cases of justified criminal punishment and war, and even in cases of balancing competing interests. As with actions that punish other persons, rightness or wrongness depends on the strength of one's justification for the action. Perhaps even more importantly, what counts as a harm to one person may not be a harm at all to another person, because of their competing visions of what constitutes a setback to interests. We will return to this problem in the chapter on beneficence (pp. 289ff, 293ff, 301ff).

Some definitions of harm are so broad as to include setbacks to reputation, property, privacy, or liberty. Within this broad definition, trivial harms can be distinguished from serious harms by the order and magnitude of the interests affected. Other definitions with a narrower focus view harms exclusively as setbacks to physical and psychological interests, such as those in health and survival. Whether the broad or the narrow account is preferable is not critical for our discussion. We will concentrate on physical harms, including pain, disability, and death, without denying the importance of mental harms and setbacks to other interests. In particular, we will emphasize intending, causing, and permitting death or risk of death.

Rules Supported by the Principle of Nonmaleficence

Because of the many types of harm, the principle of nonmaleficence supports many more specific moral rules (although other principles will also occasionally be called on to help justify these rules). Typical examples of such rules include:[9]

1. "Do not kill."
2. "Do not cause pain or suffering to others."
3. "Do not incapacitate others."
4. "Do not cause offense to others."
5. "Do not deprive others of the goods of life."

Both the principle and its specifications in these moral rules are prima facie, not absolute. As noted above, some philosophers assign a priority in their system to principles and rules that prohibit infliction of harm, but we reject this ordering principle and all similar hierarchical arrangements.[10]

The Standard of Due Care

Obligations of nonmaleficence are obligations of not inflicting harms and not imposing risks of harm. A person can harm or place another person at risk without malicious or harmful intent, and the agent of harm may or may not be morally or legally responsible for the harms. In some cases agents are causally responsible for a harm when they do not intend or are even unaware of the harm caused. For example, if cancer rates are elevated at a chemical plant as the result of exposure to a chemical not previously suspected as a carcinogen, workers have been placed at risk by their employer, although the harm was not intentionally or knowingly caused.

In cases of risk imposition, law and morality recognize a standard of due care that specifies the principle of nonmaleficence. This standard can be met only if the goals sought justify the risks that must be imposed to achieve the goals. Grave risks require commensurately momentous goals for their justification, and emergencies justify risks that are not justified in nonemergency situations. For example, attempting to save lives after a major accident justifies the dangers created by speeding emergency vehicles. Negligence, a departure from the standard of due care toward others, includes intentionally imposing risks that are unreasonable as well as unintentionally but carelessly imposing risks. The term *negligence* applies to several forms of failure to meet obligations, including the failure to guard against risks of harm to others.[11] In treating negligence, we will concentrate on conduct that falls below a standard of due care that is established by law or by morality to protect others from the careless or unreasonable imposition of risks.[12]

Courts often must determine responsibility and liability for harm because a patient, client, or customer seeks compensation for setbacks to interests or punishment of a responsible party, or both. Legal liability will not be considered here, but the legal model of responsibility for harmful action suggests a general framework that can be adapted to express the idea of moral responsibility for harm caused by health care professionals. The following are essential elements in a professional model of due care:

1. The professional must have a duty to the affected party.
2. The professional must breach that duty.
3. The affected party must experience a harm.
4. The harm must be caused by the breach of duty.[13]

Professional malpractice is an instance of negligence in which professional standards of care have not been followed.

For health care professionals, legal and moral standards of due care include proper training, skills, and diligence. In making services available, physicians accept the responsibility to observe these standards. If their conduct falls below these standards, they act negligently. If the therapeutic relationship proves to be harmful or unhelpful, malpractice occurs if and only if professional standards of care are not met. For example, in *Adkins v. Ropp,* the Supreme Court of Indiana considered a patient's claim that a physician had been negligent in removing foreign matter from the patient's eye and that, as a result, the eye became infected and blinded. The court held as follows:

When a physician and surgeon assumes to treat and care for a patient, in the absence of a special agreement, he is held in law to have impliedly contracted that he possesses the reasonable and ordinary qualifications of his profession and that he will exercise at least reasonable skill, care and diligence in his treatment of him. This implied contract on the part of the physician does not include a promise to effect a cure and negligence cannot be imputed because a cure is not effected, but he does impliedly promise that he will use due diligence and ordinary skill in his treatment of the patient so that a cure may follow such care and skill, and this degree of care and skill is required of him, not only in performing an operation or administering first treatments, but he is held to the like degree of care and skill in the necessary subsequent treatments unless he is excused from further service by the patient himself, or the physician or surgeon upon due notice refuses to further treat the case.[14]

The customs, practices, and policies of the medical profession help establish applicable criteria of due care. For example, the Principles of Medical Ethics of the American Medical Association require physicians to provide "competent medical service" and to "continue to study, apply and advance scientific knowledge." In some circumstances, "a physician shall . . . obtain consultation, and use the talents of other health professionals when indicated." Although due care requirements cannot eliminate all mistakes or prevent all harms, they can reduce the probability of harmful outcomes in diagnosis and treatment.

The line between due care and care that falls below or exceeds what is due is often difficult to draw. Health risks can sometimes be reduced—in industry, say—by increased safety measures, by investing in epidemiological and toxicological studies, by educational or health promotional programs, by training programs, and the like. But a substantial question often remains about the lengths to which physicians, employers, and others must go to avoid or lower risks and thereby satisfy due care criteria. We will see below how this problem presents difficulties for determining the scope of obligations of nonmaleficence.

Traditional Distinctions and Rules Governing Nontreatment

Several guidelines have been developed in religious traditions, philosophical discourse, professional codes, and the law to specify requirements of nonmaleficence in health care, particularly with regard to treatment and nontreatment decisions. Some of these guidelines are thorough and helpful, but others should be either revised or replaced.

Several traditional guidelines draw heavily on the following distinctions:

1. Withholding and withdrawing life-sustaining treatment
2. Extraordinary (or heroic) and ordinary treatment
3. Artificial feeding and life-sustaining medical technologies
4. Intended effects and merely foreseen effects

We will argue that these distinctions are all untenable. They are distinctions without a relevant difference and should be replaced by the distinction between obligatory and optional means of treatment and by an account of the benefit–burden ratio. The venerable position that these traditional distinctions occupy in many professional codes, institutional policies, and writings in biomedical ethics does not supply an adequate reason for retaining them. Indeed, some of these distinctions are morally dangerous.

Withholding vs. Withdrawing Treatments

Much debate about the principle of nonmaleficence and forgoing life-sustaining treatments has centered on the omission–commission distinction, especially the distinction between withholding (not starting) and withdrawing (stopping) treatments. Many professionals and family members feel justified in withholding treatments they never started, but not in withdrawing treatments already initiated. They sense that decisions to stop treatments are more momentous and consequential than decisions not to start them. Stopping a respirator, for example, seems to cause the person's death, whereas not starting the respirator seems like a prudent medical decision. But are these beliefs justifiable?

Consider the following case: An elderly man suffered from several major medical problems, including cancer, with no reasonable chance of recovery. Comatose and unable to communicate, he was being kept alive by antibiotics to fight infection and by an intravenous (IV) line to provide nutrition and hydration. No evidence indicated that he had expressed his wishes about life-sustaining treatments while competent, and he had no family members to serve as proxy decisionmakers. The staff quickly agreed on a "no code" or "do not resuscitate" (DNR) order, a signed order that cardiopulmonary resuscitation not be attempted if a cardiac or respiratory arrest occurred. In the event of a cardiac arrest, the patient would be allowed to die. The staff was comfortable with this decision because of the patient's overall condition and prognosis and because not resuscitating the patient could be viewed as withholding rather than withdrawing treatment.

Some members of the health care team thought that all medical treatments, including artificial nutrition, hydration, and antibiotics, should be stopped, because they were "extraordinary" or "heroic." Others, perhaps a majority, thought it was wrong to stop these treatments once they had been started. A disagreement erupted about whether it would be permissible not to insert the IV line again if it became infiltrated—that is, if it broke through the blood vessel and began leaking fluid into surrounding tissue. Some who had opposed stopping treatment felt comfortable about not reinserting the IV line because they viewed the action as withholding rather than withdrawing. They emphatically opposed reinsertion if it required a cutdown (an incision to gain access to the deep large blood vessels) or a central line into the heart. Others viewed the provision of artificial nutrition and hydration as a single process and felt that inserting the IV line again was simply restarting or continuing what had been interrupted. For them, not restarting was equivalent to withdrawing, and thus (unlike withholding) morally wrong.[15]

Caregivers' discomfort about withdrawing life-sustaining treatments appears to reflect the view that such actions render them more responsible for, and therefore culpable for, a patient's death—whereas they are not responsible if they do not initiate a life-sustaining treatment. Another source of caregiver discomfort about withdrawing treatments is the conviction that starting a treatment often creates expectations that it will be continued, whereas stopping it appears to breach expectations, promises, or contractual obligations to the patient and family. Such wrong expectations and misleading promises can and should be avoided from the outset. The appropriate expectation or promise is that caregivers will act in accordance with the patient's interests and wishes (as limited by defensible systems for the allocation of health care and defensible social rules about killing). Withdrawing a particular treatment, including life support, need not involve abandonment of the patient. It can follow the patient's directives and can be accompanied by other modes of care after a life-sustaining treatment is stopped.

Feelings of reluctance about withdrawing treatments are understandable, but the distinction between withdrawing and withholding treatments is morally untenable. The distinction is unclear, inasmuch as withdrawing can happen through an omission (withholding) such as not recharging batteries that power respirators or not putting the infusion into a feeding tube. In multistaged treatments, decisions not to start the next stage of a treatment plan can be tantamount to stopping treatment, even if the early phases of the treatment continue. Is such termination of the overall treatment withdrawing, withholding part of the treatment, or both?

Even if the distinction were clear, starting and stopping can both be justified, depending on the circumstances. Both starting and stopping can cause the death of a patient, and both can be instances of allowing to die. Courts recognize that a crime can be committed by omission if an obligation to act is present, just as a wrong can be committed by omission in medical practice. These judgments depend on whether a physician has an obligation to act in cases of either withholding or withdrawing treatment. In the *Spring* case (Case 5), the court raised a legal problem about continuing kidney dialysis as follows: "The question presented by . . . modern technology is, once undertaken, at what point does it cease to perform its intended function?" This court held that "a physician has no duty to continue treatment, once it has proven to be ineffective." The court emphasized the need to balance benefits and burdens to determine overall effectiveness.[16] Although legal responsibility cannot be equated with moral responsibility in such cases, this conclusion is consistent with the moral conclusions for which we are presently arguing.

Paradoxically, the moral burden of proof often should be heavier when the decision is to withhold than when it is to withdraw treatments.[17] In many cases, only after starting treatments will it be possible to make a proper diagnosis and prognosis as well as to balance prospective benefits and burdens. Uncertainty about outcomes can be reduced by such a trial period. Patients and surrogates often feel less stress and more in control if a decision to treat can be reversed or otherwise changed after it has been begun. Responsible health care, then, may require proposing a trial with periodic reevaluation. Caregivers then have time to judge the effectiveness of the treatment, and the patient or surrogate has time to evaluate its benefits and burdens. Not to propose or allow the test at all is morally worse than not trying.

The distinction between withholding and withdrawing treatment also can lead to overtreatment in some cases—that is, to continuation of a treatment that is no longer beneficial or desirable for the patient. Less obviously, the distinction can lead to undertreatment. Patients and families worry about being trapped by biomedical technology that, once begun, cannot be stopped. To circumvent this problem, they become reluctant to authorize the technology, even when it could be beneficial. Health care professionals often exhibit the same reluctance. In one case, a seriously ill newborn died after several months of treatment, much of it against the parents' wishes, because a physician was unwilling to stop the respirator once it had been connected. Later it was reported that this physician was "less eager to attach babies to respirators now." [18] The distinction between withholding and withdrawing therefore can prevent patients from receiving medical benefits they should have.

We conclude that the distinction between withholding and withdrawing is morally irrelevant. Treatment can always permissibly be withdrawn if it can permissibly be withheld. This distinction, when combined with a reluctance to stop or a reluctance to start treatments under the assumption that they cannot then be stopped, creates dangerous situations for some patients. It also follows from the arguments in Chapter 3 that the patient has a right to forgo treatment at any time. Decisions about beginning or ending treatment should be based on considerations of the patient's rights and welfare, and, therefore, on the benefits and burdens of the treatment as judged by a patient or surrogate. Moreover, if a caregiver makes decisions about treatment using this irrelevant distinction, or allows a surrogate (without efforts at dissuasion) to make such a decision, the caregiver is morally blameworthy for any negative outcomes.

The felt importance of the distinction between not starting and stopping undoubtedly accounts for, although it does not justify, the ease with which hospitals and health care professionals have accepted "no code" or DNR orders. Hospital policies regarding cardiopulmonary resuscitation (CPR), a variety of interventions aimed at restoring function when a cardiac or respiratory arrest occurs, are particularly consequential, because cardiac arrest inevitably occurs in the dying process regardless of the underlying cause of death. CPR is commonly used in an attempt to prolong, at least briefly, the lives of patients who die in hospitals.

Policies regarding CPR are often independent of other policies about life-sustaining technologies, such as respirators, in part because many health care professionals view not providing CPR as withholding rather than withdrawing treatment. Their decisions to provide or not provide CPR are especially problematic when made without advance consultation with patients or their families. [19] DNR orders are often appropriate, and the option of such orders should be provided to patients or surrogates in a variety of circumstances, including terminal illness, irreversible loss of consciousness, and the likelihood of unmanageable cardiac or respiratory arrest. However, it is often unclear to hospital staffs, as well as to patients or their families, what, if anything, DNR orders imply about other levels of care and other technologies. For example, some patients with DNR orders still receive chemotherapy, surgery, and admission to the intensive care unit, whereas others do not. (Providing CPR where it is futile will be examined in Chapter 5.)

It is not justifiable to view decisions about CPR as different from decisions about other life-sustaining technologies. Neither the distinction between withholding and withdrawing treatments nor the distinction between ordinary and extraordinary means of treatment, as we will now argue, provides a justification.

Ordinary vs. Extraordinary Treatments

The distinction between ordinary and extraordinary treatments has been widely invoked both to justify and to condemn decisions to use or forgo life-sustaining treatments. The traditional rule is that extraordinary treatments can legitimately be forgone, but that ordinary treatments cannot legitimately be forgone. It has a prominent history in medical practice, judicial decisions, and Roman Catholic casuistry. This distinction has also been employed to determine whether an act that results in death counts as killing, especially as culpable killing. As developed by Roman Catholic theologians to deal with problems of surgery (prior to the development of antisepsis and anesthesia), this distinction has been used to determine whether a patient's refusal of treatment should be classified as suicide. Refusal of ordinary means of treatment was long considered suicide, but refusal of extraordinary means was not. Likewise, families and physicians did not commit homicide if they withheld or withdrew extraordinary means of treatment from patients.

Unfortunately, neither a long history nor contemporary precedent guarantees clarity or acceptability, and the distinction between ordinary and extraordinary means of treatment is both vague and morally unacceptable. Several problems surround the nature and purpose of the distinction. Throughout its history, several meanings and functions have been assigned to the distinction. *Ordinary* has often been taken to mean "usual" or "customary," whereas *extraordinary* has often been taken to mean "unusual" or "uncustomary." The ordinary has then been interpreted as the customary in medical practice, under either the professional practice standard discussed in Chapter 3 or the due care standard discussed earlier in this chapter. Treatments have been considered extraordinary if they are unusual or uncustomary for physicians to use in the relevant contexts. The terms thereby became attached to particular technologies.

The customary or usual in medical practice can be relevant to a moral judgment, but is not by itself sufficient or decisive. It is customary medical practice to treat a disease by a specific means, but whether this treatment should be repeated for a particular patient depends on the patient's wishes and condition as a whole, not alone on what is customary.[20] For example, treating pneumonia with antibiotics is usual, but it is morally optional for a patient who is irreversibly and imminently dying from cancer or AIDS. Ethical judgment is not reducible to professional custom, consensus, traditional codes, or oaths, as indispensable as these are for some professional contexts.

Criteria other than usual and unusual medical practice have also been proposed for the extraordinary procedures. These criteria include whether the treatment is simple or complex, natural or artificial, noninvasive or highly invasive, inexpensive or expensive, and routine or heroic. These substitutions are rarely analyzed with care and usually reduce to or mark no advance over *usual* and *unusual*. If a treatment is simple, natural, noninvasive, inexpensive, or routine, it is more likely to be viewed as ordinary (and thus obligatory) than if it is complex, artificial, invasive, expensive, or heroic (and thus optional). But these criteria are relevant only if some deeper moral considerations make them relevant. For instance, if a complex treatment is available and in accordance with the patient's wishes and interests, it is difficult to see why morally it should be distinguished from a simple treatment in accordance with the patient's wishes and interests. Similar confusions surround the criteria of the natural and the artificial. According to one study, physicians typically view respirators, dialyzers, and resuscitators as artificial; but they split evenly on intravenous feeding, and two-thirds view insulin, antibiotics, and chemotherapy as natural. They usually view mechanical systems as more artificial than drugs and other treatments.[21]

More consequential than these conceptual problems is whether such distinctions give sound moral guidance for treatment and nontreatment decisions. All treatments that fall into these classifications are sometimes beneficial for patients, sometimes burdensome; the principal consideration is whether a treatment is beneficial or burdensome, not its form. Thus, these distinctions appear irrelevant except insofar as they point to a quality-of-life criterion that requires balancing benefits against burdens. The need to balance benefits and burdens of treatments appears in the following influential exposition of the ordinary-extraordinary distinction:

Ordinary means are all medicines, treatments, and operations which offer a reasonable hope of benefit and which can be obtained and used without excessive expense, pain, or other inconvenience. Extraordinary means are all medicines, treatments, and operations, which cannot be obtained or used without excessive expense, pain, or other inconvenience, or which, if used, would not offer a reasonable hope of benefit.[22]

If excessiveness is to be determined by the probability and magnitude of the benefit, as weighed against the likely burdens, this distinction will in the end reduce to the balance of burdens and benefits. If no reasonable hope of benefit exists, then any expense, pain, or other inconvenience is excessive, and it is sometimes obligatory not to treat. If a reasonable hope of benefit exists, along with significant burdensomeness, the treatment is optional. Competent patients have a right to make decisions about treatment in light of their assessment of burdens and benefits, and for incompetent patients the treatment is not obligatory if a high level of burdensomeness is present. The ordinary–extraordinary distinction thus collapses into the balance between benefits and burdens, where the latter category includes immediate detriment, inconvenience, risk of harm, and other costs.

We conclude that the distinction between ordinary and extraordinary treatment is morally irrelevant and should be replaced by the distinction between optional and obligatory treatment, as determined by the balance of benefits and burdens to the patient.

Sustenance Technologies vs. Medical Technologies

In recent years there has been widespread debate about whether the distinction between *medical* technologies and *sustenance* technologies that supply nutrition and hydration using needles, tubes, catheters, and the like can legitimately be used to distinguish justified and unjustified forgoing of life-sustaining treatments. Some argue that technologies of caregiving for dispensing sustenance, such as artificially administered nutrition and hydration, are *nonmedical* means of maintaining life that are unlike optional forms of medical life-sustaining treatment, such as respirators and dialysis machines. To determine whether this distinction is more acceptable than the previous distinctions, we begin with three cases.

First, consider the case of a seventy-nine-year-old widow who had been a resident of a nursing home for several years. In the past she had experienced repeated transient ischemic attacks (caused by reductions or stoppages of blood flow to the brain). Because of progressive organic brain syndrome, she had lost most of her mental abilities and had become disoriented. She also had thrombophlebitis (inflammation of a vein associated with clotting) and congestive heart failure. Her daughter and grandchildren visited her frequently and loved her deeply. One day she suffered a massive stroke. She made no recovery, remaining obtunded and nonverbal, but she continued to manifest a withdrawal reaction to painful stimuli and exhibited some purposeful behaviors. She strongly resisted a nasogastric tube being placed in her stomach to introduce nutritional formulas and water. At each attempt she thrashed about violently and pushed the tube away. When the tube was finally placed, she managed to remove it. After several days on intravenous lines, the sites for inserting IV lines were exhausted. The staff debated whether to take further "extraordinary" measures to maintain fluid and nutritional intake for this elderly patient who had failed to improve and was largely unaware and unresponsive. After lengthy discussions with nurses on the floor and with the patient's family, the physicians in charge reached the conclusion that they should not provide further IVs, cutdowns, or a feeding tube. The patient had minimal oral intake and died quietly the following week.[23]

Second, in a ground-breaking case in 1976 the New Jersey Supreme Court held that it was permissible for a guardian to disconnect Karen Ann Quinlan's respirator and allow her to die.[24] After the respirator was removed, she lived for almost ten years, protected by antibiotics and sustained by nutrition and hydration provided through a nasogastric tube. Unable to communicate, she lay comatose in a fetal position, with increasing respiratory problems, bedsores, and weight loss (from 115 to 70 pounds). A moral issue developed over the course of those ten years. If it is permissible to remove the respirator, is it permissible for the same reasons to remove the feeding tube? Several Roman Catholic moral theologians advised the parents that they were not morally required to continue medically administered nutrition and hydration (MN&H) or antibiotics to fight infections. Nevertheless, the Quinlans continued MN&H because they believed that the feeding tube did not cause pain, whereas the respirator had.

Third, while Karen Quinlan lingered, the same state supreme court faced another case involving artificial nutrition and hydration in which a guardian requested withdrawal of MN&H for an eighty-four-year-old nursing home resident. The court held that the provision of nutrition and hydration through nasogastric tubes and other medical means is not always legally required.[25] A similar decision was soon reached in the Brophy case in Massachusetts, involving a forty-nine-year-old man who had been in a persistent vegetative state for more than three years.[26] Courts have since increasingly maintained that no relevant difference distinguishes MN&H from other life-support measures. They have viewed MN&H as a medical procedure subject to the same standards as other medical procedures and thus sometimes unjustifiably burdensome.[27] A similar discussion about MN&H has surfaced in treatment decisions about newborns who are seriously ill or severely disabled.

Whether one is confronted with an elderly woman, a twenty-year-old youth, or an infant, the same moral question is present: Should such medical procedures be construed as obligatory or as optional, and under which circumstances?[28] We maintain that MN&H may justifiably be forgone in some circumstances, as is true of other life-sustaining technologies. The chief premises in our argument are (1) that no morally relevant difference exists between various life-sustaining technologies and (2) that the right to refuse medical treatment is not contingent on the type of treatment. We find no reason to believe that MN&H is always an essential part of palliative care or that it necessarily constitutes, on balance, a beneficial medical treatment.

Although our view is consistent with many recent court decisions, professional codes, and philosophical arguments, it remains controversial. Philosopher G. E. M. Anscombe contends that, "For wilful starvation there can be no excuse. The same can't be said quite without qualification about failing to operate or to adopt some course of treatment." [29] C. Everett Koop, former Surgeon General of the United States, denounces practices of allowing newborns to die (including by omitting MN&H) as infanticide by "starving a child to death;" [30] he likewise condemns similar practices for adults as intentional acts of killing that amount to active euthanasia because they cause a preventable death. [31] Others maintain that MN&H are not relevantly similar to other treatments in medicine and that no moral principle requires or permits the judgments about MN&H that are legitimately made about other medical procedures. From this perspective, although it is legitimate to omit some forms of treatment, MN&H cannot justifiably be omitted.

Three main arguments have been advanced in defense of this position, and each directly challenges our position. The first argument holds that MN&H are required because they are necessary for the patient's comfort and dignity. This view underlies the controversial rule once proposed by the U.S. Department of Health and Human Services for treatment of disabled newborns: "The basic provision of nourishment, fluids, and routine nursing care is a fundamental matter of human dignity, not an option for medical judgment." [32] This rule includes all means of providing nutrition and hydration. A similar conviction about patient comfort and dignity underlies the exclusionary clause in several natural death acts that disallow advance directives about artificial nutrition and hydration, while permitting advance directives for nonsustenance procedures that prolong life. [33]

A second argument that MN&H are never optional focuses on symbolic significance. Medical professionals generally find it intuitively devastating to "starve" someone. Provision of nutrition and hydration symbolizes the essence of care and compassion in medical as well as nonmedical contexts. As Daniel Callahan puts it, feeding the hungry and nursing by nourishing are "the rudimentary healing gesture" and "the perfect symbol of the fact that human life is inescapably social and communal." [34] Our experiences of thirst and hunger enhance this symbol. Thirst and hunger are uncomfortable, and we infer that severe malnutrition and dehydration must involve extreme agony.

The third argument is a version of the wedge or slippery slope argument considered later in this chapter. The controlling idea is that policies of not providing MN&H will lead to adverse consequences because society will not be able to limit decisions about MN&H to legitimate cases, especially under pressures for cost containment in health care. Whereas "death with dignity" first emerged as a compassionate response to the threat of overtreatment, patients now face the threat of undertreatment because of pressures to contain the escalating costs of health care. Such concerns about psychological and social barriers focus on a slide from acting in the patient's interests to acting in the society's interests, from considering the patient's quality of life to considering the patient's value for society, from decisions about terminally ill patients to decisions about nondying patients, from letting die to killing, and from cessation of artificial feeding to cessation of natural feeding. The fear is that the "right to die" will be transformed into the "obligation to die," perhaps against the patient's wishes and interests.[35]

We have several reservations about these three arguments. Whether the rationale is life prolongation or patient comfort and dignity, an absolute requirement to provide medically assisted nutrition and hydration has serious drawbacks. Procedures of MN&H themselves sometimes involve risks of harm, discomfort, and indignity, such as pain from a central IV and physical restraints that prevent patients from removing the lines or tubes. Evidence also indicates that patients who are allowed to die without artificial hydration sometimes die more comfortably than patients who receive such hydration. It is often misleading to project the common experience of hunger and thirst on a dying patient who is malnourished and dehydrated. Malnutrition is not identical with hunger; dehydration is not identical with thirst; and starvation is very different from acute dehydration in a medical setting. Feelings of hunger, thirst, dryness of the mouth, and related problems also can be alleviated by other means, such as ice on the lips, without introducing MN&H.[36]

For some patients the burdens of MN&H outweigh their benefits, and no one should deprive them of the right to refuse treatment. The obligation to care for patients entails provision of treatments that are in accordance with their preferences and interests (within the limits set by just allocation policies), not the provision of treatments because of what they symbolize in the larger society. In an approach that represents a compromise for physicians who want to engage in symbolically significant actions, while also acting in accord with the patient's wishes and interests, some physicians start and continue IV lines at a rate that will result in dehydration over time.[37] This approach is both risky and deceptive. These physicians fail to acknowledge their final objective, which is that the patient will become dehydrated and malnourished, and die as a result. The act resulting in death is intentional, and death at the time it occurs is a foreseen and avoidable consequence.

The fears underlying the third argument about the slippery slope are legitimate and troubling because of uncertainties about whether lines can be drawn and maintained in order to prevent abuses. Perhaps eighty percent of the over two million people who die each year in the United States die in nursing homes or hospitals under the care of strangers, often at considerable cost to their families and to the society.[38] These and other patients in long-term care are vulnerable, and we should be concerned about the potential loss of broad moral commitments that form the cement of our social universe. However, no evidence exists that the protection of these patients requires that MN&H be provided in all circumstances or that the emotions underlying the symbol of providing nutrition and hydration are either necessary or sufficient to avert social disaster.

We conclude that it is sometimes legitimate to remove MN&H, paving the way for death and that the presumption in favor of MN&H can be successfully rebutted under the following conditions: (1) The procedures are highly unlikely to improve nutritional and fluid levels. (2) The procedures will improve nutritional and fluid levels, but the patient will not benefit (for example, in cases of anencephaly or permanent vegetative state). (3) The procedures will improve nutritional and fluid levels and the patient will benefit, but the burdens of MN&H outweigh the benefits. For example, for a severely demented patient, essential physical restraints can cause fear and discomfort, especially as the patient struggles to break free of the restraints.

Intended Effects vs. Merely Foreseen Effects

We have thus far rejected or revised several traditional rules and distinctions in medical ethics. Another venerable attempt to specify the principle of nonmaleficence appears in the rule of double effect (RDE), often called the principle or doctrine of double effect. This rule too has a pivotal distinction, viz. between intended effects (or consequences) and foreseen effects (or consequences). The RDE is invoked to justify claims that a single act having two foreseen effects, one good and one harmful (such as death), is not always morally prohibited if the harmful effect is not intended.[39]

Functions and conditions of the RDE. The RDE finds its natural setting in ethical theories that view certain actions as intrinsically and absolutely wrong, including theories that prohibit the direct infliction of harm on innocent persons.[40] The RDE is one attempt to specify the conditions of the principle of nonmaleficence for situations in which an agent cannot avoid all harms and still achieve important goods.

As an example of the use of the RDE, consider a patient experiencing terrible pain and suffering who asks a physician for help in ending his life. If the physician directly kills the patient to end the patient's pain and suffering, the patient's death is caused intentionally as a means to relieve pain and suffering. But suppose that the physician could provide medication to relieve the patient's pain and suffering at a substantial risk that the patient will die earlier as a result of the medication. If the physician refuses to administer the toxic analgesia, the patient will be harmed by continuing pain and suffering; if the physician provides the medication, the patient's death may be hastened. Under the RDE, the physician's provision of medication must be intended to relieve grave pain and suffering and must not be intended to hasten death. If no intention of a lethal effect exists, this act is not prohibited by the principle "Do not directly and intentionally harm the innocent."

According to classical formulations of the RDE, four conditions or elements must be satisfied for an act with a double effect to be justified. Each is a necessary condition, and together they form sufficient conditions of morally permissible action: [41]

1. *The nature of the act.* The act must be good, or at least morally neutral (independent of its consequences).
2. *The agent's intention.* The agent intends only the good effect. The bad effect can be foreseen, tolerated, and permitted, but it must not be intended.
3. *The distinction between means and effects.* The bad effect must not be a means to the good effect. If the good effect were the direct causal result of the bad effect, the agent would intend the bad effect in pursuit of the good effect.
4. *Proportionality between the good effect and the bad effect.* The good effect must outweigh the bad effect. The bad effect is permissible only if a proportionate reason is present that compensates for permitting the foreseen bad effect.

Controversy has surrounded all four of these traditional conditions. We begin our analysis by considering four cases of what many call therapeutic abortion (limited to protection of maternal life in these examples). (A) A pregnant woman has cancer of the cervix; a hysterectomy is needed to save her life, but it will result in the death of the fetus. (B) A pregnant woman has an ectopic pregnancy—the nonviable fetus is in the fallopian tube—and removal of the tube, which will result in the death of the fetus, is medically indicated to prevent hemorrhage. (C) A pregnant woman has a serious heart disease that will probably result in her death if she attempts to carry the pregnancy to term. (D) A pregnant woman in difficult labor will die unless a craniotomy (crushing the head of the unborn fetus) is performed. Official Roman Catholic teaching and many moral philosophers and theologians hold that actions that produce fetal deaths in cases A and B sometimes satisfy the four conditions of the RDE and therefore are morally acceptable, whereas the actions that produce fetal deaths in cases C and D never meet the conditions of the RDE and therefore are morally unacceptable. [42]

In the first two cases, according to the RDE, a physician undertakes a legitimate medical procedure aimed at saving the pregnant woman's life with the foreseen, but unintended, result of fetal death. Viewed as side effects that are not intended (rather than as ends or means), these fetal deaths can be justified by a proportionately grave reason (saving the pregnant woman). In both cases

C and D, the action of killing the fetus as a means to save the pregnant woman's life requires intending the death (even if the death is not desired). Therefore, in those cases it is not permissible to consider proportionality.

Critics of the RDE contend that it is difficult and perhaps impossible to establish a morally relevant difference between cases such as A (hysterectomy) and D (craniotomy) through RDE conditions. In neither case does the agent want or desire the death of the fetus, and the descriptions of the acts in these cases do not indicate morally relevant differences. It is not clear why craniotomy is killing the fetus rather than crushing the skull of the fetus with the unintended result that the fetus dies. It is also not clear why in the hysterectomy case the death is foreseen but not intended. A proponent of the RDE must have a practicable way to distinguish the intended from the merely foreseen, but it has proved difficult to draw defensible moral lines between various cases like the hysterectomy and craniotomy cases. Some modern reformulations of the RDE (especially those emphasizing the fourth condition) even permit craniotomies to save the pregnant woman's life because of the proportional value of the woman's life.[43]

Critique of the RDE. Adherents of the RDE need an account of intentional actions and intended effects of action (intentionally causing or allowing) that properly distinguishes them from nonintentional actions and unintended effects (foreseeably causing or allowing). The literature on intentional action is itself highly controversial and focuses on diverse conditions such as volition, deliberateness, willing, reasoning, and planning. One of the few widely shared views in this literature is that intentional actions require an agent's plan—a blueprint, map, or representation of the means and ends proposed for the execution of an action.[44] For an action to be intentional, it must correspond to the agent's conception of how it was planned to be performed.

Alvin Goldman uses the following example in an attempt to prove that merely foreseen effects are unintentional.[45] Imagine that Mr. G is taking a driver's test to prove competence. He comes to an intersection that requires a right turn and extends his arm to signal for a turn, although he knows it is raining and his hand will become wet. According to Goldman, Mr. G's signaling for a turn is an intentional act. By contrast, his getting a wet hand is an unintended effect or "incidental by-product." The defender of the RDE elects a similarly narrow conception of what is intended in order to avoid the unacceptable conclusion that an agent intentionally brings about all the consequences of an action that the agent foresees. The defender distinguishes between acts and effects, and then between (1) effects that are desired or wanted and (2) effects that are foreseen but not desired or wanted. The latter effects are viewed in RDE as foreseen, but not intended.

However, it is better to discard the language of desiring and wanting altogether, and to say that these effects are "tolerated."[46] These effects are not so undesirable that the actor would choose not to perform the act that results in them, and they are a part of the plan of an intentional action. If we use a model of intentionality based on what is *willed* rather than what is *wanted,* intentional actions and intentional effects include any action and any effect willed in accordance with a plan, including tolerated as well as wanted effects.[47] On this conception, a physician can desire not to do what he intends to do, in the same way that we can be willing to do something but, at the same time, be reluctant to do it or even detest doing it. Undesirable effects or risks of harm that attend particular procedures usually fall into this category. Under this conception of intentional acts and intended effects, the distinction between what is intended and what is merely foreseen is not viable.[48]

Thus, a person who knowingly and voluntarily acts to bring about an effect brings about that effect intentionally. The effect is intended, although the person did not desire it, did not will it for its own sake, or did not intend it as the goal of the action. For example, if a man enters a room and flips a switch that he knows turns on both a light and a fan, but desires only to activate the light, he cannot say that he activates the fan unintentionally. Although the fan makes an obnoxious whirring that he desires to avoid, it would be conceptually mistaken to say that he unintentionally brought about the obnoxious sound by flipping the switch.

Finally, the moral relevance of the RDE and its distinctions must be considered. Is it plausible to distinguish morally between intentionally causing the death of a fetus by craniotomy and intentionally removing a cancerous uterus that causes the death of a fetus? In both actions, the intention is to save the woman's life with knowledge that the fetus will be lost. No agent desires a bad result (the fetus's death) for its own sake, and none would have tolerated the bad result if its avoidance were morally preferable. Each party accepts the bad effect only because it cannot be eliminated without losing the good effect. Accordingly, the agents in our various examples above do not appear to want, will, or intend in ways that make a moral difference.

In the standard interpretation of the RDE, the fetus's death is a *means* to saving a woman's life in the unacceptable case, but merely a *side effect* in the acceptable case; a means is intended, whereas a side effect need not be. But this approach seems to allow almost anything to be foreseen as a side effect rather than intended as a means (although this is not to claim that we can create or direct intentions as we please). For example, in the craniotomy case, the surgeon might not intend the death of the fetus but only intend to remove it from the birth canal. The fetus will die, but is this outcome more than an unwanted and (in double effect theory) unintended consequence?[49]

There may be a way out of these puzzles for defenders of the RDE, but it is doubtful that the way has yet been found.[50] Meanwhile, other criticisms need to be answered. Critics who accept a broadly consequentialist approach argue that unacceptable consequences must be deemed acceptable in the doctrine of double effect. For example, slowly causing death by administering medication to reduce pain can involve painful days or weeks of a life that a patient wishes to end, whereas a more active means to death, such as a larger and lethal dose of the same painkiller, would end life more quickly and with less pain. Critics charge that the RDE forces its exponents to accept less humane methods of ending human life than should be provided.

One constructive effort to retain an emphasis on intention without entirely abandoning or neglecting the point of the RDE focuses on the way actions display a person's motives and character. From this perspective, the core issue is whether a person's conduct flows from a proper motivational structure and a good character. Often in evaluating persons we are more concerned with their *motivation* to perform an action (why they performed the action) than with their *intention* in performing the action (what they planned to do). The intention to kill another person may be less relevant morally than the motive in doing so— for example, self-defense or defense of an innocent third party. When juries hear cases of mercy killing, the intention to kill is morally and legally pertinent, but the crucial moral assessment is often the motive behind the killing, not the intention to kill. The motive to relieve suffering is, of course, entirely consistent with the intention to kill.

In the case of performing a craniotomy to save a pregnant woman's life, the action need not be motivated by a disregard for human life or by a positive desire to end it. A physician may not *want* or *desire* the death of the fetus in this case and may regret performing a craniotomy, just as much as in the case of removing a cancerous uterus. Such facts about the physician's motivation and character can make a decisive difference to a moral assessment of the action and the agent. But the RDE is unable to reach this conclusion on its own. In effect, our proposal to focus on motivation transforms the RDE into another moral framework. We develop the acceptable features of this framework in Chapter 8.

Even if one accepts the RDE, it will be irrelevant in many pressing problems about harm and killing that are currently under discussion in biomedical ethics, including the issues surrounding assisted suicide and euthanasia that we consider later in this chapter. The RDE is fashioned exclusively for cases with both a bad and a good effect, but often the central matter in dispute is whether an effect such as death is bad. Nothing in the RDE decides this issue. For example, one cannot decide from the RDE whether voluntary active euthanasia produces a bad effect or a good effect, because this premise must be defended or rejected on independent grounds.

Some parts of the RDE are perfectly acceptable—for example, the rule that a harmful effect is justifiably allowed only if a proportionately weighty good will probably be brought about. But as we will now see, this latter rule can be put to many uses in biomedical ethics beyond those permitted by the full RDE.

Optional Treatments and Obligatory Treatments

We have now rejected several of the leading distinctions and rules about forgoing life-sustaining treatment sanctioned by various traditions of medical ethics. We do not deny that some of these traditional distinctions are deeply embedded in the beliefs and guidelines of many health care professions, as well as in the policies and practices of many health care institutions. However, the key question is whether the health care professions and institutions need to revise their traditional beliefs to accommodate a broader and more compelling moral perspective, including patients' rights of autonomy.

We will now propose a replacement distinction—viz. between obligatory and optional treatments—and explain why this distinction is more suitable. In doing so, we will rely heavily on an analysis of quality of life that is largely incompatible with the distinctions we have rejected. The following categories are central to our arguments:

I. Obligatory to Treat (Wrong Not to Treat)
II. Optional Whether to Treat
    A. Neutral (Neither Required nor Prohibited)
    B. Supererogatory (Surpassing Obligation)
III. Obligatory Not to Treat (Wrong to Treat)

Most ethical discussions have focused on I and II, with only scant attention to different interpretations of II. A treatment is optional, under IIA, if it is morally neutral whether a physician provides it, a surrogate authorizes or refuses it, and the like. It is optional, under II B, if providing it would be supererogatory and therefore praiseworthy, while not providing it would not be morally blameworthy. These terms are used to indicate a variety of actions, including those involving expenditure of additional time, effort, energy, and resources when a very limited chance of success is present. (For a discussion of the terms *supererogatory* and *praiseworthy,* see Chapter 8.)

Under category III, is it ever wrong to treat (or obligatory not to treat)? The principles of nonmaleficence and beneficence establish a presumption in favor of providing life-sustaining treatments for sick and injured patients, but they also indicate conditions for rebutting that presumption. In addition, life-sustaining treatments sometimes violate patients' interests. For example, pain can be so severe and physical restraints so burdensome that they outweigh anticipated benefits such as brief prolongation of life. In these circumstances, providing the treatment is sometimes inhumane or cruel and therefore in violation of the principle of nonmaleficence. It will often—perhaps usually—be difficult to determine the balance of benefits and burdens to the incompetent patient, particularly when he or she has never lived as a competent person expressing values. However, the burdens can so outweigh the benefits to the incompetent patient that the treatment is wrong rather than optional, just as in the case of a competent patient who refuses treatment.

We reserve a systematic treatment of cost–benefit and risk–benefit assessment for the next chapter. Our concern at present is with substantive standards that distinguish obligatory and optional treatments. Competent patients who can make informed and voluntary choices should have more latitude than other parties in balancing benefits and burdens and in accepting and refusing treatment. As noted throughout this chapter, the incompetent patient's vulnerability to harm sometimes requires actions, based on principles of nonmaleficence and beneficence, that would violate respect for a competent patient's autonomy unless authorized by that patient.

Conditions for Overriding the Prima Facie Obligation to Treat

Several conditions justify decisions to omit treatment by patients, surrogates, or health care professionals. We introduce these conditions in this section.

Futile or pointless treatment. Treatment is not obligatory when it offers no benefit to the patient because it is pointless or futile. Several treatments fit this description. For example, if a patient is dead, although still on a respirator, he or she can no longer be harmed by cessation of treatment, and a standard of medical best interests does not dictate treatment. However, in some religious and personal belief systems, a patient is not considered dead according to the criteria recognized in health care institutions. For example, if heart and lung function can be maintained, some religious traditions hold that the person is not dead, and the treatment is therefore not futile, even if it is deemed futile by health care professionals. This is the tip of an iceberg of controversies that surround the notion of futility.

Typically we think of the term *futile* as referring to a situation in which patients who are irreversibly dying have reached a point at which further treatment provides no physiological benefit or is hopeless and becomes optional, although palliative interventions (those intended to alleviate discomfort, pain, and suffering, but not to cure) may need to be continued. This model, however, covers only a narrow range of cases that have been *labeled* futile in the literature on the subject. All of the following have been referred to as futile treatments: whatever is highly unlikely to be efficacious (statistically the odds of success are exceedingly small), a low-grade outcome that is virtually certain (qualitatively the results are expected to be exceedingly poor), whatever is highly likely to be more burdensome than beneficial, and whatever is completely speculative because it is an untried "treatment." Thus, the term *futility* is now used to cover both situations of predicted impossibility and situations in which there are competing interpretations of probabilities and competing value judgments such as a balance of probable benefits and burdens (as we discuss below and in Chapter 5).[51] This situation of equivocation and ambiguity suggests that the term *futility* generally should be avoided in favor of more precise language.

Ideally in cases involving either those who are dead or those who are irreversibly dying, objective medical factors and expert judgment are central. Realistically, though, this ideal is difficult to satisfy in setting criteria of futility and in making judgments of futility. Disagreement often exists in the medical community, and conflicts may arise from a family's belief in a possible miracle, a religious tradition's insistence on doing everything in such a circumstance, and so forth. It is sometimes difficult to know whether a judgment of futility is based on a probabilistic prediction of failure or on something closer to medical certainty. If an elderly patient has a one percent chance of surviving an arduous and painful regimen, one physician may call the procedure futile and another may view survival as an unlikely outcome but still a possibility that should be considered. We here encounter a value judgment about what is worth the effort, as well as a judgment based on scientific knowledge. "Futility" is typically used to express a combined value judgment and scientific judgment, although many people mistakenly construe judgments of futility as value free.

Writings in biomedical ethics that discuss futility often focus on the patient's or surrogate's right to refuse futile treatment. However, circumstances have increasingly appeared in which the question is whether the physician may or should refuse to provide some treatment. The fact that a treatment is futile is often said to change the physician's moral relationship to patients or surrogates. The physician is not required to provide such treatment and sometimes is not required to discuss the treatment. These circumstances commonly involve incompetent persons, especially patients in a persistent vegetative state (PVS), where physicians or hospital policies impose decisions to forgo life-support on patients or surrogates. Increasingly hospitals are adopting policies explicitly aimed at denying therapies that are judged futile by physicians, especially after the therapy has been tried for a reasonable period of time.

The possibility of judgmental error by physicians should lead to caution in formulating these policies, but, at the same time, unreasonable demands by patients and families should not preclude reasonable policies by health care institutions. Here, as well as elsewhere, respect for the autonomy of patients is not a trump that allows them alone to determine whether a treatment is required or is futile. In one case, Mr. C. was irreversibly dying from emphysema and insisted on having his life prolonged as long as possible by all available means. He demanded aggressive treatment, although the staff considered the treatment futile. When he became unconscious, his family and the staff had to decide whether to respect their earlier agreement with him or let him die. Without a prior statement of Mr. C.'s wishes, there would be no moral difficulty in terminating treatment that was only prolonging his dying. But even with the prior agreement, following Mr. C.'s previous wishes might not be justified because of the combination of futility and limited health care resources.[52] For instance, if other patients who were not irreversibly dying could not otherwise gain access to the ventilator and space in the intensive care unit, we would not be obligated to continue treatment.

The upshot is that a pointless or futile treatment, in the sense of a treatment that has no chance of being efficacious, is morally optional but that other putatively futile treatments are often not optional.

Burdens of treatment outweigh benefits. A mistaken assumption about law and ethics sometimes found in medical codes is that life-sustaining treatments may be terminated only if a patient is terminally ill. If the patient is not terminally ill, life-sustaining medical treatment is still not obligatory if its burdens outweigh its benefits to the patient. Medical treatment for those not terminally ill is sometimes optional, although it could prolong life for an indefinite period and the patient is incompetent and has left no advance directive.[53]

The principle of nonmaleficence does not imply the maintenance of biological life, nor does it require the initiation or continuation of treatment without regard to the patient's pain, suffering, and discomfort. In Case 5, seventy-eight-year-old Earle Spring developed numerous medical problems, including chronic organic brain syndrome and kidney failure. The latter problem was controlled by hemodialysis. Although several aspects of this case are in dispute—such as whether Spring was conscious, aware, and able to express his wishes—there is at least a plausible argument that the family and health care professionals were not morally obligated to continue hemodialysis, because of the balance of benefits and burdens to the patient. This case, like many others, is complicated by the fact that the family had a conflict of interest because of their obligations both to pay mounting and burdensome health care costs and to make judgments about the patient's best interests.

Few decisions are more momentous than those to withhold or withdraw a medical procedure that sustains life. But in some cases it is unjustified for surrogates and clinicians to begin or to continue therapy knowing that it will produce a greater balance of pain and suffering for a patient incapable of choosing for or against such therapy. As the supreme judicial court of Massachusetts once held, "the 'best interests' of an incompetent person are not necessarily served by imposing on such persons results not mandated as to competent persons similarly situated."[54]

The Centrality of Quality-of-Life Judgments

Controversies about quality-of-life judgments. Our arguments thus far give considerable weight to quality-of-life judgments in determining whether treatments are optional or obligatory. When quality of life is sufficiently low that an intervention produces more harm than benefit for the patient, it is justifiable to withhold or to withdraw treatment. Such judgments require justified criteria of benefits and burdens, so that quality of life is not reduced to arbitrary judgments of personal preference and the social worth of the patient.

In a landmark case involving quality-of-life judgments, sixty-eight-year-old Joseph Saikewicz, who had an IQ of 10 and a mental age of approximately two years and eight months, suffered from acute myeloblastic monocytic leukemia. Chemotherapy would have produced extensive suffering and possibly serious side effects. Remission under chemotherapy occurs in only thirty to fifty percent of such cases and typically only for between two and thirteen months. Without chemotherapy, Saikewicz could be expected to live for several weeks or perhaps several months, during which he would not experience severe pain or suffering. In not ordering treatment, the lower court considered "the quality of life available to him [Saikewicz] even if the treatment does bring about remission." The supreme judicial court of Massachusetts, however, rejected this formulation if construed to equate the value of life with a measure of the quality of life—in particular, with Saikewicz's lower quality of life because of mental retardation. The court interpreted "the vague, and perhaps ill-chosen, term 'quality of life' . . . as a reference to the continuing state of pain and disorientation precipitated by the chemotherapy treatment."[55] It thus balanced prospective benefit against pain and suffering, finally determining that the patient's interests supported a decision not to provide chemotherapy. From a moral standpoint, we agree with the reasoning and conclusion reached in this legal opinion.

Slogans such as "quality of life" sometimes are more misleading than illuminating and thus need careful analysis. Some writers propose that we reject *moral* judgments about quality of life and rely exclusively on *medical* indications for treatment decisions. Paul Ramsey, for example, argues that for incompetent patients we need only determine which treatment is medically indicated to know which treatment is obligatory and which is optional. For dying patients, responsibilities are not fixed by obligations to provide treatments that serve only to extend the dying process, but rather by obligations to provide appropriate care in dying. The choices are thus between further palliative treatments and no treatments. Ramsey worries that unless we use these guidelines we will gradually move toward a policy of active, involuntary euthanasia for unconscious or incompetent, nondying patients, based on quality-of-life judgments.[56]

However, putatively objective medical factors—such as general criteria used to determine medical indications for treatment—cannot provide what Ramsey envisions. It is impossible to determine what will benefit a patient without presupposing some quality-of-life standard and some conception of the life the patient will live after a medical intervention. Good examples are patients in a condition of permanent unconsciousness, such as Karen Ann Quinlan and Nancy Cruzan. Accurate medical diagnosis and prognosis are indispensable, but a judgment about whether to use life-prolonging measures rests unavoidably on the anticipated quality of life. The benefits of life-prolonging treatment to a permanently unconscious patient are often so limited as to render the treatment optional.[57] Unless the maintenance of mere biological life is a benefit, any benefit to the patient would appear to reside in the possibility of a diagnostic or prognostic error or of a medical breakthrough, rather than in the quality of the life that is prolonged.

Ramsey has objected that a quality-of-life approach wrongly shifts the focus from whether treatments are beneficial to patients to whether patients' lives are beneficial to them. Questioning the latter, he insists, opens the door to active, involuntary euthanasia.[58] But the principal issue is whether criteria of quality of life can be stated with sufficient precision and cogency to avoid the dangers envisioned by wedge arguments. We think they can, but the vagueness surrounding terms such as *dignity* and *meaningful life* is a cause for concern, and cases in which seriously ill or disabled newborn infants have been "allowed to die" under questionable justifications provide a reason for caution.

Several conditions of patients should be excluded from consideration. For example, mental retardation is irrelevant in determining whether treatment is in the patient's best interest. Quality of life for the patient should also not be confused with the quality or the value of life for others, and proxies should not refuse treatment against the incompetent patient's interests to avoid burdens to the family or costs to society. The incompetent patient's best medical interests generally should be the decisive criterion for a proxy, even if these interests conflict with familial interests.

The President's Commission for the Study of Ethical Problems in Medicine and Biomedical and Behavioral Research recognized a broader conception of best interests that includes the welfare of the family: "The impact of a decision on an incapacitated patient's loved ones may be taken into account in determining someone's best interests, for most people do have an important interest in the well-being of their families or close associates."[59] True, a patient sometimes has an interest in the family's welfare, but it is a long step from this premise to a conclusion about whose interests should be overriding. When the incompetent patient has never been competent or never expressed his or her wishes while competent, it is not proper to impute altruism—a desire to relieve the family of its burdens—to that patient against his or her medical best interests.[60]

Children with serious illnesses or disabilities. Some of the most difficult questions about quality of life and treatment omission involve endangered near-term fetuses, seriously ill newborns, and young children. Prenatal obstetric management and neonatal intensive care can now salvage the lives of many anomalous fetuses and disabled newborns with physical conditions that would have been fatal two decades ago. However, the resultant quality of life is sometimes so low that it raises questions about whether the aggressive obstetric management or intensive care has produced more harm than benefit for the patient. Some commentators argue that avoidance of harm (including iatrogenic harm) is the best guide to decisions on behalf of fetuses and infants in neonatal nurseries,[61] whereas others argue that aggressive intervention violates the obligation of nonmaleficence if any one of three conditions is present: "inability to survive infancy, inability to live without severe pain, and inability to participate, at least minimally, in human experience."[62]

We accept the conclusion that nonaggressive management of high-risk pregnancies and allowing seriously disabled newborns to die are under some conditions morally permissible actions, because they do not violate obligations of nonmaleficence and satisfy other justifying conditions. When quality of life is so low that aggressive intervention or intensive care produces more harm than benefit for the patient, it is justifiable to withhold or to withdraw treatment from fetuses, newborns, or infants with a variety of problems. These problems include a number of antenatal conditions that commonly eventuate in stillbirth, severe brain damage caused by birth asphyxia, Tay-Sachs disease, which involves increasing spasticity and dementia and usually results in death by age three or four, and Lesch-Nyhan disease, which involves uncontrollable spasms, mental retardation, compulsive self-mutilation, and early death. In severe cases of neural tube defects, newborns lack all or most of the brain, and death is inevitable. More problematic is meningomyelocele (protrusion of part of the covering and substance of the spinal cord because of a defect in the vertebral column). The wide range of possible outcomes from this condition makes it difficult to know whether to treat vigorously. Some children can have a meaningful life, while the chances are slim for others.

The debate about treatment or nontreatment of seriously ill and disabled newborns was stimulated in the United States by a 1973 article in which Raymond S. Duff and A. G. M. Campbell reported that forty-three of two-hundred ninety-nine consecutive deaths in the intensive care nursery at the Yale-New

Haven Hospital had occurred following a decision for nontreatment based on the infants' extremely poor prognosis for meaningful life.[63] This and similar reports led to a public debate that went unaccompanied by government intervention for almost a decade. Vigorous government action then occurred in response to the Infant Doe case, in which Infant Doe died six days after he was born with Down syndrome and respiratory and digestive complications requiring major surgery, which his parents refused to authorize. Subsequently, Congress passed amendments to the Child Abuse and Treatment Act that defined as child abuse the "withholding of medically indicated treatment" from children.[64] This law and subsequent regulations define "medically indicated treatment" as all treatment that is likely to ameliorate life-threatening conditions, including nutrition and hydration. However, three conditions are recognized under each of which life-sustaining treatment is optional.

1. The infant is chronically and irreversibly comatose
2. Provision of such treatment would merely prolong dying or not be effective in ameliorating or correcting the infant's life-threatening conditions
3. Provision of such treatment would be futile and the treatment would be inhumane

This approach has been interpreted by some influential government officials as involving reasonable *medical* judgments, rather than *quality-of-life* judgments. This strategy attempts to keep judgments in line with sound professional practice, but it is problematic on several grounds. We have already argued that "medically indicated treatments" themselves presuppose values and, often, standards of quality of life. Conditions 1 through 3 cannot be reduced to nonevaluative, medically indicated exceptive conditions to otherwise medically indicated treatments. Rather, these conditions express Congress's view of ethically indicated exceptions, and they incorporate quality-of-life judgments about which lives should be saved.[65] The judgment in condition 1 that a human life in an irreversible coma need not be prolonged is a quality-of-life judgment, and the conclusion in condition 3 requires consideration of the inhumaneness of treatment in relation to the limited prospects of success.

Consistent with our arguments in Chapter 3, the most appropriate standard in cases of never-competent patients, including seriously ill newborns, is that of best interests, as judged by the best obtainable estimate of what reasonable persons would consider the highest net benefit among the available options. Such quality-of-life judgments need to be restricted by justifiable criteria of benefits and burdens, so that quality of life is not reduced to arbitrary and partial judgments of personal preference or of the social worth of a child. For example, as we suggested previously, Down syndrome is not by itself a sufficient reason to allow a newborn to die, and usually it is not sufficient when the newborn suffers from other life-threatening conditions that require treatment.

We conclude that controlled quality-of-life considerations, together with the principle of respect for autonomy for competent patients, can legitimately determine whether treatments are optional or obligatory. These categories should replace the traditional distinctions and rules considered earlier in this chapter. However, we must now consider the most difficult of all distinctions used to determine acceptable decisions about treatment and acceptable forms of professional conduct.

Killing and Letting Die

A persistent body of distinctions and rules about life-sustaining treatments derives from the distinction between killing and letting die (or allowing to die), which in turn draws on the act–omission and active–passive distinctions. The killing-letting die distinction also underlies distinctions (1) between suicide and forgoing treatment and (2) between homicide and natural death. These distinctions are unsatisfactory for many of the purposes to which they have been put, and we will again suggest replacing some of them with categories such as benefit–burden and obligatory–optional.

However, unlike the distinctions previously discarded, we do not recommend complete abandonment of this group of distinctions. Considerations of public policy argue against a full-scale rejection. Otherwise, we risk inadequate protections for vulnerable patients, for health professionals who care for patients, and for other social groups. More than other distinctions we have criticized, distinctions centering on killing and letting die deserve some place in our moral scheme. At the same time, these distinctions are vague and need significant reformulatation, both in biomedical ethics and in public policy. To achieve an adequate moral resolution of these issues requires appeals to both beneficence and nonmaleficence that specify precisely what constitutes a harm, what constitutes a benefit, and how they are to be balanced.

Four questions need to be addressed. (1) "What conceptually is the difference between killing and letting die?" (2) "Is forgoing life-sustaining treatment sometimes a form of killing, and if so, is it sometimes suicide and sometimes homicide?" (3) "Is killing in itself no different morally than allowing to die?" (4) "Under what conditions, if any, is it permissible for patients, health professionals, or surrogates to forgo treatment so that the patient dies, to arrange for assisted suicide, or to arrange for some other cause of death?" We consider these questions in this order.

Conceptual Differences between Killing and Letting Die

Can *killing* and *letting die* be defined so that they are conceptually distinct and without overlap? The following case illustrates the problem: A newborn with Down syndrome needed an operation to correct a tracheoesophageal fistula.

The parents and physicians maintained that survival was not in this infant's best interests and decided to let the infant die rather than perform an operation. They did not consider this *omission* of treatment an act of killing the infant. However, a public outcry occurred over the case, and critics charged that the parents and physicians had killed the child by negligently allowing the child to die.[66]

In such cases, can actions that involve intentionally not treating a patient legitimately be described as "allowing to die" or "letting die," rather than "killing"? Do at least some of these actions involve both killing and allowing to die? Is "allowing to die" a euphemism for "killing"? These conceptual questions have moral implications. Unfortunately, both ordinary discourse and legal concepts are as misleading as they are helpful in our effort to understand these concepts. In ordinary language, *killing* is any form of deprivation or destruction of life, including animal and plant life. It can even mean "bringing an end to something," as in the expression "killing a legislative bill." Neither in ordinary language nor in law does the word *killing* entail a wrongful act or a crime. Ordinary language also does not require an intentional action for killing; it permits us to say that in automobile accidents one driver killed another even when no awareness, intent, or negligence was present.

Killing represents a family of ideas whose central condition is direct causation of another's death, whereas *allowing to die* represents another family of ideas whose central condition is intentional avoidance of causal intervention so that a disease or injury causes a natural death. Nevertheless, an emotive connotation of moral wrongness commonly accompanies *killing,* even under conditions that are widely considered to warrant killing, such as killing in war, self-defense, and capital punishment. This emotive connotation does not similarly affect "letting die." A need exists, then, to sharpen these notions by stipulating more precise meanings for medical ethics.

As we will use these terms, *killing* and *letting die* are properly used only to a circumstance in which one person intentionally causes the death of another human being. Killing and letting die do not occur by accident, chance, mishap, and the like. Killing and letting die also are not mutually exclusive concepts. One person can kill another by intentionally allowing the other to die, and killing can occur by omission just as well as by commission. These more precise meanings do not derive from raw stipulation on our part. Law, medicine, ethics, and ordinary language all recognize that some forms of allowing to die constitute acts of killing. As the Supreme Court of Washington put it, "the killing of a human being [can occur] by the act, procurement [that is, instigation, contrivance], or omission of another."[67] Both killing by omission and killing by commission can be intentional. Accordingly, if either a jailer or a physician withholds nutrition and hydration with the intention of ending a person's life, and an inmate or a patient dies as result, this omission is an act of killing.

Omitting Treatment as Sometimes Killing and Sometimes Letting Die

These conceptual observations have implications for our second question. Many writers in medicine, law, and ethics have construed forgoing of treatment under good medical and moral advice as *letting die* rather than *killing,* on grounds that an underlying disease or injury is the cause of death, not the forgoing of treatment. From this perspective, one acts nonmaleficently in allowing to die, but maleficently in killing. However, in many cases this thesis is difficult to uphold.

To see why, consider the following case, sometimes referred to as the Linares case: Rudolfo Linares detached his fifteen-month-old, near brain-dead son, Samuel, from a ventilator with the intent that he die. While doing so, the father prevented health professionals from reattaching the respirator by holding them away at gunpoint. Linares allowed his son to die, but the district attorney said he also killed Samuel and therefore brought a homicide complaint, although a grand jury refused to issue a homicide indictment. What would we think in this case if Linares had protested the indictment by saying, "I did not kill him; the balloon he aspirated killed him. I merely allowed him to die." Although the balloon played a causal role in the son's death, it certainly appears that the father also caused a loss of the life that was left in his son. If so, he seems to have killed his son.

However, "killing" is such a loathsome stigma in medicine that a coroner later ruled that the death was neither a case of killing nor a case of allowing to die. The death, opined the coroner, was "accidental," because Samuel had been dead when admitted to the hospital.[68] But Samuel had been determined to be alive (in a persistent vegetative state, but not brain dead) by competent physicians. This bizarre case appears to come down to the one category almost no one seems to have considered at the time: a *justified* killing. In a parallel case that we can construct as a hypothetical, if Mr. X came into a hospital off the street and detached a PVS patient from a ventilator, we would consider the act an *unjustified* killing—even though the act might be exactly the same act that a physician was about to perform at a family's request, making it a case of "allowing to die." Mr. X, the physician, and Mr. Linares all perform the same act of detaching the respirator; yet the terms we use to describe these acts are very different, as are our judgments of maleficence. Moreover, some acts of this type are maleficent, some nonmaleficent, and some are beneficent.

These conclusions have profound implications. Suppose that physicians and hospital officials had in the beginning done what both they and Rudy Linares had in fact wanted to do: detach the respirator and allow his son to die. This would have been a typical case in medicine of "allowing to die." Such acts are generally regarded as nonmaleficent, and often as beneficent. What the physician does in these cases is *causally* no different than what Rudy Linares did: Technology is removed and the patient dies as a result. If Linares killed his son, and he did, then physicians who do the same thing with their patients likewise kill their patients. They cannot rightly say "We do not kill our patients, only the underlying diseases and injuries do so" any more than a jealous rival of a patient who detaches a respirator to ensure the patient's immediate demise could say, "It was the disease, not me, who killed him." Nor can they say that they did not intend the outcome of death. Whether the agents should be charged with and convicted of murder is a further matter for judicial judgment. Generally, the motives are proper in medicine, and both moral and legal justification exist for the action. But whether the motive is reprehensible or laudable, the act remains an intentional killing.

Why do we, like the coroner in the Linares case, resist this conclusion, which seems so straightforward? The history of the Conroy case (discussed in Chapter 3) helps to answer this question. An early appeals court found that removing the nasogastric tube from Claire Conroy was not merely a matter of forgoing treatment, because her death would be caused by dehydration and starvation. This court found that the patient "would have been actively killed" by a means independent of her medical condition, and so the act would amount to euthanasia.[69] Principal parts of this opinion were subsequently overruled by the New Jersey Supreme Court, which found that any medical treatment, including artificial nutrition and hydration, may in principle be withheld or withdrawn from an incompetent patient (under the legitimating circumstances we detailed in Chapter 3). The court held that nasogastric tubes were analytically indistinguishable from other forms of life-sustaining treatments such as respirators. No civil or criminal liability for killing is involved if appropriate conditions of refusal of treatment are present.[70]

One reason for this divergence of opinion is terminological. Some persons use the term *killing* as a *normative* term of maleficence, parallel to "unjustified homicide or murder." Justified acts involving the deaths of patients, therefore, logically cannot be instances of killing. They can only be cases of allowing to die. But, as we argued earlier, this approach risks conceptual confusion. Killing can be both morally and legally justified, despite its prima facie wrongness.

Courts have offered two primary explanations for why forgoing life-sustaining treatment should not be categorized as killing. The most prominent rationale rests on an account of causation. In acts of forgoing treatment, an underlying disease or injury is already present, and medical technology functions to prevent the natural course of the disease or injury. When the natural cause is released, a "natural death" occurs. To remove the technology, then, is to release natural conditions to do what they would have done before. Because disease or injury is the cause, rather than the physician's or surrogate's or patient's action, neither homicide nor assisted suicide occurs.

On this account, preexisting conditions alone cause the death, although this cannot be said if the technology is mischievously removed, because another cause then enters the picture. In both *Quinlan* and *Conroy,* for example, the New Jersey Supreme Court held that the respirator is only delaying the patient's inevitable death, which would be a "natural death" if the life-support apparatus were removed. The reigning medical and legal view is that withdrawing life-sustaining treatments in such cases is an act of allowing death to occur from preexisting conditions that have been temporarily held in check by death-delaying procedures.[71]

This account functions well to alleviate physician fears about moral blame and legal liability, but it does not cohere well with many of our ordinary beliefs about killing. If Mr. X with malice detaches a conscious and perfectly competent quadriplegic from a ventilator, he does more than release natural conditions. We could not correctly say, "he didn't kill the patient; he only allowed the patient to die." By letting the patient die, he killed—in this case murdered—the patient. Physicians, by contrast, often have a solid moral and legal basis for claiming that they are warranted in omitting treatment in identical ways. They act at the patient's request or with the patient's consent. They act under a social arrangement that encourages them to do all they can to alleviate their patient's suffering. Their motive is to meet their obligation to the patient, not to serve their own interests. Therefore, we have weighty reasons for commending rather than condemning physicians in these cases.

In the attempt to protect health care professionals from charges of killing, *value* judgments about what is (morally and legally) permissible often control our *factual* judgments about the cause of death. That is, moral judgments about justified and unjustified actions determine what constitutes "killing" and what constitutes "allowing to die from preexisting conditions," rather than the other way around.[72] This leads us to say that surrogate decisionmakers and physicians do not kill patients when they justifiably remove a life-sustaining treatment, and that patients do not kill themselves when they forgo treatment; whereas if they unjustifiably omit treatment, they do kill. "Killing" is here functioning more as a *moral* category than as a *causal* category.[73] Imagine that Karen Quinlan's father had detached her respirator against medical, moral, and legal advice and that she had died as a consequence (effectively this happened in the Linares case). Few would say, "preexisting conditions killed her, her father did not kill her." But when the father has good motives and medical, legal, and moral support for the same action, many come to identify with and justify or excuse the act. As a result, they consider the act one of letting die.

Part of the reason for moralizing the cause derives from the legal doctrine of *proximate cause.* To be a proximate, or primary, cause is to become legally liable for an outcome. These legal judgments about causation and liability are often decided by a person's obligations. If a physician has an obligation to treat, then treatment omission breaches that obligation and causes death (an act of unjustified homicide); but, if no obligation to treat exists, disease or injury serves as the proximate cause, and the physician is off the hook of liability. Conceptually, this dance with proximate causation obscures issues in the distinction between killing and allowing to die and further confuses issues about the cause of death. The doctrine assumes a single cause or single type of cause of death, yet physicians, guardians, and courts beyond a reasonable doubt play a significant causal role in bringing about death at the time it occurs in treatment-termination cases.

Even from a legal perspective, a better account can be provided than "The preexisting disease caused the death." The better account is that legal liability should not be imposed on physicians and surrogates unless they have an obligation to provide or continue the treatment. If no obligation to treat exists, then questions of causation and liability do not arise. If the categories of obligatory and optional are primary, we have a reason for avoiding discussions about killing and letting die altogether and for focusing instead on health care professionals' obligations and problems of moral and legal responsibility.

These observations are pertinent to suicide as well as to killing. Dan Brock has pointed to some relevant connections between suicide and refusal of treatment cases:

> The judgment of a person who competently decides to commit suicide is essentially that "my expected future life, under the best conditions possible for me, is so bad that I judge it to be worse than no further continued life at all." This seems to be in essence exactly the same judgment that some persons who decide to forego life-sustaining treatment make. The refusal of life-sustaining treatment is their means of ending life; they intend to end their life because of its grim prospects. Their death now when they otherwise would not have died *is* self-inflicted, whether they take a lethal poison or disconnect a respirator.[74]

Refusals of treatment, so described, are instances of suicide whenever the agent specifically arranges the conditions to bring about death. However, Brock's proposal fails to resolve the issue of whether suicidal intent and causation exist when a patient refuses treatment because of a bleak future, and this should give us pause about using the category of "suicide," as well as categories such as "killing" and "homicide." Consider a failing dialysis patient for whom the treatment has become futile: With or without treatment he is going to die in the next month. He cancels scheduled dialysis appointments in order to be at home with loved ones and die free of the machine and the hospital. This case seems to be a case lacking suicidal intent. The patient is only choosing to die under one set of circumstances rather than another. No decision is made about whether life is worth living; either way, there will soon be no life. Suicide is the wrong category, because death will, either way, be caused by untreatable conditions that are not specifically arranged by the agent for the purpose of bringing about his or her death. This is what we might call a "pure" refusal case that lacks all suicidal intent.

We conclude that the distinction between killing (suicide, homicide, etc.)

and letting die suffers from vagueness and confusion. It is conceptually impossible to classify many acts as instances of letting die without also classifying them as instances of killing. We have also seen that the language of killing is so confusing—causally, legally, and morally—that we should avoid it in discussions of euthanasia and assistance in dying. It is often morally and conceptually more satisfactory to discuss these issues exclusively in the language of optional and obligatory treatments, dispensing altogether with *killing* and *letting die.*

When Killing Is No Different Morally Than Allowing to Die

Our third question, "Is killing in itself no different morally than allowing to die?" can now be addressed. To assert (as we do) that killing is no different morally than allowing to die is simply to say that correct labeling of an act as "killing" or as "letting die" does nothing to determine if one form of action is better or worse, or more or less justified, than the other. Some particular instance of killing (a brutal murder, say) may be worse than some particular instance of allowing to die (forgoing treatment for a patient who is in a persistent vegetative state, say); but some particular instance of letting die (not resuscitating a patient who could be saved, say) also may be worse than some particular instance of killing (mercy killing at the patient's request, say). Nothing about either killing or allowing to die entails judgments about actual wrongness or rightness, or about the beneficence or nonmaleficence of the action. Rightness and wrongness depend on the merit of the justification underlying the action, not on the type of action it is. Neither killing nor letting die, therefore, is per se wrongful, and in this regard they are to be distinguished from murder, which is per se wrongful. Both killing and letting die are prima facie wrong, but can be justified under some circumstances.

It would be absurd to accept all cases of letting die as morally justified, and it is no less absurd to view all forms of killing (for example, killing in self-defense) as unjustified. A judgment that an act of either killing or letting die is justified or unjustified entails that something else be known about the act besides these characteristics. We need to know something about the actor's motive (whether it is benevolent or malicious, for example), the patients' request, and the consequences of the act. Only these additional factors will allow us to place the act on a moral map and allow us to make a normative judgment about it. All instances of killing and letting die, then, must satisfy independent criteria, such as the balance of benefits over burdens to the patient, to determine their acceptability.

The Scope of the Patient's Rights

We can now address the fourth basic question, which is formulated without the language of "killing:" Under what conditions, if any, is it permissible for patients, health professionals, or surrogates either to forgo treatment so that the patient dies or to arrange for assistance in dying?

If competent patients have a legal and moral right to refuse treatment that involves health professionals in implementing their decision and bringing about their deaths, we have a reason to suppose they have a similar right to request the assistance of willing physicians to help them control the conditions under which they die. Assuming that omission of treatment is justified by the principles of respect for autonomy and nonmaleficence, cannot the same form of justification be extended to physicians prescribing barbiturates needed by seriously ill patients, and possibly to physician-administered lethal injections? This strategy rests on the premise that reform in ethics and law is needed because of the apparent inconsistency between (1) the strong rights of autonomy that allow persons in grim circumstances to refuse treatment so as to bring about their deaths and (2) the apparent denial of a similar autonomy right to arrange for death by mutual agreement between patient and physician under equally grim circumstances.

The argument for this view seems particularly compelling when a condition has become overwhelmingly burdensome for a patient, pain management is inadequate, and only a physician can and is willing to bring relief. At present, medicine and law are in the awkward position of having to say to such patients, "If you were on life-sustaining treatment, you would have a right to withdraw the treatment and then we could let you die. But since you are not, we can only give you palliative care until you can die a natural death, however painful, undignified, and costly." This seems tantamount to condemning the patient to live a life he or she does not want.

Only a small percentage of patients face overwhelming pain and burdens because pain management and improvements in patient's environments have made circumstances at least bearable for most patients, and hospice environments have improved the care of the dying. The right to refuse nutrition and hydration also gives many patients the opportunity to control the time of their death. However, these facts do not provide a decisive reason for prohibiting increased physician assistance in dying. Some patients cannot be satisfactorily relieved, and in any event there are significant questions about autonomy rights for patients. If a right exists to stop a machine that sustains life, through an arrangement involving mutual agreement with a physician, why is there not the same right to stop the machine that *is* one's life by an arrangement with a physician?

This right has almost never been recognized in law or in codes of medical ethics. The traditional belief is that we should altogether prohibit such forms of assistance in health care while authorizing letting die in a certain range of cases. Codes of health care ethics from the time of the Hippocratic oath to the present strictly prohibit direct assistance in death, even if a patient has good reasons for wanting to die. For example, in 1991, the American Geriatrics Society opposed all physician involvement in killing or assistance in suicide.[75] In an influential statement passed in 1973 and revised in 1988 and 1991, the American Medical Association Council on Ethical and Judicial Affairs allowed forgoing life-sustaining treatments but prohibited any "intentional termination of the life of one human being by another—mercy killing." Whether letting particular patients die is morally acceptable depends on several factors in this policy, but if the deaths involve killing—even in circumstances identical to those in which a patient is allowed to die—they are never justifiable.[76]

We have already seen that the *conceptual* distinction between killing and letting die cannot bear the weight of *normative* conclusions about policies or particular cases. Many people inside and outside medicine now believe that active physician assistance for a narrow group of seriously ill and dying patients at their request can be morally justified. Many also believe that, under closely monitored supervision, such acts of assistance in dying should be made legally permissible. As a result, an increasing number of health professionals and figures in medical ethics argue that we should relax or modify our stringent rules and laws against physician involvement.

Against this pressure for reform, many health professionals insist that practices of killing patients are inconsistent with the roles of nursing, caregiving, and healing, would introduce conflicts of interest into those roles, and would taint the roles in the same way that injecting prisoners on death row taints physicians. We need, then, to assess the arguments for and against what is often called mercy killing, assisted suicide, and omitting life-sustaining treatment with the intention of causing death. Because we earlier reached a settled view on the right to forgo treatment that generally accords with contemporary medical practice, codes of ethics, and judicial decisions, we will now consider only issues of mercy killing and assisted suicide.

Our argument will proceed as follows: First, we will present a revised account of the killing–letting die distinction in which protection against certain forms of wrongfully caused death are at the center of the discussion. We then argue that merciful physician interventions in the form of voluntary active euthanasia are not inherently wrong or incompatible with the role of a health professional. Nonetheless, public policies that sanction such physician activities are unacceptable unless they are accompanied by extraordinarily careful regulation and monitoring. Second, we argue that prohibitions in biomedical ethics against certain forms of assisted suicide should be eased, making physicians more comfortable in helping certain patients achieve what for them is a comfortable and timely death. It seems likely that assisted suicide will be the driving force behind efforts to alter rules against killing in medicine, so that support of assisted suicide, which is compatible with a rejection of voluntary active euthanasia, takes on a special significance at the present time.

Recasting the Rules Governing Physician-Assisted Death

The phrase "assisted death," particularly "physician-assisted death," is now widely used, but it is ambiguous because many modes of assistance exist. Both assisted suicide and voluntary active euthanasia are instances of assistance in bringing about death. In assisted suicide, the final agent is the one whose death is brought about, and in voluntary active euthanasia the final agent is another party. At present, voluntary active euthanasia is illegal in the United States, despite some efforts for reform. Although acts of suicide or attempted suicide have been decriminalized throughout the United States, most jurisdictions continue to prohibit aiding and abetting suicide. In one early U.S. case, a woman was bedridden with advanced multiple sclerosis and asked her husband to put a cup of poison by her bed so that she could kill herself. When she consumed the poison and died, he was prosecuted and convicted of murder on grounds that he had assisted a suicide.[77] However, many acts of assisted suicide are not prosecuted. For example, to cite a case discussed in Chapter 5 (p. 287), cancer-victim Ida Rollin indicated to her daughter, Betty Rollin, that she wanted to commit suicide, and the daughter then secured the necessary pills. Although this case was reported in newspapers, a book, and a television movie, the daughter was not prosecuted.

Some writers have argued that physician-assisted deaths are unacceptable violations of nonmaleficence, whereas others have argued that many acts of this description are acceptable and even courageous actions of beneficence. In assessing these arguments, it pays dividends to focus on the scope of the claim being advanced. We believe that sufficient moral reasons exist in some cases to justify mercy killing and assisted suicide, but these reasons are not necessarily sufficient to support revisions in either codes of ethics or public policies. In addressing whether we should retain or modify some current prohibitions, we therefore need to be clear about whether the topic of discussion is the moral justification of individual acts or the justification of institutional rules and public laws governing practices.

Acts and practices.[78] To justify an act is distinct from justifying a practice or a policy. A rule of practice or a public policy that prohibits active killing in medicine may be justifiable, even if it excludes some particular acts of causing a person's death that in themselves are morally justifiable. For example, such a rule would not permit us to use a drug overdose to cause death for a patient who suffers from terrible pain, who will probably die within three weeks, and who rationally asks for a merciful assisted death, although in an individual case the act would be justified. For policy reasons, it is sometimes necessary to prohibit such acts altogether, although they are not morally wrong.

The problem is that a practice or policy that allows killing runs risks of abuse and, on balance, might cause more harm than benefit. The argument is not that serious abuses will occur immediately, but that they will grow incrementally over time. Society might start by severely restricting the number of patients who qualify for assistance in dying, but these restrictions would later be revised and expanded to include cases of unjustified killing. Unscrupulous persons would learn how to abuse the system, just as they do now with methods of tax evasion that operate on the margins of the system of legitimate tax avoidance. In short, the slope of the trail toward unjustified killing will be so slippery and precipitous that we ought never to hike on it.

Questions about the slippery slope. Many dismiss these slippery slope or wedge arguments because of their widespread abuse in biomedical ethics, a lack of empirical evidence to support their claims, and their heavily metaphorical character ("the thin edge of the wedge," "the first step on the slippery slope," "the foot in the door," and "the camel's nose under the tent"). However, some arguments of this form should be taken with the utmost seriousness.[79] They force us to think carefully about whether unacceptable harm is likely to result from attractive and apparently innocent first steps.

Wedge or slippery slope arguments appear in two versions: (1) conceptual and (2) psychological–sociological. According to the first version, the slope is slippery because the concepts and distinctions used in moral and legal rules are vague and may lead to unanticipated outcomes. A norm or justification for a type of action that, considered in isolation, is morally acceptable winds up supporting similar acts that are unacceptable. For example, some justifications that have been offered for the moral acceptability of suicide imply a justification of some forms of voluntary active euthanasia that seem unjustifiable to proponents of the initial justification. Critics then argue that the justification that was offered for suicide is the first step on the slippery slope or the thin edge of the wedge toward voluntary, active euthanasia. This first version of the wedge or slippery slope argument, however, can also be used against its proponents. If it is morally defensible to allow patients to die under conditions *x, y,* and *z,* then (in light of our previous argument) it is morally defensible to assist them more aggressively in bringing about their deaths under those identical conditions. If it is in their interests to die, it is (prima facie) irrelevant how death is brought about.

The second or psychological–sociological version of slippery slope arguments offers a better reason for maintaining the distinction between killing and letting die. This version examines the probable impact of making exceptions to professional, social, and legal rules or changing them in a more permissive direction. If certain restraints against killing are removed, various psychological and social forces would likely make it more difficult to maintain the relevant distinctions in practice. For example, in some settings it is plausible to argue as follows: (1) To authorize killing patients for their benefit when they are suffering excruciating pain or have a bleak future risks opening the door to the encouragement of euthanasia in order to relieve personal burdens on families and in financial burdens on society. (2) *Voluntary* active euthanasia (an act of killing a person at his or her informed request) invites social changes leading to *nonvoluntary* euthanasia (an act of killing a person who is incapable of making an informed request) and perhaps to *involuntary* euthanasia (an act of killing a person who while competent opposes being killed). In assessing these possibilities, we should recall that killing and various forms of assistance in dying can occur by both omission and commission. Withheld or withdrawn treatment (such as hydration and nutrition) can cause death just as an underlying disease or injury can cause death.

This second version of the slippery slope argument becomes more compelling when we consider the effects of discrimination based on disability, the increasing number of newborns with disabilities who survive at heavy cost to the public, and the growing number of aging persons with medical problems who require larger and larger proportions of the public's financial resources. If rules permitting voluntary active euthanasia become public policy, society is at increased risk that persons in these populations will be harmed; for example, the risk is increased that families and health professionals may kill disabled newborns and severely brain-damaged adults to avoid social and familial burdens. If newborns and adults can be judged by decisionmakers to have overly burdensome conditions or lives with no value, the same logic can be extended to many other populations of feeble, debilitated, and seriously ill patients who are financial and emotional burdens on families and society.

Many of these circumstances are relevantly similar to circumstances that already provide the leading justifications for widely accepted forms of withdrawing or withholding life support. Often the patients did not request these omissions and left no advance directive. These cases differ by degree as much as by kind, which makes it easier to extend the same reasoning to other cases. It takes little imagination to suppose that many parents would, if given the opportunity, withhold life-sustaining technologies from their newborns because of a wide variety of disabilities, such as blindness, retardation, and malformed limbs.

Rules in our moral code against actively causing the death of another person are not isolated fragments. They are threads in a fabric of rules that support respect for human life. The more threads we remove, the weaker the fabric becomes. If we also focus on the modification of *attitudes*, not *rules* only, the general attitude of respect for life can also be eroded by shifts in public policy. Prohibitions are often both instrumentally and symbolically important, and their removal could weaken a set of practices, restraints, and attitudes that we cannot replace.[80]

Rules against bringing about another's death also provide a basis of trust between patients and health care professionals. We expect health care professionals to promote our welfare under all circumstances. We risk a loss of public trust if physicians become agents of active euthanasia in addition to healers and caregivers. At the same time, we risk a loss of trust if patients and families believe they are being abandoned in their suffering by physicians who lack the courage and will to offer the assistance they believe they need in the darkest hours of their lives.

The ultimate success or failure of these slippery slope arguments depends on speculative predictions of a progressive erosion of moral restraints. If dire consequences will in fact flow from the legal legitimation of assisted suicide or voluntary active euthanasia, then the argument is cogent and such practices are justifiably prohibited. But how good is the evidence that dire consequences will occur? Does the evidence indicate that we cannot maintain firm distinctions in public policies between patient-requested death and involuntary euthanasia? Scant evidence supports any of the answers that have been given to these questions, so far as we can see. Those, including the present authors, who take seriously the second version of the slippery slope argument should simply admit that the argument needs a premise on the order of "better safe than sorry." The likelihood of the projected moral erosions, then, is not something we can easily assess. Arguments on every side are speculative and analogical, and different assessors of the same evidence reach different conclusions. An intractable controversy also exists over what counts as good evidence. Although we cannot here resolve this largely empirical issue, we can assess an analogy that frequently arises in these discussions: the Nazi path to a final solution.

The Nazi analogy. The holocaust continues to serve as a powerful vision of the bottom of the slippery slope for a society that carelessly initiates killing. The holocaust left a string of inadequately answered questions about so-called euthanasia. After the Nuremberg trials of German physicians, American physician Leo Alexander argued that the Nazis moved from the "small beginnings" of euthanasia for the incurably ill to policies of genocide:

The beginnings at first were merely a subtle shift in emphasis in the basic attitude of the physicians. It started with the acceptance of the attitude, basic in the euthanasia movement, that there is such a thing as life not worthy to be lived. This attitude in its early stages concerned itself merely with the severely and chronically sick. Gradually the sphere of those to be included in this category was enlarged to encompass the socially unproductive, the ideologically unwanted, the racially unwanted and finally all non-Germans. The infinitely small wedged-in lever from which this entire trend of mind received its impetus was the attitude toward the nonrehabilitable sick.[81]

This account reappears in Robert Lifton's study of Nazi physicians, which describes the first steps as well as the final horror of the rule that "life unworthy of life" is to be eliminated.[82] Lifton notes that prior to the death camps, the

Nazis adopted a policy of direct medical killing, using injections, lethal doses of medicine, and gases. The killing was arranged within the medical system and involved medical decisionmakers. Doctors and their assistants implemented the decisions. Crucial to the program was the removal of a social and psychological barrier against killing through a "medicalization of killing" that obscured the boundaries between killing and helping. Lifton argues that although this program was called *euthanasia,* eventually the term simply "camouflaged mass murder."

Contemporary proponents of euthanasia often properly insist that the rationale of the Nazi program was racist ideology, not respect for autonomy and traditional values in health care. They dispute the Nazi analogy, because the Nazis concentrated on nonvoluntary and especially involuntary killing (inappropriately labeled *euthanasia*), and did not innocently step onto the slippery slope only to find they could not stop.[83] We accept this argument that the Nazi analogy is weak and that mercy killing is not always wrong. At the same time, society must protect its members against disastrous outcomes by designing appropriate social policies and statements of professional ethics that prevent abuse.

An example of reckless mercy killing that prohibitory rules should help deter was reported in the *Journal of the American Medical Association* in January 1988 under the provocative title "It's Over, Debbie."[84] A gynecology resident rotating through a large private hospital was awakened by a telephone call from a nurse who told him that a patient on the gynecologic-oncology unit, not the resident's usual duty station, was having difficulty getting rest. The chart at the nurses' station provided some details. A twenty-year-old woman named Debbie, who was dying of ovarian cancer, was experiencing unrelenting vomiting from the alcohol drip administered for sedation (a procedure that some have criticized). The woman was emaciated, weighed eighty pounds, had an intravenous line, was receiving nasal oxygen, and was sitting in bed suffering from severe air hunger. She had not eaten or slept in two days, and she was receiving only supportive care because she had not responded to chemotherapy. The patient's only words to the resident were, "Let's get this over with." After having the nurse draw twenty milligrams of morphine sulfate into a syringe, the resident took it into the room and injected it intravenously into the patient after telling her that it "would let her rest" and "say good-bye." The patient died within a few minutes.

If this is an actual case—and doubts have been voiced about its authenticity—the resident acted rashly. Other medications could perhaps have relieved the patient's pain and suffering and enabled her to rest comfortably. The resident's intention seems to have been to kill the patient out of "mercy," but in the absence of previous contact with the patient, the resident had no basis for interpreting her words as a request to be killed and did not consult with anyone before making a quick, momentous, and irreversible decision. Both law and ethics should deter such actions.

Merciful death in the practice of medicine. In addition to fears of abuse of individuals such as the physically and mentally disabled who cannot consent, other legitimate fears haunt active medical interventions to bring about death. Consider the following two types of wrongly diagnosed patients:[85]

1. Patients who are wrongly diagnosed as hopeless and who will survive if a treatment is ceased (in order to allow a natural death)
2. Patients who are wrongly diagnosed as hopeless and who will survive only if the treatment is *not* ceased (in order to allow a natural death).

If a social rule that allows some patients to die were in effect, doctors and families who followed it would lose patients only in the second category. But if killing were permitted, at least some of the patients in the first category would be needlessly lost. Thus, a rule prohibiting killing would save some lives that would be lost if both killing and allowing to die were permitted. This consequence is not a decisive reason for a policy of (only) allowing to die, because the numbers in categories 1 and 2 are likely to be small, and other reasons for assisting in dying, such as extreme pain and autonomous choice, might be weighty. But it is a morally relevant reason for a cautious policy that calls for careful review and monitoring of decisions.

Among the strongest reasons for mercifully helping some patients to die, of course, is the relief of unbearable and uncontrollable pain and suffering, which can so ravage and dehumanize patients that death appears to be in their best interests. Prolonging life and refusing to kill in some of these circumstances seems a cruel violation of the principle of nonmaleficence by causing people to suffer. Nevertheless, an array of alternatives can be presented to many of these patients. The physician can usually relieve pain and make a patient comfortable through medications, even if the medications hasten death. Physicians can also appropriately, and often painlessly, withdraw nutrition and hydration. In many cases the patient will view this action as the best alternative. One reason for a policy of exhausting all alternatives before allowing physicians to engage in active euthanasia is the precariousness of constructing a social or professional ethic on borderline situations and emergency cases. It is dangerous to generalize from emergencies, because hard cases may make bad social and professional ethics as well as bad law.

Clinicians also have a moral obligation to inform competent patients of alternative approaches, such as hospice care and increased medication. The risk of addiction has often been overestimated and unduly feared in the care of terminally ill patients.[86] Public policy in the United States has resisted legalizing

heroin, a powerful painkiller. Government officials fear the harmful consequences that might flow from such an act, including addiction, the legitimation
of heroin, and the possibility of abuses. Yet heroin has been used for terminally
ill cancer patients for several years in the United Kingdom without evidence of
major problems. We thus see no merit in the societal prohibition of the use of
heroin to relieve pain in terminally ill cancer patients.

An ongoing controversy surrounds one experiment in socially accepted, voluntary active euthanasia—the case of the Netherlands, where euthanasia is still
technically illegal, but where guidelines developed by courts also immunize
physicians against prosecution. Euthanasia is openly practiced, and it is supported by a substantial segment of the population. Defenders of euthanasia
contend that the experiment in the Netherlands establishes that euthanasia can
be socially accepted without the parade of horrors that many people have predicted. But critics contend that the Netherlands fails as a model for the United
States for at least two reasons. First, social conditions in the United States are
vastly different from those in the Netherlands, where a more homogeneous
population carries universal access to health care and typically has close relations to primary care providers. Second, some physicians and families in the
Netherlands have gone beyond the accepted rules by putting to death some
incompetent patients, such as infants with Down syndrome, although the rules
authorize only voluntary euthanasia. According to one nationwide study in Hol-
land, about 1.8 percent of the total deaths each year are the result of euthanasia
by physician-administered lethal drugs at the patient's request, and about 0.3
percent are the result of physician-assisted suicide; in 0.8 of all deaths, drugs
are administered to shorten a patient's life "without explicit and persistent request" and without satisfying the nation's stringent criteria for euthanasia.[87]

Although all of the above arguments deserve our deepest respect, they do
not answer every question that needs to be addressed about physician-assisted
suicide and mercy killing, for at least four reasons. First, we are already on a
slippery slope by virtue of the changes in professional ethics and law that have
occurred since *Quinlan* and the first natural death acts. If it is morally permissible to unplug respirators and detach intravenous lines knowing that death will
eventuate, the logic of our present situation is that we are struggling to preserve
as many traditional restraints against killing as we can, consistent with taking
a humane approach toward seriously suffering patients and respecting their
rights. Second, as we have seen, arguments on every side of the debate about
the slippery slope are speculative and analogical, and different assessors of the
available evidence legitimately reach different conclusions. Third, law and public policy are not likely ever to be decisive guidelines for medical ethics. We
are sometimes justified in performing actions that evade or infringe legal and
social rules, and we should never allow medical ethics to be totally determined
by sound social policy. Fourth, we often accept social policies that have some

risks, knowing that tragedies will sometimes occur. For example, we allow youths sixteen years of age to drive an automobile on public roads with minimal driver's education, although we know there will be some tragic outcomes. The rationale is that, on the whole, the results of the practice will be more beneficial for all affected than any competing policy we can fashion. Proponents of voluntary active euthanasia and patients in uncontrollable pain are now asking us to accept a similar rationale. They want a sound monitoring system under which people elect to die, even though a few tragic mistakes will result from such a system.

Is there, then, a reasonable hope that a public policy of legalized euthanasia can be properly monitored and enforced without persistent and pervasive abuse? Our apparent success in managing many cases of treatment omission that qualify as forms of passive euthanasia in health care institutions and the courts is an encouraging sign that abuses are containable, although only a weak body of data exists. There is a significant problem of inconsistency in our policies if we maintain that legalizing voluntary *active* euthanasia will lead to unacceptable practices and consequences, whereas allowing both *passive* voluntary euthanasia and termination of treatment by surrogates will not present comparable difficulties. To date, the more difficult problems have not come in cases of voluntary patient requests, where patients are available for discussion and decisionmaking, but in cases of incompetent patients, such as Earle Spring and Nancy Cruzan. However, this book is not the appropriate forum in which to work out a precise framework for legal mechanisms and public policy. We are not convinced that legalization is either the best public policy or a policy that we should reject. In any event, the basic question that confronts contemporary biomedical ethics is not the precise limits in public policy that should be placed on assisting in death (as momentous as this question is), but rather which forms of assistance in death are morally justified.

The Justification of Assistance in Dying

There are, we believe, sound reasons to accept several forms of assistance in dying that help bring about death. Some of these forms of assistance qualify as voluntary active euthanasia, others as passive euthanasia.

Why Is It Wrong to Bring about Death?

Most of us believe it is not always morally wrong, on balance, to cause someone's death. Why, then, do we believe that causing someone's death is prima facie wrong, and what could make it right?

We have encountered one answer in examining slippery slope arguments: It is wrong to kill whenever killing threatens social stability or causes harmful social consequences. But this answer does not explain the wrongness of causing death, which has little, if anything, to do with parties other than the person whose life is taken. Causing a person's death is wrong because of a harm or loss to the person killed, not because of losses that others encounter. What makes it wrong, when it is wrong, is that a person is harmed—that is, suffers a setback to interests that the person otherwise would not have experienced. In particular, one is caused the loss of the capacity to plan and choose a future, together with a deprivation of expectable goods. This explains why inflicting death both harms and wrongs a person.

This conclusion is notable for the following reason: If a person desires death rather than life's more typical goods and projects, then causing that person's death at his or her autonomous request does not either harm or wrong the person (though it might still harm others—or society—by setting back their interests, which might be a reason against the *practice*). To the contrary, not to help such persons in their dying will frustrate their plans and cause them a loss, thereby harming them. It can also bring them indignity and despair. Furthermore, if *passive* allowing to die does not harm or wrong a patient because it does not violate the patient's rights, then assisted suicide and voluntary active euthanasia similarly do not harm or wrong the person who dies. Those who believe it is sometimes morally acceptable to let people die but not to take active steps to help them die must therefore give a different account of the wrongfulness of killing persons than the one we have suggested. The burden of justification, then, seems to rest on those who would refuse assistance to those who wish to die, rather than on those who would help them.

Justified Breaches of Legal Rules

Juries often excuse those who kill their suffering relatives by finding them not guilty by reason of temporary insanity. As we suggested in the section above on the rule of double effect, excusability is usually based on a judgment of the person's motive of mercy, not an assessment of the person's intentions. Consider a once famous case in New Jersey.[88] George Zygmaniak was in a motorcycle accident that left him paralyzed from the neck down. The paralysis was considered irreversible, and George begged his brother to kill him. Three days later, his brother brought a sawed-off shotgun to the hospital and shot George in the head after saying, "Close your eyes now, I'm going to shoot you." A judgment of temporary insanity in this case is a veiled moral judgment of acceptable killing. The judgment of "insanity" springs from the lack of a legal channel to say the act was, under the circumstances, justifiable. Verdicts such as "not guilty by reason of temporary insanity" function under law to excuse the agent by finding (sometimes implausibly) that he or she lacked the conditions of responsibility necessary for legal guilt. George Zygmaniak's brother was not temporarily insane, but the jury found the act morally excusable nonetheless.

Physicians (and others) on occasion find that it is morally permissible to engage in justified conscientious or civil disobedience of laws against killing and assisting in dying. This is another way of acknowledging that there are justified moral exceptions to enforceable rules against killing. The conditions that justify conscientious refusals to follow rules against killing patients are too complex to be considered here, but the key point is this: If pain and suffering of a certain magnitude can in principle justify active interventions to cause death, then acts of conscientious refusal to follow laws will sometimes be justified (as long as certain other conditions are met). It may or may not be justified to introduce parallel changes in the law. The language of "conscientious refusal" is not used to evade acceptance of the justifiability of active euthanasia in the difficult cases. We accept its justifiability for reasons now to be explained. (We discuss "conscientious refusal" in Chapter 8.)

Physician-Assisted Suicide

Debates about suicide have long occurred in medical practice, particularly psychiatric practice, because physicians have usually intervened to prevent suicides and to treat patients who attempt suicide (see Chapter 5 pp. 284–287). Physicians have also assisted patients in committing suicide, despite legal and professional prohibitions. But should physicians be given a more extensive role in facilitating suicide than medical ethics and social convention have traditionally permitted?

Jack Kevorkian's first use of his now famous suicide machine offers an example of *unjustified* physician-assisted suicide that medical ethics should discourage. In his first case, Janet Adkins, an Oregon grandmother with Alzheimer's disease, had reached a decision that she wanted to take her life rather than lose her cognitive capacities, which she was convinced were slowly deteriorating. After Adkins read about Kevorkian's machine in the news media, she communicated with him by phone and then flew from Oregon to Michigan to meet with him. Following brief discussions over a weekend, she and Kevorkian drove to a park in north Oakland County. He inserted a tube in her arm and started saline flow. His machine was constructed so that Adkins could then press a button to inject other drugs, eventuating in potassium chloride, which physically caused her death.[89] She then pressed the button.

This case raises several concerns. Janet Adkins was in the fairly early stages of the crippling effects of Alzheimer's and was not yet debilitated. Her death was on the distant horizon. At fifty-four years of age, she was still capable of enjoying a full schedule of activities with her husband and playing tennis with her son, and she might have been able to live a meaningful life for several more years. There was a slight possibility that the Alzheimer's diagnosis was incorrect, and she might have been more psychologically depressed than Kevorkian appreciated. More importantly, she had limited contact with him before they collaborated in her death, and he had not administered examinations to confirm either her diagnosis or her level of competence to commit suicide. He also lacked the professional expertise to evaluate her. The glare of media attention also raises the question whether Kevorkian acted imprudently in order to generate publicity for his suicide machine and for his forthcoming book.

Jack Kevorkian's actions have been almost universally condemned by lawyers, physicians, and writers in ethics. The case raises all the fears present in the arguments mentioned previously about killing in medicine: abuse, lack of social control, physicians acting without accountability, and unverifiable circumstances of a patient's death. Although this approach to assisted suicide is improper, Kevorkian's "patients" do raise profoundly distressing questions about the lack of a support system in medicine or elsewhere for handling their problems. Having thought for over a year about her future, Janet Adkins decided that the suffering of continued existence exceeded the benefits. Judging from her friends' reports, she knew exactly what she wanted and appreciated both the costs and the benefits. Her family supported her decision, however much they disagreed with it. She faced a bleak future from the perspective of a person who had lived an unusually vigorous life, both physically and mentally. She believed that her brain would be slowly destroyed, with progressive and devastating cognitive loss and confusion, fading memory, immense frustration, and lack of all capacity to take care of herself. She also believed that the full burden of responsibility for her care would be placed on her family. From her perspective, what Kevorkian offered was preferable to what other physicians offered.

Current social institutions, including the medical system, are inadequate to help many patients in a similar condition who have reached a similar conclusion about their fates. Many dying persons face inadequate counseling, emotional support, and pain control. To them their condition is intolerable, and no avenue of hope exists. They would rather kill themselves or be killed than face what they understand to be a bleak future without relief. To say that these persons act immorally by arranging for death at their own hand or with a physician's assistance is a harsh judgment that needs to be backed by persuasive argument. Is it, then, justifiable for physicians to assist in their suicides?

Several prominent cases of *justified* assisted suicide have emerged in medicine in recent years, despite its widespread illegality. First, consider the case of Larry McAfee, in which a court as well as physicians faced a dilemma about legitimate forms of assistance. McAfee was a competent adult paralyzed from the neck down as the result of an automobile accident. He was not terminally ill, but he found his life as a quadriplegic intolerable. A professional engineer, he devised a self-disconnecting, mouth-controlled mechanism that would separate him from his ventilator, thereby causing his death. A Georgia court found that McAfee's right to refuse treatment and disconnect himself outweighed the state's interest in the preservation of life and in preventing suicide. This finding is an endorsement of the right of a competent patient to refuse customary life-sustaining treatment.

But McAfee wanted more, from the courts and from his physicians. He had previously attempted to disconnect himself from the respirator, but had been unable to follow through with the act because he was incapacitated from loss of oxygen. He therefore asked for a physician's assistance in administering a sedative just before he attempted to disconnect himself. The court found in 1989 that no criminal or civil liability would be attached to a physician who helped him by administering the sedative, but this court hinted (agreeing with a trial court) that courts could not order a physician to administer the sedative. Nevertheless, the court found that "McAfee's right to have a sedative (a medication that in no way causes or accelerates death) administered before the ventilator is disconnected is a part of his right to control his medical treatment."[90]

These confusing and troublesome cases should never reach a court. The right acknowledged is a right that health care facilities should recognize without the patient having to meet repeated refusals of assistance from physicians. We do not propose a right that requires coercion of the conscience of physicians, a troubled area of medical ethics. We are recommending instead that medical professionals themselves confront these issues more directly and acknowledge that it is permissible to assist patients. It would then not be necessary to *require* assistance. The problem is that law and medicine (and to some extent ethics) have conspired to block this option for patients by insisting on the maintenance of traditional sanctions against physician-assisted suicide. Larry McAfee is a striking example of how the current system drives patients who need medical attention to physicians like Jack Kevorkian who are willing to take more aggressive actions.

The appellate court in the case of Elizabeth Bouvia pushed matters further. The court suggested that there is a right of privacy to commit suicide and that courts and physicians morally should make it possible for physicians to assist patients in bringing about the end of their lives in dignity and comfort. This court expressly attempted to widen the boundaries of justifiable active assistance by physicians in bringing about a patient's death. In a concurring opinion, Associate Justice Compton exhorted physicians to rethink their traditional objections to assisting such patients to die. The right to die, he said, includes the right to secure assistance from members of the medical profession.[91]

Finally, we turn to a case that many find troublesome but that we believe to be a case of justified assisted suicide. This case involves physician Timothy Quill, who prescribed the barbiturates desired by a 45–year-old patient who had refused a risky, painful, and often unsuccessful treatment for leukemia. She had been his patient for many years, and members of her family had, as a group, come to this decision with the counsel of the physician. The patient was competent, and all reasonable alternatives for the relief of suffering had been discussed and rejected. Several of the conditions that the present authors consider sufficient for justified assisted suicide were satisfied. These conditions include:

1. A voluntary request by a competent patient
2. An ongoing patient–physician relationship
3. Mutual and informed decisionmaking by patient and physician
4. A supportive yet critical and probing environment of decisionmaking
5. A considered rejection of alternatives
6. Structured consultation with other parties in medicine
7. A durable preference for death expressed by the patient
8. Unacceptable suffering by the patient
9. Use of a means that is as painless and comfortable as possible

Even though Quill's actions satisfied most of these conditions, some people find his involvement as a physician unsettling and unjustified. The wedge argument has been mentioned, because so many patients, especially in elderly populations, are potentially affected if acts like Quill's are legalized. Others are troubled by the fact that Quill potentially violated a New York State law against assisted suicide. (After he wrote an article on the case, a grand jury in Rochester, New York, where the events occurred, declined to indict him, apparently because jurors sympathized with his motives and possibly his action.) Furthermore, to reduce the risks of criminal liability, Quill lied to the medical examiner by informing him that a hospice patient had died of acute leukemia.[92]

Despite these problems, we do not oppose Quill's act, his patient's decision, or their relationship. Suffering and loss of cognitive capacity can ravage and dehumanize patients so that death is in their best interests. In these tragic situations physicians such as Quill do not act wrongly in assisting competent patients to bring about their deaths. Public policy issues regarding how to avoid abuses and discourage unjustified acts[93] should be part of our discussion about assisted suicide, but these issues are not problems about the justifiability of the physician's act.

In general we have thus far been able to respect the line between unjustifiable and justifiable passive euthanasia in medical practice, and we should similarly be able to hold the line between justified and unjustified assistance for suicide. However, we are aware that this observation is not entirely free of conflict with our earlier comments on wedge or slippery slope arguments. We therefore need to reconcile—that is, bring into reflective equilibrium—these two points of view.

The view we recommend is the following: Physicians have traditionally maintained that they have no obligation to assist in suicide, only an obligation to care for patients in the process of their dying and an obligation to "do no harm." This position suggests that the act of assisting, if justifiable, is never obligatory; at best, it is a merciful form of nonrequired assistance. This attitude needs to change in medicine. We need to reconceive certain forms of assisting in dying as part of the responsibility of caring for the patient, while rejecting other forms of assistance as outside that obligation. The focus of the discussion about euthanasia and assisted suicide in upcoming years should be on traditional attitudes in medicine, the policies they have generated, and ways to redraw the unstable and often indefensible lines in these policies. As these policies are reconsidered for competent patients, we will also need to reconsider policies for incompetent patients.

Decisionmaking for Incompetent Patients

We discussed standards for surrogate decisions for incompetent patients in Chapter 3. We will now consult those standards in order to discuss *who* should decide for the incompetent patient.

Typically, we think of families who care deeply about their elderly and incompetent members. However, this focus is too narrow. We need an approach that includes incompetent individuals who lack family members and the many residents of nursing homes, psychiatric hospitals, and facilities for the disabled and mentally retarded who rarely, if ever, see a family member. The appropriate roles of families and courts, guardians, conservators, hospital committees, and health professionals all merit consideration.

All we can hope for in treatment and nontreatment decisions for incompetent patients is imperfect procedural justice[94]—that is, a procedure that is just but cannot ensure or guarantee the right outcome (as judged by some independent standard). For example, in criminal trials an independent standard of a right verdict exists (conviction of the guilty and only the guilty), but it is impossible to design a procedure that will guarantee the right verdict in every case. We must, then, evaluate procedures for decisionmaking for incompetent patients according to their fairness and reliable (but imperfect) production of right outcomes.

Advance Directives

In an increasingly popular procedure rooted more in autonomy than in nonmaleficence, a person while competent either writes a directive for health care professionals or selects a surrogate to make decisions about life-sustaining treatments during periods of incompetence.[95] Both actions are appropriate exercises of autonomy. We need, then, to distinguish two types of *advance directive* aimed at governing future decisionmaking: (1) *living wills,* which are specific substantive directives regarding medical procedures that should be provided or forgone in specific circumstances, and (2) *durable power of attorney* (DPA) for health care, or proxy directives. A DPA is a legal document in which one person assigns another person authority to perform specified actions on behalf of the signer. The power is "durable" because, unlike the usual power of attorney, it continues in effect if the signer of the document becomes incompetent.

Much of the early legislative action on this topic (principally involving natural death acts) focused on the agent's decisions through living wills, in the form of advance directives to physicians that specify the treatment a person welcomes or declines in foreseeable circumstances such as a persistent vegetative state (PVS), irreversible loss of cognitive capacities, and incompetence. However, it has proved difficult to specify decisions or guidelines that adequately anticipate the full range of medical situations that might occur, and recently the trend has been to designate surrogates. Both kinds of advance directive can be combined in some legal jurisdictions in a single document,[96] and both can be used for refusal of life-sustaining treatment.

Living wills and DPAs protect autonomy interests and may reduce stress for families and health professionals who fear making the wrong decision, but they also generate both practical and moral problems.[97] First, relatively few persons compose them or leave explicit instructions.[98] This situation is unlikely to change with increased public awareness and patient education. Second, a designated decisionmaker might be unavailable when needed, might be incompetent to make good decisions for the patient, or might have a conflict of interest (for example, because of a prospective inheritance or an improved position in a family-owned business). Third, some patients who change their preferences about treatment fail to change their directives, and a few who become legally incompetent protest a surrogate's decision. Fourth, state laws are often written to severely restrict the use of advance directives. For example, they have legal effect in some states if and only if death is imminent and the patient is terminally ill and incompetent. But decisions must be made in some cases when death is not imminent or the medical condition cannot appropriately be described as a terminal illness. Fifth, living wills provide no basis for health professionals to overturn instructions that turn out not to be in the patient's best medical interest, although the patient could not have reasonably anticipated this circumstance while competent. Surrogate decisionmakers too make decisions with which physicians sharply disagree, in some cases asking the physician to act against his or her conscience. Sixth, some patients do not have an adequate understanding of the range of decisions a health professional or a surrogate might be called upon to make, and even with an adequate understanding it is frequently difficult to foresee clinical situations and possible future experiences.

Many living wills are phrased in vague terms, such as (to approximate AMA language cited earlier), "In the event of a terminal illness where irrefutable evidence exists that biological death is imminent, all extraordinary means of life support should be discontinued." For example, The Pennsylvania Advance Directive for Health Care "declares" as follows: "I direct my attending physician to withhold or withdraw life-sustaining treatment that serves only to prolong the process of my dying, if I should be in a terminal condition or in a state of permanent unconsciousness."[99] Additional questions often must be answered later, such as "Is this condition terminal?," "Is NG-feeding (nasogastric feeding) extraordinary means?," "Is CPR heroic?," and "Is death imminent?" Inference and discretion are involved in answering such questions. The DPA therefore is a more practical instrument than a living will.

Many of these problems can be handled through more carefully worded documents and through proper counseling and skillful explanations by physicians of medical possibilities and treatment options, but some problems of interpretation will remain despite increased physician involvement and educational tools such as videotapes. The need for resourceful interpretation is illustrated in the following case: Mrs. Z., a fifty-five-year-old teacher of foreign languages, developed aspiration pneumonia, which required admission to the intensive care unit. Her condition was probably caused by a diminished gag reflex, the result of twenty years of multiple sclerosis. To prevent future occurrence, the staff discussed oversewing the patient's epiglottis (part of the larynx), which would require a permanent tracheostomy and entail loss of laryngeal speech capability. Because of her multiple sclerosis, Mrs. Z. was confined to bed at home. Her only interaction with friends involved speech, and she tutored students at home. Without the medical procedure, a future episode of aspiration pneumonia would probably be fatal. Mrs. Z. stated that she would rather die than be unable to speak, but she was not clearly competent at the time, in part because of what was believed to be a mild organic brain syndrome. Mrs. Z.'s prior living will was then submitted by her sister. The document contained Mrs. Z.'s directive not to be kept alive artificially if she could not lead a "useful life." The sister—in effect serving as a proxy, as if there were a DPA—interpreted Mrs. Z.'s use of the phrase "useful life" to include the ability to relate to others meaningfully by verbal communication. The staff felt comfortable in accepting this judgment and in refraining from performing procedures they had been considering.[100]

Despite the questionable interpretation of "useful life" in this case, and despite the six problems cited previously, the advance directive is a promising way for competent persons to exercise their autonomy. From the perspective of ethical theory, none of these problems is theoretically untroubled. The problems are primarily practical, and some can be overcome by adequate methods of implementation that follow the outlines of procedures for informed consent in Chapter 3.

Surrogate Decisionmaking without Advance Directives

When an incompetent patient has not left an advance directive, who should make the decision, and with whom should the decisionmaker consult?

Qualifications of surrogate decisionmakers. We propose the following list of qualifications for decisionmakers for incompetent patients (including newborns):

1. Ability to make reasoned judgments (competence)
2. Adequate knowledge and information
3. Emotional stability
4. A commitment to the incompetent patient's interests that is free of conflicts of interest and free of controlling influence by those who might not act in the patient's best interests.

The first three conditions are familiar from the discussion of informed consent in Chapter 3. The only potentially controversial condition is the fourth. Here we are endorsing a criterion of *partiality,* acting as an advocate in the incompetent patient's best interests, rather than *impartiality,* which requires neutrality in the consideration of the interests of the various affected parties.[101]

Four classes of decisionmakers have been proposed and used in cases of withholding and terminating treatment for incompetent patients: families, physicians and other health care professionals, institutional committees, and courts. If a court-appointed guardian exists, that person will be the primary responsible party. But absent the intervention of a court, we need a defeasible structure of decisionmaking authority that places the family as the presumptive authority when the patient cannot make the decision and has not previously designated a decisionmaker.

The role of the family. It is now widely agreed that the patient's closest family member is the first choice as a surrogate. The family's role should be presumptively primary because of expectable identification with the patient's interests, intimate knowledge of his or her wishes, depth of concern about the patient, and the traditional role of the family in society. However, the patient's closest family member(s) are demonstrably unsatisfactory in some cases, and the authority of the family is not final or ultimate.[102] Circumstances occur in which physicians rightly feel compelled to reject a family's decision or to require its review by an ethics committee or the courts. Even the closest family member can have a conflict of interest, can be poorly informed, or can be too distant personally (even estranged). Challenges to family authority of course need to be supported by evidence of the potentially unreasonable or harmful character of their decisions.[103]

Unfortunately the term *family* is imprecise, especially if the extended family is included. Our reasons for assigning presumptive priority to the patient's closest family member also support assignment of priority to other family members, as most state statutes now require. The ranking varies in these statutes, but an example we find acceptable is the ordering in the Virginia Natural Death Act. If the patient is incompetent and has not specified standards through an advance directive, a decision to withhold or withdraw life-prolonging treatment must involve consultation and agreement between the attending physician and "any of the following individuals in the following order of priority if no individual in a prior class is reasonably available, willing and competent to act:" judicially appointed guardian (if necessary in the circumstances), patient-designated decisionmaker, spouse, adult child or a majority of the adult children reasonably available, parents of the patient, and nearest living relative of the patient.[104]

For a previously competent patient, this serial arrangement of family members—spouse, adult children, parents, etc.—rests on their presumed ability to use the person's expressed preferences or values to make the decision or to interpret the standard of best interests, as well as their presumed willingness to do so. For a newborn, the parents generally should be the primary decisionmakers, because they have engaged in a series of actions that resulted in the birth of the infant and may be presumed to seek the newborn's best interests. But they should be disqualified under conditions of child abuse, abandonment, neglect, and the like.

This suggested ranking should on occasion be reordered because of a decisionmaker's personal interest, ignorance, or bad faith. Serious conflicts of interest in the family may be more common than has generally been appreciated by either physicians or the courts. Many family members simultaneously have interests both in the patient's welfare and in the patient's death. A clear example is Case 5: Earle Spring's family was devoted to him but also was under a burdensome financial arrangement in paying for his care. As the debts mounted, a lien was placed on a family home. The court eventually appointed a guardian *ad litem* to investigate and protect Spring's interests. This case and many like it raise profound issues about valid familial decisionmaking under conflict of interest.

In many cases family members decline the decisionmaking role. Among the more difficult circumstances are those in which no party is available, willing, or obligated to make decisions for incompetent persons. A health professional must either make the decision (with or without consultation) or wait until the patient's condition worsens so that an emergency can be declared or possibly seek judicial authorization or appointment of a guardian *ad litem*. Despite many distressing circumstances with few checks and little accountability, contemporary medicine has become accustomed to patients who have no surrogate and no hope for one. However, society has not yet come to grips with the problem. Below we consider a few approaches (ethics committees, ombudsmen, and the like) that should help alleviate this problem.

The role of health care professionals. Physicians and other health care professionals can help the family become adequate decisionmakers and can safeguard the patient's interests and preferences (where known) by monitoring the quality of surrogate decisionmaking. Physicians can sometimes discharge those obligations by withdrawing from the case or transferring the patient, but typically they have obligations to help patients and to ensure that surrogates do not violate those obligations. If a surrogate's decision is contested and differences cannot be resolved, the caregiver will need an independent source of review, a hospital ethics committee or the judicial system. In the event that a surrogate, a member of the health care team, or an independent reviewer asks a caregiver to perform an act that the caregiver regards as futile or unconscionable, the caregiver is not obligated to perform the act, but may still be obligated help the surrogate or patient make other arrangements for care.

In examining the role of physicians and other health care professionals, we need more empirical evidence about their willingness to override familial decisions and their reasons for doing so. Much of the available evidence is derived from parental decisions about neonates and is not accurate beyond this class of patients.[105] Some of this evidence indicates that physicians occasionally displace parents as decisionmakers to protect the parents rather than the infants.[106] Such paternalistic actions toward the parents of seriously ill newborns usually involve nondisclosure or manipulation of information rather than coercion. For example, physicians sometimes do not adequately inform parents on grounds that the information would overburden them, upset them, or make them feel guilty. These actions may be justified, but alternatives such as counseling also may alleviate the problems.

Institutional ethics committees. Surrogates or parents sometimes refuse treatments that are in the interests of those they should protect, and physicians sometimes too readily acquiesce. In other cases, decisionmakers need help in reaching difficult decisions. In both circumstances, a mechanism or procedure is needed to help make a decision or to break a closed, private circle of refusal and acquiescence. A similar need exists for assistance in decisions regarding residents of nursing homes and hospices, psychiatric hospitals, and many residential facilities in which families often play no significant role. One promising, but loosely structured mechanism is the institutional ethics committee. Some state laws now mandate or legally empower these committees.[107]

Institutional committees were often established to allocate time on kidney machines, and for approximately three decades they have been required for research involving human subjects. However, their use for decisionmaking about treatment or nontreatment for incompetent patients is more recent and more controversial. According to a survey in 1981, ethics committees existed in only one percent of all hospitals, in less than five percent of the hospitals with more than two-hundred beds, and in no hospitals with fewer than two-hundred beds.[108] These committees grew dramatically in the 1980s to over sixty percent of all hospitals with two-hundred beds or more.[109] These committees differ widely in their composition and function. Many create and recommend explicit policies to govern actions such as withholding and withdrawing treatment, and many serve educational functions in the hospital. Controversy centers on additional functions such as whether, apart from evidence of abuse of incompetent patients, committees should make, facilitate, or monitor decisions about patients in particular cases.

Many people argue that informal de facto committees already exist because decisions about treatment and nontreatment are not private if numerous caregivers are involved, as is typical in institutions. Several cases have reached the courts because some member of the health care team, often a nurse, believed that a decision not to provide treatment violated legal obligations. From this perspective, committees are unnecessary in decisionmaking: They diffuse responsibility, impose another layer of bureaucratic delay if they are not convened in a timely way, and sometimes they become pawns of powerful groups.

The decisions of committees on occasion need to be reviewed or criticized, perhaps by an auditor or impartial fourth party. This procedural check is similar to the legal use of ''neutral factfinders'' appointed to monitor medical decisions made by parents for children who reject parental judgments.[110] Checks are needed because these committees are informal in their deliberations, and yet can have profound effects on families, institutions, and courts. The committees do not have formal procedures of evidence or legal representation, and checks help protect confidentiality, ensure fair representation, and provide for equal consideration.[111]

Nonetheless, the benefits of good committee review generally outweigh its risks. These committees help resolve disagreements, generate reasoned options, and help the parties conform to institutional guidelines and federal regulations. The committees also can help protect incompetent persons by facilitating treatment when it has been unjustifiably refused, and by denying treatment when it should not have been authorized. Consider, for example, the following case, in which the committee was empowered to make a final decision:[112]

[The review committee] found that the risks of the treatment outweighed its benefits [in the case of] an 85-year-old resident of a center for the developmentally disabled for whom a right inguinal hernia repair, cystoscopy, transurethral resection of the prostate, and right urethral-stone basketing were proposed. Citing the patient's frailty and the high risks of surgery for such a patient, the panel refused to consent to the procedures.

A major justification for committee review has been that open discussion and debate foster better thinking than can be expected of parties with a narrower perspective. The same justification is often given for clinical consultation. However, more research is needed on the role and functioning of these committees. We need to learn, for example, when committees satisfactorily serve as a forum for discussion without having a power of veto, when they should be empowered to make final decisions, and when they might engage in retrospective rather than prospective review of cases or in prospective review without veto power.

These committees have a particularly robust role to play in circumstances in which physicians acquiesce too readily to parental, familial, or guardian wishes. Until we better understand the extent to which families or guardians and physicians act or fail to act to pursue the best interests of infants, minors, or incompetent individuals, it is prudent and morally appropriate to require internal committee review whenever parents, families, or guardians decide that life-sustaining therapy should be forgone (whether or not the physician concurs with the surrogate's decision).[113] In some cases, it is appropriate to threaten parents with a possible court order to obtain necessary parental consent for a procedure that is clearly in a child's best interests.[114]

Surrogate review committees also can serve as a viable alternative to costly court review in the judicial system, especially when no clear legal conflict exists among the various parties to the decision. In some cases, committee advice can help the parties avoid threatened legal difficulties. However, these committees cannot be expected to settle serious legal disputes between parties, for reasons now to be discussed.

The judicial system. Courts have sometimes been unduly intrusive as final decisionmakers, but in many cases courts are the last recourse and the fairest decisionmaker. In a widely discussed declaration by a court, the supreme judicial court of Massachusetts held in *Saikewicz* that questions of life and death require the "process of detached but passionate investigation and decision that forms the ideal on which the judicial branch of government was created." This was expressly a departure from the *Quinlan* decision in New Jersey. The view from

Massachusetts was that the court has a responsibility for making these decisions that is "not to be entrusted to any other group." The court held that probate courts should make these decisions after considering all viewpoints and alternatives, including, if possible and appropriate, those of an ethics committee.[115]

In cases like *Saikewicz,* in which there is no involved family, another decisionmaker—physicians, a committee, or a court—is essential. Nothing is inherently objectionable about an appeal to probate courts as decisionmakers in such cases, but no solid evidence exists to indicate that physicians and hospital ethics committees would be less satisfactory than the courts in many cases. The courts should be invoked when there are good reasons to seek to disqualify the family or health care professionals in order to protect an incompetent patient's interests or to adjudicate conflicts over those interests. The courts also sometimes need to intervene in nontreatment decisions for salvageable incompetent patients in mental institutions, nursing homes, and the like. If no family members are available or willing to be involved, and if the patient is confined to a state mental institution or is in a nursing home, it may be appropriate to establish safeguards beyond the health care team and the institutional ethics committee. For example, the New Jersey Supreme Court in *Conroy* recommended the involvement of the state ombudsman, created several years earlier as an established administrative office for the surveillance of nursing homes.[116]

Conclusion

In this chapter we have concentrated on specifying the principle of nonmaleficence, particularly for actions that eventuate in death. Implicit throughout the chapter is the premise that morality is concerned with the harmfulness of harms *per se,* and not merely with responsibility for causing harm. If it is conceded that we can and should protect persons against some types and levels of harm, as well as avoid causing harm to them, it is a short step to the conclusion that a positive obligation exists to provide benefits such as health care. The step may be shorter still because of the conceptual and moral uncertainty that surrounds the distinctions between the obligation to avoid harm to others, the obligation to benefit them, and the obligation to treat them justly. These topics are engaged in Chapters 5 and 6.

Notes

1. W. H. S. Jones, *Hippocrates,* vol. I (Cambridge, MA: Harvard University Press, 1923), p. 165. See also Ludwig Edelstein, *Ancient Medicine,* ed. O. Temkin and C. L. Temkin (Baltimore: Johns Hopkins University Press, 1967); and Albert R.

Jonsen, "Do No Harm: Axiom of Medical Ethics," in *Philosophical and Medical Ethics: Its Nature and Significance,* ed. Stuart F. Spicker and H. Tristram Engelhardt, Jr. (Dordrecht, the Netherlands: D. Reidel, 1977), pp. 27–41.

2. See H. L. A. Hart, *The Concept of Law* (Oxford: Clarendon Press, 1961), p. 190.

3. See, for example, W. D. Ross, *The Right and the Good* (Oxford: Clarendon Press, 1930), pp. 21–26; and John Rawls, *A Theory of Justice* (Cambridge, MA: Harvard University Press, 1971), p. 114.

4. William Frankena, *Ethics,* 2d Ed. (Englewood Cliffs, NJ: Prentice-Hall, 1973), p. 47.

5. *McFall v. Shimp,* no. 78–1771 in Equity (C. P. Allegheny County, Pa., July 26, 1978). See also Barbara J. Culliton, "Court Upholds Refusal to Be Medical Good Samaritan," *Science* 201 (August 18, 1978): 596–97; "Bone Marrow Transplant Plea Rejected," *American Medical News* 21 (August 11, 1978): 13; "Anemia Victim Dies, Asks Forgiveness for Cousin," *International Herald Tribune,* August 12–13, 1978; "Judge Upholds Transplant Denial," *New York Times,* July 27, 1978, p. A10; Dennis A. William and Lawrence Walsh, "The Law: Bad Samaritan," *Newsweek* 92 (August 7, 1978): 35.

6. Alan Meisel and Loren H. Roth, "Must a Man Be His Cousin's Keeper?" *Hastings Center Report* 8 (October 1978): 5–6.

7. W. D. Ross, for example, regards "not injuring others" as a synonym of "nonmaleficence" and includes under the duty of nonmaleficence several of the Decalogue's prohibitions of harmful actions, such as killing, stealing, committing adultery, and bearing false witness. Ross, *The Right and the Good,* pp. 21–22.

8. See Joel Feinberg, *Harm to Others,* vol. I of *The Moral Limits of the Criminal Law* (New York: Oxford University Press, 1984), pp. 32–36.

9. For rules of nonmaleficence, see Bernard Gert, *Morality: A New Justification of Morality* (New York: Oxford University Press, 1988), ch. 6–7. He offers a different account of justificatory support for moral rules.

10. For a careful criticism of the priority of avoiding harm, see Nancy Davis, "The Priority of Avoiding Harm," in *Killing and Letting Die,* ed. Bonnie Steinbock (Englewood Cliffs, NJ: Prentice-Hall, 1980), pp. 172–214.

11. See Eric D'Arcy, *Human Acts: An Essay in their Moral Evaluation* (Oxford: Clarendon Press, 1963), p. 121.

12. Cf. William L. Prosser, *Handbook of the Law of Torts,* 4th Ed. (St. Paul, MN: West Publishing, 1971), pp. 145–46. For a broad view that includes "moral negligence," see Ronald D. Milo, *Immorality* (Princeton, NJ: Princeton University Press, 1984).

13. See "Physician's Duty to Inform of Risks," *American Law Reports,* 3d, 88 (1986): 1010–25; and Martin Curd and Larry May, *Professional Responsibility for Harmful Actions* (Dubuque, IA: Kendall/Hunt, 1984).

14. Quoted in Angela Roddy Holder, *Medical Malpractice Law* (New York: John Wiley & Sons, 1975), p. 42.

15. This case was presented to one of the authors during a consultation.

16. *In the matter of Spring,* Mass. 405 N.E. 2d 115 (1980), at 488–89.

17. See President's Commission, *Deciding to Forego Life-Sustaining Treatment,* pp. 73–77.

18. Robert Stinson and Peggy Stinson, *The Long Dying of Baby Andrew* (Boston: Little, Brown and Co., 1983), p. 355.

19. Susanna E. Bedell and Thomas L. Delbanco, "Choices about Cardiopulmonary

Resuscitation in the Hospital: When Do Physicians Talk with Patients?,'' *New England Journal of Medicine* 310 (April 26, 1984): 1089–93. See also Marcia Angell, ''Respecting the Autonomy of Competent Patients,'' *New England Journal of Medicine* 310 (April 26, 1984): 1115–16.

20. See Paul Ramsey, *The Patient as Person* (New Haven: Yale University Press, 1970), p. 120.

21. See Diane Lynn Redleaf, Suzanne Baillie Schmitt, and William Charles Thompson, ''The California Natural Death Act: An Empirical Study of Physicians' Practices,'' *Stanford Law Review* 31 (May 1979): 913–47.

22. Gerald Kelly, S.J., ''The Duty to Preserve Life,'' *Theological Studies* 12 (December 1951): 550.

23. This case has been adapted with permission from a case presented by Dr. Martin P. Albert of Charlottesville, VA.

24. In the matter of *Quinlan*, 70 N.J. 10, 355 A.2d 647, *cert. denied*, 429 U.S. 922 (1976).

25. In re *Conroy*, 486 A.2d 1209 (N.J. 1985).

26. *Brophy v. New England Sinai Hospital, Inc.*, 398 Mass. 417, 497 N.E. 2d 626 (1986).

27. These issues were first raised in 1982, in *Barber v. Superior Court*, 147 Cal. App. 3d 1006, 195 Cal. Rptr. 484 (1983). By 1988, many courts accepted this trend as determinative [see, e.g., *Gray v. Romeo*, 697 F.Supp. 580 (D.R.I. 1988) and *McConnell v. Beverly Enterprises*, 209 Conn. 692 (Conn. Sup. Ct. 1989), 553 A.2d 596]. For a review of the massive court literature during this formative period, see Alan Meisel, *The Right to Die* (New York: John Wiley and Sons, 1989), § 5.10. In *Cruzan v. Director, Missouri Department of Health*, 110 S.Ct. 2841 (1990), the U.S. Supreme Court focused on procedural requirements for termination of life-sustaining treatment for incompetent patients. The court assumed that a competent person has a constitutionally protected right to refuse lifesaving hydration and nutrition. Its dicta reflected no distinction between medical and sustenance treatments.

28. See Joanne Lynn and James F. Childress, ''Must Patients Always Be Given Food and Water?'' *Hastings Center Report* 13 (October 1983): 17–21. See also the essays in Joanne Lynn, ed., *By No Extraordinary Means* (Bloomington: Indiana University Press, 1986).

29. G. E. M. Anscombe, ''Ethical Problems in the Management of Some Severely Handicapped Children: Commentary,'' *Journal of Medical Ethics* 7 (1981): 122.

30. Koop, ''Ethical and Surgical Considerations in the Care of the Newborn with Congenital Abnormalities,'' in *Infanticide and the Handicapped Newborn*, ed. Dennis J. Horan and Melinda Delahoyde (Provo, UT: Brigham Young University Press, 1982), pp. 89–106, esp. 105.

31. C. Everett Koop and Edward R. Grant, ''The 'Small Beginnings' of Euthanasia,'' *Journal of Law, Ethics & Public Policy* 2 (1986): 607–32.

32. *Federal Register* 48, No. 129, July 5, 1983.

33. See the summary of living will legislation in *The Physician and the Hopelessly Ill Patient* (New York: Society for the Right to Die, 1985), pp. 39–80, and *1988 Supplement*, pp. 17–34.

34. Daniel Callahan, ''On Feeding the Dying,'' *Hastings Center Report* 13 (October 1983): 22, and see Ronald A. Carson, ''The Symbolic Significance of Giving to Eat and Drink,'' in *By No Extraordinary Means*, pp. 85, 87.

35. See Mark Siegler and Alan J. Weisbard, "Against the Emerging Stream: Should Fluids and Nutritional Support Be Discontinued?" *Archives of Internal Medicine* 145 (January 1985): 129–32; and Patrick Derr, "Why Food and Fluids Can Never Be Denied," *Hastings Center Report* 16 (February 1986): 28–30.

36. Joyce V. Zerwekh, "The Dehydration Question," *Nursing '83* (January 1983): 47–51, reprinted in Lynn, ed., *By No Extraordinary Means,* ch. 2; Ronald Cranford, "Neurologic Syndromes and Prolonged Survival: When Can Artificial Nutrition and Hydration be Foregone?" *Law, Medicine, and Health Care* 19 (1991): 13–22, esp. 18–19.

37. Kenneth C. Micetich, Patricia H. Steinecker, and David C. Thomasma, "Are Intravenous Fluids Morally Required for Dying Patients?" *Archives of Internal Medicine* 143 (May, 1983): 975–78.

38. President's Commission, *Deciding to Forego Life-Sustaining Treatment,* pp. 17–18.

39. The rule of double effect has precedents that predate the writings of St. Thomas Aquinas (e.g., in Augustine and Abelard). However, the history primarily flows from Aquinas in traditions such as that of the Jesuits. See Anthony Kenny, "The History of Intention in Ethics," *Anatomy of the Soul* (Oxford: Basil Blackwell, 1973), Appendix; and Joseph T. Mangan, S.J., "An Historical Analysis of the Principle of Double Effect," *Theological Studies* 10 (1949): 41–61.

40. However, the RDE is defended by some as having only a prima facie moral force that can be overridden by competing moral considerations. See Warren S. Quinn, "Actions, Intentions, and Consequences: The Doctrine of Double Effect," *Philosophy and Public Affairs* 18 (1989): 334–51, esp. 344–45.

41. Joseph Boyle reduces the RDE to two conditions: intention and proportionality. "Who Is Entitled to Double Effect?" *Journal of Medicine and Philosophy* 16 (1991): 475–94, and "Toward Understanding the Principle of Double Effect," *Ethics* 90 (1980): 527–38. For an emphasis on intention, see Charles Fried, *Right and Wrong* (Cambridge, MA: Harvard University Press, 1978) and Thomas Nagel, *The View from Nowhere* (New York: Oxford University Press, 1986). For an emphasis on proportionality, see Richard McCormick, *Ambiguity in Moral Choice* (Milwaukee, WI: Marquette University, 1973) and his contribution to Paul Ramsey and Richard A. McCormick, S.J., eds., *Doing Evil to Achieve Good: Moral Choice in Conflict Situations* (Chicago: Loyola University Press, 1978). For guides to the large literature, see works cited in this section and several essays in the *Journal of Medicine and Philosophy* 16 (1991).

42. For these cases, see David Granfield, *The Abortion Decision* (Garden City, NY: Image Books, 1971), which defends the RDE, and Susan Nicholson, *Abortion and the Roman Catholic Church* (Knoxville, TN: Religious Ethics, Inc., 1978), which criticizes it. See also the criticisms in Donald Marquis, "Four Versions of Double Effect," *Journal of Medicine and Philosophy* 16 (1991): 515–44.

43. For a critique with special reference to Richard McCormick, see G. E. M. Anscombe, "Action, Intention, and 'Double Effect,' " *Proceedings of the American Catholic Philosophical Association* 56 (1982): 21–24.

44. The most developed analysis is Bratman, *Intention, Plans, and Practical Reason* (Cambridge, MA: Harvard University Press, 1987).

45. Alvin I. Goldman, *A Theory of Human Action* (Englewood Cliffs, NJ: Prentice-Hall, 1970), pp. 49–85.

46. See Hector-Neri Castañeda, "Intensionality and Identity in Human Action and Philosophical Method," *Nous* 13 (1979): 235–60, esp. 255.

47. Our analysis here borrows from Ruth R. Faden and Tom L. Beauchamp, *A History and Theory of Informed Consent* (New York: Oxford University Press, 1986), chap. 7.

48. We follow John Searle in thinking that we cannot reliably distinguish in many situations among acts, effects, consequences, and events. Searle, "The Intentionality of Intention and Action," *Cognitive Science* 4 (1980): 65.

49. Such an interpretation of double effect is defended by Boyle, "Who Is Entitled to Double Effect?"

50. See the synoptic argument to this conclusion in Helga Kuhse, *The Sanctity-of-Life Doctrine in Medicine: A Critique* (Oxford: Clarendon Press, 1987), esp. pp. 93–103.

51. For debates about futility, see Stuart J. Youngner, "Who Defines Futility?," *Journal of the American Medical Association* 260 (October 14, 1988): 2094–95 and "Futility in Context," *Journal of the American Medical Association* 264 (September 12, 1990): 1295–96; Steven H. Miles, "Informed Demand for 'Non-Beneficial' Medical Treatment," *New England Journal of Medicine* 325 (Aug. 15, 1991): 512–15; John D. Lantos et al., "The Illusion of Futility in Clinical Practice," *The American Journal of Medicine* 87 (July 1989): 81–84; and Nancy Jecker, "Are Physicians Obligated to Provide Futile Treatment?," *Medical Ethics* 7 (December 1992): 9–11.

52. This case was recorded by Robert Baker in his project on Moral Methodologies in ICUs.

53. Many judicial opinions accept this conclusion. Competent patients have the legal right to refuse treatment in the United States, even if not terminally ill, as a result of *Cruzan v. Director,* 110 S.Ct. 2841, at 2851 (1990). See also *Bouvia* and *McAfee,* as discussed later in this chapter. For statements regarding incompetent patients, see *In re Browning,* 543 So.2d 258 (Fla. Dist. Ct. App. 1989), *aff'd* 568 So.2d 4 (Fla. 1990) and *McConnell v. Beverly Enterprises,* 209 Conn. 692, 553 A.2d 596 (1989).

54. *Superintendent of Belchertown State School v. Saikewicz,* Mass., 370 N.E. 2d 417 (1977), at 428.

55. Ibid.

56. Ramsey, *Ethics at the Edges of Life* (New Haven: Yale University Press, 1978), p. 155.

57. See President's Commission, *Deciding to Forego Life-Sustaining Treatment,* ch. 5, and the articles on "The Persistent Problem of PVS," *Hastings Center Report* 18 (February/March 1988): 26–47.

58. Ramsey, *Ethics at the Edges of Life,* p. 172.

59. President's Commission, *Deciding to Forego Life-Sustaining Treatment.*

60. See Norman L. Cantor, *Legal Frontiers of Death and Dying* (Bloomington: Indiana University Press, 1987), pp. 87–91.

61. See Frank A. Chervenak and Laurence B. McCullough, "Nonaggressive Obstetric Management," *Journal of the American Medical Association* 261 (June 16, 1989): 3439–40. For issues about decisions regarding seriously ill newborns, see Hastings Center Newborn Project, "Imperiled Newborns," *Hastings Center Report* 17 (December 1987): 5–32; Richard C. McMillan, H. Tristram Engelhardt, Jr., and Stuart

F. Spicker, eds., *Euthanasia and the Newborn: Conflicts Regarding Saving Lives* (Dordrecht, the Netherlands: D. Reidel, 1987); and Arthur L. Caplan and Robert H. Blank, eds., *Compassion: Government Intervention in the Treatment of Critically Ill Newborns* (Totowa, NJ: The Humana Press, 1992).

62. Albert R. Jonsen and Michael J. Garland, "A Moral Policy for Life/Death Decisions in the Intensive Care Nursery," in *Ethics of Newborn Intensive Care,* ed. Albert R. Jonsen and Michael J. Garland (Berkeley: University of California, Institute of Governmental Studies, 1976), p. 148.

63. Raymond S. Duff and A. G. M. Campbell, "Moral and Ethical Dilemmas in the Special-Care Nursery," *New England Journal of Medicine* 289 (October 25, 1973): 890–94.

64. "Child Abuse Prevention and Treatment and Adoption Reform Act Amendments of 1984," Public Law 98–457, 42 U.S.C. 5101ff (1984); "Child Abuse and Neglect Prevention and Treatment Program: Final Rule," *Federal Register* 50 (April 15, 1985): 14878–901. The American Medical Association, the American Hospital Association and other professional groups challenged these regulations in *United States v. University Hospital,* 729 F.2d 144 (1984) and *American Hospital Association v. Heckler,* 585 F. Supp. 541, App. to Pet. for Cert. 50a (1984). Lower courts found the regulations invalid, and this ruling was upheld by the U.S. Supreme Court on June 9, 1986 (*Bowen v. American Hospital Association et al.,* No. 84-1529, 54 LW 4579 (June 9, 1986). For stages in the evolution of the government's action, see Nancy M. P. King, "Federal and State Regulation of Neonatal Decision-Making," and Mary Ann Gardell and H. Tristram Engelhardt, Jr., "The Baby Doe Controversy: An Outline of Some Points in Its Development," in McMillan, Engelhardt, and Spicker, eds., *Euthanasia and the Newborn,* pp. 89–116, 293–99.

65. See Helga Kuhse and Peter Singer, *Should the Baby Live?* (Oxford: Oxford University Press, 1985), p. 46.

66. See Fred Barbash and Christina Russell, "The Demise of 'Infant . . .': Permitted Death Gives Life to an Old Debate," *Washington Post,* April 17, 1982.

67. *In re Colyer,* 660 P.2d 738 (1983), at 751.

68. A special issue of *Law, Medicine, and Health Care* 17 (Winter 1989) is devoted to the Linares case. See also Steven H. Miles, "Taking Hostages: The Linares Case," *Hastings Center Report* 19 (July/August 1989): 4.

69. In the matter of *Claire C. Conroy,* 190 N.J. Sup. 453, 464 A.2d 303 (App. Div. 1983). See the analysis in several articles in Joanne Lynn, ed., *By No Extraordinary Means,* pp. 227–66.

70. In the matter of *Claire C. Conroy,* 486 A.2d 1209 (New Jersey Supreme Court, 1985), at 1222–23, 1236.

71. See *In re Estate of Greenspan,* 558 N.E.2d 1194, at 1203 (Ill. 1990).

72. Causal judgments are *commonly* controlled by forms of practical judgment as well as by causal explanation. See H. L. A. Hart and A. M. Honore, *Causation in the Law* (Oxford: Clarendon Press, 1959), and Samuel Gorovitz, "Causal Judgments and Causal Explanations," *Journal of Philosophy* 62 (1965): 695–711.

73. For an example of one author who straightforwardly uses "killing" as a moral notion entailing culpability, see Daniel Callahan, "When Self-Determination Runs Amok," *Hastings Center Report* 22 (March–April 1992): 53–54.

74. Dan Brock, "Death and Dying," in *Medical Ethics,* ed. Robert M. Veatch (Boston: Jones and Bartlett Publishers, 1989), p. 345.

75. American Geriatrics Society, Public Policy Committee, "Voluntary Active Euthanasia," *Journal of the American Geriatrics Society* 39 (August 1991): 826.

76. American Medical Association, Council on Ethical and Judicial Affairs, *Euthanasia: Report C,* in *Proceedings of the House of Delegates* (Chicago: American Medical Association, June, 1988): 258–60 (and see *Current Opinions,* § 2.20, p. 13, 1989); "Decisions Near the End of Life," *Report B,* adopted by the House of Delegates (1991), pp. 11–15, and see the abridged version in "Decisions Near the End of Life," *Journal of the American Medical Association* 267 (April 22/29, 1992): 2229–33. In March 1986 the AMA amended an earlier statement so that "life-prolonging medical treatment includes medication and artificially or technologically supplied respiration, nutrition or hydration." *Current Opinions* (Chicago: AMA, 1986), § 2.18, pp. 12–13.

77. *People v. Roberts,* 211 Mich. 187, 178 N.W. 690 (1920).

78. This distinction and our arguments are indebted to John Rawls, "Two Concepts of Rules," *Philosophical Review* 64 (1955): 3–32.

79. For fuller discussions, see Douglas Walton, *Slippery Slope Arguments* (Oxford: Clarendon Press, 1992); Trudy Govier, "What's Wrong with Slippery Slope Arguments?" *Canadian Journal of Philosophy* 12 (June 1982): 303–16; Frederick Schauer, "Slippery Slopes," *Harvard Law Review* 99 (1985): 361–83; Bernard Williams, "Which Slopes Are Slippery?" in *Moral Dilemmas in Modern Medicine,* ed. Michael Lockwood (Oxford: Oxford University Press, 1985), pp. 126–37; David Lamb, *Down the Slippery Slope: Arguing in Applied Ethics* (London: Croom Helm, 1988); Wibren van der Burg, "The Slippery Slope Arguments," *Ethics* 102 (October 1991): 42–65; and James Rachels, *The End of Life: Euthanasia and Morality* (Oxford: Oxford University Press, 1986), ch. 10.

80. See Gerald J. Hughes, S.J., "Killing and Letting Die," *The Month* 8 (February 1975): 42–45; and David Louisell, "Euthanasia and Biathanasia: On Dying and Killing," *Linacre Quarterly* 40 (November 1973): 234–58.

81. Leo Alexander, "Medical Science under Dictatorship," *New England Journal of Medicine* 241 (1949): 39–47.

82. Robert Jay Lifton, *The Nazi Doctors: Medical Killing and the Psychology of Genocide* (New York: Basic Books, 1986).

83. See Rachels, *The End of Life,* and the special supplement on "Biomedical Ethics and the Shadow of Nazism," *Hastings Center Report* 6 (August 1976), Supp., esp. the article by Lucy Dawidowicz. See also Arthur L. Caplan, ed., *When Medicine Went Mad: Bioethics and the Holocaust* (Totowa, NJ: Humana Press, 1992); and George J. Annas and Michael Grodin, *The Nazi Doctors and the Nuremberg Code* (New York: Oxford University Press, 1992).

84. "It's Over, Debbie," *Journal of the American Medical Association* 259 (1988): 272. A substantial controversy followed publication of this article. The pro and con positions are quoted and much of the literature summarized in Victor Cohn, "Is It Time for Mercy Killing?," *Washington Post,* Health Section (Aug. 15, 1989), pp. 12–15.

85. We owe much in this argument to James Rachels (personal correspondence).

86. Marcia Angell, "The Quality of Mercy," *New England Journal of Medicine* 306 (January 14, 1982): 98–99.

87. Paul J. van der Maas et al., "Euthanasia and Other Medical Decisions Concerning the End of Life," *The Lancet* 338 (September 14, 1991): 669–74. Defenders and critics of euthanasia interpret the evidence differently. For a critic's interpretation,

see Carlos Gomez, *Regulating Death: The Case of the Netherlands* (New York: The Free Press, 1991); for a defender's interpretation, see Margaret Battin, "Voluntary Euthanasia and the Risks of Abuse: Can We Learn Anything from the Netherlands?" *Law, Medicine & Health Care* 20 (Spring–Summer, 1992): 135.

88. For a discussion of this case, see Paige Mitchell, *Act of Love: The Killing of George Zygmaniak* (New York: Alfred A. Knopf, 1976).

89. Based on: *New York Times,* June 6, pp. A1, B6; June 7, 1990, pp. A1, D22; June 9, p. A6; June 12, p. C3; *Newsweek,* June 18, 1990, p. 46. For Kevorkian's description of the events, see his *Prescription: Medicide* (Buffalo, NY: Prometheus Books, 1991), pp. 221–31.

90. *State of Georgia v. McAfee,* 385 S.E.2d 651 (Ga. 1989).

91. *Bouvia v. Superior Court,* 179 Cal. App. 3d 1127, at 1146–47. 225 Cal. Rptr. 297 (1986). See also Lorna A. Voboril, *"Bouvia v. Superior Court:* The Death Option," *Pacific Law Journal* 18 (1987): 1029–53.

92. See Timothy E. Quill, "Death and Dignity: A Case of Individualized Decision Making," *New England Journal of Medicine* 324 (March 7, 1991): 691–94, reprinted with additional analysis in Quill, *Death and Dignity* (New York: W. W. Norton & Co., 1993); Lawrence K. Altman, "A Doctor Agonized but Provided Drugs To Help End a Life," *New York Times,* March 3, 1991, pp. A1, B8; Altman, "Jury Declines to Indict a Doctor Who Said He Aided in a Suicide," *New York Times,* July 27, 1991, pp. A1, A10.

93. For a recommendation that we should emphasize good palliative care and sensitive laws for termination of treatment as our public policy, while rejecting active killing, see Joanne Lynn, "The Health Care Professional's Role When Active Euthanasia Is Sought," *Journal of Palliative Care* 4 (1988): 100–102, and Susan Wolf, "Holding the Line on Euthanasia," *Hastings Center Report* 19 (January–February 1989): S13–S15.

94. See Rawls, *A Theory of Justice,* pp. 85–86.

95. In 1991, forty-nine states and the District of Columbia had some form of advance-directive law that anticipates decisions and decisionmaking authority regarding use of life-sustaining treatment. Of these, twenty states acknowledged durable power of attorney permitting the appointment of a surrogate to make treatment decisions; this figure showed a dramatic increase, since only nine acknowledged durable power of attorney in 1989. See Advance Directives Seminar Group, "Advance Directives: Are They an Advance?," *Canadian Medical Association Journal* 146 (January 15, 1992): 127–34. For a helpful discussion, see Nancy M. P. King, *Making Sense of Advance Directives* (Dordrecht, the Netherlands: Kluwer Academic Publishers, 1991).

96. For an attempt to combine the two forms in a single document, see Robert Olick, "Approximating Informed Consent and Fostering Communication: The Anatomy of an Advance Directive," *Journal of Clinical Ethics* 2 (1991): 181–95.

97. For a balanced account of problems and promise in advance directives, see Dan Brock, "Trumping Advance Directives," *Hastings Center Report* 21 (September–October 1991): S5–S6.

98. See E. R. Gamble et al., "Knowledge, Attitudes, and Behavior of Elderly Persons Regarding Living Wills," *Archives of Internal Medicine* 151 (February 1991): 277–80.

99. General Assembly of Pennsylvania, Senate Bill No. 3, Session of 1991, as amended April 6, 1992, as published in *Philadelphia Medicine* 88 (August 1992): 329–33.

100. Stuart J. Eisendrath and Albert R. Jonsen, "The Living Will," *Journal of the American Medical Association* 249 (April 15, 1983): 2054–58.

101. See the somewhat different set of qualifications proposed by Robert Weir, *Selective Nontreatment of Handicapped Newborns* (New York: Oxford University Press, 1984), ch. 9. He uses the criterion of impartiality, rather than partiality.

102. See Judith Areen, "The Legal Status of Consent Obtained from Families of Adult Patients to Withhold or Withdraw Treatment," *Journal of the American Medical Association* 258 (July 10, 1987): 229–35; and John W. Warren et al., "Informed Consent by Proxy: An Issue in Research with Elderly Patients," *New England Journal of Medicine* 315 (October, 1986): 1124–28, as discussed in Chapter 3, this volume (p. 177).

103. Nancy Rhoden has proposed that physicians who reject family's choices should be placed under a burden of adducing evidence in court as to the unreasonableness of the decision. "Litigating Life and Death," *Harvard Law Review* 102 (1988): 437. Patricia King has argued that some family interests other than those that support the patient's best medical interests should be considered legitimate. "The Authority of Families to Make Medical Decisions for Incompetent Patients after the *Cruzan* Decision," *Law, Medicine & Health Care* 19 (1991): 76–79.

104. Virginia Natural Death Act, Va. Code §§ 54–325.8:1–13 (1983).

105. See A. Shaw, J. G. Randolph, and B. Manard, "Ethical Issues in Pediatric Surgery: A National Survey of Pediatricians and Pediatric Surgeons," *Pediatrics* 60 (1977): 588–99; and David Todres, "Pediatricians' Attitudes Affecting Decision-Making in Defective Infants," *Pediatrics* 60 (1977): 197. Even though there is debate about the available survey data, such data played a role in the efforts by the U.S. Department of Health and Human Services to establish a mechanism for protecting handicapped infants from discrimination. See *Federal Register* 49 (January 12, 1984): 1645.

106. See President's Commission, *Deciding to Forego Life-Sustaining Treatment,* pp. 210–11.

107. See Clarence J. Sundram, "Informed Consent for Major Medical Treatment of Mentally Disabled People," *New England Journal of Medicine* 318 (May 26, 1988): 1368–73.

108. President's Commission, *Deciding to Forego Life-Sustaining Treatment,* p. 446.

109. See American Academy of Pediatrics Infant Bioethics Task Force and Consultants, Guidelines for Infant Bioethics Committees, *Pediatrics* 74 (August 1984): 306–310; American Medical Association, Judicial Council, "Guidelines for Ethics Committees in Health Care Institutions," *Journal of the American Medical Association* 253 (May 10, 1985): 2698–99; Fred Rosner, "Hospital Medical Ethics Committees: A Review of Their Development," *Journal of the American Medical Association* 253 (May 10, 1985); Tracy Miller and Anna Maria Cugliari, "Withdrawing and Withholding Treatment: Policies in Long-Term Care Facilities," *Gerontologist* 30 (August 1990): 462–68.

110. See *Parham v. J.R.,* 442 U.S. 584, 602 (1979).

111. See Susan M. Wolf, "Ethics Committees and Due Process: Nesting Rights in a Community of Caring," *Maryland Law Review* 50 (1991): 798–858.

112. Sundram, "Informed Consent for Major Medical Treatment of Mentally Disabled People," p. 1372.

113. Cf. President's Commission, *Deciding to Forego Life-Sustaining Treatment,* p. 227. Contrast Raymond S. Duff and A. G. M. Campbell, "Moral Communities

and Tragic Choice,'' in McMillan, Engelhardt, and Spicker, eds., *Euthanasia and the Newborn,* pp. 273–80.

114. For a case in which this expedient was necessary, see Mary B. Mahowald, ''Baby Doe Committees: A Critical Evaluation,'' Ethical and Legal Issues in Perinatology, *Clinics in Perinatology* 15 (December 1988): 792–93.

115. *Superintendent of Belchertown State School v. Saikewicz,* Mass., 370 N.E. 2d 417 (1977).

116. *In re Conroy,* 486 A.2d 1209 (N.J. 1985), at 1239–42.

5

Beneficence

Morality requires not only that we treat persons autonomously and refrain from harming them, but also that we contribute to their welfare. Such beneficial actions fall under the heading of beneficence. No sharp breaks exist on the continuum from the noninfliction of harm to the provision of benefit, but principles of beneficence potentially demand more than the principle of nonmaleficence because agents must take positive steps to help others, not merely refrain from harmful acts. The word *nonmaleficence* is sometimes used broadly to include the prevention of harm and the removal of harmful conditions. However, prevention and removal require positive acts to benefit others, and therefore belong under beneficence rather than nonmaleficence.

In the present chapter we examine two principles of beneficence: positive beneficence and utility. *Positive beneficence* requires the provision of benefits. *Utility* requires that benefits and drawbacks be balanced. Both together are distinguished from the virtue of benevolence, from various forms of care, and from nonobligatory ideals of beneficence. Building on these distinctions and our analysis of them, we discuss conflicts between beneficence and respect for autonomy in paternalistic refusals to acquiesce in a patient's wishes or choices. The remainder of the chapter focuses on balancing benefits, risks, and costs, especially through analytical methods designed to implement the principle of utility in health policy and clinical care. We conclude that these methods have a useful, although limited, role as aids to decisionmaking, and that they need

259

to be constrained by moral norms, especially justice in the distribution of benefits, risks, and costs.

The Concept of Beneficence

In ordinary English the term *beneficence* connotes acts of mercy, kindness, and charity. Altruism, love, and humanity are also sometimes considered forms of beneficence. We will understand beneficent action even more broadly, so that it includes all forms of action intended to benefit other persons. *Beneficence* refers to an action done for the benefit of others; *benevolence* refers to the character trait or virtue of being disposed to act for the benefit of others; and *principle of beneficence* refers to a moral obligation to act for the benefit of others. Many acts of beneficence are not obligatory, but a principle of beneficence, in our usage, asserts an obligation to help others further their important and legitimate interests.

Beneficence and benevolence have played central roles in some ethical theories. Utilitarianism, for example, is systematically arranged on a principle of beneficence (the principle of utility), and during the Scottish Enlightenment, major figures such as Francis Hutcheson and David Hume made benevolence the centerpiece of their common-morality theories. In all of these theories, beneficence is central, in part because it is conceived as an aspect of human nature that motivates us to act in the interests of others, and this goal is closely associated in these theories with the goal of morality itself.

We will argue, somewhat similarly, that obligations to confer benefits, to prevent and remove harms, and to weigh and balance the possible goods against the costs and possible harms of an action are central to biomedical ethics, although principles of beneficence are not broad enough to include all other principles. Because the moral life typically does not provide the opportunity to produce benefits or eliminate harms without creating risks or incurring costs, the principle of utility is an essential extension of the principle of positive beneficence. For example, in our discussion in Chapter 4 of withholding and withdrawing life-sustaining treatment from incompetent patients, we noted the importance of considering a treatment's probable chance of success and then balancing its probable benefits against its probable costs or risks to the patient. And, as we saw in Chapter 2, utilitarians and nonutilitarians both need a principle for balancing benefits and harms, balancing benefits against alternative benefits, and balancing harms against alternative harms.

This principle of utility is not identical, in our analysis, to the classical utilitarian principle of utility, which is an absolute or preeminent principle. Our principle should be construed neither as the sole principle of ethics nor as one that justifies or overrides all other principles. It is one among a number of prima facie principles. This principle is also limited to balancing benefits, risks, and costs (outcomes of actions), and does not determine the overall balancing of obligations. The principle of utility (sometimes called proportionality) is often criticized because it appears to allow the interests of society to override individual interests and rights. In medical research, for example, the principle of utility suggests that dangerous research on human subjects can be undertaken, and ought to be undertaken, if a likely benefit to society outweighs the danger of the research to the individual. Although it is true that an *unconstrained* principle of utilitarian balancing carries this danger, we do not defend such a principle. To the contrary, we propose several constraints on utility.[1]

Obligatory and Ideal Beneficence

Although philosophers as different as Jeremy Bentham and W. D. Ross have employed the term *beneficence* to identify positive obligations to others, many critics are suspicious of the claim that we have these positive obligations. They hold that beneficence is purely a virtuous ideal or an act of charity, and thus that persons are not morally deficient if they fail to act beneficently. These concerns rightly point to a need to clarify and specify beneficence, taking care to note the limits of our obligations and the points at which beneficence is optional rather than obligatory.

The most famous example of beneficence is found in the New Testament parable of the Good Samaritan, which illustrates several problems in interpreting beneficence. In this parable, a man traveling from Jerusalem to Jericho was beaten by robbers who left him "half-dead." After two other travelers passed by the injured man without rendering help, a Samaritan who saw him "had compassion, and went to him and bound up his wounds, . . . brought him to an inn, and took care of him." In having compassion and showing mercy, the Good Samaritan expressed an attitude of caring for the injured man and also took care of him. Both his motives and his actions were beneficent. However, the parable suggests that positive beneficence is more an ideal than an obligation, because the Samaritan's act seems to exceed ordinary morality. Moreover, suppose that the injured man, when encountered by the Samaritan, had pulled out an advance directive indicating that he wanted to die if wounded on the dangerous road from Jerusalem to Jericho. Then the Samaritan would have faced a dilemma: to respect the injured man's wishes or to take care of him against his wishes. Our beneficence, then, is sometimes an admirable ideal of action that exceeds obligations, and at other times it is appropriately limited by other moral obligations. But are we ever *obligated* to act beneficently?

We can begin to address this question by noting that acts of beneficence play a vital role in the moral life quite apart from a principle of *obligatory* beneficence. No one denies that many beneficent acts, such as the donation of a kidney to a stranger, are morally praiseworthy and not obligatory. Similarly, virtually everyone agrees that the common morality does not contain a principle of beneficence that requires severe sacrifice and extreme altruism in the moral life—for example, giving both of one's kidneys for transplantation. Only *ideals* of beneficence incorporate such extreme generosity. We are likewise not morally required to benefit persons on all occasions, even if we are in a position to do so. For example, we are not morally required to perform all possible acts of generosity or charity that would benefit others. We can readily grant, then, that much is ideal rather than obligatory in beneficent behavior, and that the line between an obligation and a moral ideal is difficult to establish in the case of beneficence.

Nonetheless, several rules of obligatory beneficence form an important part of morality. Because of the range of types of benefit, the principle of positive beneficence supports an array of more specific moral rules—including some that we have already noted without referring to them as rules. Examples of these rules of beneficence are

1. Protect and defend the rights of others.
2. Prevent harm from occurring to others.
3. Remove conditions that will cause harm to others.
4. Help persons with disabilities.
5. Rescue persons in danger.

Distinguishing Rules of Beneficence from Rules of Nonmaleficence

Principles and rules of beneficence are distinguishable in several ways from those of nonmaleficence. As we mentioned in Chapter 4, rules of nonmaleficence (i) are negative prohibitions of action that (ii) must be obeyed impartially, and (iii) provide reasons for legal prohibitions of certain forms of conduct. By contrast, rules of beneficence (i) present positive requirements of action, (ii) do not always need to be obeyed impartially, and (iii) rarely, if ever, provide reasons for legal punishment when one fails to abide by the rules. The second condition, impartial obedience, is especially important and merits additional attention.

We are morally prohibited from causing harm to anyone (a perfect obligation). However, we are morally permitted to help or benefit those with whom we have special relationships, and we are not similarly required to help or benefit those with whom we have no such special relationship. Morality thus allows us to exhibit our beneficence with partiality in regard to those with whom we have special relationships (an imperfect obligation). These distinctions are not arbitrary. It is possible to act nonmaleficently toward all persons, but it would be impossible to act beneficently toward all persons. We cannot have obligations to do the impossible, as it is morally incoherent to require what cannot be done. Failing to act nonmaleficently toward any party is (prima facie) immoral, but failing to act beneficently toward any party is often not immoral. Arguably, some rules of beneficence, such as those requiring the rescue of strangers under conditions of minimal risk, must be followed impartially; and some legal punishments for failure to rescue strangers may be justifiable. But, with rare exceptions, obligations of nonmaleficence must be discharged impartially and obligations of beneficence need not be discharged impartially.

However, and very importantly, from the fact that morally recommended actions are not strong enough to support legal sanctions or to satisfy a requirement of impartiality, it does not follow that they are merely moral ideals and not obligations in the moral life. Not only are various norms of beneficence obligations, but they can be sufficiently strong obligations that they *override obligations of nonmaleficence*. For example, they can be overriding obligations by fulfilling the demands of the principle of utility: When a major benefit can be produced by causing a minor harm or when a major benefit for many people can be produced with a harm being caused for only a few, the requirement to benefit is overriding. For example, many public health programs, such as vaccinations, cause harm to a certain percentage of the population while providing a major benefit to other parts of the population. Coercive taxation schemes that fund health care for the indigent justifiably set back the interests of those taxed to benefit the indigent. If there were no obligations of beneficence—only moral ideals—this overriding would be unjustified. Thus, even though nonmaleficence requires impartial treatment, it does not necessarily override or take priority over beneficence.

General Beneficence

These differences between beneficence and nonmaleficence have led to confusion in moral theory about the distinction between obligatory beneficence and nonobligatory moral ideals. Some of this confusion can be eliminated by a distinction between *specific* and *general* beneficence. Specific beneficence is directed at specific parties, such as children, friends, and patients; whereas general beneficence is directed beyond these special relationships to all persons. A significant moral dispute underlies these categories. Virtually everyone agrees that all morally decent persons should act in the interests of their children, friends, and all such special parties. Advocates of a principle of general beneficence, however, argue the far more demanding thesis that we are obligated to act impartially to promote the interests of persons beyond our limited sphere of relationships and influence.

Those who defend a strong principle of general beneficence (utilitarians and some Christian moralists, for example) do not maintain the implausible *psychological* thesis that persons have a natural moral disposition to act beneficently beyond their specific relationships. Rather, they defend the *normative* thesis that we ought to act on a principle of general beneficence. As we saw in Chapter 2, some moral theories favor principles of general beneficence, whereas others tend to recoil from them while acknowledging that a moral ideal of general beneficence is acceptable and sometimes laudable. The various types and rules of obligatory beneficence include cases of both general beneficence and specific beneficence. In the category of obligations of specific beneficence we include the obligation to rescue identifiable persons in need and obligations grounded in special moral relations, such as parenthood, friendship, and role relations in health care. We will address these categories of specific beneficence momentarily, but first we will treat obligations of general beneficence.

Ross suggests that obligations of general beneficence "rest on the mere fact that there are other beings in the world whose condition we can make better." [2] Such an unqualified form of general beneficence obligates us to benefit even persons who we do not know and with whose views we are not ourselves sympathetic. Obligation of beneficence, so understood, are potentially very demanding. To take an example in ethical theory, in a recent work directed at promoting the overall good, Shelly Kagan has argued that we should recognize no limits, in principle, to the sacrifice that morality can demand of us. [3] The thesis that we have the same impartial obligation to persons we do not know as we have to our own families is both overly romantic and impractical. It is also perilous because it imposes an unrealistic and alien standard that may divert attention from our obligations to those to whom we are close or indebted, and where our responsibilities are clear rather than clouded. The more widely we generalize obligations of beneficence, the less likely we will be to meet our primary responsibilities, which many of us already find difficult to meet. In part for this reason, we believe that the common morality does recognize limits to the demands of moral obligation and that the limits on obligatory beneficence many writers in ethical theory have incorporated into their accounts of obligations of beneficence are defensible. [4]

Some writers set limits by distinguishing the removal of harm, the prevention of harm, and the promotion of benefit (see Chapter 4, pp. 190–192). For instance, in developing "the obligation to assist," Peter Singer distinguishes preventing evil from promoting good, and contends that "if it is in our power to prevent something bad from happening, without thereby sacrificing anything of comparable moral importance, we ought, morally, to do it." [5] Singer's criterion of comparable importance sets a limit on sacrifice: We ought to donate time and resources until we reach a level at which, by giving more, we would cause as much suffering to ourselves as we would relieve through our gift. This argument implies that morality sometimes requires us to make large sacrifices and to reduce our standard of living substantially in the effort to rescue needy persons around the world.

However, Singer's proposed obligation of beneficence and his limit on the obligation are still overly demanding. If a person's life plans must be seriously disrupted in order to benefit those who are sick or starving, then the limits to common-morality obligations have been exceeded. Standards in the common morality assume that the level of cost or risk that Singer seeks to make obligatory is beyond moral obligation—again, a commendable moral ideal, but not an obligation. Michael Slote has argued against Singer that beneficent prevention of evil or harm must not require the sacrifice of a "basic life plan." He formulates the "principle of positive obligation" in this way: "One has an obligation to prevent serious evil or harm when one can do so without seriously interfering with one's life plans or style and without doing any wrongs of commission."[6]

There may be ambiguities and serious moral problems in Slote's formulation,[7] but the common morality (by contrast to the act-utilitarian perspective defended by Singer) does not seem to demand much more beneficence than Slote's statement suggests. It is also not clear that moral standards could demand more beneficence without requiring sacrifice beyond the capability of most agents. If so, Singer puts most agents in the precarious position of moral disenfranchisement. Whenever the standards of morality are too high for some persons to achieve, those persons cannot participate in that domain of the moral life.

Singer later attempted to take account of the objection that his principle sets "too high a standard." He came to agree that his principle requires a more guarded formulation. To the question "What level of assistance should we advocate?," he now offers a more realistic answer:

Any figure will be arbitrary, but there may be something to be said for a round percentage of one's income like, say, 10 per cent—more than a token donation, yet not so high as to be beyond all but saints. . . . No figure should be advocated as a rigid minimum or maximum; . . . [but by] any reasonable ethical standards this is the minimum we ought to do, and we do wrong if we do less.[8]

It is difficult to assess a percentage of income as an expression of one's obligation, especially in light of vast differences in income and wealth and also in light of conditions we identify below. But Singer's revised thesis rightly attempts to set additional limits on the scope of the obligation of beneficence—limits that reduce required costs and impacts on the agent's life plans. As Singer notes, his proposal also reflects a strand in some forms of Western morality, particularly in religious traditions that identify tithing (providing one-tenth) as obligatory.

Specific Beneficence: The Obligation to Rescue

In some circumstances the discretion allowed by general beneficence is eliminated or reduced, and the agent has an obligation of specific beneficence toward particular persons. Consider the stock example of a passerby who observes someone drowning, but stands in no special moral relationship with the victim. The obligation of beneficence is not strong enough, in our view, to require that a passerby who is a very poor swimmer to risk his or her life by trying to swim a hundred yards to rescue someone who is drowning in deep water. But if the passerby does nothing—for example, fails to run several yards to alert a lifeguard—the omission is morally culpable.

Apart from special moral relationships such as contracts, a person X has a determinate obligation of beneficence toward person Y if and only if each of the following conditions is satisfied (assuming X is aware of the relevant facts):

1. Y is at risk of significant loss of or damage to life or health or some other major interest.
2. X's action is needed (singly or in concert with others) to prevent this loss or damage.
3. X's action (singly or in concert with others) has a high probability of preventing it.
4. X's action would not present significant risks, costs, or burdens to X.
5. The benefit that Y can be expected to gain outweighs any harms, costs, or burdens that X is likely to incur.[9]

A person can have an *obligation* of beneficence under these five conditions, even apart from special moral relationships such as professional roles. The fourth condition is critical because it enables us to engage the problems that surround formulations of the obligation of beneficence. Although it is difficult to specify "significant risks, costs, or burdens," the implication of the fourth condition is clear: Even if X's action would probably save Y's life and would meet all conditions except the fourth, the action would not be obligatory on grounds of beneficence.

We shall now test these theses about the demands of beneficence with two cases. The first is a borderline case of specific obligatory beneficence, involving rescue, whereas the second presents a clear-cut case of specific obligatory beneficence. In one case, first introduced in Chapter 4, Robert McFall was diagnosed as having aplastic anemia, which is usually fatal, but his physician believed that a bone marrow transplant from a genetically compatible donor could increase his chances of surviving one year from twenty-five percent to between forty and sixty percent. David Shimp, McFall's cousin, was the only relative willing to undergo the first test, which established tissue compatibility.

However, Shimp then refused to undergo the second test for genetic compatibility. When McFall sued to force his cousin to undergo the second test and to donate bone marrow if he turned out to be compatible, the judge ruled that the *law* did not allow him to force Shimp to engage in such acts of positive beneficence, but added that Shimp's refusal was "*morally* indefensible."

Conditions (1) and (2) above were met for an obligation of specific beneficence, but condition (3) was not as clearly satisfied. McFall's chance of surviving one year would have only increased from twenty-five to between forty and sixty percent. These contingencies make it difficult to determine whether principles of beneficence demanded a particular course of action. Although most medical commentators agreed that the risks to the donor were minimal, Shimp was especially concerned about the fourth condition. Bone marrow transplants require one hundred to one hundred and fifty punctures of the pelvic bone. These punctures can be painlessly performed under anesthesia, and the major risk is a one-in-ten-thousand chance of death from anesthesia. Shimp, however, believed that the risks were greater ("What if I become a cripple?," he said) and that they outweighed the probability and magnitude of benefit to McFall, despite the lack of medical evidence to support his fears. This case, then, is a borderline case of obligatory specific beneficence.

Second, in the *Tarasoff* case (Case 1), upon learning of his patient's intention to kill an identified woman, the therapist notified the police but not the intended victim because of constraints of confidentiality. Suppose we modify the actual circumstances in this case in order to create the following hypothetical situation: A psychiatrist has informed his patient that he does not believe in keeping information of any sort confidential. The patient agrees to treatment under these conditions and subsequently reveals a clearly serious intention to kill an identified woman. The psychiatrist may now either remain aloof or make some move to protect the woman (by notifying her or the police). What does morality—and specifically beneficence—demand of the psychiatrist in this case?

Only a remarkably narrow view of moral obligation would hold that the psychiatrist is under no obligation to protect the woman by contacting her. The psychiatrist is not at risk (and, moreover, will suffer virtually no inconvenience or interference with his life plan). If morality does not demand this much beneficence, it is hard to see how morality imposes any positive obligations at all. Moreover, if a competing obligation exists, such as protection of confidentiality, requirements of beneficence will still sometimes override it. Similar conclusions can be reached about the obligations of professionals to warn spouses or lovers of HIV-infected patients who refuse to disclose their status and who refuse to engage in safe sex.

Nevertheless, the limits of obligatory, specific beneficence can crumble when an ethics of individual obligation confronts large-scale social problems. Even if we assume only that we are obligated to save a human life without making major sacrifices, James Fishkin argues that this principle will lead us step by step to enormous burdens. We have only to consider the large number of obligation-determining situations and the large number of recipients who could benefit.[10] For example, an individual could provide food for a starving person for a small amount of money, but if numerous starving people exist, each of whom could be rescued by a small additional contribution, the burden would quickly surpass an individual's resources.

This conclusion is both practically and theoretically puzzling. It is *practically* puzzling because it becomes extremely difficult to pin down and discharge obligations of beneficence. We bounce back and forth between viewing actions as charitable and as obligatory; and we sometimes feel guilty for not doing more, at the same time doubting that we are obligated to do more. The conclusion is *theoretically* puzzling because every time we try to formulate the limits of obligatory specific beneficence through general conditions, the problem of incremental obligations tends to undermine the analysis. For example, a one-dollar gift to a famine relief organization would not make a noticeable dent in our standard of living. At each point in the chain of needs and contributions, only one more dollar from our pockets would make no substantial dent in our standard of living. But if we gave away everything in our savings and investment accounts, most of us would regard the sacrifice as immense. It is therefore doubtful that ethical theory can set precise, determinate conditions of beneficence, so that apparently faultless assumptions about obligations of minimal giving do not engulf us in a morass of obligations that exceed defensible limits.

No doubt there can be a more refined analysis than the one we have presented of the limits of obligatory beneficence, but it is certain to be a revisionary analysis in the sense that it will inevitably draw a new boundary for our obligations—a line that is more explicit than any in common morality. For example, Singer's ten percent criterion is a revisionary line, despite its faint presence in Western morality. Any attempt to specify the limits of our obligations of positive beneficence will both sharpen and alter the common morality, which is not sufficiently refined to supply an answer, perhaps because most of our obligations of beneficence rest on specific role (and other special) relations.

Specific Beneficence: Role and Other Special Relations

Obligations of specific beneficence usually rest on special moral relations (for example, in families and friendships) or on special commitments, such as explicit promises and roles with attendant responsibilities. These special moral relationships and role relationships may not appear to generate the problems about specifying limits of obligatory beneficent risk-taking and cost-bearing that we have encountered thus far. However, there are limits in these contexts as well. For instance: How far are parents obligated to go in providing expensive care for their severely ill children?[11] Are physicians and other health care professionals obligated to accept extraordinary risks while caring for difficult or contagious patients?

At this stage in the discussion, we will note only the implicit assumption of beneficence that exists in medical and health care professions and their institutional contexts. Promoting the welfare of patients—not merely avoiding harm—expresses medicine's goal, rationale, and justification. As the American Nurses' Association puts it, "The nurse's primary commitment is to the health, welfare, and safety of the client."[12] Likewise in the Hippocratic oath, physicians pledge that they will "come for the benefit of the sick," will apply treatments "for the benefit of the sick according to [their] ability and judgment," and "will keep [patients] from harm and injustice."[13] Preventive medicine and active public health interventions have also long embraced concerted social actions of beneficence such as vaccination distribution and health education as obligatory rather than optional. We will return to these role responsibilities and their limits in Chapter 8.

A Reciprocity-Based Justification of Obligations of Beneficence

Several justifications have been proposed for obligations of general and specific beneficence. We will defend a reciprocity-based account, with particular reference to health care ethics, although we do not believe that reciprocity can account for the full range of obligations of beneficence.

Utilitarians recognize obligations of beneficence as flowing directly from the principle of utility, and Kant and Ross recognize these obligations as central to their deontological systems of ethics. David Hume, by contrast, argued that the obligation to benefit others arises from social interactions: "All our obligations to do good to society seem to imply something reciprocal. I receive the benefits of society, and therefore ought to promote its interests."[14] Reciprocity is the act or practice of making an appropriate (often proportional) return—for example, returning benefit by proportional benefit, harm by proportional criminal sentencing, and friendliness by gratitude. Hume's reciprocity account rightly maintains that we incur obligations to help or benefit others at least in part because we have received or will receive beneficial assistance from them (understood as assistance that they intended in good faith to provide). As he and others recognize, reciprocity functions in circumstances of justice and friendship, as well as in relationships of benefit. Reciprocity is therefore a pervasive feature of social life, although not so pervasive that all of the moral life can be reduced to obligations of reciprocity. Certainly, not all forms of benevolence can be justified in terms of reciprocity (for example, the loving care of children).

It is even doubtful that *all obligations* of beneficence can be so justified. For example, a physician may have a moral obligation to take care of an indigent stranger at the scene of an automobile accident. We therefore do not hold that persons devoid of reciprocal relationships of benefit never have an obligation to act beneficently. Nonetheless, obligations of beneficence to society (as distinct from those to identified individuals) are typically derived from some form of reciprocity. It is implausible to maintain that we are largely free of or can free ourselves of a broad range of indebtednesses to our parents, to researchers in medicine and public health, to educators, and to social institutions such as schools. The claim that we make our way independent of our benefactors is as unrealistic as the idea that we can always act autonomously without affecting others. Accordingly, many obligations of beneficence are appropriately justified by implicit arrangements underlying the necessary give-and-take of social life. Even some obligations of specific beneficence to rescue people in severe need who stand outside special moral relations or institutional relationships can be so justified.[15]

Traditionally, codes of medical ethics have inappropriately viewed physicians as independent, self-sufficient philanthropists whose beneficence is analogous to generous acts of giving. According to the Hippocratic oath, for example, physicians' obligations to patients represent philanthropy and service, whereas their obligations to teachers represent debts incurred in becoming physicians. However, physicians and many other health care professionals are today deeply indebted to society (e.g., for education and privileges) and to patients, past and present (e.g., for research and "practice"). Because of this indebtedness, the medical profession's role of beneficent care of patients is misconstrued if modeled primarily on philanthropy, altruism, and personal commitment. Rather, their care is rooted in what William May calls the "reciprocity of giving and receiving."[16] This reciprocity creates an obligation of general beneficence both to patients and to society, although the precise terms of the obligation are rarely specified (and are very difficult to specify).

Obligations of specific beneficence, by contrast, typically derive from special moral relationships with persons, frequently through institutional roles and contractual arrangements. These obligations derive from implicit and explicit commitments such as promises and roles as well as from the acceptance of specific benefits. Thus, both our "station and its duties" and our promises impose obligations. For example, a lifeguard on duty is obligated to try to rescue a drowning swimmer, despite personal risk, just as a physician is obligated to meet the needs of his or her patients despite potential health risks. The claims that we make on each other as parents, spouses, and friends stem not only from interpersonal encounters, but from settled rules, roles, and relations that constitute the matrix of social obligations and role-derived obligations.

When a patient contracts with a physician for services, the latter assumes a role-specific obligation of beneficent treatment that would not be present apart from the relationship. Although physicians in private practice typically have no legal obligation to see patients in emergencies or to help those injured in an automobile accident, moral obligations of beneficence do on occasion require such acts of physicians. The obligation to render assistance in extraordinary circumstances such as an automobile accident is not limited to physicians or to health care professionals. If a lawyer or student, say, had happened on the scene of an accident in the same way, then he or she too would have had an obligation to assist. Anyone who falls under our five-condition analysis of the general obligation of beneficence has an obligation to provide such assistance, as he or she is able.

Of course, physicians are typically able to lend more assistance in an emergency than other citizens, and we can therefore ask whether the physician has a specific obligation of assistance unique to persons with the skills and training of a medical professional. Here we encounter a gray area between a role-specific obligation and a non-role-specific obligation. The physician at the scene of an accident is obligated to do more than the lawyer or student to aid the injured, in accordance with the need for the skills of the medical profession; yet a physician-stranger is not morally required to assume the same level of commitment and risk that is legally and morally required in a prior contractual relationship with a patient or hospital. This analysis suggests that we need to be careful in using the language of role or professional obligations. It also suggests, as health professionals and parents have long believed, that specific role obligations can take priority over more general obligations in cases of conflict.

If the parable of the Good Samaritan is interpreted to present ideal rather than obligatory standards of action, then a physician is not morally obligated to emulate the good Samaritan. However, a physician may still be obligated to be what Judith Thomson calls a *minimally decent* Samaritan.[17] Controversy exists about the extent to which society should enforce obligations of general and specific beneficence that are not based on explicit contracts and agreements. So-called Good Samaritan laws are perhaps most effective when they do not require assistance by physicians or other health care professionals under threat of a sanction, but rather protect them from civil or criminal liability when they act in good faith and render aid in emergencies. For example, if a threat of liability exists for rendering medical assistance in an emergency, the professional may view the legal risk of intervening as a valid excuse for not fulfilling a moral obligation to intervene (based on the five conditions identified earlier).

Paternalism: Conflicts between Beneficence and Autonomy

In an inchoate form, the idea that beneficence expresses the primary obligation in health care is ancient. Throughout the history of health care, the profes-

sional's obligations and virtues have been interpreted as commitments of beneficence. We find perhaps the most celebrated expression in the Hippocratic
work *Epidemics:* "As to disease, make a habit of two things—*to help, or at
least to do no harm.*"[18] Traditionally, physicians were able to rely almost
exclusively on their own judgments about their patients' needs for treatment,
information, and consultation. However, medicine has increasingly been confronted—especially in the last thirty years—with assertions of the patient's
right to make an independent judgment about his or her medical fate. As assertions of autonomy rights have increased, the problem of paternalism has
loomed larger.

Disputes about the Primacy of Beneficence

Whether respect for the autonomy of patients should have priority over professional beneficence has become a central problem in biomedical ethics. For proponents of autonomy rights for patients, the physician's obligations to the patient of disclosure, seeking consent, confidentiality, and privacy are established
primarily (and perhaps exclusively) by the principle of respect for autonomy.
Others, by contrast, ground such obligations on the professional's obligatory
beneficence. The physician's primary obligation is to act for the patient's medical benefit, not to promote autonomous decisionmaking. However, autonomy
rights have become so influential that it is today difficult to find clear affirma-
tions of traditional models of medical beneficence.

The debate between proponents of the autonomy model and proponents of
the beneficence model—as we will refer to these two contrasting paradigms—
has often been confused by a failure to distinguish between a principle of beneficence that *competes* with a principle of respect for autonomy and a principle
of beneficence that *incorporates* the patient's autonomy (in the sense that the
patient's preferences help to determine what counts as a medical benefit). For
example, two exponents of the preeminence of the beneficence model—Edmund Pellegrino and David Thomasma—argue that "the best interests of the
patients are intimately linked with their preferences," from which "are derived
our primary duties toward them."[19] This formulation of the beneficence model
appears to be little more than a dressed-up defense of the autonomy model. If
the content of the physician's obligation to be beneficent is set exclusively by
the patient's preferences, respect for autonomy rather than beneficence has tri-
umphed.

Elsewhere, however, Pellegrino and Thomasma interpret the meaning and
authority of beneficence as independent of—and potentially in conflict with—
the patient's preferences: "Both autonomy and paternalism are superseded by
the obligation to act beneficently. . . . In the real world of clinical medicine,
there are no absolute moral principles except the injunction to act in the pa-

tient's best interest." They then present several circumstances in which medical beneficence appropriately overrides the patient's autonomy because the patient has made irresponsible choices. For example, "autonomy would be wrongly exercised if [the patient] rejected penicillin treatment for pneumococcal or meningococcal meningitis."[20] The latter infections are life-threatening and can produce serious central nervous system damage; refusal of treatment would be irresponsible, and a caring physician therefore should override the patient's irresponsible refusal of necessary treatment. Here we find a defense of a beneficence model with backbone.

However, we will argue that debate about which principle or model should be overriding in medical practice cannot be solved in this streamlined manner by defending one principle against the other principle, or by making one principle absolute. No premier and overriding authority exists in either the patient or the physician, and no preeminent principle exists in biomedical ethics, not even the admonition to act in the patient's best interest. This position is consistent with our earlier claim that beneficence provides the primary goal and rationale of medicine and health care, whereas respect for autonomy (and nonmaleficence and justice) sets moral limits on the professional's actions in pursuit of this goal. To demonstrate the consistency between these two theses requires us to examine several aspects of the problem of paternalism, beginning with some conceptual problems.

The Nature of Paternalism

Philosophical analyses of paternalism are at least as old as Immanuel Kant, who denounced paternalistic government ("imperium paternale," he called it) for benevolently restricting the freedoms of its subjects. Kant was concerned about a government that "cancels freedom." He never considered the possibility that a parental model of benevolent intervention—one that likens the state to a protective parent caring for an incompetent minor—might be considered paternalistic. Nor did John Stuart Mill contemplate the possibility that paternalism might encompass interventions with those who have limited or no autonomy.[21] However, what they never anticipated came to pass. Intervention in the life of a substantially nonautonomous dependent became and remains the most widely accepted model of justified paternalism. That is, the paradigmatic form of justified paternalism starts with incompetent children in need of parental supervision and extends to other incompetents in need of treatment analogous to beneficent parental guidance.

The *O.E.D.* dates the term *paternalism* from the 1880s (after Kant and Mill), giving its root meaning as "the principle and practice of paternal administration; government as by a father; the claim or attempt to supply the needs or to regulate the life of a nation or community in the same way a father does those of his children.'' The analogy with the father presupposes two features of the paternal role: that the father acts beneficently (that is, in accordance with his conception of the interests of his children) and that he makes all or at least some of the decisions relating to his children's welfare, rather than letting them make those decisions. In health care relationships, the analogy is extended further: A professional has superior training, knowledge, and insight and is in an authoritative position to determine the patient's best interests. From this perspective, a health care professional is like a loving parent with dependent and often ignorant and fearful children.

Paternalism always involves some form of interference with or refusal to conform to another person's preferences regarding their own good. Paternalistic acts typically involve force or coercion, on the one hand, or deception, lying, manipulation of information, or nondisclosure of information on the other. According to some definitions in the literature, a paternalistic action necessarily places a limit on autonomous choice. Although one author of this text prefers this conception,[22] we will here follow the current mainstream of the literature on paternalism and accept the broader definition suggested by the *O.E.D.*: intentional nonacquiescence or intervention in another person's preferences, desires, or actions with the intention of either avoiding harm to or benefiting the person. If a person's desires, intentional actions, and the like do not derive from a substantially autonomous choice, then overriding them can still be paternalistic under this definition.[23] For example, if a man ignorant of his fragile, life-threatening condition and sick with a raging fever attempts to leave a hospital, it would be paternalistic to detain him, even if his attempt to leave did not derive from a substantially autonomous choice.

Paternalism, then, is the intentional overriding of one person's known preferences or actions by another person, where the person who overrides justifies the action by the goal of benefiting or avoiding harm to the person whose will is overridden. This definition is normatively neutral, and therefore it does not presume that paternalism is either justified or unjustified. Although the definition assumes an act of beneficence analogous to parental beneficence, it does not assume whether the beneficence is justified, misplaced, obligatory, etc.

Sometimes an action may appear to be paternalistic under this definition, when in fact it is nonpaternalistic. An example is found in biomedical research involving prisoners. In its report on research involving prisoners, the National Commission for the Protection of Human Subjects of Biomedical and Behavioral Research argued that the closed nature of prison environments creates a potential for abuse of authority and therefore invites the exploitation and coercion of prisoners.[24] Although a commission study indicated that most prisoners do not regard their consent to research as compromised by coercion or undue influence, the commission argued that the coercive and exploitative possibilities in prisons justify regulations prohibiting the use of prisoners in research, even if they wish to participate.

This restriction appears to be paternalistic, but closer analysis shows that it is not. The commission maintained that if an environment were not exploitative or coercive (and if a few other conditions were met), then prisoners should be allowed to choose to participate in research. The commission's justifying ground was the factual premise that most prisons could not be rendered sufficiently free of coercion arid exploitation by drug companies and prison officials, not the paternalistic perspective that prisoners should be protected from their wishes and choices. The argument is that we cannot predict whether prisoners will be exploited in settings that render them vulnerable, but that research to which they might validly consent should nonetheless be prohibited because we cannot adequately monitor the consent process and subsequent uses of the subjects.

Many circumstances in biomedical ethics suggest a need to examine carefully whether classes of persons are being exploited, but special restrictions placed on members of those classes may or may not be paternalistic. Healthy, nonrelated organ donors and cancer patients solicited for research, for example, are in this respect sometimes treated like the prisoners just mentioned; but even stringent protective requirements aimed at their welfare may not be paternalistic. In some cases, the justification of an act, policy, or practice of nonacquiescence or intervention in a person's preferences is partially but not purely paternalistic because it is intermixed with nonpaternalistic reasons such as protection of third parties. Such impure or mixed paternalism is common in public policy debates.

Moral Problems of Medical Paternalism

Throughout the history of medical ethics the principle of nonmaleficence as well as principles of beneficence have been viewed as providing a basis for paternalistic treatment of patients. For example, physicians have traditionally taken the view that disclosing certain forms of information can cause harm to patients under their care and that medical ethics obligates them not to cause such harm.

In Case 3, a man brings his father, who is in his late sixties, to his physician because he has a suspicion that his father's problems in interpreting and responding to daily events indicate Alzheimer's disease. The man also makes an "impassioned plea" that the physician not tell his father whether the tests suggest Alzheimer's. Tests subsequently indicate that the father probably does have the disease. The physician now faces a dilemma, because of the conflict between demands of respect for autonomy and demands of beneficence. The

physician first considers the now widely recognized obligation to inform patients of a diagnosis of cancer. This obligation typically presupposes accuracy
in the diagnosis, a relatively clear course of the disease, and a competent patient—none of which is clearly present in this case. The physician also notes
that disclosure of Alzheimer's disease adversely affects patients' coping mechanisms, and thus could harm the patient, particularly by causing further decline,
depression, agitation, and paranoia.

Some patients—for example, those who are depressed or addicted to potentially harmful drugs—are unlikely to reach adequately reasoned decisions.
Other patients who are competent and deliberative may make poor choices
about courses of action recommended by their physicians. When patients of
either type choose harmful courses of action, some health care professionals
respect autonomy by not interfering beyond attempts at persuasion, whereas
others act beneficently by protecting patients against the potentially harmful
consequences of their own choices. Problems of how to specify the principles,
which principle to follow under which conditions, and how to intervene in the
decisions and affairs of such patients when intervention is warranted are all
central to debates about medical paternalism.[25]

In a classic article, L. J. Henderson argued that "the best physicians" use
the following as their primary guide: "So far as possible, 'Do No Harm.' You
can do harm by the process that is quaintly called telling the truth. You can do
harm by lying. . . . But try to do as little harm as possible, not only in treatment with drugs, or with the knife, but also in treatment with words." Henderson argued that, for the patient's good, some information should be withheld
or should be disclosed only to the family and that deference to the autonomy
rights of patients is dangerous because it compromises clinical judgment and
presents a hazard to the patient's health.[26]

An example appears in Case 2. Here an inoperable, incurable carcinoma is
discovered in a sixty-nine-year-old man. Because of a long relationship with
this patient, the physician knew that the patient was fragile in several respects.
The patient was neurotic, had a history of psychiatric disease, and had recently
suffered a severe depressive reaction, during which he had behaved irrationally
and attempted suicide. When he blurted out, "Am I OK?" and, "I don't have
cancer, do I?" the physician answered, "You're as good as you were ten years
ago," knowing that the response was a paternalistic lie but also believing it
was justified. The physician was worried that a truthful disclosure would seriously disrupt the man's life plans—he was undergoing this routine physical
examination in preparation for a brief but greatly anticipated trip to Australia—
and would possibly cause mental instability or lead to suicide. The physician
planned to disclose the diagnosis to the patient later—after the trip to Australia,
when attention could be given to the man's mental condition.

Despite his stringent opposition to paternalism, Mill considered temporary beneficent interventions in a person's actions to be justified on some occasions. He argued, for example, that a person who is ignorant of a significant risk— for example, in starting to cross a dangerous bridge—may justifiably be restrained in order to ensure that he or she is acting intentionally and with adequate knowledge of the consequences of the action. Once warned, the person should be free to choose whatever course he or she desires. Because Mill did not regard this temporary intervention as a "real infringement" of liberty, he did not view it as paternalistic. However, under the definition of paternalism we have accepted, such a temporary intervention is paternalistic.

If a paternalistic intervention does not override autonomy because no substantial autonomy is present, it is easier to justify the intervention than it would be if a comparable preference or action were autonomous. However, in contrast to much of the literature on paternalism, we will argue that autonomous actions as well as nonautonomous ones are sometimes justifiably restricted on grounds of beneficence.

Weak (Soft) and Strong (Hard) Paternalism

This analysis of paternalism can be further clarified by a distinction Joel Feinberg introduced between strong and weak paternalism, which he later referred to as hard and soft paternalism.[27] In weak paternalism, an agent intervenes on grounds of beneficence or nonmaleficence only to prevent *substantially nonvoluntary* conduct—that is, to protect persons against their own substantially nonautonomous action(s). Substantially nonvoluntary or nonautonomous actions include cases of consent that is not adequately informed, severe depression that precludes rational deliberation, and severe addiction that prevents free choice and action. Weak paternalism requires that some such form of compromised ability be present.

Strong paternalism, by contrast, involves interventions intended to benefit a person despite the fact that the person's risky choices and actions are informed, voluntary, and autonomous. A strong paternalist refuses to acquiesce in a person's autonomous wishes, choices, and actions in order to protect that person, often by restricting the information available to the person and by overriding that person's informed and voluntary choices. These choices need not be *fully* informed or voluntary, but for the interventions to qualify as strong paternalism, the choices must be *substantially* autonomous. Unlike weak paternalism, strong paternalism does not depend on a conception of compromised ability, dysfunctional incompetence, or encumbrance in deciding, willing, or acting.

As we will see, reasons exist to doubt that weak paternalism qualifies as a form of paternalism that needs a defense. That persons deserve to be protected from harm caused *to* an individual by conditions *beyond* his or her self-control is not a disputed premise. Paternalism is largely a problem about the conditions under which persons can and should be protected against *self*-caused harm, but weak paternalists leave a strong residue of doubt about whether the position they espouse prevents truly self-caused harm. The weak paternalist seems to straddle fences without defending a controversial position. As Feinberg has bluntly argued, "it is severely misleading to think of [weak paternalism] as any kind of [real] paternalism."[28]

The Justification of Paternalism and Antipaternalism

Three main positions have been defended on the justifiability of paternalism: (1) antipaternalism, (2) a justified paternalism that appeals primarily to some form of the principle of respect for autonomy, and (3) a justified paternalism that appeals primarily to principles of beneficence. All three positions agree that some acts of weak paternalism are justified, such as preventing a man under the influence of an hallucinogenic drug from killing himself. Even antipaternalists will not object to these interventions because substantially autonomous actions are not at stake. By contrast, strong paternalism is rejected by most writers who espouse all three of these positions.

Antipaternalism. Antipaternalists believe that (strong) paternalistic intervention cannot be justified because it violates individual rights and unduly restricts free choice. The serious adverse consequences of giving paternalistic authority to the state or to a class of individuals such as physicians forms one basis for the antipaternalistic rejection of (strong) paternalism, but another and more influential basis is that rightful authority resides in the individual. The argument for this conclusion rests on in the analysis of autonomy rights in Chapter 3: Strong paternalistic interventions display disrespect toward autonomous agents and fail to treat them as moral equals, treating them as less than independent determiners of their own good. If others impose their conception of the good on us, we are denied the respect that we are owed even if the other agent is in fact providing us with a benefit and has a better conception of our needs than we do.[29]

Antipaternalists also argue that paternalistic standards are too broad and therefore would authorize and institutionalize too much intervention if made the basis of policy. Using an extreme example, Robert Harris argues that paternalism would in principle "justify the imposition of a Spartan-like regimen requiring rigorous physical exercise and abstention from smoking, drinking, and hazardous pastimes,"[30] subject to the threat of criminal sanctions. Careful defenses of paternalism would disallow these extreme interventions, and at best these antipaternalist arguments establish only a rebuttable presumption against paternalistic intervention.

Nonetheless, antipaternalists are convinced that an unacceptable latitude of judgment would remain in contexts in which power is subject to abuse. For example, suppose a woman risks her life for the advancement of medicine by submitting to a highly risky experiment, an act most would think not in her best interests. Are we to commend her, ignore her, or coercively restrain her? Strong paternalism suggests that it would be permissible and perhaps obligatory to restrain her. If so, antipaternalists argue, the state is permitted, in principle, to coerce its morally heroic citizens if they act in a manner "harmful" to themselves. More generally, the state would be empowered to take away from persons the right to make any decision over their lives when officials view risks as excessive. Similarly, in health care institutions physicians and nurses would be authorized to override the plans and preferences of patients.

The medical example with the most extensive antipaternalistic literature is the involuntary hospitalization of persons who have neither been harmed by others nor actually harmed themselves, but who are thought to be at risk of such harm. These cases involve a double paternalism: a paternalistic justification for both therapy and commitment. For example, Catherine Lake suffered from arteriosclerosis, which caused temporary confusion and mild loss of memory. Her condition was interspersed with periods of mental alertness and rationality. All parties agreed that Lake had never harmed anyone or presented a threat of danger, but she was committed to a mental institution because she often seemed confused and defenseless. At her trial, while apparently rational, she testified that she knew the risks of living outside the hospital and preferred to assume those risks rather than remain in the hospital environment. The court of appeals denied her petition, arguing that she is "mentally ill," a "danger to herself," and "not competent to care for herself." The legal justification cited by the court was a statute that "provides for involuntary hospitalization of a person who is 'mentally ill and, because of that illness is likely to injure himself'."[31] Antipaternalists argue that since Lake did not harm others and understood the dangers under which she placed herself, her freedom should not have been restricted.

Antipaternalists would view this case differently if Lake had not been substantially autonomous. The antipaternalist would then regard the intervention as justified by the intent to benefit, and would note that in these cases beneficence is not in conflict with respect for autonomy because no substantial autonomy exists. It is therefore doubtful that weak paternalism as a moral position can be distinguished from antipaternalism; and if no substantive disagreement exists, no grounds favor one position over the other. (There is often a related and vigorous debate about whether a patient is substantially autonomous or substantially nonautonomous, but this is a conceptual or empirical problem about the nature and conditions of autonomy, not a problem about the moral grounds of intervention.)

Is paternalism justified by consent or by benefit? Some influential supporters of paternalistic intervention hold that a paternalistic action can be justified only if

(1) the harms prevented from occurring or the benefits provided to the person outweigh the loss of independence and the sense of invasion caused by the intervention, (2) the person's condition seriously limits his or her ability to make an autonomous choice, (3) the intervention is universally justified under relevantly similar circumstances, and (4) the beneficiary of the paternalistic actions has consented, will consent, or would, if rational, consent to those actions on his or her behalf.

The following case presents an example of a paternalistic action that some would view as satisfying these criteria of justified paternalism. An involuntarily committed mental patient wishes to leave the hospital, although his family is opposed to his release. The patient argues that his mental condition does not justify confinement. However, after one previous release, he plucked out his right eye, and after another release he severed his right hand. The patient functions competently in the state hospital, where he sells news materials to fellow patients and handles limited financial affairs. The source of his "problems" is his religious beliefs. He regards himself as a true prophet of God and believes that "it is far better for one man to believe and accept an appropriate message from God to sacrifice an eye or a hand according to the sacred scriptures rather than for the present course of the world to cause even greater loss of human life." Acting on this belief, he engages in self-mutilation. According to the paternalist, this person functions rationally from day to day, yet at times needs and deserves help. His capacities are too diminished and his dangerousness to himself too severe to allow complete independence without custodial care.[32]

Several prominent theories appeal to *consent* to justify paternalistic interventions in such cases—be it rational consent, subsequent consent, hypothetical consent, or some other type of consent. As Gerald Dworkin puts it, "the basic notion of consent is important and seems to me the only acceptable way to try to delimit an area of justified paternalism." Rosemary Carter agrees, arguing that "consent plays the central role in justifying paternalism, and indeed . . . no other concepts are relevant." Donald VanDeVeer similarly justifies paternalistic interventions for persons "acting in a seriously encumbered manner [where] it is highly probable that they would give valid consent to the intervention if the opportunity were available."[33]

For some who support a consent-based theory, paternalism is a "social insurance policy" to which fully rational persons would subscribe in order to protect themselves.[34] Such persons would know, for example, that they might be tempted at times to make decisions that are far-reaching, potentially dangerous, and irreversible. At other times they might suffer irresistible psychological or social pressures to take actions that are unjustifiably risky, such as placing their honor in question by a challenge to fight. In still other cases, persons might not sufficiently understand dangers, such as medical facts about the effects of smoking, although they might believe they have a sufficient understanding.

Consent theorists thus conclude that we would consent to a limited authorization for others to control our actions by paternalistic policies and interventions.

John Rawls and Gerald Dworkin espouse a form of justified paternalism based on the premise that completely rational agents (those fully aware of their circumstances) would consent to paternalism and would even consent to a system of penalties to motivate them to avoid foolish actions. According to the theory of consent that supports this position, those whose autonomy is defective are unable to make the prudent decision that they would otherwise make. Rawls and Dworkin do not propose a *predictive* consent theory, according to which a consent would be given if the present impairment were removed. Rather, they argue from a Kantian conception of what the rational and autonomous agent would agree to in a hypothetical circumstance of consent.[35]

A theory that appeals to rational consent to justify paternalistic interventions has attractive features, particularly its attempt to harmonize principles of beneficence and respect for autonomy so that paternalistic interventions respect autonomy rather than override it. However, this approach does not incorporate an individual's actual *consent,* and, without additional specification, this position will also likely justify more paternalism than the original defenders of the position anticipated. Almost any risk accepted by an agent can form the basis of an intervention on grounds that no rational person would assume the risk.

More importantly, consent in this or any form is not necessary to justify paternalistic interventions, and appeals to consent obscure more than they clarify the issues. It is best to keep autonomy-based justifications at arm's length from paternalism. Beneficence alone justifies truly paternalistic actions, just as it does in the justification of parental actions that override the preferences of children.[36] We do not control children because we believe that they will subsequently consent to or would rationally approve our interventions. We interfere because we believe they will have better (or at least less risky) lives, whether they know it or not. Even if we hope for subsequent consent or approval by our children and patients, the justification of our intervention rests on their welfare, not on their autonomous choices.

The most plausible justification of paternalism views benefit as resting on a scale with autonomy interests, where both must be balanced: As a person's interests in autonomy increase and the benefits for the person decrease, the justification of paternalism is rendered less likely; conversely, as the benefits for a person increase and the person's interests in autonomy decrease, the plausibility of an act of paternalism being justified increases. Thus, preventing minor harms or providing minor benefits while deeply disrespecting autonomy has no plausible justification; but preventing major harms or providing major benefits while only trivially disrespecting autonomy has a highly plausible paternalistic justification. However, this claim is contested in contemporary biomedical ethics—especially for strong paternalism.

Justified Strong Paternalism

Although strong paternalism is a dangerous position that is subject to abuse, conditions can be specified that restrict the range of interventions and that justify only a narrow range of acts. In reaching this conclusion, we do not defend public and institutional *policies* of strong paternalism, but only certain *acts* of strong paternalism.

Two cases provide starting points for reflection on the conditions of justified strong paternalism. In the first, a physician has obtained the results of a myelogram (a graph of the spinal region) following examination of a patient. Even though the results are inconclusive and need to be repeated, the tests nonetheless suggest a serious pathology. When the patient asks about the test results, the physician decides on grounds of beneficence to withhold potentially negative information, knowing that upon disclosure the patient would be distressed and anxious. Based on her experience with other patients and her ten-year knowledge of this patient, the physician is confident that the information would not affect the patient's decision to consent to another myelogram. Her sole motivation in withholding the information is to spare the patient the emotional distress of thinking through a painful decision prematurely and perhaps unnecessarily. However, the physician intends to be completely truthful with the patient about the results of the second test, no matter how negative the findings, and will disclose the information well before the patient will need to make a decision about surgery. This physician's act of temporary nondisclosure seems to us morally justified, though beneficence is (temporarily) given priority over respect for autonomy.

A more commonplace example of justified strong paternalism appears in the following case reported by Mary Silva:

After receiving his preoperative medicine, C, a 23-year-old male athlete scheduled for a hernia repair, states that he does not want the side rails up. C is of clear mind and understands why the rule is required; however, C does not feel the rule should apply to him because he is not the least bit drowsy from the preoperative medication and he has no intention of falling out of bed. After considerable discussion between the nurse and patient, the nurse responsible for C's care puts the side rails up. Her justification is as follows: C is not drowsy because he has just received the preoperative medication, and its effects have not occurred. Furthermore, if he follows the typical pattern of patients receiving this medication in this dosage, he will become drowsy very quickly. A drowsy patient is at risk for a fall. Since there is no family at the hospital to remain with the patient, and since the nurses on the unit are exceptionally busy, no one can constantly stay with C to monitor his level of alertness. Under these circumstances the patient must be protected from the potential harm of a fall, despite the fact that he does not want this protection. . . . The nurse restricted this autonomous patient's liberty based on . . . protection of the patient from potential harm . . . and *not* as a hedge against liability or for protection from criticism.[37]

Such minor strong paternalistic actions are common in hospitals. If there is no reasonable alternative or if, for example, dying patients are spared totally point-less grief and suffering, these actions are cases of justified strong paternalism. Normally, they are appropriate and justified in health care only if the following limiting conditions are satisfied:

1. A patient is at risk of a significant, preventable harm.
2. The paternalistic action will probably prevent the harm.
3. The projected benefits to the patient of the paternalistic action outweigh its risks to the patient.
4. The least autonomy-restrictive alternative that will secure the benefits and reduce the risks is adopted.

These conditions typically justify strong paternalism, but their interpretation and limits need more analysis than we can provide here. We are tempted to add a fifth condition requiring that a paternalistic action not substantially re-strict autonomy. This condition could be satisfied only if vital or substantial autonomy interests are not at stake. For example, if a Jehovah's Witness re-fuses a blood transfusion because of a deeply held conviction, a vital autonomy interest is at stake. To intervene coercively by providing the transfusion would be a substantial infringement of autonomy and thus unjustifiable under this additional condition. However, some rare cases of justified strong paternalism cross this line of minimal infringement. In general, as the risk to a patient's welfare increases or the likelihood of an irreversible harm increases, the likeli-hood of a justified paternalistic intervention correspondingly increases.[38] Condi-tion (3) above therefore affects our willingness to relax our normal expectations that paternalistic acts should not substantially restrict autonomy.

The following case plausibly supports strong paternalistic intervention, even though there is more than minimal infringement of respect for autonomy: A psychiatrist is treating a patient similar to the patient discussed above who plucked out his eye and cut off his hand for religious reasons. Presume, now, that this patient is not insane and acts conscientiously on his unique religious views. Suppose further that this patient asks the psychiatrist a question about his condition, a question that has a definite answer but which, if answered, would lead the patient to engage in self-maiming behavior in order to fulfill what he believes to be the requirements of his religion. Many, including the present authors, would maintain that the doctor acts paternalistically, but justi-fiably, by concealing information from the patient, even if the patient is rational and otherwise informed. Because the infringement of the principle of respect for autonomy is more than minimal in this case, a condition requiring no substantial infringement of autonomy cannot be a necessary condition for all cases of justified strong paternalism.

Finally, at times we may seem to have suggested in this section that a decision about the justifiability of paternalism is a matter of giving overriding status to some principle of respect for autonomy or beneficence—that is, a matter of choosing one principle over another. However, framing the issues in such a way is overly simplistic and can be seriously misleading. A better strategy is to return to the arguments about specification, balancing, and coherence presented in Chapter 1. Developing a position on issues of paternalism is a matter of appreciating the limits of principles and the need to give them additional content, while attempting to render one's consequent rules and judgments as coherent with other commitments as possible. The problem of medical paternalism is the problem of putting just the right specification and balance of physician beneficence and patient autonomy in the patient–physician relationship. It is a messy and complicated problem, and coherence is difficult to achieve. Paternalistic intervention requires persons of good judgment as well as persons with well-developed principles able to confront contingent conflicts.

Problems of Suicide Intervention

Both strong and weak paternalism are present in certain forms of suicide intervention. The state, religious institutions, and health care facilities have all traditionally assumed some jurisdiction to intervene with suicide. Those who intervene do not always attempt to justify their actions on paternalistic grounds, but paternalism has been the primary justification.

Approximately thirty thousand certified suicides occur in the United States each year, and many other suicides are routinely classified as accidental deaths, in part because too little is known about the decedents' intentions. Several conceptual questions about the term *suicide* also make it difficult to classify acts as suicides.[39] For example, when Barney Clark became the first human to receive an artificial heart, he was given a key that he could use to turn off the compressor if he wanted to die. As Dr. Willem Kolff noted, if the patient "suffers and feels it isn't worth it any more, he has a key that he can apply. . . . I think it is entirely legitimate that this man whose life has been extended should have the right to cut it off if he doesn't want it, if [his] life ceases to be enjoyable."[40] Would Clark's use of the key to turn off the artificial heart have been an act of suicide? If he had refused to accept the artificial heart in the first place, few would have labeled his act a suicide. His overall condition was extremely poor, the artificial heart was experimental, and no suicidal intention was evident. If, on the other hand, Clark had intentionally shot himself with a gun while on the artificial heart, the act would have been classified as suicide. If Clark had used the key to turn off his artificial heart, controversy would have erupted about whether to characterize his act as forgoing life-sustaining treatment, as withdrawing from an experiment, as suicide, or as all of the above.

It would take us too far from our topic to pursue conceptual problems about the vagueness of *suicide*. We will concentrate instead on paternalistic interventions in cases that are generally agreed to be acts of suicide or attempted suicide. The primary moral issue is the following: Do individuals have a moral right to decide about the acceptability of suicide and to act unimpeded on their convictions? If suicide is a protected moral right, then the state and other individuals such as health professionals have no legitimate grounds for intervention in autonomous suicide attempts. No one seriously doubts that we should intervene to prevent suicide by nonautonomous persons, and few people wish to return to the days when suicide was a criminal act. But if we accept an autonomy right, then the imprudent suicide who would want to live under more favorable circumstances could not legitimately be prevented from committing suicide.

A clear and relevant example of attempted suicide appears in the following case, involving John K., a thirty-two-year-old lawyer. Two neurologists independently confirmed that his facial twitching, which had been evident for three months, is an early sign of Huntington's disease, a neurological disorder that progressively worsens, leads to irreversible dementia, and is uniformly fatal in approximately ten years. His mother suffered a horrible death from the same disease, and John K. had often said that he would prefer to die than to suffer the way his mother suffered. Over several years he had been anxious, had drunk heavily, and had sought psychiatric help for intermittent depression. Following a confirming diagnosis, John K. told his psychiatrist about his situation and asked for help in committing suicide. After the psychiatrist refused to help, he attempted to take his own life by ingesting his antidepressant medication, leaving a note of explanation to his wife and child.[41]

Several interventions occurred or were possible in this case. First, the psychiatrist refused to assist John K.'s suicide and would have sought to have him involuntarily committed if he had not assured the psychiatrist that he did not plan to attempt suicide anytime soon. The psychiatrist probably thought that he could provide appropriate psychotherapy over time. Second, John K.'s wife found him unconscious and rushed him to the emergency room. Third, the emergency room staff decided to treat him despite the suicide note. Which, if any, of these possible or actual interventions is justifiable?

One widely accepted account of our obligations is based on a modification of the strategy of temporary intervention defended by Mill: Intervention is justified to ascertain or to establish the quality of autonomy in the person; further intervention is unjustified once it is determined that the person's actions are substantially autonomous. Glanville Williams used this strategy in an influential statement:

If one suddenly comes upon another person attempting suicide, the natural and humane thing to do is to try to stop him, for the purpose of ascertaining the cause of his distress and attempting to remedy it, or else of attempting moral dissuasion if it seems that the act of suicide shows lack of consideration for others, or else again from the purpose of trying to persuade him to accept psychiatric help if this seems to be called for. . . . But nothing longer than a temporary restraint could be defended. I would gravely doubt whether a suicide attempt should be a factor leading to a diagnosis of psychosis or to compulsory admissions to a hospital. Psychiatrists are too ready to assume that an attempt to commit suicide is the act of mentally sick persons.[42]

This antipaternalist stance is vulnerable to criticism on two grounds. First, failure to intervene symbolically communicates to potential suicides a lack of communal concern and works to diminish our sense of communal responsibility. Second, many persons who commit suicide are either mentally ill, clinically depressed, or destabilized by a crisis and are therefore not acting autonomously. From a clinical perspective, many suicidal persons are beset with ambivalence, simply wish to reduce or interrupt anxiety, or are under the influence of drugs, alcohol, or intense pressure. Many mental health professionals believe that suicides are almost always the result of maladaptive attitudes or illnesses needing therapeutic attention and social support.[43]

In a typical circumstance, the potential suicide plans how to end life while simultaneously holding fantasies about how rescue will occur, not only rescue from death but from the negative circumstances prompting the suicide. If the suicide springs from clinical depression or is a call for help, a failure to intervene seems to show disrespect for the person's deepest autonomous wishes, including his or her hopes for the future. Surface intentions do not always capture deeper desires or inclinations, and in a matter as serious as suicide, deeper motives should receive a heavy weighting in the justification of intervention.

Several public policy problems are connected to these claims. Many people are concerned that changes in suicide laws either to legalize physician-assisted suicide or to discourage suicide intervention will have the effect of encouraging suicides by persons who are not substantially autonomous, especially those who are terminally ill and in need of both care and resources. Recent studies indicate that people who have been diagnosed with AIDS commit suicide at a rate many times greater—one study suggests thirty-five times greater—than the general population.[44] Some AIDS patients want to commit suicide rather than face the process of suffering and dying from their disease, but their medical condition also causes central nervous system complications such as delirium or dementia that may render them unable to make a substantially autonomous choice. While recognizing the case for "rational suicide" by patients with AIDS, one physician contends that "from the clinical point of view, careful evaluations of suicides, even in terminally ill patients, almost invariably reveal evidence that the suicide occurred as a manifestation of a psychiatric disorder rather than as a rational choice."[45]

Another worry is that new suicide laws would have the effect of encouraging insensitive attitudes on the part of health care professionals and patients, especially in a medical system organized around cost reduction. Some institutions devoted to caring for the ill and elderly, such as the modern nursing home, already communicate a message of indifference to various forms of suffering that lead patients to end their lives. These institutions contrast sharply with the ethos of a hospice, which is a prime example of an institution established to care for suffering patients and to provide a supportive community. Hospices are but one of many concrete examples of social institutions that counterbalance an undue social emphasis on rights of autonomy and self-reliance.

However, caution is also needed in calls for communal beneficence, which may express itself paternalistically through forceful interventions or criminal sanctions. Although suicide has been decriminalized, a suicide attempt, irrespective of motive, almost universally provides a legal basis for intervention by public officers, as well as grounds for involuntary hospitalization.[46] Often the burden of proof is more appropriately placed on those who claim that the patient's judgment is not autonomous. For example, Ida Rollin, seventy-four years old, suffered from ovarian cancer, and her physicians told her that she had only a few months to live and that her dying would be very painful and upsetting. Rollin indicated to her daughter that she wanted to commit suicide and requested her assistance. The daughter secured some pills and conveyed a doctor's instructions about how they should be taken. When the daughter expressed reservations about these plans, her husband reminded her that they "weren't driving, she [Ida Rollin] was" and that they were only "navigators."[47]

This metaphor-laden reference to rightful authority is a reminder that those who propose suicide intervention require a solid moral justification that fits the context. There are occasions in health care (and elsewhere) when it is appropriate to step aside and allow a suicide, and even to assist in a person's suicide, just as there are occasions under which it is appropriate to intervene. (See Chapter 4, pp. 235–241.)

Denying Requests for Nonbeneficial Procedures

Patients or their surrogates occasionally request medical procedures that the clinician is convinced will not be beneficial. The clinician may believe that the procedure is ineffective or futile or that its harms or risks will prevent a net benefit. Often, though not always, denials of such requests are paternalistic.

Passive paternalism. Debates about paternalism typically focus on active paternalistic interventions when the patient prefers nonintervention. A comparatively neglected form of paternalism appears in the professional's refusal to execute the positive preferences of a patient for paternalistic reasons—a passive paternalism.[48] The following case illustrates passive paternalism. Elizabeth Stanley, a sexually active 26-year-old intern, requests a tubal ligation, insisting that she has thought about this request for months, dislikes available contraceptives, does not want children, and understands that tubal ligation is irreversible. When the gynecologist suggests that she might someday want to get married and have children, she responds that she would either find a husband who did not want children or adopt children. She thinks that she is not likely to change her mind and wants the tubal ligation to make it impossible for her to reconsider. She has scheduled a vacation in two weeks and wants the surgery then.[49]

If a physician justifies a refusal to perform the tubal ligation on grounds of the patient's benefit, the action is paternalistic. Such actions typically are more easily justified than active paternalism because physicians generally do not have a moral obligation to satisfy the patient's desires when they are incompatible with acceptable standards of medical practice or are against the physicians' conscience. If physicians believe that providing a requested treatment, such as antibiotics for a cold or laetrile for cancer, is not in the patient's best interests, they are not compelled to violate their conscience, even when the patient is substantially autonomous. Of course, setting a professional standard of practice may itself be a paternalistic effort to protect patients' interests, but that is a separate problem.

Medical futility. Passive paternalism has been central to recent debates about medical futility, a topic we introduced in Chapter 4. Consider the case of 85-year-old Helga Wanglie, who was maintained on a respirator in a persistent vegetative state (Case 6 in the appendix). The hospital sought to stop the respirator on grounds that it was " 'nonbeneficial,' in that it could not heal her lungs, palliate her suffering, or enable this unconscious and permanently respirator-dependent woman to experience the benefit of the life afforded by respirator support." The surrogate decisionmakers—her husband, a son, and a daughter—wanted life support continued on grounds that Mrs. Wanglie would not be better off dead, that a miracle could occur, that physicians should not play God, and that efforts to remove her life support indicated "moral decay in our civilization."

If life support for such patients is futile, denials of requests for treatment are warranted. Even the restrictive Baby Doe regulations (see p. 218) allow physicians to withhold treatment that is considered "futile in terms of the survival of the infant" or "virtually futile." A justified claim that a medical procedure is futile removes it from the range of otherwise beneficial acts among which patients or their surrogates may choose. The claim is typically not that an intervention will harm the patient (in violation of the principle of nonmaleficence), but only that it will not produce the benefit sought by the patient or the surrogate. The obligation to provide a medical benefit is effectively cancelled by a justified claim of futility. But does the language of futility illuminate these issues, and is there a bona fide issue of passive paternalism or only an issue about wasted resources and coercion of the conscience of health professionals?

As noted in Chapter 4, "medical futility" has several distinguishable meanings in the literature, including the following: (1) the procedure cannot be performed because of a patient's biological condition, (2) the procedure cannot produce the intended physiological effect, (3) the procedure cannot be expected to produce the benefit that is sought, and (4) the anticipated benefits of the procedure will be outweighed by the burdens, harms, and costs. In our judgment, only the first three are bona fide instances of "medical futility," because the fourth is an on-balance judgment having nothing to do with futility. Claims of medical futility are often presented as objective and value-free, when in fact they are subjective and value-laden. For example, some clinicians insist that a treatment is futile only if there is no chance it will work, while others label a treatment as futile if it has a thirteen percent or lower chance of success.[50]

Claims of futility involve the prediction and evaluation of outcomes, which are usually probable rather than certain. Determining a statistical threshold is in part evaluative; that is, a line must be fixed in light of values. Even if we assume consensus among clinicians about the statistical threshold, problems will still occur in clinical estimates of the probability that an intervention will be successful.[51] Some contend that a medical procedure is reasonably judged futile when physicians determine through personal experiences and reported empirical data that "in the last 100 cases, a medical treatment has been useless."[52] However, dissimilarities among otherwise similar patients may call this sweeping conclusion into question.

It is always appropriate to ask for a specification of the objectives with respect to which a procedure is said to be futile. An inquiry may reveal that the benefit the physician doubts can be achieved may not be the same benefit the patient seeks. For example, it is often assumed that a legitimate objective of cardiopulmonary resuscitation (CPR) is survival to discharge from the hospital; CPR is deemed futile for patients in the categories that statistically do not survive to discharge.[53] However, short-term survival may be the main objective for the patient or the family. Hence, it is not simply a medical judgment whether efforts should be undertaken to gain several days or weeks of additional time, even if survival to discharge cannot be reasonably expected.

Furthermore, some acts, such as providing artificial nutrition and hydration, may have symbolic significance in expressing commitments of care, while accomplishing no other medical benefit for patients. Lantos and colleagues argue that "feeding patients in a persistent vegetative state may be futile if the goal is to restore cognition, but it may provide emotional and symbolic benefits to the patient's family or to society. These goals may be relevant to futility determinations and should not be automatically excluded."[54] In short, the debate about futility is often at bottom a debate about goals, and disputes about appropriate goals involve conflicts of values.

One physician in the Wanglie case (Case 6) described her treatment as "nonbeneficial" and identified the goals it could not realize. The question is in part whether the prolongation of life is a sufficient goal for a patient in PVS in the absence of other benefits. This debate too is best interpreted as a dispute about the legitimacy of goals, rather than as a dispute about futility, in the sense of utter hopelessness. Nothing is gained—and much is obscured—by using the label *futility*. The rhetorical power of claims of medical futility derives from the supposition that these judgments are objective and value-free. However, as we have seen, it is a fiction to describe many judgments of medical futility in this way, and such appeals risk unwarranted paternalism.

Nevertheless, it is at times a justifiable act of paternalism to withhold procedures *without* the consent of patients or their surrogates. It may be misleading and may diminish autonomy to provide information about a useless procedure. Consider in-hospital CPR as an example. Hospital policies usually require that CPR be attempted, unless a written do-not-resuscitate (DNR) order exists that includes patient or family consent. However, some argue that when resuscitation would clearly provide no medical benefit to the patient, hospitals should not require that options be discussed with either the patient or the family.[55] Both beneficence and nonmaleficence support a paternalistic policy of not presenting nonbeneficial interventions as an option for decisionmaking. Clinicians would put families in a difficult emotional position by informing them about CPR and then attempting to convince them that it would produce no medical benefit. In addition, such an approach could reduce rather than enhance autonomous decisionmaking by implying that a meaningful choice exists when in fact there is none. A moral judgment is therefore required that takes account of different contextual factors in deciding whether it is appropriate or obligatory to inform patients and families that CPR or other nonbeneficial interventions will not be undertaken.[56]

Some interpreters believe that "futility judgments can be endorsed on nonpaternalistic grounds and that indeed it may be the failure to make such judgments that truly undermines autonomous choices by patients and surrogates.''[57] This claim is correct, but there is no reason to be suspicious of the argument that some professional standards of care aimed at promoting the interests of patients are paternalistic and are justified. If health professionals *cannot* provide medical (or nonmedical) benefits, no obligation exists to follow patient or surrogate demands for interventions.

Finally, conceptions of medical futility are usually presented as independent of considerations of financial costs. Nevertheless, much of the interest in medical futility has been fueled by the need to control costs. We develop a framework for the just allocation of health care in Chapter 6, but first we need to examine formal analyses of benefits, costs, and risks to determine whether they can play a legitimate role in judgments about acceptable care and the distribution of care.

Balancing Benefits, Costs, and Risks

Thus far we have concentrated on the role of the principle of beneficence in clinical medicine. But many public and institutional policies are also developed from reasoned choices about appropriate benefits relative to costs and risks. Particularly prominent are various forms of cost- and risk-benefit analysis that implement the principle of utility in health policies. These tools are morally unobjectionable and may be morally required if they can illuminate trade-offs and enhance our ability to make reasoned assessments and wise judgments about trade-offs.

Questions commonly arise about the comparison and relative weights of costs, risks, and benefits. Judgments about the most suitable medical treatments are routinely based on probable benefits and harms, and judgments about the ethical acceptability of research involving human subjects reflect, in part, judgments about whether the risks to subjects are outweighed by the probable overall benefits. For example, in submitting a research protocol involving human subjects to an institutional review board (IRB) for approval, an investigator is expected to array the risks to subjects and probable benefits to both subjects and society, and then to explain why the probable benefits outweigh the risks. The IRB then offers a reasoned assessment. If the research is approved, the investigator is expected to describe the risks and probable benefits to potential subjects so that they can make an informed decision about participation in the research. This appeal to beneficence in research can, with only slight reformulation, be extended to the treatment of patients, the delivery of health services, and the assessment of medical technologies.

Various informal strategies have evolved to help make decisions about costs, risks, and benefits. These strategies include expert judgments based on the most reliable data that can be assembled and analogical reasoning based on precedents. The latter strategy attempts to establish new policies on the basis of policies that have already proved their value. When IRBs array risks and benefits, determine their respective weights, and reach decisions on this basis, they typically use *informal* techniques. They virtually never use formal techniques that manipulate numbers in order to express the objective probability that an event will result in a benefit or a harm. However, our focus in this section is on techniques that employ *formal, quantitative* analysis of costs, risks, and benefits.

The Nature of Costs, Risks, and Benefits

Costs are the resources required to bring about a benefit, as well as the negative effects of pursuing and realizing that benefit. They represent, in effect, sacrifices made in the attempt to reach some important objective. We will concentrate on costs expressed in monetary terms—the primary interpretation of costs in cost–benefit and cost–effectiveness analysis. The term *risk,* by contrast, refers to a possible future harm, where harm is defined as a setback to interests in life, health, and welfare. Expressions such as *minimal risk, reasonable risk,* and *high risk* usually refer to the chance of experiencing a harm—its *probability*—but sometimes they refer to the severity of the harm if it occurs—its *magnitude*.

Statements of risk are descriptive inasmuch as they state the probability that harmful events will occur. However, statements of risk are also evaluative, inasmuch as a value is necessarily attached to the occurrence or prevention of the events. No risk exists unless a prior negative evaluation of some condition has taken place. Thus, risk is both a descriptive and an evaluative concept. At its core, a circumstance of risk is one in which there is both a possible occurrence of something that has been evaluated as harmful and an uncertainty about its occurrence that can be expressed in terms of its probability.

Several types of risks exist: physical, psychological, financial, legal, among others. The following case illustrates the range of types of risk that correlate with human interests that may be set back. In this case, a baby girl suffers from Seckel or "bird-headed" dwarfism, a recessive genetic disease, as well as multiple other medical complications. The child is at risk of starvation if an operation is not performed, but she also is at risk of severe suffering and serious medical complications if the operation is performed. The family is at further risk of psychological harm and economic harm because of the extremely low per capita funding for state institutions that house the mentally retarded. Eventually, the parents decide against the surgery, a decision that in some jurisdictions would place them at legal risk.[58]

The term *benefit* sometimes refers to cost avoidance and risk reduction, but more commonly in biomedicine it refers to something of positive value such as life or health. Unlike *risk, benefit* is not a probabilistic term. Probability of benefit is the proper contrast to risk, and benefits are comparable to harms rather than to risks of harm. Thus, risk–benefit relations are best conceived in terms of a ratio between the probability and magnitude of an anticipated benefit and the probability and magnitude of an anticipated harm.

Use of the terms *cost, risk,* and *benefit* necessarily involves an evaluation. Values determine *what* will count as costs, harms, and benefits as well as *how much* particular costs, harms, and benefits will count—that is, how much weight they will have in our calculations.

Cost-Effectiveness and Cost-Benefit Analysis

Cost-effectiveness analysis (CEA) and cost-benefit analysis (CBA) are two controversial but widely used tools of formal analysis. They have been increasingly employed in setting public policies regarding health, safety, and medical technologies. Often these policies are responses to burgeoning demands for expensive medical care and the need to contain the costs of health care. CEA and CBA present trade-offs with as much rigor and objectivity as possible, using quantified terms. These techniques have been praised as ways of reducing intuitive weighing of options and avoiding subjective and political decisions. However, these tools have also been sharply criticized. Critics claim that these methods of analysis are not sufficiently comprehensive to include all relevant values and options, that they are often themselves subjective and biased, and that they are sometimes ad hoc. Critics also charge that these techniques concentrate decisionmaking authority in the hands of narrow, technical professionals who fail to understand moral, legal, and political constraints that legitimately limit use of these methods.

Both CEA and CBA aim to identify, measure, compare, and evaluate all relevant costs and consequences of policies, programs, and technologies in quantitative terms.[59] However, the two can be distinguished by the terms in which they state the value of outcomes. In CBA both the benefits and the costs are measured in monetary terms. In CEA the benefits are measured in nonmonetary terms, such as years of life, quality-adjusted life-years, or cases of disease. CEA offers a bottom line such as "cost per year of life saved," whereas CBA offers a bottom line of a benefit-cost ratio stated in monetary figures that express the common measurement. Although CBA often begins by measuring different quantitative units—such as number of accidents, statistical deaths, number of persons treated, and dollars expended—it attempts in the end to convert and express these seemingly incommensurable units of measurement into a common one.

Consider as an example of these approaches the debate about the use of low-osmolality contrast agents (LOCAs). These agents are used in intravascular radiographic studies, especially in cardiac angiography, because they offer reduced risks of serious adverse reactions, including death. Even though LOCAs do not appear to offer a diagnostic advantage over older, high-osmolality contrast agents, LOCAs would be adopted universally if costs were not a factor, because of their superior safety. However, LOCAs are very expensive and cost between twelve and twenty times more than alternative agents. Over ten million intravascular contrast studies are performed in the United States each year. If LOCAs were used universally, the total additional cost would be over $1 billion (using a conservative twelvefold incremental cost over traditional agents).

The relative merits of the available agents have been stated in terms of the (monetary) value of life (as would be appropriate in CBA), but more often in terms of the value of life-years (as is often the case in CEA). Conventional contrast agents are estimated to cause one fatal reaction per 30,000 uses, while LOCAs are estimated to cause only one fatal reaction per 250,000 uses. Universal adoption of LOCAs would result in a net reduction of 293 fatalities (per year)—an expenditure of $3.4 million for each death prevented. For purposes of CEA, the figures are developed to reflect life-years. If patients undergoing these examinations have a mean age of 46 years and a life expectancy of 32 additional years, the cost for each year of life saved would be $106,000. This cost is much higher than, for example, treatment of hypertension ($30,000) and dialysis for end-stage renal disease ($32,000). However, if LOCAs were provided only to the 15%–20% of patients who have high risks for serious adverse reactions—e.g., because they are elderly—the cost per death prevented would be $1 million and the cost per year of life saved would be $31,250, which is in line with the two treatments just identified.

From the standpoint of marginal costs of preventing deaths in the low-risk group (80%–85%), analysts calculate that the additional cost of extending LOCAs from high-risk patients to all patients undergoing contrast injections would be $878 million, which would result in a reduction of 117 additional deaths each year, at a cost of $7.8 million for each death averted and $234,000 for each life-year saved. Some analysts have noticed that this cost-effectiveness ratio is far higher than that of the bulk of medical programs in the United States.[60] While the CEA of LOCAs focuses on the cost of saving lives and especially on the cost per life-year saved, it does not include what is taken as a primary end point of many CEAs in health policy and health care: *Quality-adjusted* life-years (see below, pp. 308–313). This omission is understandable because these diagnostic procedures are used for many patients with a wide range of conditions and variable prognoses, as well as variably successful treatments.

This case illustrates the role and importance of some analytic tools and categories that will be prominent in the remainder of this chapter. Using the common metric of money, CBA permits a comparison of programs that save lives with programs that reduce disability. By contrast, CEA functions best to compare and evaluate different programs sharing an identical aim, such as saving years of life. It does not permit an evaluation of the inherent worth of programs or a comparative evaluation of programs with different aims. The point of CEA is to display which among the possible alternatives either maximizes the desirable consequences, given a fixed set of resources such as money, or minimizes the costs in order to achieve a desired consequence.

Thus, many CEAs involve comparing alternative courses of action that have similar health benefits in order to determine which is most cost-effective. A good example in medical practice is the use of the guaiac test, an inexpensive test for detecting minute amounts of blood in the stool. Such blood may result from several problems, including hemorrhoids, benign intestinal polyps, or colonic cancer. (The last problem is a major killer, but it may be curable if diagnosed very early.) A guaiac test cannot identify the cause of the bleeding, but if there is a positive stool guaiac and no other obvious cause for the bleeding, physicians undertake other tests. The American Cancer Society in 1974 proposed that six sequential stool guaiac tests be used to screen for colorectal cancer. This proposal was based on the fact that any single stool guaiac detects only approximately ninety-two percent of the colorectal cancers. Two analysts prepared a careful CEA of the six stool guaiac tests. They assumed that the initial test costs four dollars, that each additional test costs one dollar, and that many fewer cases of cancer are detected with each successive test. They then determined that the marginal cost per case of detected cancer increased dramatically: $1,175 for one test; $5,492 for two tests; $49,150 for three tests; $469,534 for four tests; $4.7 million for five tests; and $47 million for the full six-test screen.[61]

These findings do not dictate a conclusion, but the analysis is relevant for a society allocating resources, for insurance companies and hospitals setting policies, for physicians making recommendations to patients, and for patients considering diagnostic procedures. This analysis is a CEA rather than a CBA because it does not attempt to convert the benefit of detection of colorectal cancer into a measure, such as dollars, that can then be compared with the costs. It also does not include effects such as the reassurance given to patients that may be hard to measure.

Conceptual confusion has surrounded the meaning of CEA. According to some analysts, CEA should not be confused with either a reduction of costs or an increase of effectiveness alone, because it often depends on an examination of both together. In some cases, when two programs are compared, the cost savings offered by one may be sufficient to view it as more cost-effective than the other. However, a program may be more cost-effective than another even if it (1) *costs more*—because it may increase medical effectiveness—or (2) leads to a *decrease in medical effectiveness*—because it may greatly reduce the costs. For these reasons, some analysts argue that the term *cost-effective* should be used for cases in which "one strategy is more 'cost effective' than another if it is (a) less costly and at least as effective; (b) more effective and more costly, its additional benefit being worth its additional cost; or (c) less effective and less costly, the added benefit of the rival strategy not being worth its extra cost."[62]

However, many analysts accept only (a), holding that one strategy is more cost-effective than another if it costs less and achieves the same goal. In this conception, CEA presupposes a uniform goal already established by an independent assessment of the benefits of reaching that goal. Diagnostic or therapeutic procedures may be more or less cost-effective in comparison with others that have the same outcome. If both procedures produce an equal outcome— in, say, life-years—but one is less expensive, then that procedure is more cost-effective. To say that it is cost-effective, apart from such a comparison, is to presuppose a value placed on the health outcome relative to the monetary cost. This evaluation takes a step in the direction of CBA, though perhaps without converting the benefit into a measure common to the costs, such as dollars.

For instance, according to a study of leukocyte transfusion during chemotherapy for acute leukemia, prophylactic transfusion costs $2,431 more than therapeutic transfusion and increases the patient's life expectancy by 0.0285 years.[63] But whether it is appropriate to say that prophylactic transfusion is more or less cost-effective than therapeutic transfusion depends on the value assigned to the additional benefit relative to the additional cost. Put bluntly, is it worth $85,300 for an additional statistical year of life gained? Without answering this question, one cannot determine whether prophylactic transfusion is cost-effective.

The principle of utility does not dictate a medical procedure simply because it has the lowest cost-effectiveness ratio (e.g., because it provides the greatest benefit for each dollar). To assign priority to the lowest cost-effectiveness ratio is to endorse a minimalist approach to medical diagnosis and therapy.[64] For example, such an approach would stop with the first stool guaiac test, because the cost-effectiveness ratio is the lowest for that first test and increases for subsequent tests. This approach to decision analysis is too narrow, because it excludes from the calculation the value of the additional health benefits, including psychological reassurance, provided by the additional tests.

Prevention of accident, disease, and illness has often been touted as the best way to contain the costs of health care. However, prevention is not always better than cure from the standpoint of CEA. Prevention may produce savings in particular treatments, but it may also add medical expenditures for other health problems.[65] Similarly, successful strategies to reduce risky lifestyles and behavioral patterns generally result in an increase rather than a decrease in social expenditures, because people who live longer often need a wide array of social assistance and services.[66] However, an exclusive focus on costs will downplay the value of health itself, because preventive strategies, if effective, have the advantage of maintaining health over time, even if they have an increased net cost.

Risk Assessment

Risk assessment is another important technique of analysis that we need to consider before offering an overall evaluation of CBA. As already noted, risk involves probability and magnitude of negative outcome. Hence, risk *assessment* involves the analysis and evaluation of probabilities of negative outcomes, especially harms. Risk *identification* involves locating some hazard. Risk *estimation* involves determining the probability and magnitude of harms from that hazard. Risk *evaluation* determines the acceptability of the identified and estimated risks, often in relation to other objectives. Evaluation of risk in relation to probable benefits is often labeled *risk–benefit analysis* (RBA), which may be formulated in terms of a ratio of expected benefits to risks and may lead to a judgment about the acceptability of the risk under assessment. Risk identification, estimation, and evaluation are all stages in risk assessment. The next stage in the process is risk *management*—the set of individual or institutional responses to the analysis and assessment of risk, including decisions to reduce or control risks. For example, risk management in hospitals includes setting policies to reduce the risk of medical malpractice suits.

   In this section we focus on risk assessment, which is frequently used for technology assessment, environmental impact statements, and public policies protecting health and safety. Risk assessment may be charted in the following schema of magnitude and probability of harm:

		Magnitude of Harm	
		Major	*Minor*
	High	1	2
Probability of Harm			
	Low	3	4

For purposes of medical decisionmaking and public policy, the acceptability of risks should be determined through the most objective estimates of probability and magnitude of harm that are possible, together with all of the relevant values, including desired benefits.

   As category 4 suggests, a question exists about whether some risks are so insignificant, in terms of either probability or magnitude of harm or both, as not to merit attention. So-called *de minimis* risks are acceptable because they can be construed as effectively zero. For example, according to the Food and

Drug Administration (FDA), a risk of less than one cancer per million persons exposed is *de minimis*. Yet the quantitative threshold or cutoff point used in a *de minimis* approach is problematic. For instance, an annual risk of one cancer per million persons for the U.S. population would produce the same number of fatalities—240—as a risk of one per one hundred in a town with a population of 24,000. Furthermore, in focusing on the annual risk of cancer or death to one individual per million, the *de minimis* approach may neglect the cumulative, overall level of risk created for individuals over their lifetimes by the addition of several one-per-million risks.[67]

Risk assessment also focuses on the acceptability of risks relative to benefits that are sought. With the possible exception of *de minimis* risks, most risks will be considered acceptable or unacceptable in relation to the benefits that can be derived from the actions that carry those risks—for example, the benefits of radiation or a surgical procedure in health care, or the benefits of nuclear power or of toxic chemicals in the workplace.[68]

The problem of uncertainty. Risk is to be distinguished from uncertainty, although both assume a lack of predictability or knowledge of future events. *Risk* refers to the probability and magnitude of a setback to interests. *Uncertainty,* by contrast, refers to a lack of predictability or knowledge because of insufficient evidence. Risk assessment and management are fraught with uncertainty. There may be large margins of error in quantifying risks, and it may be difficult to extrapolate information about the effects of a chemical on human beings, even though the chemical is demonstrably carcinogenic at high dose levels in rodents. A fundamental question, then, is which way to err in situations of uncertainty. Whether uncertainty will be resolved optimistically or pessimistically depends on the value judgments of those who perform the analysis. Regulators, for example, typically assume the most conservative estimate by taking a worst-case scenario.[69]

In trying to reduce uncertainty, the same standards of evidence—for example, that a particular substance is carcinogenic—typically do not apply in all settings. For example, debates arise about where to set evidentiary standards in policies to protect the environment and to protect patients from unsafe drugs, medical devices, and the like. In general, the standard of proof sets forth the risk of error that is acceptable. Acceptance of any confidence level presupposes normative moral, social, and political considerations. For instance, whether a regulatory agency should set a standard of evidence that a substance is toxic or carcinogenic at a ninety-five percent confidence level is a matter of normative judgment, not merely scientific judgment, and it will have an impact on both commercial interests and potential victims of a substance. Where there are small samples and relatively rare diseases, use of the ninety-five-percent rule will often protect commercial manufacturers and sellers of a substance more effectively than its potential victims.[70] Accepting any standard of evidence, then, involves moral, social, and political judgments.

A related issue concerns which side has the burden of proof. In moral and political decisions, as in legal decisions, justifying a judgment may hinge on who must bear the burden of proof—or example, in the debate about the safety of silicone-gel breast implants, which is discussed below. Far from a matter of neutral decisionmaking, locating the burden of proof reflects certain values. In the example of criminal law, the state has the burden of proof to establish the guilt of an alleged criminal beyond a reasonable doubt; rather than having to prove his or her innocence, the alleged criminal has only to establish reasonable doubt that he or she committed the crime. In technology assessment, we must decide whether supporters or opponents of a technology have the burden of proof. Making this judgment will depend on premises about which way we should err in cases of uncertainty and doubt. For instance, should we be more concerned that a technology will be environmentally unsafe when it is thought to be safe or that it will be environmentally safe when it is thought to be unsafe? Convictions about the value of the environment and of technological progress will generally figure in assignments of the burden of proof.

A common uncertainty is whether and how a technology will interact with other technologies to produce unanticipatable effects.[71] For example, it may be uncertain which effects simultaneous exposure to several chemicals will have on individuals, because the interaction of the chemicals may produce synergistic rather than additive effects. Other uncertainties about technologies include how they will be used—for example, how physicians will manage them and whether patients will follow instructions. Proposals for safer sex in the AIDS crisis hinge not only on the quality of the condoms used but also on care by users. Thus, evidence based on laboratory studies of the effectiveness of condoms in preventing the transmission of HIV (human immunodeficiency virus) is insufficient for a predictive judgment about the effectiveness of condoms in actual sexual intercourse.

Other uncertainties stem from the social and cultural context of technological advances. For example, Lynn White insists that technology assessment requires social analysis, because the impact of a technology is filtered through the society and its culture, often in unpredictable ways. One of his case studies focuses on alcohol, which was distilled from wine as a pharmaceutical in the twelfth century at Salerno, the site of Europe's most famous medical school. Widely heralded initially as a pharmaceutical with beneficial effects for chronic headaches, stomach trouble, cancer, arthritis, sterility, falling or graying hair, bad breath, and a "cold temperament," it gradually led to widespread drunkenness and disorder and then in the twentieth century to alcohol-related diseases and automobile accidents, none of which could have been predicted by a technology assessment panel in the twelfth century.[72]

Similar uncertainties arise about the interaction of society, culture, and new technologies for sex selection. Whether prospective parents, for instance, would prefer more male or more female children or prefer to have a male or female firstborn may depend on cultural attitudes and on social policies such as whether males or females have more or equal opportunities and rewards. Some of the main risks of techniques for sex selection are their social effects. For example, widespread sex selection could reinforce sexual stereotypes and sex discrimination, while setting back social policies of equal opportunity.

Risk perception. An individual's perception of risks may differ from an expert's assessment. Variations may reflect not only different goals and "risk budgets," but also different qualitative assessments of particular risks, including whether the risks in question are voluntary, controllable, highly salient, novel, or dreaded.[73] Consider the possible impact of personal life plans and risk budgets on patients' perceptions and assessments of the risks of coronary artery bypass surgery. Of every one hundred patients who undergo the operation, one to two die. An active sportsperson might view this risk of death from surgery as insignificant in view of the active life sought; another person might choose medical treatment because of a fear of dying on the operating table.[74] In addition, as we saw in Chapter 3 (p. 158), a patient's perception of risks and benefits may depend in part on how the physician presents them—for example, whether in terms of the probability of dying or the probability of surviving.

Public and professional responses to accidental exposure to the blood of patients infected with the human immunodeficiency virus (HIV) provides an illustration. Such exposure produces greater fear than did accidental exposure to the blood of patients with hepatitis B a few years ago, even though statistically both exposures carried an approximately equal overall risk of death. The probability of infection by HIV is lower (apparently less than 1%), but death from the infection is virtually certain over time; the probability of infection by the hepatitis B virus is higher, at approximately twenty-five percent, but the death rate is conservatively estimated to be only five percent. According to one study, the fear of certain death if one is infected with HIV appears to account for the greater fear of HIV infection through accidental exposure.[75] Other factors include the social stigma attached to HIV infection and AIDS.

Differences in risk perception suggest limitations in attempts to use only objective, quantitative statements of probability and magnitude in reaching conclusions about the acceptability of risk. The public's informed but subjective perception of a harm needs to be considered and given equal weight when formulating public policy. Experts sometimes charge the public with inconsistency and irrationality in voluntarily assuming major risks while strenuously objecting to low, externally imposed risks.[76] These charges are not always fair to reasonable public perceptions, but analysts can helpfully identify different perceptions of risk and communicate accurate information about risks. To reject such information altogether would be to capitulate to an unwarranted cultural or individual-relativist view that fails to appreciate that views about risk can be mistaken and can be corrected.[77]

Risk-Benefit Analysis in the Regulation of Drugs and Medical Devices

Some of the conceptual, normative, and empirical issues in risk assessment and, specifically, RBA, are evident in the regulation by the FDA of drugs and medical devices. The FDA's regulatory activities protect the public's health, while sacrificing some patient freedom to make choices about the use of drugs and medical devices that could possibly benefit them. Its approval of drugs for commercial marketing is contingent upon both safety and efficacy. In a rigorous procedure following preclinical animal studies, the FDA requires three phases of human trials. Each stage involves RBA to determine whether to proceed to the next stage and, finally, whether to approve a drug for wider use. (Related issues in clinical trials are examined in Chapter 7.)

This process in the United States has been criticized by patients, physicians, and other health care professionals because of the length of time required for approval—an average of eight years from synthesis of the drug, which is several years longer than in European countries. Critics contend that the standard of evidence for a favorable risk-benefit ratio is too high, with the result that patients' access to promising new drugs is severely limited, often in times of dire need imposed by serious, even fatal, medical conditions.

Over the last few years, particularly in response to the AIDS epidemic and the demands of AIDS activists, the FDA has developed formal mechanisms to provide expanded access to experimental drugs, especially for patients with seriously debilitating or life-threatening conditions and with no satisfactory alternative treatments.[78] In a shift of tradition, the agency has authorized treatment uses (in contrast to investigational uses) of unapproved experimental drugs for patients with an illness that is serious or poses an imminent threat to life and that has no other satisfactory alternative therapy if those drugs are also being tested in clinical trials. Other FDA initiatives include a "fast track" (expedited approval) and a "parallel track." The fast track allows patients with "seriously debilitating" or "life-threatening" conditions to accept greater risks in new drugs in the absence of acceptable alternatives. This approach was used in the approval of zidovudine (AZT). In its medical risk-benefit analysis for expedited approval, the FDA sought to determine whether the benefits of the drug outweighed its risks, both known and unknown, and the need to have more evidence about those benefits and risks, in view of the disease's "seriously debilitating" or "life-threatening" conditions. The parallel track, by contrast, allows limited access to experimental AIDS drugs that, according to early studies, are reasonably safe and promising, while clinical investigations continue.

These modes of expanded access resulted in part from vigorous efforts by AIDS protesters, whose civil disobedience and other dramatic actions drew attention to the needs of AIDS patients. These actions have raised questions about the role of advocates in securing access for special groups of patients to new drugs. A tension exists between scientific evidence about risks and benefits and patients' desires for access to certain drugs for certain conditions, and there are major concerns about the commercial exploitation of these desires if scientific standards of evidence are not maintained. Early and wide access may limit researchers' and the FDA's efforts to complete important double-blind, placebo-controlled clinical trials to establish a firmer RBA of the treatments. Some critics predict that the major beneficiaries of FDA's beneficent efforts to expand patient access to new drugs will not be the patients themselves, but rather drug companies who enjoy increased sales.[79]

The primary ethical issue is whether and how society, through a regulatory mechanism that reflects several stages of RBA, should control access to the new drugs that companies want to offer, professionals want to prescribe, and patients seek to use. According to our conception of the balance between societal beneficence and patient autonomy, expanded access to experimental drugs is warranted in response to serious and particularly life-threatening medical conditions, where no effective alternative treatments are available. In these circumstances allowing considerable latitude for patients' values regarding risks and benefits is entirely appropriate. Nevertheless, it is important not to subvert the important role for regulation of new drugs to protect the public.

A controversial decision by the FDA to severely restrict the use of silicone-gel breast implants exemplifies societal controversies about RBA in the context of health care. Issues include who should make the decisions, which values are relevant, what constitutes an acceptable risk-benefit ratio, and which standard of evidence should be adopted. Women have elected implants for over thirty years, either to augment their breast size or to reconstruct their breasts following mastectomies for cancer or other surgery. Each year in the United States, prior to this decision, approximately 150,000 implants occur, eighty percent for augmentation and twenty percent for reconstruction. Over two million women in the United States have had these implants (three million worldwide). Since legislation in 1976,[80] manufacturers have had the burden of proof in establishing that their medical devices are safe and effective before they may be distributed and used, but many manufacturers, such as those making silicone-gel breast implants, have had additional time to meet this standard because their products were already on the market.

In April 1992, after extensive discussion and debate, the FDA severely restricted the use of silicone-gel breast implants until additional studies could be conducted to establish their safety. Use was restricted to patients enrolled in clinical studies. Concerns have centered on the implants' longevity, rate of rupture, and link with various diseases. Those who defend complete prohibition contend that no woman should be allowed to take a risk of unknown, but potentially serious magnitude because her consent could not be informed. However, FDA Commissioner David Kessler defends a restrictive policy, rather than prohibition. He argues that for "patients with cancer and others with a need for breast reconstruction," there can be a favorable risk–benefit ratio in carefully controlled circumstances.[81] Kessler and the FDA distinguish sharply between reconstruction candidates and augmentation candidates, arguing that the favorable risk-benefit ratio is confined to reconstruction candidates.

Critics of this decision charge that the government's decision to restrict women's access to silicone-gel breast implants is inappropriately paternalistic, especially by contrast to the permissive public decisions reached in European countries. Europeans have relied heavily on the strong historical evidence indicating a low rate of health problems among the hundreds of thousands of recipients. We concur with Marcia Angell that the FDA has overweighed the unknown risks, in part because it has viewed the benefits of breast implants as subjective and limited, or even nonexistent, except in cases of reconstruction. The agency then concluded that these implants must be held to a high standard of safety, instead of allowing women to decide for themselves whether they want to take the risks for their own subjectively defined benefits—a clear act of strong paternalism. Regarding FDA's risk-benefit analysis, Angell writes that:

Demonstrating the safety and effectiveness of a drug or device does not, of course, mean showing that there are no side effects or risks. If that were the standard, we would have no drugs or devices, since nearly all of them have possible adverse effects. The issue is the balance between risks and benefits. Greater risks are permitted for greater benefits. In evaluation of the balance, risks and benefits are usually considered separately, then weighed.[82]

The benefits of implants, particularly for women who seek augmentation, cannot be measured in terms of the value of increased life expectancy, but the benefits may still be significant for quality of life. Subjective benefits for many women outweigh the risks that have been identified, and opinion surveys indicate that ninety percent of women receiving the implants are satisfied with the results. The risks of the implants are themselves controversial in light of available data. If the evidence had indicated high risk relative to benefit, as well as unwarranted risk-taking by patients, a different conclusion might be sustained. But present evidence points in the other direction.[83] Given the considerable range of both scientific and policy disagreement, the FDA policy seems unjustifiably paternalistic.

The FDA decision makes a judgment about different women's needs and desires for implants, giving greater value to reconstructive surgery for women who have had mastectomies than to breast augmentation for women with small or asymmetrical breasts. Interpretations of the needs and desires of both groups of women are all value-laden, but in the FDA decision breast argumentation is viewed as other than a treatment or a component of treatment for a disease. The benefits from either reconstructive or augmentation surgery could be viewed as primarily "cosmetic benefits," but Kessler construes reconstructive surgery to be an integral and accepted part of the treatment of the disease that led to mastectomy, which is covered by most health insurers who tend not to cover cosmetic surgery.

Kessler insists that the FDA's decision did not involve "any judgment about values," but simply focused on the "higher risk" presented for women receiving augmentation implants. This controversial claim is based on the fact that women with augmentation implants still have breast tissue. One central argument is that in the presence of an implant, it will be difficult to use mammography to detect breast cancer in the breast tissue, and, further, that the use of mammography creates a risk of radiation exposure in healthy young women with breast tissue who have silent ruptures of the gel implant without symptoms. "In the end, it comes down to this," Kessler writes, "in our opinion the risk-benefit ratio does not at this time favor the unrestricted use of silicone breast implants in healthy women."

However, a more defensible policy is to permit the continuing use of silicone-gel breast implants, regardless of the recipient's problems and aims, while requiring adequate disclosure of information about risks (known and unknown) that would be involved in a clinical trial. This is an antipaternalist strategy that would allow women to make their own decisions, an approach recommended by the fact that no evidence of major risks to health has appeared in thirty years of use of silicone-gel implants.[84] Raising the level of disclosure standards is, from this perspective, more appropriate than raising the level of restraints on choice. The FDA itself took a similar course of action subsequent to the 1992 decision when two 1993-released studies confirmed that silicone gel had caused problems in the immune system of laboratory rats. Rather than further upgrading its restrictions on implants, the FDA elected to require breast implant manufacturers to inform women who are considering implants of the new studies.[85]

The FDA's decision has also raised disproportionate fears among the more than one million women now alive with breast implants. Many have sought to have their implants removed, but they are unable to pay the approximately $5,000 required for removal. At least two women have cut their breasts either to force hospitals to remove the implants or to have their insurance companies pay for explantation.[86] Women's fears are understandable, and the FDA's recommendation to women not to have their implants removed unless they have medical problems rings hollow, because its policy implies that breast implants are dangerous based on the available evidence regarding their safety.[87]

Finally, the RBA of implants by the FDA occurs within a social context that includes sexist attitudes and practices that have encouraged certain body images and desires. It is not inconsistent to affirm a woman's right to decide and at the same time criticize the sexist standards of beauty that promote breast augmentation. Sexist attitudes may also be reflected in targeting a device used by many women, because of lack of evidence about its safety, while the society permits riskier actions, such as smoking cigarettes, that involve men as well as women.

We reach two general conclusions from this examination of FDA decisionmaking. First, it is morally legitimate and often obligatory for society to act beneficently through the government and its agencies to protect citizens from harmful medical drugs and devices and those of unproven safety and efficacy. The FDA plays an important role in setting minimum standards of safety and efficacy for drugs and devices, in the face of commercial interests in selling drugs and devices and the impossibility that individual physicians and patients can independently assess each drug or device. Our conclusion that the FDA should not have severely restricted or prohibited the use of breast implants should not be interpreted as an argument against the role of the FDA as society's guardian. Second, no value-free risk assessments or RBAs exist. Values are evident in the FDA's expanded access to drugs for AIDS and, despite Kessler's disavowal, in its decision to restrict access to silicone-gel breast implants. To hold that risks to women seeking implants for augmentation are significant and more important than subjective cosmetic benefits is a value-laden position, and it raises the question of which moral and nonmoral values should be used.

Both the value of life and the quality of life are at stake in many controversies about risk, as we will now see.

The Value and Quality of Life

We now turn to controversies regarding how a value might be placed on life—which have centered on CBAs—and to controversies over the value of quality-adjusted life-years (QALYs)—which have centered on CEAs.

Valuing Lives

A dramatic and controversial version of analysis assigns an economic value to human life. Analysts try to determine the monetary value of human life in order to state benefits in terms that can be balanced against the costs, hoping to develop consistency across practices and policies. As analysts note, a society may spend x number of dollars to save a life (e.g., by reducing the risk of death from causes such as cancer and mining accidents) in one setting but only spend *y* to save a life in another setting. These different expenditures are inconsistent only if life has a certain value and death a certain disvalue that can be quantitatively compared across the two settings.[88]

Methods for valuing lives. Several methods have been developed to determine the value of human life. According to the discounted future earnings (DFE), or human capital approach, the value of life can be determined by considering what people at risk of some disease or accident could be expected to earn if they survived. Future income is discounted, because money earned now could be invested and thus is worth more than future income. In the simplest terms, the value of a life is equivalent to the sum of money that would have to be invested at the present time in order to pay dividends equal to the sum the person would earn over the course of an expected lifetime. On these economic assumptions, those who have no income have no value, and those who drain society's resources have a negative value (e.g., thieves, the institutionalized mentally ill, unemployed, and retirees).

This approach can help measure the economic costs of diseases, accidents, and death, but it biases health policy in favor of classes such as young adult white men and people with wealth, because they can be expected to earn more. Thus, a public health policy to encourage motorcyclists to wear helmets might be selected over a cervical cancer detection program. This approach also raises moral questions because it gauges, for policy purposes, the social value of human lives in terms of economic value—a problem we discuss as an issue of justice in Chapter 6.

The moral problems associated with the DFE approach have contributed to the popularity of a second, more defensible approach, known as willingness to pay (WTP). It considers how much individuals would be willing to pay to reduce the risks of death (first by summing up the amounts reported by individuals, and then dividing by the anticipated number of deaths that could be prevented). One version of WTP focuses on *revealed preferences* by analyzing preferences that are well established in society and that can be identified by empirical research. This research attempts to determine how much risk individuals now assume—for example, in their decisions about work hazards—in order to obtain certain benefits. Their preferences, as exhibited in their balancing of risks and benefits, become the basis for establishing the level of risk that should be permitted in that group when a new technology is introduced or a new hazard is discovered. This approach is reliable only if individuals actually understand the risks and voluntarily assume them. For example, if workers do not understand and appreciate the risks of their work, and if they have few choices in employment, then this version of WTP is unreliable. This approach also takes what is desired or accepted by individuals as the measure of what is desirable or acceptable, and this methodological assumption can be criticized as normatively flawed.

Another version of WTP focuses on *expressed preferences* by considering how people respond to hypothetical questions designed to determine how much they are willing to pay to reduce the risk of death. One study asked members of the public how much they would be willing to spend in taxes to put ambulances and other life-saving devices in communities around the country in order to save twenty people from heart attacks each year.[89] Such questions are relevant in decisions about developing and funding expensive technologies through community resources. However, individuals' answers to hypothetical questions may not adequately indicate how much they would be willing to spend on an actual program to reduce their (and others') risk of death.

Moral apraisal of valuing lives. Moral objections have been registered to these various efforts to place a value on human life. Some deontological writers are skeptical of these approaches, because they hold, with Kant, that persons have dignity but not a price.[90] Utilitarian theories that take a broad view of the range of consequences also raise questions about putting a purely economic value on human life. However, these reservations must be put in perspective or they will appear trifling and unduly obstructive for social policy.

Obligations of beneficence do not require individuals or society to do everything possible, regardless of the costs, to reduce risks to human life. Such requirements would be self-defeating. Even the slogan that human life has infinite value or sanctity does not imply that it must be preserved irrespective of other values. An examination of individual risk budgets indicates that people are willing to risk their lives for various possible benefits, including recreation, friendship, fame, and fortune. Religious traditions recognize the possibility, in some cases the obligation, of martyrdom in preserving faith. Many kinds of trade-offs are also involved in determining the value to be placed on human life. There is nothing intrinsically wrong with *economic* analysis to clarify the nature of such trade-offs.

However, a monetary value does not always need to be placed on human life for purposes of health policy. In many cases qualitative factors are far more important than the purely economic factors operative in CBA. For example, how certain deaths occur, by what means, and with what symbolic features may legitimately lead a society to allocate its resources differently in order to reduce various risks of death. Studies of subjective perceptions of risk, as we have seen, reflect many qualitative factors, such as dread and unfamiliarity, that justifiably play a role in some determinations of acceptable risk.

A society also may justifiably expend time, energy, and money to rescue individuals from peril. Such unstinting acts of communal beneficence as rescuing trapped coal miners symbolize society's benevolence and affirm the value to society of the victims. The social value of acts of rescue focuses on "identified lives" in peril, whereas preventive measures to reduce the risk of death are aimed at "statistical lives"—that is, unknown persons who will be in future danger. We do not know in these cases whose death will be prevented, but we know statistically that some people will be saved by reducing their risk of death. Concentrating resources on identified individuals in peril may turn out to be less efficient than a preventive strategy, but this priority is not necessarily irrational. Policies may also be rational *because* they express or symbolize significant values.

It has been argued that the symbolic value of rescuing identified individuals accounts in part for the 1972 U.S. congressional decision—following widespread publicity in the media about particular individuals who were dying of renal failure—to make funds available for virtually all citizens who need renal dialysis or renal transplantation.[91] This decision also reflected the moral importance of equal consideration and treatment. Earlier, hospital committees had decided which identified individuals suffering from end-stage renal failure would receive access to scarce kidney dialysis machines, and thus which ones would live and which ones would die. The end-stage renal disease program now costs over $3 billion a year, and serious questions have been raised about its justifiability from the standpoint of CBA.[92] However, it is not necessarily unreasonable or unethical to violate efficiency criteria in order to express a societal commitment to a precious value.

Probable consequences of the use of CBA should also be considered. For example, putting a price on a nonmarket entity such as human life can reduce its perceived value, and society may choose to value human life more highly in collective decisions than some individuals would in their private decisions. It is not, then, legitimate to infer from individuals' conduct or from their answers to hypothetical questions precisely how much human life should be valued in social policies.[93] Data gathered by these techniques are relevant to the formation of public policies, but they provide only one set of premises about beneficence, among others, in a complex process of specifying and balancing values.

It is often unnecessary to put a specific economic value on human life in order to evaluate possible risk-reduction policies and to compare their costs. Evaluation may reasonably focus on the life-years or quality-adjusted life-years saved, without attempting a conversion into monetary measures. In the evaluation of health care, CBA is now less common than CEA, which often assumes the goal of maximizing quality-adjusted life-years.

Valuing Quality-Adjusted Life-Years

Quality of life and QALYs. In both health policy and health care everyone is interested not only in saving lives and years of life, but also in the quality of those lives, however long. We agree with the President's Commission for the Study of Ethical Problems in Medicine and Biomedical and Behavioral Research that "quality of life [is] an ethically essential concept that focuses on the good of the individual, what kind of life is possible given the person's condition, and whether that condition will allow the individual to have a life that he or she views as worth living."[94] Improving the quality of a patient's life is an especially important goal in chronic and rehabilitative care. For example, few people appear to be interested in living life in a persistent vegetative state, and it is common for individuals contemplating different modes of treatment for a particular condition to trade some life-years for improved quality of life during their remaining life-years.

The basic idea of quality-adjusted life-years or QALYs is that "if an extra year of healthy (i.e., good quality) life-expectancy is worth one, then an extra year of unhealthy (i.e., poor quality) life-expectancy must be worth less than one (for why otherwise do people seek to be healthy?)."[95] QALYs represent trade-offs between quality and quantity of life, and thus can be used to measure the net health effectiveness of programs or activities. QALYs represent an attempt to bring the two dimensions of *length* of life and *quality* of life into a single framework of evaluation.[96] Among their various functions, QALYs can be used to monitor the effects of treatments on patients in clinical practice or in clinical trials, to determine what to recommend to patients, and to provide information to patients about the effects of different treatments. In some contexts, it may be sufficient to consider only the net effectiveness of treatments in terms of their QALYs. However, in many contexts, including the allocation of health care resources, costs must be examined relative to the QALYs provided by different treatments. Only then can efficiency be determined together with effectiveness.

In a widely noted study, British health economist Alan Williams examined the cost-effectiveness of coronary artery bypass grafting in terms of QALYs. According to his analysis, bypass grafting compares favorably with pacemakers for heart block. It is superior to heart transplantation and the treatment of end-stage renal failure, but it appears to be less cost-effective than hip replacement. He also found that bypass grafting for severe angina and extensive coronary artery disease is more cost-effective than for less severe cases. The rate of survival can be misleading for coronary artery bypass grafting and many other therapeutic procedures that have a major impact on quality of life. On the basis of his analysis, Williams recommended that resources "be redeployed at the margin to procedures for which the benefits to patients are high in relation to the costs."[97]

Measurements of quality of life. How can we determine quality of life? Analysts often start with rough measures such as physical mobility, freedom from pain and distress, and the capacity to perform the activities of daily life and to engage in social interactions. Quality of life thus may appear to be one way to talk about the ingredients of a good life. However, this description renders the notion so amorphous and so variable as to be unusable in health policy and health care. We need to identify a certain level of goods that are vital for an individual's fulfillment of his or her life plans.[98] Some negative conditions thwart the realization of individual life plans, whatever their content. These positive and negative conditions provide the needed content for the notion of "health-related quality of life."[99] For purposes of this section, QALYs will refer only to "health-related quality of life."

We cannot here consider all the various psychometric and decision-analytic methods of determining what people value in health-related quality of life, but some methods are analogous to those used for determining the value of life. In one example, in which respondents were asked to make explicit trade-offs between quality and quantity of life, Barbara McNeil and colleagues used principles of expected-utility theory to study hypothetical trade-offs between quantity (longevity) and quality of life (voice preservation) in the treatment of cancer of the larynx. In their hypothetical choices among treatments for cancer of the larynx, "most subjects were willing to accept some decrease in long-term survival to maintain normal speech, [but] virtually none would ever accept any decrease below 5 years." These healthy subjects were informed that sixty percent could expect to survive three years with laryngectomy, and thirty to forty percent could expect to survive three years with radiation. Virtually all would accept surgery if radiation offered only a thirty percent chance of three-year survival, nineteen percent would choose radiation alone if it offered a forty percent chance of three-year survival, and twenty-four percent would choose radiation with delayed laryngectomy if necessary. The researchers concluded that treatment choices should be based on patients' attitudes toward both the quality of life and the length of the period of survival.[100]

Through such methods, it may be possible to develop, for example, "average population preferences" for health outcomes and, by implication, for health services that can then be used in health care and health policy, including allocation decisions.[101] However, the different approaches do not always yield the same result or dominant values. Some variations stem from the "framing" effects of different questions or descriptions of health states (see pp. 159–160), as well as from the ages and current health status of the respondents. Attitudes toward risk and toward the time in life of good and bad health also may not be adequately reflected in these different methods.[102]

Despite methodological variations and limits, we will assume for purposes of the present discussion that instruments can be developed and refined to present meaningful and accurate measures of health-related quality of life for use in QALY assessment. Without an explicit and examined approach to the public's preferences, we are likely to operate with implicit and unexamined views about trade-offs between quantity and quality of life in relation to cost. However, we do need to address further the ethical assumptions involved in QALY-based CEA.

Ethical assumptions of QALYs. Implicit in QALY-based CEA is the idea that the only objective of health services is health maximization. But some non-health benefits or utilities of health services also contribute to quality of life. As was evident in our discussion of silicone-gel breast implants, conditions such as asymmetrical breasts may affect a person's subjective estimate of quality of life and may merit inclusion as a source of distress. Other issues of quality of life are relevant, including information about patients' health status. Furthermore, a health intervention's transient adverse consequences, such as discomfort and nausea associated with use of high-osmolality contrast agents in the diagnostic tests discussed above, may justifiably be excluded because of their limited effect on quality of life, and yet these interventions may prove to be relevant to the overall assessment of particular health care interventions. Certain values are also neglected in QALY-based CEA, which attaches utility only to selected outcomes. These additional values include how care is provided (e.g., whether it is personal care) and how it is distributed (e.g., whether universal access is provided).[103] QALY-based CEA therefore must be conceived as broadly as possible, but it will still require supplementation.

Debates about equity often focus on whether the use of QALYs in CEA is egalitarian. In general, proponents of QALY-based CEA hold that each healthy life-year is equally valuable for everyone. Thus, a QALY is a QALY, regardless of who possesses it.[104] However, it appears that QALY-based CEA will often discriminate against older people, because, *ceteris paribus,* saving the life of a younger person is likely to produce more QALYs than saving the life of an older person. Age will also play a role in considerations of quality of life, which is often more compromised among the elderly. (We return to issues of equity and age discrimination when we assess the range of analytic techniques later in this chapter and in Chapter 6.)

QALY-based CEA does not try to realize the greatest good for the greatest number of individuals, or even the greatest medical good for the greatest number of patients. It also does not matter in QALY-based CEA how life-years are distributed among numbers of patients, and QALY-based CEA may not entail efforts to reduce the number of individual victims in its attempts to increase the number of life-years. From this standpoint, no difference exists between saving one person who can be expected to have forty QALYs and saving two people who can be expected to have twenty QALYs each. In principle, priority *should* be given to saving one person with forty expected QALYs over two with only fifteen expected QALYs each.

Critics also charge that QALY-based CEA favors life-years over individual lives, the number of life-years over the number of individual lives, and quality of life over quantity of life, while failing to recognize that societal and professional obligations of beneficence require rescuing individual lives, rather than maximizing the number of QALYs salvaged. John Harris, for example, condemns QALYs as a ''life-threatening device,'' because they suggest that life-years rather than individual lives are valuable.[105]

QALY-based CEA also neglects obligations of beneficence to rescue endangered individual lives. A tension exists between QALY-based CEA and a duty to rescue, although both are grounded on beneficence. This tension appears in a widely discussed effort by the Oregon Health Services Commission, consisting of eleven government-appointed health care providers and lay people, to develop a prioritized list of health services. The State of Oregon wanted to expand Medicaid coverage to *all* of its poor citizens, but it could only accomplish that goal by limiting its coverage to services considered to have a relatively high priority. (For a fuller explanation, see pp. 367–369.) A draft priority list in May 1990 evoked vigorous criticisms by physicians and other citizens because it ranked some life-saving procedures below some routine procedures. Faulty data may have played a role in the controversy, but David Hadorn rightly contends that another, more systemic factor was significant: ''The cost-effectiveness analysis approach used to create the initial list conflicted directly with the powerful 'Rule of Rescue'—people's perceived duty to save endangered life whenever possible.''[106] One example from the initial priority list indicates the tension between QALY-based CEA and the duty to rescue. Surgery for ectopic pregnancy was ranked in the priority line at 372, just below tooth-capping, at 371; and surgery for appendicitis was ranked, at 377, just below splints for temporomandibular joint disorder, at 376. Ectopic pregnancy and appendicitis are life-threatening if untreated, and treatment is virtually always efficacious. By contrast, problems treated by tooth-capping and temporomandibular joint disorder are minor and may even improve without treatment.[107]

Hadorn argues that ''Setting priorities first on the basis of net expected health benefit, followed by a determination of the degree of benefit required before services are deemed necessary (e.g., how close to the top of the list they must be for coverage) provides a reasonable compromise between a public-good, utilitarian framework and the need to accommodate the Rule of Rescue.''[108] This approach determines *effectiveness,* possibly using QALYs, but not *cost-effectiveness.* It thus may be able to avoid the problem that Oregon faced in the late 1980s when, after it dropped Medicaid coverage for various transplants, Coby Howard, a 7-year-old boy, died of acute lymphocytic leukemia without a chance for a bone marrow transplant because in the absence of Medicaid funds he was not able to raise enough money from voluntary contributions to cover the cost of the procedure. Such a dramatic case creates both personal and social distress, in part because an identified life appears to be sacrificed in order to save money.

In our examination of QALY-based CEA, several questions have emerged about the adequacy and value of this tool of analysis for health policy and health care. In particular, we have noted methodological problems in the assignment of priority to life-years over individual lives. The implication of this assignment of priority is that beneficence-based rescue (especially life saving) is less significant than cost-utility, that the distribution of life-years is unimportant, that saving more lives is less critical than maximizing the number of life-years, and that quality of life is more important than quantity of life. We have rejected some aspect of each of these implications. With these conclusions behind us, we can now examine two central questions about the decisionmaking process and about distributive justice.

The Decisionmaking Process: Who Decides and How?

Which and whose values should be considered in the calculus of CEA, CBA, and RBA? The surest guarantee that a set of values will be represented is to incorporate its proponents into the decisionmaking process. Those who emphasize decisionmaking by experts engaged in putatively objective analyses often disagree with those who put a premium on public participation. Experts have an important role to play, particularly in arraying the costs, risks, and benefits involved, but legitimate reasons often exist for not allowing experts to make the final decision. Our reservations about experts are grounded, in part, on the recognition that value judgments pervade the entire process. For example, in RBA value judgments are involved in risk identification and estimation, as well as in risk assessment and management.

Many proponents of CEA, CBA, and RBA who support expert judgment deny that they are nondemocratic or antidemocratic. They argue that experts respect consumer sovereignty and derive values from expressed, revealed, or implied preferences of consumers; costs, risks, and benefits are then assessed in relation to those values. Defenders of CBA also contend that their methods make it possible for the government to regulate risks ''by finding, developing, and legitimating methods for making centralized decisions.'' [109] They note that the public's perception is sometimes unpredictable and erratic and often reflects the ''whims of the moment.'' Although there is much to commend the corrective powers of these analytic techniques and the insights of experts who use them, we should respect individuals' values when expressed politically no less than economically. Appropriate mechanisms for public participation in decisions that incorporate CEA, CBA, and RBA are at least as socially valuable as the methods themselves. Considerations of justice often support specific procedures of public participation—such as adversary hearings and testimony at pub-

lic forums. A fair and acceptable process of decisionmaking is defensible because of the principles it embodies as well as the prospect that it will produce
a good decision or outcome. At the same time, society should address the
implications of CEA, CBA, and RBA through democratic processes.

Despite the flurry of public involvement in Oregon's efforts to set priorities
in the allocation of health care, critics have charged that the community meeting process did not reach a representative cross section of the population, because approximately fifty percent of participants were health professionals.
White, college-educated, and higher socioeconomic groups were disproportionately represented, and the uninsured were not proportionately represented. Furthermore, the values announced in the community meetings were not ranked
and not specific enough to set priorities for health services. It is, therefore,
difficult to know whether the public process was fair and effective in practice
and whether values were generated that actually reflected the community's
views and also shaped the list of priorities.[110] Similar questions can be raised
about the public's participation in the development of policies for human genetic interventions through, for example, the Human Gene Therapy Subcom-
mittee and the Recombinant DNA Advisory Committee of the National Institutes of Health, and in the development of policies for the distribution and
allocation of cadaveric organs for transplantation through the United Network
for Organ Sharing (UNOS).

Formal techniques are therefore most appropriately viewed not as methods
of decisionmaking, but rather as aids to help decisionmakers specify obligations
of beneficence directed at the welfare of citizens. It would be misleading in
many contexts to view these methods of analysis as more than aids, especially
if other interpretations of beneficence or other moral principles point to different conclusions. Formal methods of analysis are fashioned for specific goals
and should be evaluated strictly in light of their service to those goals. These
goals include both clarification of the assumptions of decisionmaking and the
trade-offs among costs, risks, and benefits.

In practice, analytic techniques tend to attach exaggerated importance to
quantifiable values while ignoring nonquantifiable values, such as relief of pain
and suffering and the symbolic significance of actions and policies. For instance, a hospice program caring for dying patients may be defensible because
of its intangible benefits, including dying with dignity and without pain and
suffering, but a formal CEA/CBA based solely on economic considerations
may dismiss these considerations.[111] A related concern is the possible impact
of analytic techniques, especially CBA, on personal and social values, perspectives, and attitudes. One issue is whether ''large-scale computations in modern
politics and social planning bring with them a coarseness and grossness of
moral feeling, a blunting of sensibility, and a suppression of individual discrimination and gentleness.''[112] There are also legitimate fears that economic lan-

guage, already evident in the discussions of "the health care industry," "providers," and "consumers," as well as in CEA and CBA, will corrupt or even replace the traditional moral language of the doctor–patient relationship, especially under pressures of cost containment.[113]

In view of these legitimate fears, close attention should be paid to the social (as well as the economic) costs of such approaches. These negative effects can be avoided if the analytic techniques are limited in the ways we have proposed. These techniques are acceptable and often useful, as long as their limitations and limits are recognized, especially the limits set by respect for autonomy and justice.

Constraints of Distributive Justice

We discuss justice comprehensively in the next chapter, but the above argument leads to a consideration of some problems of justice at this point. Utilitarianism and analytic techniques are commonly said to fail to take account of problems of justice because they focus on the net balance of benefits over costs, without considering the distribution of those benefits and costs. For example, a study of the costs and benefits of treating mental retardation in small institutions emphasizing advanced individual training might show that the costs outweigh the benefits, but justice might demand that special benefits be extended to mentally retarded persons. In both examples, justice may require a different distribution of resources than CBA or CEA would support.

RBA is also subject to constraints of justice. Consider four possible patterns of distribution of risks and benefits: (1) The risks and benefits may fall on the same party. For example, in most therapy, the patient bears the major risks and stands to gain the major benefits. (2) One party may bear the risks, while another party gains the benefits. For example, one generation may gain the benefits of technologies that will adversely affect future generations. (3) Both parties may bear the risks, but only one party stands to benefit. For example, a nuclear-powered artificial heart would primarily benefit the user, but its risks would also be imposed on other parties in contact with the user. (4) Both parties may gain the benefits, while only one party bears the risks. For example, persons in the vicinity of a nuclear power plant may bear significantly greater risks than other persons who also benefit from the plant.

Although it is unacceptable to consider utility without simultaneously considering patterns of distribution, principles of justice also do not always triumph over economic efficiency. Here our views stand in contrast to theories that assign principles of justice an absolute priority over consequentialist principles such as utility. A practical judgment is required that takes into consideration, specifies, and balances all morally relevant factors—without giving any one an a priori advantage.

316   PRINCIPLES OF BIOMEDICAL ETHICS

As an example of the balancing required between beneficence and distributive justice in programs of risk reduction, consider the use of genetic screening and monitoring in the workplace. Workers may be screened for a genetic predisposition toward diseases that may be more likely to occur as a result of exposure to chemicals in a plant, and their health may be periodically monitored during their employment. There is nothing inherently objectionable about surveillance to determine workers' susceptibility to and development of diseases. These tests may be justified by benefits for workers, as well as by the reduction of costs to the company and the society. However, the company may be able to reduce risks in several different ways, some of which are morally preferable to others. The options may include (1) barring workers from certain jobs by not hiring them or by assigning them to other jobs, (2) devising protective equipment for the workers, or (3) altering the work environment.[114]

It is tempting for corporations to dismiss the latter two options on grounds that they are too costly for the benefits to be derived in the reduction of risks, and the first option does suggest ways in which fair access to jobs might be balanced against reduction of risks. If a worker's condition either interferes with job performance or endangers others, no serious ethical problem is present for option (1). But if health risks are present for a broad array of workers, the ethical problems can be prominent and knotty. Here it is often morally appropriate (although, we acknowledge, not always feasible) to require the company to reduce the risk for all workers (perhaps by options 2 and 3), rather than denying employment to those whose risks may be increased by their genetic predisposition.

Related questions of beneficence and justice have arisen in debates about reproductive risk in the workplace. A complex set of obligations of nonmaleficence and beneficence exists in the workplace, including the society's and the employers' obligations to workers and to workers' offspring, as well as the workers' obligations to their offspring.[115] Workers may believe that the health hazards to a fetus or future offspring are outweighed by benefits they can provide for their offspring through their income, such as housing, food, and health care. Faced with the options identified above for reducing risk exposure in the workplace, some employers accepted a policy of excluding women of childbearing age from certain jobs or, in some cases, made "voluntary" sterilization a condition of employment. Although a U.S. Supreme Court ruling struck down these particular policies on grounds of unlawful sex discrimination,[116] the ethical issues did not disappear in the American workplace because the circumstances of reproductive risk did not change.

Similar questions emerge about hiring practices toward people with the sickle-cell trait, which affects approximately seven to thirteen percent of the black population but rarely appears in the rest of the population. Those with the sickle-cell trait do not have sickle-cell disease, but they are sometimes barred from occupations because of the possibility that they are at greater risk from exposure to substances that might compromise the oxygen-carrying capacity of blood. Nevertheless, before anyone is denied work because of general evidence of high risks, scientific evidence should establish that the individual person is hypersusceptible to the hazards and that there is no reasonable way to protect him or her against the hazards.[117]

It is sometimes argued that monetary compensation for voluntarily assuming risks can satisfy the demands of justice in circumstances in which benefits and risks are unequally distributed. For example, some hold that fair compensation for employment—or even additional compensation for risky assignments—makes the imposition of risks on workers fair. To be acceptable, this argument must require the premise that these workers have voluntarily assumed the risks of their jobs and that the conditions for autonomous choice are met, including adequate understanding in addition to substantial voluntariness. There is often less adequate understanding of health hazards than safety hazards, in part because health problems such as cancer typically develop over time and may result from several factors. It may also be difficult to disclose what is known in a way that facilitates an informed choice, and the worker's voluntariness may be compromised by a lack of available alternative jobs. Thus, in the context of employment, voluntary acceptance of a job and hazard pay may be unjust substitutes for what should be done—namely, correcting dangerous working conditions.[118]

A second argument is that retrospective monetary *compensation*—for example, through tort claims—is a valid substitute for prospective *prevention* of exposure to hazards. The proposal is again that an adequate system of compensation for injury satisfies the conditions of fairness. However, even if a CBA supports the compensation scheme, fairness requires both employers and society to undertake to reduce the hazards to the lowest level that is feasible or practicable, because compensation cannot restore victims to the health they enjoyed prior to their exposure.[119] This example indicates how a norm of justice constrains CBA, even though the constraint is prima facie rather than absolute.

Conclusion

We have reached several conclusions in this chapter that build on conclusions reached in previous chapters. We first established that two principles of beneficence need to be distinguished and that both should be distinguished from negative obligations to avoid causing harm. We then defended a version of paternalism that justifies strong paternalistic interventions under some conditions. However, we acknowledged that a policy or rule permitting strong paternalism in professional practice is often not worth the risk of abuse that it invites. Finally, we argued that formal techniques of analysis—CEA, CBA, and RBA—can be morally unobjectionable appeals to the principle of utility. However, limits to these techniques are set by principles of respect for autonomy and justice, and they should conform to social procedures to resolve conflicts and assign weights to different benefits, costs, and risks. Chapter 6 further considers the issues of justice that concluded the present chapter.

Notes

1. Utilitarianism does not offer the only basis on which this principle might be justified. It can be and has been defended on the basis of several different theories, such as Kantian theories of hypothetical consent and theories of individual rights. See Douglas MacLean, "Risk and Consent: Philosophical Issues for Centralized Decisions," in *Values at Risk,* ed. D. MacLean (Totowa, NJ: Rowman and Allanheld, 1986), pp. 17–30.
2. W. D. Ross, *The Right and the Good* (Oxford: Clarendon Press, 1930), p. 21.
3. Shelly Kagan, *The Limits of Morality* (Oxford: Clarendon Press, 1989), pp. 1–2, 402–3. This claim is tempered by a recognition that agents can make a greater contribution to the overall good by not recklessly and foolishly sacrificing themselves.
4. One limit is that agents often have discretion about when, where, how, and toward whom to act beneficently. As we saw in Chapter 2, Mill argued that we are obligated to practice beneficence, "but not toward any definite person, nor at any prescribed time." However, we believe the principles of beneficence create *some* perfect and *some* imperfect obligations. If a person never acted beneficently, he or she would be morally *blameworthy* and *defective* in character. This claim sharply contrasts with the views of philosophers who contend that beneficence is merely an ideal. However, we acknowledge that it is difficult to draw lines to indicate that one has adequately discharged this duty. This is bound to be true because the obligation of general beneficence in the common morality is indeterminate. See K. Danner Clouser and Bernard Gert, "A Critique of Principlism," *Journal of Medicine and Philosophy* 15 (1990): 228. They rely almost exclusively on nonmaleficence in their ethical theory.
5. Peter Singer, "Famine, Affluence, and Morality," *Philosophy and Public Affairs* 1 (1972): 229–43.
6. Michael A. Slote, "The Morality of Wealth," in *World Hunger and Moral Obligation,* ed. W. Aiken and H. LaFollette (Englewood Cliffs, NJ: Prentice-Hall, 1977), p. 127.
7. For a defense of a demanding but restricted maximizing principle, see Michael Otsuka, "The Paradox of Group Beneficence," *Philosophy and Public Affairs* 20 (Spring 1991): 132–49.
8. Peter Singer, *Practical Ethics,* 2nd Ed. (Cambridge: Cambridge University Press, 1993), p. 246.
9. Our formulation is indebted to Eric D'Arcy, *Human Acts: An Essay in Their Moral Evaluation* (Oxford: Clarendon Press, 1963), pp. 56–57. We have added the fourth

condition and altered others. See also Ernest J. Weinrib, "The Case for a Duty to Rescue," *Yale Law Journal* 90 (December 1980): 247–93; and Joel Feinberg, *Harm to Others,* vol. I of *The Moral Limits of the Criminal Law* (New York: Oxford University Press, 1984), ch. 4.

10. James S. Fishkin, *The Limits of Obligation* (New Haven, CT: Yale University Press, 1982). See pp. 4–9 for a summary of the full argument.

11. See Arthur L. Caplan, Robert H. Blank, and Janna C. Merrick, eds., *Compelled Compassion: Government Intervention in the Treatment of Critically Ill Newborns* (Totowa, NJ: The Humana Press Inc., 1992).

12. American Nurses' Association, *Code for Nurses with Interpretive Statements* (Kansas City, MO: American Nurses Association, 1985), sec. 3.1, p. 6.

13. Ludwig Edelstein, *Ancient Medicine,* ed. Oswei Temkin and C. Lillian Temkin (Baltimore: Johns Hopkins University Press, 1967).

14. David Hume, "Of Suicide," in *Essays Moral, Political, and Literary,* ed. Eugene Miller (Indianapolis, IN: Liberty Classics, 1985): 577–89.

15. See David A. J. Richards, *A Theory of Reasons for Action* (Oxford: Clarendon Press, 1971), p. 186 (a contractarian account); Lawrence Becker, *Reciprocity* (Chicago: University of Chicago Press, 1990); Aristotle, *Nicomachean Ethics,* bks. 8–9.

16. William F. May, "Code and Covenant or Philanthropy and Contract?" in *Ethics in Medicine,* ed. S. Reiser, A. Dyck, and W. Curran (Cambridge, MA: MIT Press, 1977), pp. 65–76.

17. Judith Jarvis Thomson, "A Defense of Abortion," *Philosophy and Public Affairs* 1 (1971): 47–66.

18. *Epidemics,* 1:11, from W. H. S. Jones, ed., *Hippocrates* (Cambridge, MA: Harvard University Press, 1923), vol. I, p. 165.

19. Edmund Pellegrino and David Thomasma, *For the Patient's Good: The Restoration of Beneficence in Health Care* (New York: Oxford University Press, 1988), p. 29.

20. Ibid., pp. 25, 32, 46–47. See also Pellegrino and Thomasma, "The Conflict between Autonomy and Beneficence in Medical Ethics," *Journal of Contemporary Health Law and Policy* 3 (1987): 23–46.

21. Immanuel Kant, *On the Old Saw: That May Be Right in Theory But It Won't Work in Practice,* trans. E. B. Ashton (Philadelphia: University of Pennsylvania Press, 1974), pp. 290–91; John Stuart Mill, *On Liberty, Collected Works of John Stuart Mill,* vol. 18 (Toronto: University of Toronto Press, 1977).

22. See Tom L. Beauchamp and Laurence B. McCullough, *Medical Ethics: The Moral Responsibilities of Physicians* (Englewood Cliffs, NJ: Prentice-Hall, 1984), p. 84.

23. See Donald VanDeVeer, *Paternalistic Intervention: The Moral Bounds on Benevolence* (Princeton, NJ: Princeton University Press, 1986), pp. 16–40; John Kleinig, *Paternalism* (Totowa, NJ: Rowman and Allanheld, 1983), pp. 6–14.

24. National Commission for the Protection of Human Subjects of Biomedical and Behavioral Research, *Report and Recommendations: Research Involving Prisoners* (Washington, DC: DHEW Publication No. OS 76-131, 1976).

25. The term *paternalism* is not wholly felicitous, especially because it is sex-linked. Although it might seem desirable to use *parentalism,* the term *paternalism* is now well established by usage and philosophical discussion. Also, some feminists in bioethics have argued that this usage is a rare case in which gendered language should be retained, because an appropriate link is made between the privileges of a father in a patriarchical family and the privileges of physicians in an authoritarian

320 PRINCIPLES OF BIOMEDICAL ETHICS

medical system. The thesis is that just as hierarchical arrangements have long been the norm in the family, so paternalism has been the norm in medicine. See Susan Sherwin, *No Longer Patient: Feminist Ethics and Health Care* (Philadelphia: Temple University Press, 1992), ch. 7.

26. L. J. Henderson, "Physician and Patient as a Social System," *New England Journal of Medicine* 212 (1935): 819–23.

27. See Joel Feinberg, "Legal Paternalism," *Canadian Journal of Philosophy* 1 (1971): 105–24, esp. 113, 116. See also, *Harm to Self,* vol. III of *The Moral Limits of the Criminal Law* (New York: Oxford University Press, 1986), esp. pp. 12ff.

28. Feinberg, *Harm to Self,* p. 14.

29. For interpretations of (strong) paternalism as insult, disrespect, and treatment of individual as unequals, see Ronald Dworkin, *Taking Rights Seriously* (Cambridge, MA: Harvard University Press, 1978), pp. 262–63, and Childress, *Who Should Decide? Paternalism in Health Care* (New York: Oxford University Press, 1982), ch. 3.

30. Robert Harris, "Private Consensual Adult Behavior: The Requirement of Harm to Others in the Enforcement of Morality," *UCLA Law Review* 14 (1967): 585n. Similar complaints in political philosophy are registered in Isaiah Berlin, *Four Essays on Liberty* (Oxford: Oxford University Press, 1969), pp. lxi–lxii, 132–33, 137–38, 149–51, 157.

31. See Jay Katz, Joseph Goldstein, and Alan M. Dershowitz, eds., *Psychoanalysis, Psychiatry, and the Law* (New York: The Free Press, 1967), pp. 552–54, 710–13; and Robert A. Burt, *Taking Care of Strangers: The Rule of Law in Doctor–Patient Relations* (New York: The Free Press, 1979), ch. 2.

32. This case was prepared by Browning Hoffman for a "Medicine and Society," conference at the University of Virginia.

33. Gerald Dworkin, "Paternalism," *The Monist* 56 (January 1972): 64–84; Rosemary Carter, "Justifying Paternalism," *Canadian Journal of Philosophy* 7 (1977): 133–45, esp. 135; Donald VanDeVeer, *Paternalistic Intervention: The Moral Bounds on Benevolence* (Princeton, NJ: Princeton University Press, 1986), p. 424.

34. Dworkin, "Paternalism," p. 65.

35. See Dworkin, "Paternalism"; and John Rawls, *A Theory of Justice* (Cambridge, MA: Harvard University Press, 1971), pp. 209, 248–49.

36. It should be noted that Dworkin himself says, "The reasons which support paternalism are those which support any altruistic action—the welfare of another person." "Paternalism," in *Encyclopedia of Ethics,* ed. Lawrence Becker (New York: Garland Publishing: 1992), p. 940. For a wide variety of consent and nonconsent defenses of paternalism, see Kleinig, *Paternalism,* pp. 38–73, and VanDeVeer, *Paternalistic Intervention, passim.*

37. Mary C. Silva, *Ethical Decisionmaking in Nursing Administration* (Norwalk, CT: Appleton and Lange, 1989), ch. 3, p. 64.

38. Compare Kleinig's similar conclusion, *Paternalism,* p. 76.

39. We do not here address the many problems surrounding the definition of suicide. See Tom L. Beauchamp, "Suicide," in *Matters of Life and Death,* ed. Tom Regan, 3rd Ed.(New York: Random House, 1993), esp. part I; and the articles in John Donnelly, ed., *Suicide: Right or Wrong?* (Buffalo, NY: Prometheus Books, 1991).

40. See James Rachels, "Barney Clark's Key," *Hastings Center Report* 13 (April 1983): 17–19, esp. p.17.

41. This case has been adapted from Marc Basson, ed., *Rights and Responsibilities in Modern Medicine* (New York: Alan R. Liss, 1981), pp. 183–84.

42. Glanville Williams, "Euthanasia," *Medico-Legal Journal* 41 (1973): 27.
43. See, e.g., three articles by psychiatrists Alan L. Berman, Robert E. Litman, and Seymour Perlin in *Non-Natural Death—Coming to Terms with Suicide, Euthanasia, Withholding or Withdrawing Treatment* (Denver: Center for Applied Biomedical Ethics at Rose Medical Center, 1986). A useful discussion of "Criteria for Rational Suicide" is found in Margaret Pabst Battin, *Ethical Issues in Suicide* (Englewood Cliffs, NJ: Prentice-Hall, 1982), pp. 132–53.
44. See Peter M. Marzuk et al., "Increased Risk of Suicide in Persons with AIDS," *Journal of the American Medical Association* 259 (March 4, 1988): 1333–37. The figures reported in this article are exclusively for *men* with AIDS.
45. See Richard M. Glass, "AIDS and Suicide," *Journal of the American Medical Association* 259 (March 4, 1988): 1369–70.
46. See President's Commission for the Study of Ethical Problems in Medicine and Biomedical and Behavioral Research, *Deciding to Forego Life-Sustaining Treatment,* p. 37.
47. Betty Rollin, *Last Wish* (New York: Linden Press/Simon and Schuster, 1985).
48. Childress, *Who Should Decide? Paternalism in Health Care* (New York: Oxford University Press, 1982), ch. 1. On the issues in this section, see Allan S. Brett and Laurence B. McCullough, "When Patients Request Specific Interventions: Defining the Limits of the Physician's Obligation," *New England Journal of Medicine* 315 (Nov. 20, 1986): 1347–51.
49. This case is adapted from "The Refusal to Sterilize: A Paternalistic Decision," in *Rights and Responsibilities in Modern Medicine,* ed. Basson, pp. 135–36, where it is discussed by Tom L. Beauchamp and Eric Cassell.
50. John D. Lantos, Peter A. Singer, Robert M. Walker, et al., "The Illusion of Futility in Clinical Practice," *The American Journal of Medicine* 87 (July 1989): 82.
51. Robert D. Truog, Allan S. Brett, and Joel Frader, "The Problem with Futility," *New England Journal of Medicine* 326 (June 4, 1992): 1561, which has influenced these paragraphs.
52. Lawrence J. Schneiderman, Nancy S. Jecker, and Albert R. Jonsen, "Medical Futility: Its Meaning and Ethical Implications," *Annals of Internal Medicine* 112 (June 15, 1990): 951.
53. S. E. Bedell, T. L. Delbanco, E. F. Cook, and F. H. Epstein, "Survival after Cardiopulmonary Resuscitation in the Hospital," *New England Journal of Medicine* 309 (September 8, 1983): 569–76.
54. Lantos et al., "The Illusion of Futility in Clinical Practice," p. 83.
55. J. Chris Hackler and F. Charles Hiller, "Family Consent to Orders Not to Resuscitate," *Journal of the American Medical Association* 264 (September 12, 1990): 1282.
56. This paragraph is indebted to Stuart J. Youngner, "Futility in Context," *Journal of the American Medical Association* 264 (September 12, 1990): 1295–96.
57. Tom Tomlinson and Howard Brody, "Futility and the Ethics of Resuscitation," *Journal of the American Medical Association* 264 (September 12, 1990): 1279, and see Brody, *The Healer's Power* (New Haven: Yale University Press, 1992), p. 175. See also Nancy S. Jecker and Robert A. Pearlman, "Medical Futility," *Archives of Internal Medicine* 152 (June 1992): 1140–44.
58. This case was prepared by Robert M. Veatch and is used by permission.
59. U.S. Congress, Office of Technology Assessment, *The Implications of Cost-Effectiveness Analysis of Medical Technology: Summary* (Washington, DC: U.S. Government Printing Office, 1980). We have drawn on this document in this para-

graph as well as Kenneth E. Warner and Bryan R. Luce, *Cost-Benefit and Cost-Effectiveness Analysis in Health Care* (Ann Arbor, MI: Health Administration Press, 1982), and David Eddy, "Cost-Effectiveness Analysis" *Journal of the American Medical Association* 267 (March 25, 1992): 1669–75; 267 (June 24, 1992): 3342–48; and 268 (July 1, 1992): 132–36.

60. This case study has been drawn largely from Peter D. Jacobson and John Rosenquist, "The Introduction of Low-Osmolar Contrast Agents in Radiology: Medical, Economic, Legal, and Public Policy Issues," *Journal of the American Medical Association* 260 (September 16, 1988): 1586–92, with some input from Earl P. Steinberg, Richard D. Moore, Neil R. Powe, et al., "Safety and Cost-Effectiveness of High-Osmolality as Compared with Low-Osmolality Contrast Material in Patients Undergoing Cardiac Angiography," *New England Journal of Medicine* 326 (February 13, 1992): 425–30, and John W. Hirshfield, Jr., "Low-Osmolality Contrast Agents—Who Needs Them?" *New England Journal of Medicine* 326 (February 13, 1992): 482–84.

61. Duncan Neuhauser and Ann M. Lewicki, "What Do We Gain from the Sixth Stool Guaiac?" *New England Journal of Medicine* 293 (July 31, 1975): 226–28. See also "American Cancer Society Report on the Cancer-related Checkup," *CA—A Cancer Journal for Clinicians* 30 (1980): 193–240, which recommends the full six stool guaiac tests.

62. Peter Doubilet, Milton C. Weinstein, and Barbara J. McNeil, "Use and Misuse of the Term 'Cost Effective' in Medicine," *New England Journal of Medicine* 314 (January 23, 1986): 253–56, which has influenced this paragraph and the next two paragraphs.

63. M. S. Rosenshein et al., "The Cost Effectiveness of Therapeutic and Prophylactic Leukocyte Transfusion," *New England Journal of Medicine* 302 (May 8, 1980): 1058–62.

64. Doubilet et al., "Use and Misuse of the Term 'Cost Effective,' " p. 255.

65. Louise Russell, *Is Prevention Better Than Cure?* (Washington, DC: Brookings Institution, 1986), p. 111.

66. See Howard Leichter, "Public Policy and the British Experience," *Hastings Center Report* 11 (October 1981): 32–39.

67. See Sheila Jasanoff, "Acceptable Evidence in a Pluralistic Society," in *Acceptable Evidence: Science and Values in Risk Management,* ed. Deborah G. Mayo and Rachelle D. Hollander (New York: Oxford University Press, 1991), "An Analysis of the de Minimis Strategy for Risk Management," *Risk Analysis* 6 (1986). See also Nicholas Rescher, *Risk* (Washington, DC: University Press of America, 1983), pp. 35–40.

68. See Richard Wilson and E. A. C. Crouch, "Risk Assessment and Comparisons: An Introduction," *Science* 236 (April 17, 1987): 267–70.

69. Lester B. Lave, "Health and Safety Risk Analyses: Information for Better Decisions," *Science* 236 (April 17, 1987): 292–93. See also Kristin Shrader-Frechette, *Risk and Rationality: Philosophical Foundations for Populist Reforms* (Berkeley: University of California Press, 1991), ch. 8.

70. See Carl F. Cranor, "Some Moral Issues in Risk Assessment," *Ethics* 101 (October 1990): 123–43, which has influenced this paragraph. See also Shrader-Frechette, *Risk and Rationality,* and Mayo and Hollander, eds., *Acceptable Evidence.*

71. Ian Hacking, "Culpable Ignorance of Interference Effects," in *Values at Risk,* ed. MacLean, ch. 7.

72. Lynn White, Jr., "Technology Assessment from the Stance of a Medieval Historian," *Medieval Religion and Technology: Collected Essays* (Berkeley: University of California Press, 1978), pp. 261–76.

73. See Paul Slovic, "Perception of Risk," *Science* 236 (April 17, 1987): 280–85; Slovic, "Beyond Numbers: A Broader Perspective on Risk Perception and Risk Communication," in *Acceptable Evidence,* pp. 48–65, esp. 34–35; and Richard J. Zeckhauser and W. Kip Viscusi, "Risk Within Reason," *Science* 248 (May 4, 1990): 559–64.

74. Lave, "Health and Safety Risk Analyses," p. 291.

75. Lawrence J. Schneiderman and Robert M. Kaplan, "Fear of Dying and HIV Infection vs Hepatitis B Infection," *American Journal of Public Health* 82 (April 1992): 584–89.

76. Zeckhauser and Viscusi, "Risk Within Reason." The judgments that experts offer of risks tend to correlate closely with the technical estimates of annual deaths. See Paul Slovic, "Beyond Numbers: A Broader Perspective on Risk Perception and Risk Communication," p. 56.

77. For the cultural relativist view, see Mary Douglas and Aaron Wildavsky, *Risk and Culture: An Essay on the Selection of Technology and Environmental Dangers* (Berkeley: University of California Press, 1982), and Aaron Wildavsky and Karl Drake, "Theories of Risk Perception: Who Fears What and Why?" *Daedalus* 119, vol. 4 (Fall 1990): 41–60.

78. On the significant role of AIDS activists, see Robert M. Wachter, "Sounding Board: AIDS, Activism and the Politics of Health," *New England Journal of Medicine* 326 (January 9, 1992): 128–31.

79. See George Annas, "FDA's Compassion for Desperate Drug Companies," *Hastings Center Report* 20 (January/ February 1990): 35–37.

80. Medical Device Amendments to the Food, Drug, and Cosmetic Act.

81. David A. Kessler, "Special Report: The Basis of the FDA's Decision on Breast Implants," *New England Journal of Medicine* 326 (June 18, 1992): 1713–15. Hereafter in the discussion of implants, all references in the text to Kessler's views are to this article.

82. Marcia Angell, "Breast Implants—Protection or Paternalism?," *New England Journal of Medicine* 326 (June 18, 1992): 1695–96. Hereafter in the discussion of implants, all references to Angell's views are to this article.

83. See Lisa S. Parker, "Social Justice, Federal Paternalism, and Feminism: Breast Implantation in the Cultural Context of Female Beauty," *Kennedy Institute of Ethics Journal* 3 (1993): 57–76; and Jack C. Fisher, "The Silicone Controversy: When Will Science Prevail?" *New England Journal of Medicine* 326 (1992): 1696–98.

84. Ibid.

85. "U.S. Orders Breast Implant Makers to Cite New Studies," *The Washington Post,* March 21, 1993, p. A26.

86. Sandra G. Boodman, "Breast Implants: Now Women Are Having A Hard Time Getting Them Out," *The Washington Post,* June 23, 1992, *Health* Section, pp. 10–14.

87. Angell, "Breast Implants—Protection or Paternalism?"

88. Rescher, *Risk.*

89. Quoted in Steven E. Rhoads, "How Much Should We Spend to Save a Life?" in *Valuing Life: Public Policy Dilemmas,* ed. Rhoads (Boulder, CO: Westview Press, 1980), p. 293.

90. Barbara MacKinnon, "Pricing Human Life," *Science, Technology & Human Values* 11 (Spring 1986): 29–39.

91. Richard Zeckhauser, "Procedures for Valuing Lives," *Public Policy* (Fall 1975): 447–48. Contrast Richard A. Rettig, "Valuing Lives: The Policy Debate on Patient Care Financing for Victims of End-Stage Renal Disease," *The Rand Paper Series* (Santa Monica, CA: Rand Corporation, 1976). See also Rettig, "Origins of the Medicare Kidney Disease Entitlement: The Social Security Amendments of 1972," in *Biomedical Politics,* ed. Kathi Hanna (Washington, DC: National Academy Press, 1991).

92. John Moskop, "The Moral Limits to Federal Funding for Kidney Disease," *Hastings Center Report* 17 (April 1987): 11–15.

93. Steven Kelman, "Cost-Benefit Analysis: An Ethical Critique," *Regulation* (January–February 1981).

94. Quoted in John LaPuma and Edward F. Lawlor, "Quality-Adjusted Life-Years: Ethical Implications for Physicians and Policy-Makers," *Journal of the American Medical Association* 263 (June 6, 1990): 2917–21.

95. Alan Williams, "The Importance of Quality of Life in Policy Decisions," in *Quality of Life: Assessment and Application,* ed. Stuart R. Walker and Rachel M. Rosser (Boston: MTP Press Limited, 1988), p. 285.

96. See David Eddy, "Cost-Effectiveness Analysis: Is It Up to the Task?" *Journal of the American Medical Association* 267 (June 24, 1992): 3344.

97. Alan Williams, "Economics of Coronary Artery Bypass Grafting," *British Medical Journal* 291 (August 3, 1985): 326–29. See also M. C. Weinstein and W. B. Stason, "Cost-Effectiveness of Coronary Artery Bypass Surgery," *Circulation* 66, Suppl. 5, pt. 2 (1982): III, 56–66.

98. John Rawls included "health and vigor" as primary natural goods, in contrast to primary social goods. See *A Theory of Justice* (Cambridge, MA: Harvard University Press, 1971), p. 62.

99. Cf. Donald L. Patrick and Pennifer Erickson, "Assessing Health-Related Quality of Life for Clinical Decision Making," in *Quality of Life,* ed., Walker and Rosser, p. 11.

100. B. J. McNeil, R. Weichselbaum, and S. G. Pauker, "Speech and Survival: Tradeoffs Between Quality and Quantity of Life in Laryngeal Cancer," *New England Journal of Medicine* 305 (October 22, 1981): 982–87.

101. See David C. Hadorn, "The Role of Public Values in Setting Health Care Priorities," *Social Science and Medicine* 32 (1991): 773–81.

102. For a discussion of systematic disparities among and deficiencies of these methods, see Mooney and Olsen, "QALYs: Where Next?" and Drummond, "Output Measurement for Resource-Allocation Decisions in Health Care," in *Providing Health Care,* ed., McGuire, Fenn, and Mayhew. On "framing" effects, see Daniel Kahneman and Amos Tversky, "Prospect Theory: An Analysis of Decision Under Risk," *Econometrica* 47 (1979): 263–91.

103. Gavin Mooney, "QALYs: Are They Enough? A Health Economist's Perspective," *Journal of Medical Ethics* 15 (1989): 148–52.

104. Alan Williams, "The Importance of Quality of Life in Policy Decisions," in *Quality of Life,* ed. Walker and Rosser, p. 286.

105. John Harris, "QALYfying the Value of Life," *Journal of Medical Ethics* 13 (1987): 117.

106. David C. Hadorn, "Setting Health Care Priorities in Oregon: Cost-Effectiveness

Meets the Rule of Rescue,'' *Journal of the American Medical Association* 265 (May 1, 1991): 2218. Hadorn draws the "rule of rescue" from Albert Jonsen, "Bentham in a Box: Technology Assessment and Health Care Allocation," *Law, Medicine and Health Care* 14 (1986): 172–74. See also Hadorn's discussion in "The Oregon Priority-Setting Exercise: Quality of Life and Public Policy," along with Charles J. Dougherty, "Setting Health Care Priorities: Oregon's Next Steps," *Hastings Center Report* 21 (May–June 1991), Supplement, A Conference Report: 1–15.

107. David C. Hadorn, "Setting Health Care Priorities in Oregon: Cost-Effectiveness Meets the Rule of Rescue," p. 2219.

108. Ibid., p. 2221.

109. Herman B. Leonard and Richard J. Zeckhauser, "Cost-Benefit Analysis Applied to Risks: Its Philosophy and Legitimacy," in *Values at Risk,* ed. MacLean, p. 34.

110. For a perceptive analysis, see Norman Daniels, "Is the Oregon Rationing Plan Fair?" *Journal of the American Medical Association* 265 (May 1, 1991): 2232–35.

111. U.S. Congress, Office of Technology Assessment, *The Implications of Cost-Effectiveness Analysis.*

112. Stuart Hampshire, "Morality and Pessimism," in *Public and Private Morality,* ed. Stuart Hampshire (Cambridge: Cambridge University Press, 1978), pp. 5–6.

113. See Rashi Fein, "What Is Wrong with the Language of Medicine?" *New England Journal of Medicine* 306 (1982): 863f.

114. U.S. Congress, Office of Technology Assessment, *The Role of Genetic Testing in the Prevention of Occupational Disease* (Washington, DC: U.S. Government Printing Office, 1983), p. 146. For fuller ethical assessments, see U.S. Congress, Office of Technology Assessment, *Genetic Monitoring and Screening in the Workplace,* OTA-BA-455 (Washington, DC: U.S. Government Printing Office, October 1990), and Elaine Draper, *Risky Business: Genetic Testing and Exclusionary Practices in the Hazardous Workplace* (New York: Cambridge University Press, 1991).

115. U.S. Congress, Office of Technology Assessment, *Reproductive Hazards in the Workplace* (Washington, DC: U.S. Government Printing Office, 1985).

116. *International Union, UAW v. Johnson Controls,* 111 S.Ct. 1196 (1991).

117. Eula Bingham, "Hypersusceptibility to Occupational Hazards," in National Academy of Engineering, *Hazards: Technology and Fairness* (Washington, DC: National Academy Press, 1986), p. 80.

118. A pioneering argument for this conclusion appears in Nicholas Ashford, *Crisis in the Workplace: Occupational Disease and Injury* (Cambridge, MA: MIT Press, 1976).

119. Roger E. Kasperson, "Hazardous Waste Facility Siting: Community, Firm, and Governmental Perspectives," in National Academy of Engineering, *Hazards: Technology and Fairness,* pp. 118–44.

6

Justice

Inequalities in access to health care and health insurance, combined with dramatic increases in the costs of health care, have fueled debates about social justice in the United States and in many other countries. But is *inequality* in access a serious moral problem? Should all age groups, for example, have equal access to health care resources? In attempting to answer such questions, we often encounter uncertainty over how to balance and reconcile goals such as the freedom to choose a health plan, equal access to health care, health promotion, a free-market economy, social efficiency, and the beneficent state. Which of these goals and which principles express what justice demands in the distribution of health care and in the funding of research on disease and injury?

In a short story titled "The Lottery in Babylon," Jorge Luis Borges depicts a society in which all social benefits and burdens are distributed solely on the basis of a periodic lottery.[1] Each person is assigned a social role such as a slave, a factory owner, a priest, or an executioner, purely by the lottery. This random selection system disregards achievement, training, merit, experience, contribution, need, and effort. The ethical and political oddity of the system described in Borges's story is jolting because assigning positions in this way fails so noticeably to cohere with conventional standards. Borges's system appears capricious and unfair, because we expect valid principles of justice to determine how social burdens, benefits, and positions ought to be allocated.

However, if we attempt to expound principles of justice, they seem as elusive as the lottery method seems capricious; and the construction of a comprehensive and unified theory of justice that captures our diverse conceptions may be impossible. (We will see later, for example, that a lottery is a justifiable mechanism for distributing health care under certain conditions.) Moreover, many proposed principles of justice are not distinct from and independent of other principles, such as nonmaleficence and beneficence. We begin to explore these problems in this chapter by analyzing the terms *justice* and *distributive justice*. Later we will examine substantive problems of social justice, including problems in the allocation of resources for and within the health care system.

The Concept of Justice

The terms *fairness, desert* (what is deserved), and *entitlement* (that to which one is entitled) have been used by various philosophers in attempts to explicate *justice*.[2] These accounts all interpret justice as fair, equitable, and appropriate treatment in light of what is due or owed to persons. A situation of justice is present whenever persons are due benefits or burdens because of their particular properties or circumstances, such as being productive or having been harmed by another person's acts. One who has a valid claim based in justice has a right, and therefore is due something. An injustice therefore involves a wrongful act or omission that denies people benefits to which they have a right or fails to distribute burdens fairly.

The term *distributive justice* refers to fair, equitable, and appropriate distribution in society determined by justified norms that structure the terms of social cooperation. Its scope includes policies that allot diverse benefits and burdens such as property, resources, taxation, privileges, and opportunities. Various public and private institutions are involved, including the government and the health care system. The term *distributive justice* is sometimes used broadly to refer to the distribution of all rights and responsibilities in society, including, for example, civil and political rights such as the rights to vote and to freedom of speech. (Distributive justice is commonly distinguished from other types of justice, including *criminal* justice, which refers to the just infliction of punishment, usually through the criminal law, and *rectificatory* justice, which refers to just compensation for transactional problems such as breaches of contracts and malpractice, usually through the civil law.)

Problems of distributive justice arise under conditions of scarcity and competition. If ample fresh water existed for industrial disposal of waste materials, and no subsequent harm to human beings or other forms of life occurred from this disposal, it would not be necessary to restrict use. Only if, for example, the supply of drinking water is endangered or if pollutants create public health problems or threaten wildlife do we need to limit the amounts of permissible discharge. Trade-offs are inevitably involved. The goal of pollution reduction is to protect the public health and the environment, but the task of reduction itself requires resources that might be used elsewhere. Many contemporary discussions of just benefits in prepaid health maintenance programs, just programs of care for the mentally retarded, and appropriate sources of funds for national health insurance similarly involve trade-offs.

A compelling example of distributive justice in the context of trade-offs appears in the following case. An interdisciplinary panel of distinguished physicians, ethicists, and lawyers considered the merits and demerits of using modern technology to produce an artificial heart—the so-called totally implantable artificial heart. The panel narrowed the alternatives to three possibilities: (1) Produce no heart because it is too expensive; (2) produce a heart powered by nuclear energy; or (3) produce a heart with an electric motor and rechargeable batteries. Eventually the panel decided that, on balance, the battery-powered heart posed fewer risks to the recipient, to his or her family, and to other members of society than the nuclear-powered heart. In assessing each alternative, the panel considered its implications for the quality of life of recipients, its cost to society, and its relative expense in comparison with other medical needs that could be met instead. The panel concluded that, despite the substantial costs, it would be unjust not to allocate money to develop the artificial heart for those in need of it (on grounds that distributive justice requires it), but that the nuclear-powered heart would create greater risk to society than could be justified.[3]

Weighing such alternatives is typical of circumstances of distributive justice and concerns not only aggregate risks, costs, and benefits of various alternatives but also their distribution throughout society. The fairness of a distribution, as we saw in the example of the lottery, generates questions about principles of justice. No single principle of justice is capable of addressing such problems. Somewhat like our division of principles under the general heading of beneficence, several principles of justice are worthy of acceptance, each requiring specification and balancing in particular contexts. One of these principles is *formal,* the others *material.*

The Principle of Formal Justice

Common to all theories of justice is a minimal requirement traditionally attributed to Aristotle: Equals must be treated equally, and unequals must be treated unequally. This principle of formal justice (sometimes called the *principle of formal equality*) is "formal" because it states no particular respects in which equals ought to be treated equally and provides no criteria for determining whether two or more individuals are in fact equals. It merely asserts that whatever respects are under consideration as relevant, persons equal in those respects should be treated equally. That is, no person should be treated unequally, despite all differences with other persons, unless some difference between them is relevant to the treatment at stake.

An obvious problem with the formal principle is its lack of substance. That equals ought to be treated equally does not provoke debate. But how shall we define *equality,* and who is equal and who unequal? Which differences are relevant in comparing individuals or groups? Presumably all citizens should have equal political rights, equal access to public services, and equal treatment under the law. But how far does equality reach? A typical problem is the following. Virtually all accounts of justice in health care hold that delivery programs and services designed to assist persons of a certain class, such as the poor or the elderly, should be made available to all members of that class. To deny access to some when others in the same class receive the benefits is unjust. But is it also unjust to deny access to equally needy persons outside of the delineated class?

In one test case, a woman in labor, Hattie Mae Campbell, was denied access to an emergency room on grounds that she was at the wrong hospital and should have gone to a hospital in which she had been provided with prenatal care. She and her sister retreated to the hospital parking lot, where she gave birth to a son in their car. She then brought suit against the hospital, charging that its policy of not admitting patients who are not referred by local physicians is a capricious and arbitrary denial of the constitutional right to use a government facility.[4] The hospital's policy classified patients according to a criterion of referral by a local physician. This classification system resulted in the differential treatment of individuals based on the categories (or class) to which they belonged. Equals were treated equally, and unequals were treated unequally.

Although the hospital's classification and treatment system is just under the formal principle of justice, are the criteria used by the hospital to establish the differences (inequalities) between people just? The hospital must be able to justify treating two candidates for admission differently. Some courts have affirmed that the hospital's criteria are proper under law.[5] But does the classification scheme employed by the hospital in this case identify morally relevant differences between persons for differential access to health care? Any answer to this question will presuppose an account of justice that contains material principles in addition to the formal principle.

Material Principles of Justice

Principles that specify the relevant characteristics for equal treatment are *material* because they identify the substantive properties for distribution. Consider the principle of need, which declares that distribution based on need is just. To say that a person needs something is to say that without it the person will be harmed, or at least detrimentally affected. However, we are not required to distribute all goods and services to satisfy all needs, such as needs for bed-boards, athletic equipment, and antilock brakes (unless a radical form of egali-tarianism is defensible). Presumably we are interested only in *fundamental needs*. To say that someone has a fundamental need for something is to say that the person will be harmed or detrimentally affected in a fundamental way if that need is not fulfilled. For example, the person might be harmed through malnutrition, bodily injury, or nondisclosure of critical information.

If we were to analyze further the notions of fundamental needs and primary goods, the material principle of need could be progressively specified and shaped into a public policy for purposes of distribution. We will turn to public policy later. For the moment we are emphasizing the significance of the argu-ment's first step: acceptance of the principle of need as a valid material princi-ple of justice. By contrast, if one were to accept only a principle of free-market distribution, then one would oppose a principle of need as a basis for public policy. All public and institutional policies based on distributive justice ulti-mately derive from the acceptance (or rejection) of some material principles and some procedures for specifying and refining them, and many disputes over the right policy or distribution spring from rival, or at least alternative, starting points with different material principles.

The following principles have each been proposed by some writers as valid material principles of distributive justice (although other principles have also been proposed[6]).

1. To each person an equal share
2. To each person according to need
3. To each person according to effort
4. To each person according to contribution
5. To each person according to merit
6. To each person according to free-market exchanges

There is no obvious barrier to acceptance of more than one of these principles, and some theories of justice accept all six as valid. A plausible moral thesis is that each of these material principles identifies a prima facie obligation whose weight cannot be assessed independently of particular circumstances or spheres in which they are especially applicable. Additional specification may also es-tablish the relevance of these principles to spheres in which they formerly had not been judged applicable.

In treating principles in the three previous chapters, we have noted the many ways principles can be made effective in the moral life by their support of more specific moral rules (and we noted that several principles may be called on to help justify a single rule). One might argue that each of the above material principles of justice is parallel to the moral rules we have listed in each previ-ous chapter. However, this claim is more controversial in the case of justice because the acceptability of these material principles is in each case more disputed than the rules cited in previous chapters. Nonetheless, we will here accept the validity of each of the above material principles, at least for some contexts.

Most societies invoke several of these material principles in framing public policies, appealing to different principles in different spheres and contexts. In the United States, for example, unemployment subsidies, welfare payments, and many health care programs are distributed on the basis of need (and to some extent on other criteria such as previous length of employment); jobs and promotions in many sectors are awarded (distributed) on the basis of demonstrated achievement and merit; the higher incomes of some professionals are allowed and often encouraged on grounds of free-market wage scales, superior effort, merit, or potential social contribution; and, at least theoretically, the opportunity for elementary and secondary education is distributed equally to all citizens.

It seems attractive, then, to include each of the above-listed principles in a theory of justice. Conflicts among them, however, create a serious priority problem as well as a challenge to a moral system that aims for a coherent framework of principles. These conflicts indicate the need for both specification and balancing, as is illustrated by the case of Mark Dalton, a histology technician employed by a large chemical company.[7] Dalton was an excellent worker, but after a week of sick leave, a company nurse discovered that he had a chronic renal disease. The company determined that the permissible levels of chemical vapor exposure in Dalton's job might exacerbate his renal condition. Management found him another job, with the same salary, but two other employees eligible for promotion were also interested in the job. Both employees had more seniority and better training than Dalton, and one was a woman. In this situation, each of the three employees could legitimately appeal to a different material principle of justice to support his or her claim to the available position. Dalton could cite the material principle of need, arguing that his medical condition required that he either be offered the new position or be dismissed from the company with compensation. With their superior experience and training, the other two employees could invoke material principles of merit, societal contribution, and perhaps individual effort in support of their claims. Considerations of equal opportunity also gave the woman valid grounds for claiming that justice entitles her to the position. Without further specification and balancing of these material principles, such conflicts are not resolvable.

Relevant Properties

Material principles identify relevant properties that persons must possess to qualify for a particular distribution. Several theoretical and practical difficulties plague the justification of alleged relevant properties. Ambivalence over which properties to emphasize, and in which contexts, accounts in part for the patch-work character of government regulation and health policy in many countries.

In some contexts relevant properties are firmly established by tradition, by moral or legal principle, or by policy. For example, trophies are awarded (dis-tributed) at the end of a tennis tournament on the basis of achievement; and achievement is determined by the tradition-bound rules of tournament tennis. Similarly, prison terms are distributed in principle only to those found guilty of crimes; guilt is relevant to conviction and sentencing as a matter of law and morality. However, in many contexts it is appropriate either to institute a policy establishing relevant properties where none previously existed or to develop a new policy that revises entrenched criteria. For example, the question has been raised whether nonresident aliens should be included on waiting lists in the United States for cadaveric organ transplantation. Whether being a resident or a citizen of a country is a relevant property for access to some medical care is among the issues discussed later in this chapter.

Courts often mandate new policies that revise entrenched notions about rele-vant properties. For example, in 1991 the United States Supreme Court de-cided, in the case of *Auto Workers v. Johnson Controls, Inc.*,[8] that employers cannot legally adopt ''fetal protection policies'' that specifically exclude women of childbearing age from a hazardous workplace, because these policies discriminate illegally based on sex. Under these policies, only fertile men could choose whether they wished to assume reproductive risks. The majority of jus-tices held that this gender-based policy used the irrelevant property of being a woman, despite the fact that mutagenic substances affect sperm as well as eggs.

When an irrelevant property is detected, we sometimes need not abandon a policy altogether. For example, we might still be able to formulate an accept-able, nondiscriminatory policy for protecting fetuses from reproductive haz-ards. We might respond by shifting some operative set of ''relevant'' properties to a better set of relevant properties. Certain properties previously accepted as relevant will then become irrelevant, or certain properties formerly presumed irrelevant will be relevant in the new or revised policy.

A contemporary illustration of this problem is demonstrated by Case 4, which involves an incompetent organ donor: A forty-year-old woman's life depends on a kidney transplant, which her fourteen-year-old daughter offers to supply. The kidney is a fairly good match. However, the woman has a thirty-five-year-old mentally retarded brother who is a better match. An informal sur-vey of nurses, social workers, and physicians who work with such patients indicated that the majority of these health care professionals would seek a court order to take the kidney from the thirty-five-year-old, institutionalized, men-tally retarded brother.[9] Here we have a straightforward dilemma regarding which criteria should be used to select among three options: selecting one of these two potential donors or waiting for a cadaveric donor (an unlikely prospect at the time). The closeness of the match is considered a relevant property favoring use of the brother, but the impossibility of obtaining consent from the brother and the apparently knowledgeable consent of the minor introduces a reason favoring use of the child. There are also reasons against using either potential donor. The child might be overwhelmingly influenced by the fact that her *mother* needs her kidney. The closeness of their relationship creates an emotion-laden situation that exerts pressure on the child, perhaps to a degree that renders the quality of consent problematic. How, then, are decisions about relevant and irrelevant properties—such as quality of match, age, and competence—connected to problems of justice?

Decisions, rules, and laws tend to be unjust when they make distinctions between classes of persons who are actually similar in relevant respects, or fail to make distinctions between classes of persons who are actually different in relevant respects. A longstanding issue about justice and classes of persons concerns the selection of human subjects of research. Two primary questions need an answer. First, should a particular class of subjects be used at all? For example, should prisoners, fetuses, children, and those institutionalized for mental disability be used as subjects in research, and, if so, for what reasons and under what conditions? Second, if it is permissible to involve these subjects, should there be a hierarchy for selecting subjects within that class, based on relevantly different properties possessed by members of the class? For example, it seems morally relevant to distinguish within the class of children between older and younger children—or, better, between (1) children who comprehend what is proposed and report their feelings with clarity and (2) children with limited capacity to do so. Typically, these distinctions have policy implications. For example, a policy might be adopted that competent adults, older children, and younger children be ranked in that order of priority as potential subjects of biomedical research.

Several of these problems of justice are illustrated by Case 7, a case popularly known as Willowbrook. At a state institution for mentally retarded children, some of the children were used as research subjects in order to develop an effective prophylactic agent against the strains of hepatitis prevalent in the institution. The research involved intentionally exposing children to the resident strains. Studies were carried out in a special unit that isolated the children and protected them from other infectious diseases. The use of these mentally retarded children precipitated a series of debates about the moral permissibility of using children, institutionalized persons, and those with mental disabilities in research. If it is permissible to involve members of each of these three classes, is it also permissible to use as subjects those who belong to all three classes—namely, children who are both institutionalized and retarded? If it is permissible, under which conditions may they be used, and should there be a ranking, such as older children first or those most severely retarded last?

These cases illustrate how abstract principles of justice provide only rough guidelines when specific policies must be formed or actions taken, so that further moral argument, including specification of principles and balancing of competing claims, is needed to determine which specific aspects of a situation are morally relevant and decisive in forming a reasoned judgment. We can reasonably expect that agreement will often be difficult to achieve, and some philosophers have for this reason concluded that abstract material distributive principles are not the right instruments for resolving social problems of justice. In *Utilitarianism*,[10] John Stuart Mill argued that common sense precepts or principles such as ''to each according to effort'' or ''to each according to need'' lead to intractable conflicts among principles and to conflicting moral injunctions. The principles assign no relative weight to their demands when they conflict, and, consequently, offer little help when a judgment of relative merit must be made. Mill maintained that the whole set of such precepts would fall short of a theory of justice, and would only result in unhelpful pluralism. John Rawls joined Mill in this conclusion, arguing that ''None of these precepts can be plausibly raised to a first principle. . . . Common sense precepts are at the wrong level of generality. In order to find suitable first principles one must step behind them'' and develop a theory.[11]

If Rawls and Mill are right, abstract material principles of justice offer little help until they have been integrated into a systematic framework or theory. But how much help will theories themselves provide?

Theories of Justice

Theories of distributive justice have been developed to specify and render coherent our diverse principles, rules, and judgments. A theory attempts to connect the characteristics of persons with morally justifiable distributions of benefits and burdens. For example, a person's service, effort, or misfortune might be the basis of distribution. Several systematic theories have been proposed to determine how social burdens and goods and services, including health care goods and services, should be distributed—or, as some insist, redistributed. These theories differ with respect to the specific material criteria they emphasize and the forms of justification they employ.

The following are influential types of theory: *Utilitarian* theories emphasize a mixture of criteria for the purpose of maximizing public utility; *libertarian* theories emphasize rights to social and economic liberty (invoking fair procedures rather than substantive outcomes); *communitarian* theories stress the principles and practices of justice that evolve through traditions in a community; and *egalitarian* theories emphasize equal access to the goods in life that every rational person values (often invoking material criteria of need and equality). The acceptability of any theory of justice is determined by the strength of its moral argument that one or more selected principles ought to be given priority over other principles.

We can expect only partial success from these theories in bringing coherence and comprehensiveness to our fragmented visions of social justice. Policies for health care access and distribution in many capitalist countries provide an example of the problems that confront these theories. We seek to provide the best possible health care for all citizens, while promoting the public interest through cost-containment programs. We promote the ideal of equal access to health care for everyone, including care for indigents, while maintaining a free-market competitive environment. These desirable goals of superior care, equality of access, freedom of choice, and social efficiency are difficult to render coherent in a social system. Different conceptions of the just society underlie them, and one goal is likely to diminish another.

Nonetheless, several theories of justice try either to achieve a balance between competing social goals or to eliminate some social objectives while retaining others.

Utilitarian Theories

Utilitarian theories were discussed in Chapter 2, where we saw that utilitarians regard distributive justice as one among several problems of maximizing value. They argue that the standard of justice is not independent of the principle of utility. Rather, *justice* is the name for the paramount and most stringent forms of obligation created by the principle of utility. Typically, utilitarian obligations of justice are correlative rights for individuals that should be enforced by law, if necessary. These rights are contingent upon social arrangements that maximize net social utility in the circumstances. Rights have no other basis, which generates disputes even among utilitarians as to whether they are genuine rights. However, if the justification of a system of rights is that its protections *over time* maximize utility, then these rights can in principle override short-term utility calculations.

In the distribution of health care, utilitarians commonly see justice as involving trade-offs—for instance, in establishing benefits in prepaid health maintenance programs. Many utilitarians favor social programs that protect public health and distribute basic health care equally to all citizens, on grounds that these programs maximize utility. However, problems emerge if utilitarian principles of justice are accepted as sufficient by themselves. For example, individual rights, such as the right to health care, have an indefinite and tenuous foundation when they rest on overall utility maximization, which could change at any time. Another problem is that utilitarian approaches neglect considerations of justice that focus on how benefits and burdens are distributed, apart from aggregate welfare. For example, social utility might be maximized by not allowing access to health care for some of society's sickest and most vulnerable populations.

Nevertheless, as we will see, principles of utilitarian justice have a legitimate role in the formation of policies of both macroallocation and microallocation.

Libertarian Theories

The United States has traditionally, though not exclusively, accepted the free-market ideal that distributions of health care services and goods are best left to the marketplace, which operates on the material principle of ability to pay either directly or indirectly through insurance. Health care is not a right under this conception, and privatization in the health care system is a protected value. These standards are accepted by a libertarian interpretation of justice that consists not in a *result* such as increased public utility or meeting the health needs of citizens, but in the unfettered operation of fair *procedures*. The just society protects rights of property and liberty, allowing persons to improve their circumstances on their own initiative. Social intervention in the market therefore undermines justice by placing unwarranted constraints on individual liberty.

In regarding free choice and privatization as central to justice in economic distribution, contemporary libertarian writers, as well as classical exponents such as John Locke and Adam Smith, assume an individualist conception of economic production and value. Libertarians grant that people deserve equal treatment in various morally significant respects (for example, in the right to vote), but they believe that other theories of justice entail practices of coercive and immoral expropriation of financial resources through taxation, which amounts to an unjust redistribution of private property as if it were public property. Principles of equality and utility, from this perspective, sacrifice basic liberties to the larger public interest. However, a libertarian is not opposed to utilitarian or egalitarian modes of distribution if they are freely chosen. Any distribution scheme, such as for health care, is just and justified if (and only if) it is freely chosen by the relevant group. (It is sometimes left unclear whether the group decision must be unanimous to qualify as binding.)

Libertarians support a system in which health care insurance is privately and voluntarily purchased. In this system, no one's personal property is coercively extracted by the state to benefit another. Investors in health care and insured persons have property rights, physicians have liberty rights, and society is not morally obligated to provide funds to cover health care. Indeed, the society is morally obligated to refrain from providing funds or assigning physicians if the mechanism is coercive taxation or conscription. We discussed earlier a case in which Hattie Mae Campbell was denied admission to the Marshall County Hospital and gave birth to her baby in her car. She had freely made an arrangement with another physician and health care facility, but had not made any arrangement with the county hospital. From the libertarian's point of view, a hospital might grant her admission as an act of charity and kindness, but unless she has a valid contractual entitlement she has no right of access or entitlement to care. (The libertarian sees the strongest case for these conclusions in a private hospital's policies; Campbell's case involved a public facility.)

The libertarian theory has been defended in an influential book by Robert Nozick, who refers to his conclusions as an "entitlement theory" of justice in which government action is justified if and only if it protects the rights or entitlements of citizens, in particular rights to liberty and private property.[12] He argues that a theory of justice should affirm individual rights rather than create "patterns" of economic distribution in which governments act to redistribute the wealth acquired by persons under the free market. In these countries the wealthy are taxed at a progressively higher rate than those who are less wealthy, and the proceeds are used to underwrite state support of the indigent through welfare payments and unemployment compensation. The libertarian condemns all such visions of justice as coercive and unfair.

Nozick accepts a form of procedural justice with three and only three principles: justice in acquisition, justice in transfer, and justice in rectification. No pattern of just distribution exists independent of free-market procedures of acquiring property, legitimately transferring that property, and providing rectification for those who had property illegitimately extracted or otherwise were illegitimately obstructed in the free market. Justice consists in the operation of just procedures (such as fair play), not in the production of just outcomes (such as an equal distribution of resources). There are no welfare rights, and therefore no rights to health care or claims to health care based on justice.

Health policy proposals in the United States have often been influenced by libertarianism. For instance, market strategies and managed competition have recently been touted as ways to further enhance the quality of health care in the United States while controlling its escalating costs. More controversially, proposals exist to increase the supply of cadaveric organs for transplantation by overturning the federal ban on the transfer of organs for monetary payments. However, many competing theories of justice reject the libertarian's uncompromising commitment to liberty and pure procedural justice. The leading competitors to libertarian theories in recent years have been communitarianism and egalitarianism.

Communitarian Theories

Communitarian theories were discussed in Chapter 2, but little was said about their accounts of justice. Communitarians react negatively to liberal models of society (such as those of Mill, Rawls, and Nozick) that base human relationships on rights and contracts and that attempt to construct a single theory of justice by which to judge every society. Communitarians regard principles of justice as pluralistic, deriving from as many different conceptions of the good as there are diverse moral communities. They regard what is due individuals and groups as depending on these community-derived standards.[13] A communitarian can therefore be expected to oppose conceptions of distributing health care through individual contracts. For example, communitarians would reject the American Medical Association's policy on access to health care—both the AMA's traditional endorsement of free-market premises and the AMA's current policy of supporting "a pluralist delivery system" that encourages several funding mechanisms, none of which derive from a conception of the common good or the values of community.[14]

Communitarians emphasize either the responsibility of the community to the individual or, increasingly in contemporary policy, the responsibility of the individual to the community. Some communitarians eschew the language of justice and adopt the language of *solidarity,* which is both a personal virtue of commitment and a principle of social morality based on the shared values of a group. For example, in the Netherlands solidarity is sometimes viewed as a collective obligation to take care of citizens. The 1991 report of a Committee for Choices in Health Care, assembled under the Dutch Secretary for Public Health, established that certain services or procedures are vital to ensure the "adequate functioning of society as a whole," and that they should be "consonant with the basic values of Dutch society." The report assigned an "absolute priority . . . to care for the elderly, the handicapped, and psychiatric patients."[15]

Some moderate communitarian writers in biomedical ethics have attempted to incorporate parts of liberalism into their theories. As discussed in Chapter 2, Ezekiel J. Emanuel envisions small deliberative democratic communities that develop shared conceptions of the good life and justice.[16] He proposes thousands of community health programs (CHPs), each involving citizen-members who join in a federation. Each family would receive a voucher for participation, and the CHP would determine democratically which benefits to provide, which care is most important, and whether expensive services such as heart transplants will be included or excluded. Justice is located in the guarantee that services will be provided to fulfill a particular community-endorsed conception of social goals. However, this proposal faces serious practical obstacles, and moral questions arise about the criteria CHPs may use to admit and exclude applicants and about the moral adequacy of a group's selecting a system of inferior coverage that likely would shift certain uncovered costs to other social units.

Michael Walzer's communitarianism, by contrast, focuses on past and present socio-moral practices. According to Walzer, no single principle of distributive justice governs all social goods and their distribution. Rather, a series of principles constructed by human societies constitute distinct "spheres of justice." Notions of justice are not derived from some "rational" or "natural" foundation external to the society, but rather from standards developed internally, as a political community evolves. Walzer holds that community traditions in the United States include developed commitments of equal access to health care. He argues that a "distinctive logic" in the practice of medicine already exists in this social context: "Care should be proportionate to illness and not to wealth." While conceding that a two-tiered health care system—a decent minimum for all and then liberty of contract for the advantaged—is not unjust in principle, Walzer contends that this system would be unjust in the United States because the "common appreciation of the importance of medical care" has already carried the American people beyond this arrangement: "So long as communal funds are spent, as they currently are, to finance research, build hospitals, and pay the fees of doctors in private practice, the services that these expenditures underwrite must be *equally available*."[17]

Walzer's point is plausible inasmuch as Americans are typically outraged when they become aware of cases in which persons are denied access to health care because of a lack of money. At the same time, his communitarian argument for equal access to health care fails to appreciate the diversity of the American tradition and fails to argue for the superiority of one strand of the American tradition over other strands.[18] It is doubtful that equal access to health care finds stronger support throughout the American tradition than free-market principles or beliefs in the right to a decent basic minimum of health care.

Egalitarian Theories

Ideas of equal distribution of social benefits and burdens have occupied a central position in many influential ethical theories. Political equality in the right to vote is a standard example. Egalitarian theories of justice propose that persons be provided an equal distribution of certain goods such as health care, but all prominent egalitarian theories of justice are cautiously formulated to avoid making equal sharing of all possible social benefits a requirement of justice. When structuring social arrangements, qualified egalitarianism requires only some basic equalities among individuals, and permits inequalities that redound to the benefit of the least advantaged.

As we saw in Chapter 2, John Rawls's theory of justice presents an egalitarian challenge to libertarian and utilitarian theories. Rawls explicates justice as *fairness*, understood as norms of cooperation agreed to by free and equal persons who participate in social activities with mutual respect. Consistent with his views about reflective equilibrium and coherence, Rawls argues that "what justifies a conception of justice is not its being true to an order antecedent and given to us, but its congruence with our deeper understanding of ourselves and our aspirations, and our realization that, given our history and the traditions embedded in our public life, it is the most reasonable doctrine for us."[19] A theory of justice therefore matches our commonly accepted judgments of fairness with our general principles.

Rawls's theory has some widely discussed implications for health policy. Although he has not himself pursued these implications, others have. According to one interpretation and expansion of his views,[20] Rawls's theory supports the following perspective on health policy: Rational agents blinded behind a "veil of ignorance" about their personal situation would choose principles of justice that maximize the minimum level of primary goods in order to protect vital interests such as health in potentially damaging contexts. These agents would elect social allocations to meet certain health needs, as well as allowing the conventional marketplace to distribute other health care goods according to individual initiative. Health policy would guarantee a safety net or minimum floor below which citizens would not be allowed to fall. Rational agents would reject both utilitarian systems (as attempts to produce the highest possible or average level of health care) and systems that distribute equal sums to be invested in any commodity, including health care, the individual wishes.

In an influential interpretation and extension of Rawls's theory, Norman Daniels argues for a just health care system based centrally on a Rawlsian principle of "fair equality of opportunity." Although Daniels offers no explicit defense of this principle, he relies implicitly on the importance of health care needs and on a considered judgment that fair opportunity is central to any acceptable theory of justice. Daniels's thesis is that social institutions affecting health care distribution should be arranged, as far as possible, to allow each person to achieve a fair share of the normal range of opportunities present in that society. The normal range of opportunity is determined by the range of life plans that a person could reasonably hope to pursue, given his or her talents and skills.

This theory, like Rawls's, recognizes a positive societal obligation to eliminate or reduce barriers that prevent fair equality of opportunity, an obligation that extends to programs that correct or compensate for various disadvantages. Disease and disability are viewed as undeserved restrictions on persons' opportunities to meet basic goals. Health care needs are determined by whatever is necessary to achieve, maintain, or restore adequate or "species-typical" levels of functioning (or the equivalents of these levels). A health care system designed to meet these needs should attempt to prevent disease, illness, or injury from reducing the range of opportunity open to the individual. The allocation of health care resources, then, should ensure justice through fair equality of opportunity. Forms of health care that have a significant effect on preventing, limiting, or compensating for reductions in normal species functioning should receive priority in designing health care institutions and allocating health care.[21]

Both of these Rawls-inspired theories have far-reaching egalitarian implications for a national health policy. Each member of society, irrespective of wealth or position, would have equal access to an adequate, although not maximal, level of health care—the exact level of access being contingent on available social resources and public processes of decisionmaking. Better services, such as luxury hospital rooms and optional, cosmetic dental work, would be made available for purchase at personal expense, including through private insurance.

The power of Rawls's theory of justice, together with the political significance of the decent-minimum proposal, have engendered wide support for egalitarianism. One of its achievements has been to encourage discussion of the role of the rule of fair opportunity in a theory of social justice.

Fair Opportunity

Daniels's appeal to fair opportunity is only one way to use the fair-opportunity rule. To explore this rule further, we need first to consider properties that often have served as bases of distribution, although as a matter of justice they should not be considered relevant properties. Primary examples are gender, race, IQ, accent, national origin, and social status. In some anomalous contexts these properties are relevant. For example, if a script calls for an actor in a male role, then females are properly excluded (although this example is sometimes contested in contemporary film and theater). But general rules such as "To each according to gender" and "To each according to IQ" are unacceptable material principles.

A widely accepted reason why these properties are both irrelevant and discriminatory is that they permit differential treatment of persons, sometimes with devastating effects, because of differences introduced by chance, for which the affected individual is not responsible and which he or she does not deserve. This element of chance is the source of the oft-used metaphor of a lottery, suggesting that differences between persons are relevant in distributional rules only if those persons are responsible for those differences.

The Fair-Opportunity Rule

This account of fairness can be formulated as a rule of social distribution that attempts to diminish or eradicate unjust forms of distribution. The fair-opportunity rule says that no persons should be granted social benefits on the basis of undeserved advantageous properties (because no persons are responsible for having these properties) and that no persons should be denied social benefits on the basis of undeserved disadvantageous properties (because they also are not responsible for these properties). Properties distributed by the lotteries of social and biological life are not grounds for morally acceptable discrimination between persons if they are not properties that people have a fair chance to acquire or overcome.

Although in many societies properties such as social status can be altered, race, gender, and IQ—those properties that most bedevil fair treatment—are not easily altered. If IQ, for example, is a property for which a person is not responsible, and if no one should be denied the benefits of a public distributional system on the basis of such a morally irrelevant property, then it would be unjust not to provide mentally disabled or retarded persons the benefits conferred upon all who share in the system of benefits. Similarly, if people are not responsible for various diseases, it would be unjust not to provide them the social benefits available to others who do not suffer from the same health problems. The fair-opportunity rule requires that persons be given a fair chance in life when their disadvantages are not of their making.

The attempt to supply all citizens with a basic education raises some thorny moral problems that are analogous to those we encounter in attempting to provide everyone with a decent level of health care. Imagine a community that offers a high-quality education to all students with basic abilities, regardless of gender or race, but does not offer a comparable opportunity for education to students with reading difficulties or mental deficiencies. This system seems unjust. The students with disabilities lack basic skills and need special training to overcome their problems; they should receive an education that suits their needs. If these students were responsible for their learning disabilities, they might not be entitled to special training. But if they are not responsible, they are entitled to the special training, because of the fair-opportunity rule. The equal distribution of economic resources is not at stake here. The disabled or slow learners with special reading problems are not owed the same amount of money, training, or resources as other pupils. They should receive what for them is a quality education, even if it costs more. The fair-opportunity rule requires that they receive these benefits to ameliorate the unfortunate effects dispensed by life's lottery (within limits of available resources, a distinct but closely related problem of justice).

This argument for awarding larger and unequal distributional shares to disadvantaged persons in education can be similarly applied to health policy. To determine a person's entitlement exclusively on the basis of material principles such as effort and personal merit or equality of social resources would be morally wrong, because the fair-opportunity rule systematically rejects the employment of these material principles when disadvantageous properties are distributed by chance. Persons with functional disabilities lack capacity and need health care to gain a higher level of function and have a fair chance in life. If they were responsible for their disabilities, they might not be entitled to health care services. But if they were not responsible, the fair-opportunity rule demands that they receive what for them will help ameliorate the unfortunate effects dispensed by life's lottery of health. Like provisions for welfare and education, health care is often a necessity of life.

Although many debates in health policy turn on an interpretation of the fair-opportunity rule and its significance, limits exist both to its use and to the goods and services that can be provided for the disadvantaged. Comparative justice demands a fair share, not an unfairly large share. For example, children treated for myelomeningocele, a severe central nervous system anomaly, often receive partial treatment rather than total care, in the expectation that they will soon die. But some do not die, and over a period of years a series of expensive medical treatments for a variety of problems is often recommended. These children can be afflicted by blindness, severe mental disabilities, and multiple medical problems in need of constant attention. It is perplexingly difficult to determine what the fair-opportunity rule demands for these children. Our society does not provide the exceptional medical care and training that such a child would need to receive a fair opportunity by comparison to other children of the same age. Have we, then, failed to discharge our obligations?

Ameliorating the Effects of Life's Lotteries

The fair-opportunity rule offers a revisionary perspective on many contemporary practices of distribution. The rule suggests that whenever persons lack equal opportunities to advance their interests because of "disadvantageous" properties for which they are not responsible, they should not be denied important benefits because of those properties. Numerous properties might be disadvantaging—for example, a squeaky voice, an ugly face, poor command of a language, or an inadequate early education. But how far should we extend the range of undeserved properties that create a right in justice to some form of assistance?

One hypothesis is that virtually all "abilities" and "disabilities" are functions of what John Rawls refers to as "the natural lottery" and "the social lottery." *Natural lottery* refers to the distribution of advantageous and disadvantageous properties through birth, and *social lottery* refers to the distribution of social assets or deficits through family property, school systems, and the like. Suppose that all our talents and disabilities result from heredity, natural environment, family upbringing, education, and inheritance. From this perspective, even the ability to work long hours and the ability to compete are biologically, environmentally, and socially produced. If so, talents, abilities, and successes are not to our credit, just as genetic disease is acquired through no fault of the afflicted person. People do not deserve these advantageous properties any more than they deserve disadvantageous, disabling properties.

If this theory of the causal origins of advantageous and disadvantageous properties were accepted, together with the fair-opportunity rule, it would entail views about distributive justice fundamentally different from those now acknowledged. Rawls uses fair opportunity as a rule of redress. In order to overcome disadvantaging conditions (whether from biology or society) that are not deserved, the rule demands compensation for those with the disadvantages. The goal is to redress the unequal distributions created by undeserved properties to attain greater equality. Evening out disabilities in this way, Rawls claims, is a fundamental part of our shared conception of justice.

The full implications of this approach are uncertain, but the conclusions reached by Rawls are challenging:

[A free-market arrangement] permits the distribution of wealth and income to be determined by the natural distribution of abilities and talents. Within the limits allowed by the background arrangements, distributive shares are decided by the outcome of the natural lottery; and this outcome is *arbitrary from a moral perspective*. There is no more reason to permit the distribution of income and wealth to be settled by the distribution of natural assets than by historical and social fortune. Furthermore, the principle of fair opportunity can be only imperfectly carried out, at least as long as the institution of the family exists. The extent to which natural capacities develop and reach fruition is affected by *all kinds of social conditions and class attitudes*. Even the willingness to make an effort, to try, and so to be deserving in the ordinary sense is itself dependent upon happy family and social circumstances.[22]

At a minimum, our social system of distributing benefits and burdens would undergo massive revision if we accepted this approach. Rather than allowing broad inequalities in social distribution based on effort, contribution, and merit, as some Western nations do, we would regard justice as achieved only if radical inequalities are diminished. Remaining inequalities would be permissible only if "disadvantaged" persons benefited more from the remaining inequalities than from an equal distribution of benefits.

Nevertheless, at some point this process of reducing inequalities introduced by life's lotteries must stop.[23] Libertarians have rightly pointed to the impossible dimensions of a program that carried the fair-opportunity rule to conclusion without limits. Some disadvantages are properly categorized as merely *unfortunate,* whereas others are *unfair* (and therefore obligatory in justice to correct). From the libertarian perspective, as Tristram Engelhardt has argued, society should call a halt to claims of fairness or justice at the point of this distinction between the unfair and the unfortunate: "Where one draws the line between what is unfair and unfortunate will, as a result, have great consequences as to what allocations of health care resources are just or unfair as opposed to desirable or undesirable. If the natural lottery is neutral, in the sense of not creating an obligation to blunt its effects, one does not have [even] prima facie grounds for arguing for a right to health care on the basis of claims of fairness or justice.''[24] From this perspective, if a person's afflictions are unfortunate they may still be ameliorated through the benevolence or compassion of others; but only if the afflictions are unfair does the obligation of justice require compensation to the disadvantaged through the use of state force to generate the needed resources for compensation. Maleficently or negligently caused setbacks to health justify the designation unfair, but other setbacks to health are matters of misfortune.

In light of this problem of a criterion of unfairness, the implications of the Rawlsian approach and the demands of the fair-opportunity rule remain uncertain in biomedical ethics and health policy. No bright lines distinguish the unfair and the unfortunate, but the assumption that a clear distinction exists can blind us to forms of individual need and social responsibility that we might not consider to be based in an injustice.[25] As the lottery metaphor suggests, many setbacks to health are randomly distributed and not under anyone's direct control. This metaphor is problematic if it suggests in addition that no social obligation requires us to prevent, remove, control, or compensate for such harms.

It would be inappropriate to explore these theoretical problems further here. The point of exploring them as far as we have is to show that if one accepts a justification of unequal treatment based on the fair-opportunity rule, as we do, then many areas of moral reflection and social policy will potentially be affected.

Distributing Health Care on the Basis of Gender and Race

We can now sketch some implications of the fair-opportunity rule for health care distribution, with particular attention to distribution based on racial and gender properties. The fair-opportunity rule excludes policies that deprive women and racial groups of health services because of gender and race. Yet compelling evidence exists that health care has often been covertly distributed on the basis of these properties, resulting in a differential impact on women and minorities. The fair-opportunity rule requires scrutiny of these allocation policies to determine whether they unfairly discriminate.

One example has emerged from the U.S. experience with access to kidney dialysis. In the late 1960s, when dialysis was scarce, many institutions used committees to select recipients on the basis of medical and social criteria, including ability to pay. Patients receiving dialysis were then largely white, married, male high-school graduates between twenty-five and forty-five. More than forty percent were employed. Their ability to pay and their actual or potential social contribution were primary factors in their selection. With the implementation in 1972 of the End-Stage Renal Disease Program of Medicare, which ensured virtually universal access, the characteristics of the dialysis patient population changed dramatically. By the late seventies, the patient population more closely reflected the incidence of end-stage renal failure among distinct social groups. Current projections are that this trend will continue and that a greater percentage of elderly, diabetic, hypertensive, and minority patients will seek treatment in the future.[26]

Recent studies indicate that blacks and women still have less access to various forms of health care than do white males, in part because of socioeconomic factors. A large difference has been shown in the rates of coronary artery by-pass grafting (CABG) between white and black Medicare patients, as well as between male and female Medicare patients. The national CABG rate was 27.1 per 10,000 whites (40.4 for white men and 16.2 for white women), but only 7.6 for blacks (9.3 for black men and 6.4 for black women). Differences were evident across the United States, but were pronounced in the southeast's rural areas. Differences in need cannot entirely account for the variance, and it remains unclear how far the rates can be explained by physician supply, poverty, awareness of health care opportunities, less willingness among blacks and women to undergo surgery, and racial prejudice.[27]

Another controversy has focused on the use of HLA (human lymphocyte antigen) matching for the distribution of kidneys for transplantation. Evidence indicates that the degree of HLA match between donor and recipient influences the long-term survival of the transplanted graft. The United Network for Organ Sharing (UNOS) has therefore revised its criteria for the allocation of donated kidneys to give greater weight to the HLA match, thereby reducing the importance of patient sensitization and time on the waiting list (as well as logistics and urgency of need).[28] Critics charge that this allocation plan, designed to improve success rates in kidney transplantation, will have discriminatory effects. It appears that discrimination against blacks, other minorities, and women has already occurred at the point of admission to waiting lists, and assigning priority to tissue matching can produce further discriminatory effects for minorities. Most organ donors are white, and certain HLA phenotypes are different in white, black, and Hispanic populations. The identification of HLA phenotypes is less complete for blacks and Hispanics, and yet nonwhites have a higher rate of end-stage renal disease. Nonwhite populations are also disproportionately represented on dialysis rolls. However, blacks on the waiting list wait months longer than whites, almost twice as long, according to some studies, to receive a first kidney transplant.[29]

If organs are allocated on the basis of tissue match, whites appear to obtain an advantage.[30] Justice minimally requires careful monitoring of the revised point system to determine whether discriminatory effects exist, and it may be justified to sacrifice some probability of successful transplantation in order to take affirmative action, based on the fair-opportunity rule, to protect minorities. However, defenders of the primacy of tissue matching argue that the revised allocation rules simply reflect the natural lottery, which determines the spread of HLA types in the population. Still, the social context is not irrelevant. Suspicion among minorities about the justice of the health care system is a factor in their lower rate of cadaveric organ donation, because they worry about exploitation, as sources of organs for whites. Social factors also play a role in the higher rate among blacks of medical conditions such as hypertension that contribute to end-stage kidney failure and the need for both dialysis and transplantation.

Recently, the Council on Ethical and Judicial Affairs of the American Medical Association examined evidence that has raised concerns about whether women are disadvantaged because of inadequate attention to research, diagnosis, and treatment of their health problems.[31] Some studies indicate that women have more physician visits per year than men and receive more services per visit, but gender disparities appear in three areas: (1) diagnosis of lung cancer, (2) diagnosis and treatment of cardiac disease, and (3) access to kidney transplantation. These disparities cannot be accounted for entirely by biological differences. The council notes that gender bias does not always appear as overt sexual discrimination. Social attitudes involving stereotypes, prejudices, and gender-role attributions are often present, including the attribution of women's health complaints to emotional rather than physical causes.

In the use of diagnostic and therapeutic procedures for patients with coronary heart disease, good evidence exists that men and women are treated differently for reasons that appear unrelated to their medical conditions. One study found that women reported more cardiac disability than men before myocardial infarction, but they were less likely than men to undergo procedures that were known to reduce symptoms and improve cardiac function.[32] There is ongoing debate about whether these procedures are overused in men, underused in women, or both. However, at least for heart disease and perhaps for lung disease, many health care professionals and public officials may have a biased view of these diseases as male diseases. Bernadine Healy, a former Director of the National Institutes of Health, noted that "the problem is to convince both the lay and medical sectors that coronary heart disease is also a women's disease, not a man's disease in disguise. [As in Isaac B. Singer's story *Yentl*] being 'just like a man' has historically been a price women have had to pay for equality."[33]

The fair-opportunity rule, then, directs our attention to the potential discriminatory impact of policies and practices that allocate health care on the basis of gender or race. But what about the criterion of *age?* Several philosophers have argued that the fair-opportunity rule is consistent rather than inconsistent with

unequal distributions of health care on the basis of age, a criterion that has
been used both implicitly and explicitly in health policy. We will assess this
issue below in a discussion of rationing (see pp. 369–372).

The Right to a Decent Minimum of Health Care

We have seen that questions about who shall receive what share of society's
scarce resources generate controversies about a national health policy, unequal
distributions of advantages to the disadvantaged, and rationing of health care.
These questions of distributive justice recur for problems of access to and distribution of health insurance, expensive medical equipment, artificial organs, and
the like. Although more than two thousand dollars per person and over fourteen
percent of the gross national product are spent annually for health care in the
United States, the poorly insured and the uninsured often cannot afford or gain
access to adequate care. Ultimately the primary economic barrier to health care
access in the United States is the lack of adequate insurance, especially for the
roughly 37 million U.S. citizens (one in seven) who lack health insurance of
any kind. Inadequate insurance affects persons who are either uninsured, uninsurable, underinsured, or only occasionally insured.

Over sixty percent of the U.S. population has employer-based health insurance coverage, and another twenty-five percent has either private health insurance unconnected to employment or some form of publicly supported health
insurance programs (Medicaid, Medicare, and the like). The remainder of the
population has no health insurance. Many uninsured persons are employed, but
by companies offering no health insurance benefits, especially employees of
small firms for whom the costs of maintaining insurance are much higher than
for large employers; and many employee-benefit packages provide no coverage
for dependents and part-time employees. Almost half of those who are employed but uninsured work in businesses with fewer than 25 employees, and
close to two-thirds of uninsured workers are in firms with 100 or fewer employees.[34]

Other U.S. citizens are *uninsurable,* although they normally would qualify
for group coverage provided by an employer or could afford standard insurance. Roughly seven percent of the uninsured are medically uninsurable by
current underwriting practices.[35] Forms of insurance other than open-enrollment
group plans typically require physical examinations as well as family and personal medical histories as a condition of eligibility. Those with poor health or
risky preexisting conditions or family histories that suggest the potential for
expensive future claims are often denied coverage under exclusion clauses (or
are offered only inferior and more expensive coverage). Insurers use exclusionary clauses that exempt certain illnesses, treatments, or conditions from coverage, and refuse to accept persons in specified occupations or with certain life-

styles. The AIDS crisis has presented dramatic instances of these problems of insurability and underwriting practices. Insurers often appeal to actuarial fairness in defending their decisions, while neglecting social justice. Justice in access to health care depends on protecting the place of fair-opportunity rules, which in turn requires sharing financial risks in an insurance scheme. A deep flaw in the U.S. system, as Norman Daniels has argued, is that both legislators and insurers act as if the uninsured are the responsibility of the other party, while neither assumes the responsibility for rectifying the moral unfairness that results from an actuarially fair system.[36]

As a result, many are denied coverage for the primary condition for which they need coverage, including persons in employer-based plans. They constitute one subgroup of those who, though insured, are *underinsured*. Exclusionary clauses deny access for various types of treatment and exclude coverage for specific diseases, injuries, organ systems, and preexisting conditions. Other persons are *occasionally insured*, sometimes uninsured and sometimes underinsured, because they experience gaps in coverage that are virtually impossible to bridge. These persons move quickly from job to job and suffer from temporary but sometimes lengthy layoffs. Their plight is common. More than a million laborers in the United States lose their insurance for some period of time during the year while they are unemployed, and more than twenty-five percent of the U.S. population changes insurance, with the potential for a gap, during the course of each year. It has been estimated that over fifty-five million U.S. residents are uninsured at some time during any given year.[37]

Many parts of this system are unfair, especially because of the reliance on employers for financing the system. Persons with medium to large size employers are usually better covered and in part are subsidized by tax breaks in the system. By contrast, citizens employed by small employers are usually not covered, and others left with no coverage include part-time employees, unemployed persons, and widows, widowers, and divorcees who were formerly covered by policies for their spouses. When employed persons who are not covered become ill, taxpayers rather than free-riding employers usually pick up the bill. The financing of health care is also regressive. Low-income families pay premiums comparable to and often higher than the premiums paid by high-income families, and many individuals who do not qualify for group coverage pay dramatically more for the same coverage than those who qualify in a group. Finally, eligibility for Medicaid varies dramatically across states, and not one state among fifty covers all citizens who are below the poverty line.

Many proposals to alleviate this situation have been based not on claims of justice, but rather on the virtues of charity, compassion, and benevolence toward sick persons. Health care for the needy in former eras was primarily handled through institutions such as charity hospitals that had been founded on these aspirations of virtue. But in the new era of high technology and commensurately high costs, these ideals have proved inadequate to the task of meeting many health care needs. The older models of voluntary assistance have gradually given way to a widely accepted model of an enforceable right to health care based in justice.

An influential case provides an example of various circumstances of modern health care that have prompted this shift of focus. In June 1985, an uninsured worker with third-degree burns was denied admission to several Dallas-area emergency rooms because he did not have the financial resources to qualify. He could not pay a deposit ranging from five hundred dollars to fifteen hundred dollars. At the second of these several hospitals, North Texas Medical Center, doctors inserted an intravenous tube and a catheter to stabilize liquids (a critical factor for burn patients). But without a deposit, they would not admit him. After seven hours and seventy miles of travel in an automobile seeking admission to various hospitals, he gained admission to Parkland Memorial, a public teaching hospital, where he was given care at a cost of $22,189 for nineteen days of hospitalization and a skin graft. Although several facilities to which he had sought admission declared him a non-emergency case, Parkland considered him "definitely an emergency case."[38]

As a result of this incident and similar cases, a "Texas transfer law" was passed that became a model for national legislation regulating denials and transfers. Many state statutes have been passed to prevent abuses, and the Comprehensive Omnibus Budget Reconciliation Act was passed as a federal law with provisions requiring both careful screening of patients at hospitals and treatment for all patients who arrive under emergency conditions.[39] However, such laws treat only the visible effects of the health care system, not the more difficult underlying causes. Distressed health care institutions will find ways of preventing admission by indigent patients as long as a strong financial incentive exists to do so, and new health care facilities will locate in affluent neighborhoods or with legally enforced restrictions on admission. These motivations and actions will persist until a system of adequate insurance and equitable access is in place.

In the face of these problems, a broad social consensus appears to be emerging in the United States that all citizens should be able to secure equitable access to health care, including insurance coverage without temporal gaps and unjust exclusionary clauses. This consensus rejects many traditional strands of libertarianism that long formed the basis of access to health care in the United States, but the consensus is neither deep nor stable. Many U.S. citizens disagree sharply on a range of political solutions proffered to improve access, on the role of government in these solutions, and on methods of financing them. It is, therefore, unclear whether this fragile consensus will generate a secondary consensus about appropriate public policy, whether it has revolutionary potential for financing access to health care, and whether it can generate a legal right to health care. We will now address these problems, as moral issues, beginning with arguments in support of a moral right to health care.

Arguments Supporting the Right to Health Care

The history of the right to health care has been characterized more by political rhetoric than by careful analysis. The primary question has been whether the government should be involved in health care allocation and distribution, rather than leaving these matters to the marketplace. Libertarians insist that all rights to social goods based on enforced beneficence violate the principle of respect for autonomy. Society has often allowed this libertarian-supported rule of ability to pay to determine the distribution of health goods and services, but we will argue that this rule should not be allowed to serve as our only principle of distributive justice.

Two main arguments support a right to health care: (1) an argument from collective social protection and (2) an argument from fair opportunity.[40] The first argument focuses on the similarities between health needs and other needs that have conventionally been protected by government. Threats to health are relevantly similar to threats presented by crime, fire, and polluted environments. The latter threats are conventionally resisted by collective actions and resources, and many collective schemes to protect health already exist, including programs of environmental protection and sanitation. Consistency suggests that essential health care assistance in response to threats to health should likewise be a collective responsibility. This argument by analogy makes a critical appeal to coherence: If government has an obligation to provide one type of essential service, then it must have an obligation to provide another.

One can attempt to dismiss this argument by maintaining that no public good or service rests on a government obligation and that all such government responsibilities are nonessential and expendable. This line of criticism is appealing against a claim that a legal right to health care exists,[41] but it is morally unpersuasive unless one accepts a libertarian account of justice. On each of the nonlibertarian theories of justice previously explicated, the argument from government services would generate a public obligation to provide some level of goods and services to protect health, and on this basis a correlative right to health care.

However, some relevant dissimilarities between health care and many other public programs exist, including many designed to protect health.[42] In particular, these public programs pertain to social goods, such as the public health, whereas health care is largely a matter of the individual's private good. The analogy to collective social protection therefore requires supplementation. Additional premises are found in society's right to expect a decent return on the investment it has made in physicians' education, funding for biomedical research, and other parts of the medical system that pertain dominantly to health care, as distinct from public health and disease prevention. The return we expect on this taxed investment is health care protection for ourselves. We legitimately expect the scope of protection to extend beyond public health measures, because we fund more training and research in medicine than in public health.

However, we cannot reasonably expect a direct individual return on all collective investments. Some investments seek only the discovery of cures or treatments, not the dispensing of efficacious therapies once discovered. The fact that the United States funds drug research at the National Institutes of Health and drug regulation through the Food and Drug Administration does not justify the expectation that the federal government will subsidize or reimburse our drug purchases (although, in fact, the government does reimburse for drugs in some cases). In the instance of physician education, it might be argued that society invests in training physicians and protecting the public health, not in health care services themselves. This first argument in support of a moral right to health care, then, needs an account of a decent return that is not a full return or refund. We consider this problem (of a decent basic minimum) in the next section.

A second argument buttresses this first argument by appealing to the fair-opportunity rule. From this perspective, the justice of social institutions is gauged by their tendency to counteract lack of opportunity caused by unpredictable bad luck and misfortune over which the person has no meaningful control. Insofar as injury, disability, or disease creates profoundly significant disadvantages and reduces agents' capacity to function properly, justice is done if societal health care resources are used to counter these morally arbitrary, disadvantaging effects and to restore to persons a fair chance to use their capacities.[43] A society cannot discharge its obligation under the fair-opportunity rule without fairly allocating health care resources. All citizens have a right to the resources correlative to this societal obligation.

This general guideline of fair opportunity suggests a path for giving content to the idea of a decent minimum of health care and for setting priorities in the allocation of resources. The need for health care, to restore fair opportunity, is far greater among the seriously diseased and injured, because the costs of health care for them can be uncontrollable and overwhelming, particularly as their health status worsens. In the case of catastrophic illness, and often in the instance of the chronically ill and elderly, adequate private funding is unavailable. An unmanageable lack of access to health care is unjust when health care needs have a powerful effect on opportunity and functional capacity. The rule of fair opportunity asserts that collective moral obligations exist to provide health care at the level needed for persons to receive as fair a chance in life as possible.

Unless additional qualifications were introduced, acceptance of these two arguments for a right to health care would place an immense burden on society. They lead to the conclusion that society is morally obligated to funnel resources toward bringing persons ever closer to the goal of fair opportunity. However, a vast array of disabilities, injuries, and diseases limit opportunity, and many persons are so seriously affected that they could never be restored to a position of fair opportunity, even if immense sums were spent to bring them closer to that ideal. These arguments, then, need to be held in check by an account of allocation that avoids unreasonable demands on social resources in order to implement the right to health care. We will return to this problem later (see pp. 361–369). At this point, we note only that our two arguments for a general right to health care, though programmatic, are strong enough to justify the conclusion that material principles of merit, contribution, and effort are morally inappropriate for health care allocations in response to many health care needs.

Libertarians contest this conclusion and propose instead various free-market arrangements for health care. For example, Engelhardt argues that, "It may very well be unfeeling or unsympathetic not to provide [health care to those in need,] it is another thing to show that one owes others such help in a way that would morally authorize state force to redistribute resources."[44] However, some themes in libertarianism can generate a measure of agreement with the conclusions we have reached. If the libertarian holds that it is *virtuous and ideal* from the moral point of view, but not strictly a matter of *justice,* to provide collective plans of health care, there may in the end be little dispute over which health policies we should adopt—only a dispute over their moral grounding. The primary dispute seems to concern the scope and limits of *enforceable* obligation. Libertarians can insist on a right to retain property free of social compulsion and at the same time assert that morally we should be generous and provide health care services for the indigent. Nozick and Engelhardt propose that we avoid coercive redistribution of goods, but that we nonetheless attempt to achieve the same moral objectives through voluntary agreements or contributions. That is, they deny an enforceable obligation in justice (or in beneficence) but do not deny the worthiness of an unenforceable ideal of benevolence.

Although we disagree with libertarians on these issues of justification and social obligation, it is often advisable to consider whether theoretical disagreements ultimately make a practical difference (as we cautioned in Chapter 2). If a libertarian endorses a morally good outcome identical to ours, then the fact that we disagree over the enforceability of beneficence and the precise contours of (nonlibertarian) justice should not present a practical barrier in health policy. We can still agree to support a two-tiered system of health care, with society ensuring equitable access to the first level.

Even if the arguments we have presented for a *moral right* to health care are rejected on grounds that justice does not support this right, a *legal right* or *entitlement* to health care can be supported on a different moral basis such as compassion and beneficence. The current legal and political climate in the United States that tolerates a lack of equitable access to health care in the face of desperate needs for health insurance is uncaring and below what a morally just society would tolerate, but this situation can perhaps be remedied without appeal to moral rights based in justice, which frequently are disputed precisely at the point they are made legal entitlements to an increased share of social resources.

One attractive argument for a legal right to health care appeals to the role of governmental coordination in effecting charitable goals. According to the "enforced beneficence argument," as Allen Buchanan terms it, beneficent citizens who do not believe that the needy have a right to health care would still establish certain health programs for the needy while coercively requiring those with the resources to sustain the programs.[45] This argument challenges libertarian and egalitarian assumptions that coercive transfers of social resources are justified only if the persons to whom they are transferred have moral rights to the resources. If the goals are sufficiently fundamental and important, coercion can be morally justified to fulfil the goals independent of the existence of rights.

A directly related argument from societal beneficence focuses on the expression of social virtue and excellence in public policies, with an emphasis on creating a morally worthy society with which citizens can identify. This communitarian approach concentrates on compassion for victims of the various lotteries of life. Themes from this approach echo in the influential report of the President's Commission for the Study of Ethical Problems in Medicine and Biomedical Research on *Securing Access to Health Care:* "The depth of a society's concern about health care can be seen as a measure of its sense of solidarity in the face of suffering and death. . . . A society's commitment to health care reflects some of its most basic attitudes about what it means to be a member of the human community."[46]

Several different arguments, then, support the conclusion that a morally good society should ensure access to a basic level of health care. *Required* payments in an equitable system will be fairer to those already willing to cooperate and will be socially efficient. A good contemporary example of the need for a scheme of enforcement and coordination is found in the aforementioned private health insurance coverage that forms the hub of the payment system in the United States. Employers are not obligated to provide insurance, and no enforceable scheme of contributions exists, although states are permitted to regulate certain activities of insurance companies. As health and other costs increase, employers find it more difficult to offer insurance to employees. Many employers provide no health care benefits, thereby leaving their employees uninsured or only minimally insured. Firms that do provide their employees with insurance are left at a competitive disadvantage and resent competitor firms who, in effect, refuse to shoulder the burden of paying a fair share of the insurance costs. The noncontributing firms are competitively advantaged free-riders in the system of funding health care, and for this reason more and more firms that supply health insurance for their employees have come to favor mandatory contributions in an enforceable system of health care insurance.

This so-called *mandating* is a way of leveling the playing field fairly by not allowing free-riders to avoid paying a fair share while shifting costs to others. Many firms are now willing to give up their control to contract for employee health care benefits in order to achieve a more efficient and equitable system. They rightly see that such a system can be maintained only by laws that mandate.[47] This argument need not move to the conclusion that firms should be required to supply private health insurance. Economic realities such as wage levels, corporate finance, and various costs might make this approach to mandating inefficient and unfair. The appropriate conclusion is that a more efficient and equitable system is needed, but not necessarily a system exclusively featuring either public or private insurance, and not necessarily an egalitarian system either.

The Scope of the Right to Health Care

Apart from the contest between libertarian and nonlibertarian views of justice, an intractable, and ultimately the most important, problem is how to specify the entitlements and limits established by a right to health care. Two broad views have attracted wide contemporary support: a right to equal access to health care and a right to a decent minimum of health care. Both rely on egalitarian premises. The former represents a strong egalitarian perspective of equal access to *all* bona fide health care resources. The latter incorporates only a weak egalitarian point of view, viz., equal access to *fundamental* health care resources.

"Access to health care" takes on several meanings in these discussions. Sometimes it means only that no one is legitimately prevented from obtaining health care. Therefore, having a right of access does not entail that any health care must be provided by others or that a system must equitably distribute care. This interpretation is favored by libertarians. More commonly, a right of access to health care refers to a right to obtain specified goods and services to which every entitled person has an equal claim. An expansive view of the right of access requires that everyone have equal access to every treatment that is available to anyone. In none of these conceptions is it proposed that a right of access involves a right to a good health outcome. The only demand is that persons be given a fair opportunity for a good outcome.

Those who promote access to a decent minimum or adequate level of care usually do not specify where to set limits on expenditures for health care that confer precise entitlements. The right to a decent minimum of health care suggests, but need not entail, a government obligation to meet the basic health needs of all citizens, at least an obligation to function as a last resort. (None of the arguments we have presented for a right to health care is powerful enough to establish jurisdictional responsibility for funding or administration.) The societal obligation can be discharged at various levels, but the decent-minimum approach entails acceptance of the two-tiered system of health care mentioned above: enforced social coverage for basic and catastrophic health needs (tier 1), together with voluntary private coverage for other health needs and desires (tier 2). On the first tier, distribution is based on need, and needs are met by equal, universal access to basic services. Better services might be made available for purchase at personal expense at the second tier, but everyone's basic health needs would be met at the first tier. The first tier would presumably cover at least public health measures and preventive care, primary care, acute care, and special social services for those with disabilities. In this conception, society's obligations are not limitless and are regulated by a general model of a safety net for everyone, and this model must be accompanied by an account of justifiable social allocations. Otherwise "the decent minimum" is a vague abstraction.

Although some parties will be distressed to learn that the standard is "decent" care rather than "optimum" care, only the former can be justified in a socially funded policy. When we later in this chapter discuss explicit health policies such as the pioneering Oregon health plan, we will see that it is unrealistic to expect a higher level than adequate care. Rationing will also be an essential part of the process. Otherwise priorities cannot be set and maintained. (The rationing program should exclude services rather than patients.)

This proposal has the advantage of holding out the potential for compromise among libertarians, utilitarians, communitarians, and egalitarians, because it incorporates some moral concerns stressed by each of these theories. It guarantees basic health care for all on a premise of equal access, while allowing unequal additional purchase by individual initiative and contract. It mixes private and public forms of distribution, and it affirms collective as well as free-market methods of delivering health care. Utilitarians should find the proposal attractive because it serves to minimize public dissatisfaction and to maximize social utility, without demanding unduly burdensome taxation. It also permits allocation decisions based in part on such formal techniques as cost-effectiveness analysis. The egalitarian finds an opportunity to use an equal access principle and to see fair opportunity embedded in the distributional system. The communitarian perspective, too, is not neglected. A societal consensus about values, even if only rough and incomplete, is required for a practicable system. The common good is a basic point of reference for public deliberation about how to establish the decent minimum. Finally, the libertarian sees an opportunity for free-market production and distribution. The two-tiered system provides indigents with opportunities for health care that would otherwise not be available to them, and various forms of competition and incentives may be used as tools to increase the system's productivity and the quality of health care.

A health care system that finds pockets of support from each of these types of ethical theory could also turn out to be the fairest approach to democratic reform of the system. There is not now and is not likely soon to be a single viable theory of social justice. Each theory has its attractive and unattractive features, and many citizens are appropriately fearful of the social consequences of adopting one of these philosophical systems as the sole basis for justice in health policy. Experience suggests that appeals to one of these accounts of justice works well in some contexts but yields disastrous results in others. A coherent system that draws from each of these theories seems especially appropriate if only a minority is likely to agree on the nature, value, and acceptability of a general theory of justice.

Despite these attractions, the decent-minimum proposal has proved difficult to explicate and implement. It raises problems of whether society can fairly, consistently, and unambiguously devise a public policy that recognizes a right to care for primary needs without creating a right to exotic and expensive forms of treatment, such as liver transplants costing over $200,000 for what many deem to be marginal benefits in quality-adjusted life-years. More importantly, the model is purely programmatic until society defines what *decent minimum* means in operational terms. This task is, we believe, the major problem confronting health policy in the United States today.

An abstract right to health care must be specified for operational purposes through allocation decisions. Trade-offs are invariably involved in establishing precise entitlements, and no right to health care will trump all competing claims of social utility or the common good when larger questions of macroallocation are considered. This task is far too complex to be addressed by ethical theory. An acceptable system of entitlements to a decent minimum of health care must remove the gaps in health care insurance discussed above, without at the same time deeply disturbing levels of employment, employment opportunities, and incentives to employers. Health policy also should not frustrate vital social goals, such as government allocation to other entitlement programs and the system of free-market competition in the development of health care technologies. No reason exists to believe that any single plan is the only one that can be just and justified. Complex social, political, economic, and cultural beliefs therefore will all play a legitimate role in shaping how a community that recognizes a rule of fair opportunity implements an entitlement to health care.

A range of ethically acceptable policies can appropriately specify the right to health care. Within that range, good reasons sometimes exist for viewing one or more approaches as preferable in light of the overall circumstances. But ethics does not exhaust life's demands and options, and problems of feasibility are crucial. Although we cannot fix an entitlement to health care or a comprehensive public policy allocation decision in this book, we can further explore some inherent conceptual and moral problems, including the place of individual responsibility for ill health and the moral foundations of allocation decisions.

Forfeiting the Right to Health Care

If we assume that all citizens enjoy a right to a decent minimum of health care, can particular individuals forfeit that right even when they wish to preserve it? The question is not whether a person loses the full range of entitlements under the right to health care, but whether he or she forfeits the right to certain forms of care through actions that result in ill health and generate the health care needs. Examples include patients who acquired AIDS as a result of unsafe sexual activities or intravenous drug use, smokers with lung cancer, and alcoholics who develop liver disease. When people engage in such actions, does society have the same obligation to provide health care to them as it does to patients who need care because of bad luck in life's lottery of health?

Just as a person can forfeit his or her right to liberty by antisocial behavior, some argue that a person can forfeit his or her right to health care by failing to act responsibly. It is unfair, they charge, for individuals to pay higher premiums or taxes to support people who voluntarily engage in risky actions, and it is fair to withhold societal funds from needy individuals whose medical needs resulted from voluntary risk-taking.[48] This conclusion does not conflict with the rule of fair opportunity, because any lack of opportunity experienced by an individual resulted from his or her voluntary actions.

However, if principles of justice, strictly conceived, invalidate a risk-taker's claim to the full decent minimum of health care resources, several equally compelling principles raise questions about how far risk-takers can fairly be excluded from coverage. A policy of withholding societal funds cannot be justified unless several conditions are met. First, it must be possible to identify and differentiate various causal factors in morbidity, such as natural causes, the social environment, and personal activities. Then it must be confirmed that a pertinent disease or illness resulted from personal activities, rather than some other cause. It must also be shown that the personal activities in question were autonomous, in the sense that the actors were aware of the risks and accepted them. If the risks are unknown at the time of action, individuals cannot be justly held responsible for them, and if an individual is unaware of a particular risk of which other people are aware, additional questions must be addressed about whether it is fair to use the standard of what a reasonable person should have known.

Regarding the first condition, it is virtually impossible to isolate causal factors for many critical cases of ill health because of the complexity of causal links and the limitations of our knowledge. Medical needs often result from the conjunction of genetic predispositions, personal actions, and environmental and social conditions. The respective roles of these different factors will often be impossible to establish with reasonable certainty on the basis of scientific evidence. Whereas it is often possible to determine responsibility for an injury in mountain climbing or skiing, it is not possible to determine with certainty whether a particular individual's lung cancer resulted from personal cigarette smoking, passive smoking, environmental pollution, occupational conditions, or heredity (or some combination of these causal conditions). If, as many argue, ill health is broadly rooted in socially induced causes such as environmental pollutants and infant feeding practices, then the class of diseases covered by the right to a decent minimum will expand as evidence concerning the causal role of these factors increases. In the meantime, social policy may rest more on ignorance of causal factors than on knowledge.

Individuals also may not be *fully* responsible for some of their voluntary risky actions. Individual risk-taking sometimes has genetic roots or sociocultural roots. A denial of a person's right to health care would be unfair if the person could not have acted otherwise, or could have acted otherwise only with great difficulty. This point is relevant if a self-harming behavior is motivated in part by factors beyond the person's control. As in the case of criminal justice, denial of individual responsibility on the basis of genetic or environmental factors can be overplayed, and legitimate questions exist about whether particular lifestyles or behavioral patterns are substantially nonvoluntary.

Problems in policing the system are also relevant. To determine accurately the causal conditions of particular health problems and to locate voluntary risk-takers, officials would have to investigate the causes. In the worst-case scenario, these officials would be authorized to invade privacy, break confidentiality, and keep detailed records in order to document health abuses that could result in a forfeiture of the right to a particular type of health care. Such enforcement would be costly in addition to its morally unattractive features.

A major reason for the ongoing debates about forfeiture of rights to health care is rising costs, but prevention of risks through alterations in lifestyle and conduct often leads to counterintuitive outcomes. Some risk-taking requires less rather than more medical care, because it results in earlier and quicker deaths than might occur if the individual lived longer and developed a chronic debilitating condition. For example, Louise Russell used cost-effectiveness analysis to compare health care costs in groups of men of the same age who had the same blood serum cholesterol levels. She consistently found that "low-risk," non-smoking men with low blood pressure generate far higher health care costs per year of life than "high-risk" men who smoke and have high blood pressure.[49] When extended to include programs for the elderly, the cost-benefit case for denying care to individual risk-takers may disappear altogether. As noted earlier, we should expect an increase rather than a decrease in overall expenditures for both health care and social security as a result of controlling health risks.[50]

It would, nonetheless, be fair to require individuals who engage in certain risky actions that result in costly medical needs to pay higher premiums or taxes. Risk-takers might be required to contribute more to particular pools such as insurance schemes or to pay a tax on their risky conduct, such as an increased tax on cigarettes. Public-opinion surveys indicate that Americans more strongly favor increased liquor and cigarette taxes to help finance health care than any other form of tax for any purpose.[51] These requirements may fairly redistribute the burdens of the costs of health care, and they may deter risky conduct without disrespecting autonomy.

Questions about individual responsibility and the just allocation of health care have emerged with special poignancy in patients with alcohol-related end-stage liver failure who need liver transplants. Liver transplantation has recently improved the patient's chances of survival and a higher quality of life. By 1988 seventy-six percent of the liver transplant recipients survived for one year, and sixty-nine percent of liver grafts survived for one year.[52] However, despite dramatic increases in the number of liver transplants, from 15 in 1980 to 924 in 1986 to 2,946 in 1991, donated livers are scarce, and many patients suffering from end-stage liver failure (ESLF) die before they can obtain transplants. A major cause of ESLF is excessive use of alcohol that results in cirrhosis of the liver, raising the question whether patients who have alcohol-related ESLF should be excluded from waiting lists for liver transplants or should be given lower priority than other patients with ESLF. Arguments for their lower priority or total exclusion often appeal to the probability that they will resume a pattern of alcohol abuse and again experience ESLF, thereby wasting the transplanted liver. However, studies have demonstrated that patients with alcohol-related ESLF who receive a liver transplant and abstain from alcohol do as well as patients whose ESLF resulted from other causes.[53] Liver transplantation can be a sobering experience, and some centers and funding agencies already require waiting periods of a year to establish abstinence. A good case can therefore be made for not excluding alcohol-related ESLF patients altogether, but for introducing conditions that require demonstrated abstention from alcohol.

Alvin Moss and Mark Siegler would require that patients with alcohol-related ESLF (over fifty percent of the patients with ESLF) automatically receive a lower priority ranking in the allocation of donated livers than patients who develop end-stage liver disease through no fault of their own.[54] Their argument appeals to fairness, fair opportunity, and utility. They contend that it is fair to hold people responsible for their decisions, and then to allocate organs with a view to utilitarian outcomes because priorities must be set for transplantation. Although alcoholism is a chronic disease, alcoholics have a responsibility to seek effective treatment, which depends for its effectiveness on the patient's acknowledging the diagnosis and assuming responsibility for treatment. Assigning lower priority to patients with alcohol-related ESLF is unfortunate, Moss and Siegler argue, but fair: "It is fairer to give a child dying of biliary atresia an opportunity for a first normal liver than it is to give a patient with [alcohol-related ESLF] who was born with a normal liver a second one." Moss and Siegler also use the utilitarian argument that public support is indispensable for liver transplantation, both for securing funds and for securing donations of organs from the public. Transplanting donated livers into patients with alcohol-related ESLF on an equal priority basis could reduce public support for liver transplantation, and this consequence could be devastating for transplant programs.

However, this utilitarian argument may unjustly allow existing social prejudices about alcoholics to determine who receives transplants.[55] It would be unjust to allow judgments about past behavior to determine allocation criteria for those who have reformed their alcohol habits. A consensus currently exists in transplantation societies and committees that patients with alcohol-related ESLF should not be totally excluded. Ideally, they should be considered on a case-by-case basis (looking at medical need and probability of successful transplantation), rather than automatically receiving a lower priority. An individual can then receive a lower priority rating when it is warranted, as the following examples indicate: (1) If a transplant recipient fails through personal negligence to take his or her immunosuppressant medication and the transplant then fails, it would not be unjust for the transplant team to give that person a lower priority for a second transplant or to deny him or her a second transplant. (2) For the alcoholic who fails to seek effective treatment for alcoholism and develops alcohol-related ESLF, a *lower priority* is justified, although *total exclusion* needs a stronger argument than has yet been produced. Individual responsibility is therefore relevant from the standpoint of justice.

The issues raised by this debate will intensify when lung transplantation becomes more common and more cigarette smokers seek transplants, often in competition with patients who have lethal genetic conditions such as cystic fibrosis.

The Allocation of Health Care Resources

Detailed specification of the right to a decent minimum of health care encounters both theoretical and practical difficulties of just and justified social allocations. We cannot here address specific issues such as cost containment in hospitals, methods of reducing infant mortality rates, tax deductions for medical care, and incentives to employers and third-party payers. We can, however, present and assess arguments for and against different procedures, standards, and systems for allocating health care.

To allocate is to distribute by allotment. Such distribution does not presuppose either a person or a system that rations resources. A criterion of ability to pay in a competitive market, for example, is a form of allocation. "Macroallocation" decisions determine the funds to be expended and the goods made available, as well as the methods of distribution. "Microallocation" decisions, by contrast, determine who will receive particular scarce resources. This distinction between the macro and the micro levels of allocation is useful, but the line between them is not sharp, and they often interact.

Norman Daniels correctly argues that the scope and design of basic health care institutions involve allocation decisions to determine the following:

1. What kinds of health care services will exist in a society?
2. Who will receive them and on what basis?
3. Who will deliver them?
4. How will the burdens of financing them be distributed?
5. How will the power and control of those services be distributed?[56]

These decisions about the allocation of funds determine how much health care to allocate and what kind of health care to provide for which problems. Many of these decisions have far-reaching effects on other patterns of allocation. For example, the funds allocated for medical and biological research at The National Institutes of Health (NIH) affect the training programs for and distribution of physicians in the United States. Specific monetary allocations affect the choice of a profession, a specialty, an institution, a location, etc.

Problems of allocation are classifiable by types, each of which involves competition among desirable programs or alternatives. We will distinguish four distinct, yet interrelated types. The third and fourth are of particular importance for the remainder of this chapter.

1. Partitioning the Comprehensive Social Budget

Every large political unit operates with a budget, which includes allocations for health and for other social goods, including housing, education, culture, defense, and recreation. Health is not our only value or goal, and expenditures for other goods inevitably compete for limited resources with health-targeted expenditures. Some commentators argue that controversies about such competition are political rather than moral and should be resolved through political processes, as long as those processes contain morally just procedures that reflect the values, preferences, and priorities of the entire society. The thesis is that only in such a forum can we determine whether public funding for health care is adequate.[57] Under this argument, a citizen cannot complain of injustice if society uses a morally justified procedure to allocate more money to space programs or defense programs than to health programs.

This line of argument is reasonable, but a proviso must be added. If a society did not allocate sufficient funds to provide the decent minimum of health care, the system itself would not be just. Questions about the justice or injustice of particular allocation decisions—for example, to fund or not to fund heart transplants—cannot be adequately processed or resolved until a guarantee of a decent minimum has already been made.

2. Allocating within the Health Budget

The next type of allocation decision concerns how to allocate funds from within the budget segment devoted to health. We protect and promote health in many ways besides the provision of medical care, because health and disease are affected by many parts of the social system. Health services and benefits are often supplied by experts in pollution control, drug experimentation, toxicology, epidemiology, engineering, law, and the like, rather than by health care professionals. Health policies and programs for occupational safety, environmental protection, injury prevention, consumer protection, food and drug control, among others are parts of society's effort to protect and promote the health of its citizens.

The term *health resources*, then, is not a substitute for *medical resources*, and the budget for health vastly exceeds the portion for health care. Many policy questions arise as a result. For example, some commentators have rightly noted that equalizing medical care is not the most effective strategy for equalizing the opportunity for health, in view of the impact of the standard of living, housing, sanitation, and the like on health.[58]

3. Allocating within the Health Care Budget

Once society has determined its budget for health care, it still must allocate its resources within health care. Certain projects and procedures will be selected for funding and others rejected. Many decisions must be made, including whether priority should go to prevention or treatment.[59] Expenditures for treatment are far higher in the current health care system, but government officials might opt to concentrate on preventing heart disease rather than on rescuing individuals by heart transplants or artificial hearts. In many cases preventive care is more effective and more efficient than crisis medicine in saving lives, reducing suffering, raising levels of health, and lowering costs. How society might appropriately mix preventive and treatment strategies will depend in part on knowledge of causal links, such as those between disease and environmental and behavioral factors. Polio vaccine and preventive dentistry are standard examples of success in preventive care, but these models do not work well for kidney failure and heart failure, where preventive care is more speculative, in part because numerous medical problems can cause these organs to fail.

However, concentration on prevention can lead to neglect of needy persons who would benefit directly from critical care. Preventive care typically reduces morbidity and premature mortality for unknown, "statistical lives," whereas critical interventions concentrate on known, "identifiable lives."[60] Society has historically been more likely to favor identified persons and to allocate resources for critical care, even if evidence exists that preventive care is more effective and efficient. Sometimes the public becomes alarmed by its allocation patterns when it becomes aware, for example, that, despite widespread publicity, private funds cannot be raised for a leukemia victim who needs a bone marrow transplant.[61] Yet good evidence exists to show that every public health dollar targeted at poorer communities for some preventive measures, such as prenatal care, saves many times that amount in future care. Accordingly, our moral intuitions often drive us in two conflicting directions: Allocate more to rescue persons in medical need and allocate more to prevent persons from falling into such need.

Determining which categories of injury, illness, or disease (if any) should receive a priority ranking in the allocation of health care resources is another vital aspect of allocation. For example, should heart disease have priority over cancer? When discussing equal access to a decent minimum of medical care, we typically start with medical need, in contrast to geography, finances, and the like, as the proper basis for an allocation decision. But, from the standpoint of public policy, it is often essential to give categories of demonstrated medical need priority rankings in research and therapy. In trying to determine priorities among medical needs, policymakers should examine various diseases in terms of such factors as their communicability, frequency, cost, associated pain and suffering, and impact on length of life and quality of life. It might be justified, for instance, to concentrate less on killer diseases, such as some forms of cancer, and more on widespread disabling diseases, such as arthritis.

4. Allocating Scarce Treatments for Patients

Because health needs and desires are virtually limitless, every health care system faces some form of scarcity, and not everyone who needs a particular form of health care can gain access to it. Numerous medical resources and supplies such as penicillin, insulin, kidney dialysis, cardiac transplantation, and space in intensive care units have been allocated for specific patients or classes of patients. These decisions are more difficult when an illness is life-threatening and the scarce resource potentially life-saving. The question can become, "Who shall live when not everyone can live?" Such allocation occurs in the United Kingdom by several means, including queuing and the use of restrictive criteria for services,[62] and health care has often been nonsystematically allocated in the United States by ability to pay for health care or health insurance.

Allocation decisions of type 3 above and allocation decisions of type 4 interact. Type 3 decisions partially determine the necessity and extent of patient selection by determining the availability and supply of a particular resource. In contrast, distress at making difficult choices through explicit decisions of type 4 sometimes leads society to modify its macroallocation policies to increase the supply of the resource. For example, in the face of difficult allocation decisions about dialysis machines, officials in the United States provided funds to ensure near-universal access to kidney dialysis and kidney transplantation without regard for ability to pay. One plausible explanation is that the society could not tolerate explicit rationing through anonymous committees that resulted in the deaths of identified persons.[63]

In the remaining two major sections of this chapter we discuss in more detail the types of allocation decision categorized above as types 3 and 4. Both are today discussed in biomedical ethics under the topic of *rationing,* and related terms, such as *triage.* The choice of terms is not unimportant, because each term has a different history and some terms have undergone significant changes in meaning. *Rationing,* for example, originally did not suggest harshness or an emergency. It meant a form of allowance, share, or portion, as when food is divided into rations in the military.

Only recently has *rationing* been linked to limited resources, crisis management, and the setting of priorities in the health care budget. *Rationing* now has three primary meanings. The first is closely related to "denial from lack of resources." In a market economy, for example, all types of goods, including health care, are to some extent rationed by ability to pay. A second sense of *rationing* derives not from market limits but from social policy limits: The government determines an allowance or allotment, and those who can afford the good are denied access beyond the allotted amount. The rationing of gasoline and certain types of food during a war crisis are well-known examples, but any national health care system that does not allow purchases of goods or insurance beyond an allotted amount is also an example. Finally, according to a third meaning of *rationing,* an allowance or allotment is determined and distributed equitably, but those who can afford additional goods are not denied access beyond the allotted amount. In this third form, rationing involves elements of each of the first two forms: An allowance is fixed by public policy, and those who cannot afford additional units are thereby denied access. Medicare operates on this principle. All persons of a certain age receive an allotment, but those who can afford it may purchase additional insurance, goods, and services.

We will use *rationing* in each of the three senses, taking care to distinguish between them as necessary, but we will concentrate on rationing in the third sense.

Rationing through Priorities in the Health Care Budget

Many people now believe that the primary task in macroallocation of health care is to establish priorities in the health care system (type 3 above). Structuring clear priorities has been difficult in many countries, and, by many accounts, seriously inadequate in the United States. The 1965 law that established Medicare for the aged and the October 1972 extension of Medicare coverage to dialysis patients were historically and symbolically important developments. These developments reflect unprecedented change in the traditional libertarian strategy of financing health care in the United States. However, no systematic account of health care rationing has emerged.

Health care costs have risen dramatically in the United States as a result of several conditions—in particular, good insurance, new technology, and longer life in the aging population. When parties who are insured pay far less than the value of what they consume, they will consume more than they otherwise would. Insured patients typically pay between ten percent and twenty-five percent of the costs of their covered health care; insurance pays the rest. Excellent insurance, especially when provided without assessment by an employer or the government, tends to increase spending. Physicians and patients alike have an incentive to use any service, irrespective of cost, as long as it is covered. New technology and services compound this problem as they become available and are covered. Developments in expensive diagnostic equipment such as magnetic resonance imaging (MRI) and therapeutic interventions such as heart transplantation raise health care costs more rapidly than costs in other sectors. The elderly then consume more of these services and live longer. Health policy is confronted with all of these problems, and even clever plans of cost savings and waste reduction have failed to reduce inflationary pressures, to increase access to services, or to silence calls for rationing.

These problems of contemporary health policy are extraordinarily complicated, and we can here consider only a small number of the current debates. We will deal with three substantive issues, each selected because of ways in which moral reasoning is involved in health policy decisions. The three issues are (1) setting priorities in Oregon's health care budget, (2) rationing by age, and (3) allocating and funding heart transplants.

Setting Priorities in Oregon

Legislators and citizens in the State of Oregon have presented a closely watched attempt to establish priorities in allocating health care. Oregon's plan is the first for systematic rationing of health care funds in the United States, and it has become a focal point for discussion of every major aspect of national health policy, including access to care, cost-effectiveness, rationing, and the decent minimum. As such, it could mark the beginning of a new era in American medical care that brings it closer to the more systematic approaches to rationing adopted in many other countries.[64]

Faced with escalating costs and demands for more efficient and fairer access to quality health care,[65] the Oregon legislature passed a Basic Health Services Act in July 1989 designed to ensure that all citizens with a family income below the federal poverty level would receive a decent minimum of health care coverage. (The plan also included provisions for those above the poverty level by requiring workplace-based coverage for all employees and an all-payers' high-risk insurance pool.) The state established a committee charged to develop a "priority list" of hundreds of medical procedures for Medicaid (the state/federal program that provides funds to cover medical needs for financially impoverished citizens). The list ranged "from the most important to the least important" services, based in part on data about quality of well-being after treatment. State officials sought to extend coverage to a larger percentage of its citizens through its allocated Medicaid funds, and to do so both efficiently and fairly. The goal was to fund as many top priority-ranked services as possible for all eligible citizens under the principle that there is a basic social obligation to provide universal access to a decent minimum of health care.

This act also created the Oregon Health Services Commission (OHSC), which was charged with producing a ranked list of services that would define the idea of a decent minimum of coverage by Medicaid. In 1990, the OHSC issued a preliminary list of 1,600 ranked medical procedures that formed the centerpiece of the plan. The ranking was based heavily on a cost-effectiveness analysis. Later the list was reduced to 709 ranked services, and cost-effectiveness analysis was abandoned, although judgments about the expected quality of life of patients who have undergone a procedure remained a central consideration in its position in the rankings.

A treatment's rank was determined in large measure by the degree of benefit expected from the treatment. Estimates of the effect of treatments on the quality of life was the weightiest factor in determining the priority of the listed items. The following policy eventually emerged: If predetermined spending levels are insufficient to fund all desirable services when the plan is set in motion, services with the lowest priority will be eliminated from coverage. Medicaid funding will be provided for all persons needing procedures as far down the list as possible, giving priority to the higher-ranked procedures. No person's eligibility for Medicaid coverage is cut under the plan, and in this respect everyone is treated equally. However, health care is rationed because providers must limit covered services to procedures that fall within the predetermined levels.

The quality-adjusted life-years (QALY) approach discussed in Chapter 5 has played an important role in the history of Oregon's ranking of medical procedures. This approach helps rank procedures by considering both the change in health status offered by the treatment to the average patient and its associated effect on the quality of life. Because the data collected for the ranking of treatments focus on how the treatment *changes* the quality of life for the average patient receiving that treatment (the treatment's net benefit), and not on the quality of life at a given point after treatment, even disabled patients are presumably not penalized for having serious debilitating diseases or handicapping injuries. The system is designed to ensure that the very sick are not discriminated against and places them on an equal footing with the relatively healthy in this respect. (The elderly, the blind, and the disabled are excluded from the ranking scheme, as are a few long-term health services, thereby giving certain classes of persons special rights to health care.) However, utilitarian criteria are also part of the plan because final rankings consider the life-sustaining impact of a treatment.[66]

In sacrificing high-cost operations that benefit only a few patients in favor of a minimal level of health care for all residents, Oregon has implicitly relied on a theory of justice in making its determinations. Supporters of the scheme argue that only by such explicit and principled ranking and exclusion of certain treatments can the state achieve a just system that overcomes the implicit and haphazard ranking system that has characterized U.S. health care.[67]

Critics contend that the Oregon plan contains serious defects because it favors many relatively minor treatments over lifesaving treatments, fosters an "us versus them" conception of health care through its focus on benefits to the poor and on priority rankings, and lacks specificity about the conditions and treatments that will and will not be covered. Proponents of the plan, by contrast, point to the expanded access and coverage, as well as to projections of better health outcomes for the poor. The goal of a statewide system of universal health insurance without creating special burdens for the poor has been heralded by the plan's supporters, who also maintain that it will eliminate procedures deemed ineffective by the medical community or unnecessary by the general public.[68]

The sensitive issue of who will suffer a setback under the Oregon plan has proved troublesome to resolve. Clearly some groups, such as extremely premature infants, fare poorly under the plan (because treatments offer minimal to no improvement in quality of life), and some fare well by being ensured coverage. For example, the plan excludes the disabled and the elderly from loss of eligibility, and these groups should continue to receive the same benefits as before. However, some argue that the plan's use of quality-of-life criteria constitutes discrimination against persons with disabilities,[69] and others have argued that Oregon's rating of net benefit by category of treatment is intrinsically unfair, because some patients needing any given treatment will do far better on the treatment than some other patients needing the identical treatment.

In the final analysis, as Norman Daniels has noted, the basic funding must be expanded to avoid making many poor people worse off than they were prior to the plan's enactment. If current Medicaid recipients are made worse off, this fact by itself constitutes a serious objection to the plan even if a net reduction of inequality in the treatment of the poor is achieved through the plan.[70] Accordingly, the fairness of the plan depends on whether, because of its provisions, indigent persons suffer harms (setbacks to their interests); whether enough is being done for indigent persons in the state; and whether alternative policies might further improve the position of indigent persons.

Age-Based Rationing

A second issue focuses not on rationing by excluding services, as in the Oregon plan, but on rationing by excluding persons in a particular age group. Age has sometimes functioned in U.S. policy to provide advantages for the elderly— for example, in Medicare entitlements—but the elderly have also been disadvantaged by various policies. In the United Kingdom, elderly end-stage kidney patients have often been excluded from dialysis and transplantation because of their age, although a policy of rationing by age has not been explicitly formulated.[71]

Several arguments have been offered to justify the explicit use of age in allocation policies, both in assigning priorities for research and treatment and in selecting particular patients for a treatment such as dialysis. These proposals sometimes rest on judgments about the probability of successful treatment. For instance, age has been offered as an indicator of the probability of surviving a major operation. Age would then be medically relevant in selecting patients for various forms of transplantation. Determining the probability of success also can include the length of time that the recipient of an organ is expected to survive, a period that is usually shorter for an older patient than for a younger patient. If anticipated quality-adjusted life-years are used in allocation, younger patients will typically do far better than older patients.

If the age of fifty-five were used as a cut-off point for kidney dialysis in the United States (as it has been implicitly used in the United Kingdom), the population receiving this procedure would be reduced by over fifty percent, with large cost savings to the publicly supported End-Stage Renal Disease Program of Medicare. The population of patients sixty-five years and older has continually increased during the years of the program, in part because older recipients benefit substantially from dialysis, just as they do from other advanced technologies such as kidney transplantation and heart transplantation.[72]

However, some philosophers have mounted impressive arguments to justify age-based allocation of health care, both in principle and in practice. Their arguments have a particular resonance in a society in which approximately thirty million elderly U.S. citizens (sixty-five and older) receive over one-third of the national annual health care expenditures, although they represent only about twelve percent of the population. Their numbers continue to increase, particularly those eighty-five years old and older. In industrialized Western nations, a greater percentage of health care resources is spent on the elderly over age 65 than on the entire population under age 65. For example, Belgium (the lowest) spends 1.7 times more and Finland 5.5 times more on health care for citizens over age 65 than for citizens under age 65.[73] These figures make many Western societies receptive to age-based allocation.

One influential argument for viewing age as different from race and gender for purposes of health care allocation has been offered by Norman Daniels.[74] Building on his Rawlsian theory of fair equality of opportunity, Daniels constructs an argument based on prudential decisions from the perspective of an entire lifetime rather than a particular moment in time. Each age group represents a stage in a person's life span. The idea is to allocate resources prudently throughout the stages of life within a social system that provides a *fair lifetime share* of health care for each citizen. As prudent deliberators, we would choose (assuming conditions of scarcity) to distribute health care over a lifetime in a way that improved our chances of attaining a normal life span. We would, Daniels argues, reject a pattern that gave us a reduced chance of reaching a normal life span but an increased chance of living beyond a normal life span if we became elderly. By shifting resources to the treatment of younger persons that might otherwise have been consumed in prolonging the lives of the elderly, we maximize each person's chances of living a normal life span. A just system would distribute health care to protect individuals' fair shares of the normal opportunity range discussed previously.

In this argument, health policies are not unjust if they treat the young and the old differently, as long as each person is treated the same way over the course of a lifetime. This policy is consistent with fair equality of opportunity, and no basis exists for a claim of unequal treatment. Assuming appropriate conditions of scarcity, age-based rationing seems morally justified.[75] Daniels, then, justifies age-based health care allocation in a just society in terms of a prudence-driven interpretation of fair opportunity that encourages us to invest more of our resources into decreasing early death and less into extending the lives of the elderly.

However, it is questionable whether this justification can be fairly applied in current societies because of the unjustifiable inequalities in the larger health care system, which, on Daniels's own terms, would make it unjustifiable to introduce age-based distribution of health care. (One might similarly argue that the Oregon plan is acceptable only if unjustifiable inequalities are first removed from the larger health system.) Daniels, then, has made a plausible case for justifying age discrimination in a way that race and gender discrimination cannot be justified.

In contrast to the perspective of individual prudence and fair equality of opportunity over the life span, another approach to age-based health care rationing, proposed by Daniel Callahan, takes a communitarian perspective.[76] He argues that society should guarantee decent and basic care to all individuals, but not unlimited efforts to conquer illness and death. Our goal should be to help the elderly live out a full and natural life span in which life's possibilities have "on the whole been achieved" and after which death is a "relatively acceptable event." When the natural life span has been reached in the late seventies or early eighties, the goal should be to relieve suffering rather than to claim life-extending care, although long-term care and support services should be provided as part of the basic minimum of care.[77]

Both of these calls for age-based rationing face moral, political, and practical problems.[78] Ageist attitudes and practices in the United States may not be sufficiently alterable to implement strong age-based rationing while achieving solidarity and equity. Such proposals could easily perpetuate injustice by stereotyping the elderly, by treating them as scapegoats because of increases in health care costs, and by creating unnecessary conflicts between generations. Elderly persons in each succeeding generation will complain that they did not have access to new technologies that were developed (often using their taxes for funding) after they passed through their earlier years, and they will claim that it would be unfair to deny them those technologies now. These complaints would exist at the beginning of age-based allocation and would persist through new technological developments.

Some critics also contend that age-based rationing of life-extending technologies would not save substantially on resources, in part because the provision of care, including long-term care and support services, is expensive and cannot always be sharply differentiated from the care that prolongs life. Although six percent of the enrollees in Medicare who die within a year cost the program twenty-eight percent of its budget during that year, some experts argue that saving the costs of the last few weeks of life would not produce large reductions of costs overall, and they note difficulties for many diseases in predicting the final weeks of life.[79]

Nonetheless, in light of the prudential life span framework, some age-based health care allocation is both just and justified under some circumstances. We agree with Daniels that in principle, age-based allocations of health care do not violate the fair-opportunity rule. However, in the United States at this time, age-based allocation would be unjust. Until a more systematic approach is taken to ensure equitable access in U.S. health care, we are doubtful that issues about age-based rationing can be fairly decided.

Allocating and Funding Heart Transplants

We now shift to a debate about rationing that turns less on excluding services or persons in groups and more on excluding particular individuals.

Controversies over the funding of heart transplants began shortly after cardiac transplantation became increasingly effective in the 1980s as a result of medical improvements that included immunosuppressant medication. In 1980 only thirty-six heart transplants occurred in the United States, but the numbers increased dramatically in the next decade. By 1990 the figure was close to 2100.[80] This increase is somewhat surprising, because the average cost per heart transplant is well over one hundred thousand dollars, exceeding the means of most citizens (although some forms of insurance cover heart transplants). These changes have generated several public policy and private insurance questions.

One illustrative debate came from policy changes in Oregon. In 1987, legislators in Oregon ceased medicaid funding for soft-tissue transplants in order to use a limited budget for a broader and more effective array of services. They determined that the costs of approximately thirty heart, liver, bone marrow, and pancreas transplants was equivalent to the cost of regular prenatal care for 1500 pregnant women. Legislators chose the latter, declaring that they could not pay for both. They also determined that prenatal outreach programs would double the lives saved per dollar over transplant programs. The Oregon Senate president maintained that until gaps in insurance coverage are closed, it is unjust to allocate large sums for programs that serve only a few citizens. However, a different kind of inequity is introduced by this decision, because the expensive transplant (and other) technologies that are not covered are then available only to those who can afford them.

Changing medical and political circumstances have led to many similar alterations of policy that close one gap in equity only to open another. These policy shifts often reveal tensions between norms of utility and equality in determining just access. Sometimes disagreements occur about the use of social utility to specify the content and scope of a right to health care, for instance, by using cost-effectiveness analysis linked to the notion of quality-adjusted life-years (see Chapter 5). In other cases this form of analysis is shunned. As a result, the "system" for allocating funds for heart transplants in the United States is a loose, shifting, and inconsistent set of policies that cannot be recommended on grounds of either medical utility or justice.[81]

However, within a two-tiered system in which the standard at the first tier is the right to a decent minimum, there will inevitably be debate regarding appropriate allocational trade-offs between utility and equality. These debates will leave islands of uncertainty about which health services society is obligated to provide. It remains unclear whether, under the decent-minimum standard, justice requires that society provide funds to cover heart transplants or any other massively expensive form of health care.

Nonetheless, arguments have been offered for funding certain expensive procedures while also making the allocation of hearts both efficient and fair. For instance, the federal Task Force on Organ Transplantation (appointed by The Department of Health and Human Services) recommended that "a public program should be set up to cover the costs of people who are medically eligible for organ transplants but who are not covered by private insurance, Medicare, or Medicaid and who are unable to obtain an organ transplant due to the lack of funds." [82] This recommendation was limited to nonexperimental heart and liver transplants. In contrast to the federal program that ensures coverage for kidney transplants, the task force limited its proposed policy to the financially needy.

The task force based its recommendation on two arguments from justice. The first argument emphasizes the continuity between heart and liver transplants and other forms of medical care (including kidney transplants) that are already accepted as part of the decent minimum of health care that society should provide. The task force argued that transplants are comparable to other funded procedures in terms of their effectiveness in saving lives and enhancing their quality. According to the National Heart Transplantation Study, eighty percent of heart transplant recipients survived for one year, and fifty percent were alive after five years, with a good quality of life according to both objective and subjective criteria. [83] In response to the charge that heart and liver transplants are too expensive and that health care costs must be contained, the task force argued that the burden of saving public health funds should be distributed equitably rather than imposed on particular groups of patients, such as those suffering from end-stage heart or liver failure. Under the assumption that society is committed to providing funds to meet a wide variety of health-care needs, "it is arbitrary to exclude one life-saving procedure while funding others of equal life-saving potential and cost."

The task force offered a second argument for the federal government's role in guaranteeing equitable access to organ transplants, this time focusing on certain features of organ donation and procurement. Various public officials, including the president of the United States, participate in efforts to increase the supply of donated organs by appealing to all citizens to donate their organs and their dead relatives' organs. This appeal is aimed at all segments of society. However, the task force argued, it is unfair and sometimes exploitative to solicit people, rich and poor alike, to donate organs if those organs are then distributed on the basis of ability to pay; it is inconsistent to prohibit the sale of organs, as U.S. federal law does, and then to distribute donated organs according to ability to pay. It is morally problematic to distinguish buying an organ for transplantation from buying an organ transplant procedure when the organ is the centerpiece of the procedure.

Despite these two attractive arguments, the government is not required by justice to provide health care irrespective of its cost, and it is not arbitrary to use a system of rationing in which priorities are fairly established. Once a fair threshold of funding has been established, it is fair to select some procedures while excluding others when they are of equal life-saving potential and of equal cost. It would, *ceteris paribus,* be unfair to solicit people to make gifts of organs and then distribute them on the basis of ability to pay, but it would also be unfair to spend in excess of a fairly established level of funding merely because a gift has been made that would benefit another person. Of course, the system of soliciting donations might also need modification in order to avoid unjust taxation and expenditure. Potential donors need to understand the limits built into the system of procurement and distribution. But, assuming both this understanding by donors and a fair system of allocation, the government could legitimately encourage donation even if it could not pay for transplantation.

The task force did not address larger questions about trade-offs between transplants and other medical (and social) goods in the context of limited resources, but they are critical to the success of the two arguments proposed by the task force. Without addressing these issues, the task force certainly has not demonstrated a government obligation to fund all organ transplantation. Recommendations about funding heart transplants and all other expensive treatments must in the end be situated in the larger context of a social policy of macroallocation (types 1–3 discussed above).

Despite these weaknesses in the task force's arguments, we should not ignore the many unfairnesses that exist in methods of procuring and allocating organs in the United States. These injustices are dramatically highlighted by various current practices, about which donors are typically not informed. For example, some transplant centers require cash deposits that exceed what the majority of potential candidates for transplantation can raise. At a few centers, wealthy or politically influential citizens of foreign nations rank high on eligibility lists; in fact, some of them have been advanced forward on the lists for political reasons with the assistance of U.S. government officials.[84] Some centers also give priority to in-state residents, despite the massive federal support that has gone into the development of techniques of heart transplantation. These problems all point to moral unfairness that can result from the lack of a fair system of macroallocation.

The Need for a Comprehensive and Coherent System

The above examples of health policy and the previous discussion of justice in health care financing and delivery indicate that a comprehensive and coherent system is desperately needed in the United States. Unless significant change is introduced, the United States will continue on the same trail of higher costs and larger numbers of unprotected citizens. A revised system will need improvements in both utility (efficiency) and justice (fairness). Although justice and utility are often depicted as opposed values, both should be given priority positions in shaping a health care system. Creating an efficient system by cutting costs and providing appropriate incentives can conflict with the goal of universal access to health care, but many justice-based goals of universal coverage (as well as autonomy-based goals of informed consent) also tend to make the system inefficient. How, then, should a health care system be designed with a view toward both justice and utility?

An essential part of any acceptable answer to this question involves specifying the primary objectives of the plan, together with the conditions of a morally acceptable system. Four objectives should be primary. First, one key objective is unobstructed access to a decent minimum of health care through some form of universal insurance coverage that operationalizes the right to health care. The forms and sources of coverage might be pluralistic (see below), but some vulnerable parties will have to be insured by public providers.

The second objective is to alter the system of incentives for physicians and consumer-patients. Society attempts to allocate services as efficiently as possible, whereas patients and physicians look to optimize individual patients' care. Decisionmaking from one perspective undermines decisionmaking from the other perspective, creating significant tensions and inefficiencies.[85] Consumers of health care (and in some cases those who pay for health care) therefore need to become better acquainted with costs and alternatives than they are. As an example, some constraints will have to be placed on fees for services in order to meet the goal of a decent minimum. Consumers can still be offered a choice of plans, but unless cost consciousness and cost controls are introduced, expenditures will spiral out of control, and the necessity for rationing at the first tier will run the risk of undermining the goal of the decent minimum.

The third objective is to construct a fair system of rationing that will not violate the decent-minimum standard. It now seems inevitable that forms of rationing must occur at the second tier for highly desirable and sometimes lifesaving technologies; but comparable rationing at the first tier would sabotage the moral foundations of the enterprise.

Finally, the fourth objective is to implement a system that can be put into effect incrementally without drastic disruption of basic institutions that finance and deliver health care. For example, even if a system of universal access with a single payer were adopted, existing private and public insurance agencies could be retained. Legitimate fears about bureaucracy, long queues for services, and large increases in health care costs and income redistribution should be seriously considered in revising the current system.

Several carefully reasoned proposals have been introduced to meet these objectives, or at least some parts of the four objectives. Despite many differences, these proposals fall into two families: (1) *Unified systems* and (2) *Pluralist systems.* Plans of the first type have looked primarily to egalitarian justice, with utility a secondary consideration. Plans of the second type have looked primarily to utility (efficiency and broad coverage), with justice a secondary consideration. Although we cannot here consider the details of any one plan or develop an ideal plan, we can outline these two families and suggest the primary considerations that should guide us in choosing one type of plan over another, or in attempting to render the two coherent by employing them in different areas— for example, the first (a unitary system) at the first tier and the second (a pluralist system) at the second tier in a two-tier system.

Unified systems. Universal access is often presented on the model of socialized systems such as those in the United Kingdom, Canada, and the Scandinavian countries. In these plans, all citizens are covered by a unified national system without reference to age, health status, medical condition, or employment status. The justification for the system is that only government can provide universal coverage and bring increases in health care expenditures in line with the gross national product.

One widely discussed proposal for the United States is the Physician's National Health Plan (PNHP), which would be funded by the federal government and administered by the states. The plan is that each person receives a national health card, pays no charges for services, is free to choose a provider, and is eligible to receive covered services, which include long-term and chronic care services. Physicians are free to work on a salaried basis or to practice privately. Private fees are established by regional boards, and no physician is allowed to bill the government more than the amount established by the boards or to charge the patient additional fees. Other boards would regulate hospital fees and other health care charges. In this system, a single public payer replaces the more than 1500 private insurers (including Medicaid and Medicare) that provide insurance in the United States.[86]

This strategy has several drawbacks. First, it is a revolutionary proposal that many U.S. citizens and the majority of its politicians believe would be bureaucratic, inefficient, and perfunctory—eventuating in long queues for poorly delivered services. Although Canadians have done well with such a system, many people in the United States believe that the Canadian system either cannot be or should not be transplanted. Among the controversial features of the unified strategy is the elimination or near elimination of competitive aspects of the financing system. Private health insurers would have no significant function, and no incentives would be provided for consumer choice of plans. The public-sector monopoly in unified plans has been vigorously attacked on grounds of disutility. Many people have questioned the credibility of a unified plan in light of the fact that no industrialized nation that has adopted such a system has been able to create incentives to reduce waste while efficiently organizing and managing the delivery of care.

Pluralist systems. Virtually all other influential plans take a pluralist approach to financing health care. These proposals allow for a diverse array of health plans, both profit and nonprofit, both private and public. Consumers are given a choice of plans, and it is expected that each plan will be responsive to consumers because all plans, with the exception of last-resort government plans, must compete for subscribers. Employer-funded insurance is the centerpiece of health care access, and all proposals endorse minimum-benefits or decent-minimum packages. Virtually all of these plans rely on a mixture of tax incentives and disincentives that encourage employers to provide coverage, as well as on some form of public assistance in coverage. However, only one plan (Enthoven and Kronick[87]) achieves universal coverage, and it appears to create significant problems of unemployment for low-wage workers.

Pluralist plans aim to increase both utility and justice in the system, but the overriding goal has been to produce a wider and deeper social utility. Rarely in the justification of pluralist plans has a principle such as Rawls's difference principle—basic inequalities are justified only if they work to the advantage of the socially worst-off group—been seriously entertained. Even the idea of a safety net or a minimum floor below which no citizens would be allowed to fall has been a major premise in only one plan (Enthoven-Kronick). This weak egalitarian strategy contrasts sharply with unified-system plans, which often make strong appeals to egalitarian principles of justice.

Nonetheless, it is not clear that either a unified or a pluralist strategy is disqualified as such. Both could be made ethically acceptable. The major issue is how well and how fully the four objectives listed above can be met in a coherent package. Meeting these objectives will require that those who formulate policy provide adequate information to all parties about costs, benefits, and financial and political constraints—together with an explanation of the standards used in the allocation of resources. Assuming the acceptability of the dual values of utility (efficiency) and justice (fairness and equity), the best plan is likely to be the one that most coherently promotes both values and that insists on universal access to a decent minimum of health care. Any system that can meet these conditions should be morally justifiable and should serve society well in addressing questions of macroallocation. However, criteria of justice and utility must be invoked in very different ways in developing a framework for rationing scarce medical resources to patients.

Rationing Scarce Treatments to Patients

As the experiment in Oregon and the heart transplant case indicate, health care professionals and public officials often must decide who will receive an available but scarce medical resource that cannot be provided to all needy people. In discussing this form of rationing, often called *microallocation,* we will emphasize priority schemes for selecting recipients of scarce health care (often in urgent circumstances). Proposed policies of rationing (beyond ability to pay) should be assessed according to the norms of justice and the right to health care discussed earlier in this chapter, but other moral norms are also relevant.

Two broad approaches have been recommended in biomedical ethics: (1) a *utilitarian* strategy that emphasizes social efficiency and maximal benefit to patients and (2) an *egalitarian* strategy that emphasizes the equal worth of persons and fair opportunity.

Substantive Standards and Procedural Rules

We begin by recalling the distinction between just procedures and just outcomes. Often it is impossible to guarantee a just outcome by a just procedure, but whether a procedure is just is itself morally important. We are typically more secure in judgments about the justice of procedures than in judgments about just outcomes. For example, the justice of democratic decisionmaking is usually less in doubt than the justice of the outcomes reached by that procedure. Both procedures and outcomes need attention in addressing issues about the fair selection of patients under conditions of scarcity and rationing. We need to ask two questions: Who should make the decisions? and What criteria should we accept for decisionmaking? The former is a procedure-oriented question; the latter, substance-oriented. Although distinct, these questions are also interrelated. For example, if criteria of medical acceptability are prominent, then medical experts will play a central role in formulating and applying them.

We will now defend a system for selection in which two sets of substantive standards and procedural rules are required for rationing many scarce medical resources. First, criteria and procedures are needed to determine a qualifying pool of potential recipients, such as patients eligible for heart transplantation. Second, criteria and procedures are required for final selection of recipients, such as the patient to receive a particular heart. It is usually easier to secure agreement about initial screening than about final selection, in part because selecting the initial pool of potential recipients involves medical criteria, whereas final selection is more complex and includes nonmedical criteria.

Initial Screening of Potential Recipients

Criteria for screening potential recipients of care can be arranged in three basic categories, originally proposed by Nicholas Rescher: constituency, progress of science, and prospect of success.[88] We will follow this structure while using arguments from justice to fill in critical gaps.

The constituency factor. The first criterion is determined by clientele boundaries (for example, veterans served by VA medical centers), geographic or jurisdictional boundaries (for example, citizens of a state served by a state-funded hospital), and ability to pay (for example, the wealthy). These criteria are entirely nonmedical, and they involve moral judgments that often are not impartial (for example, excluding noncitizens). Such clientele boundaries are sometimes acceptable, but often they should be resisted. For example, in the United States the distribution of organs donated for transplantation has raised questions about the accidents of geography. Should specific donated organs be given to patients in the communities in which they were donated or to patients in a national system (or an international network) who most need and could most benefit from those organs? Local use is a poor system for assuring that the most suitable candidates receive available organs.

The Task Force on Organ Transplantation proposed that donated organs be considered national, public resources to be distributed, within limits, according to both the needs of patients and the probability of successful transplantation.[89] In a controversial recommendation, the task force acknowledged that foreign nationals do not have the same moral claim on organs donated in the United States as its own citizens and residents do. In conceding that national citizenship and residency are morally relevant properties for distribution, the task force nevertheless stressed that compassion should lead to the admission of some nonresident aliens. In a split vote, it recommended that nonresident aliens comprise no more than ten percent of the waiting list for cadaver kidneys donated for transplantation and that all patients on the waiting list, including nonresident aliens, have access to organs according to the same criteria of need, probability of success, and time on the waiting list.[90] The United Network for Organ Sharing has taken a similar approach. It reserves the right to audit U.S. institutions transplanting cadaveric organs into foreign nationals and will automatically audit any institution performing more than ten percent of its cadaveric transplants on foreign nationals.

Progress of science. The second criterion, advancement of scientific knowledge, is often relevant during an experimental phase in the development of a treatment such as cardiac transplantation. Patients who have other complicating diseases may justifiably be excluded in order to determine whether an experimental treatment is effective and how it can be improved. This criterion of scientific program is research-oriented, and use of this criterion rests on moral and prudential judgments about the most efficient use of resources. The criteria relevant to selection of patients for participation in such research clearly will need to be reassessed when a treatment becomes accepted.

Prospect of success. Whether a treatment is experimental or routine, likelihood of success is a relevant criterion because a scarce medical resource should be distributed only to patients who have a reasonable chance of benefit. Ignoring this factor is unjust, because it results in a waste of resources, as in the case of organs that can be transplanted only once. Although heart-transplant surgeons sometimes list their patients as urgent priority candidates for an available heart because the patients will soon die if they do not receive a transplant, some of these patients are virtually certain to die even if they do receive the heart. Good candidates are passed over in the process. A classification and queuing system that permits this form of appeal to urgent need is unjust and inefficient.

Prospect of success is commonly analyzed in terms of medical suitability, as formulated by medical experts. However, the public has a strong interest in ensuring that the formulation does not covertly incorporate irrelevant or at least undefended criteria, such as unjustified social worth criteria. In 1980, the U.S. government withheld funding for heart transplants in part because the operative screening criteria appeared to include "social" together with "medical" criteria. At the time, the criteria at Stanford, the major cardiac transplantation center, excluded patients with "a history of alcoholism, job instability, antisocial behavior, or psychiatric illness," while requiring "a stable, rewarding family and/or vocational environment to return to post transplant." Critics held that these "social" criteria are inappropriate for use in programs receiving public funds.

Controversies about the suitability of candidates have centered on whether criteria for screening and selecting recipients represent *medical* utility or *social* utility. Judgments of medical utility focus on maximizing the welfare of patients, whereas judgments of social utility focus on maximizing society's welfare.[91] For example, in distributing scarce organs for transplantation, medical utility requires that the organs be used in an effective and efficient way to maximize the welfare of patients suffering from end-stage organ failure. In judgments of social utility, however, decisionmakers consider which recipient of health care would contribute the most to society. Judgments of medical utility implicitly assume that the social value of all lives is equal, a dubious assumption, whereas judgments of social utility require assessments of the social worth of lives, a dubious enterprise.

Controversy persists about whether current operational criteria in important forms of microallocation are designed to realize medical utility, social utility, or both. The Task Force on Organ Transplantation excluded criteria such as race and gender as unjust, but it did not exclude other debatable criteria such as age, lifestyle, and a social network of support, holding instead that these criteria require constant public scrutiny through a fair and open process.[92] Because we have already discussed age and lifestyle, we will concentrate on the social network of support, but we note that age and lifestyle can help to predict medical utility and to indicate social utility.

A support network, including the family, has commonly been used as a prospect-of-success criterion in heart transplant programs. For example, it was invoked in the initial decision to deny a heart transplant at Loma Linda University Hospital to Baby Jesse, whose parents were unmarried. A network of support is often medically important in the overall success of the transplantation, particularly in post-transplant care, and can have an impact on medical utility in the sense of an effective and efficient use of a donated organ. However, rules of justice, including fair opportunity, suggest that society seek alternative support systems in some circumstances rather than use the absence of such a network as a reason for excluding a patient from transplantation.[93] Here medical utility and social utility should be distinguished. Criteria of medical utility (for example, the baby is a better candidate because of the likely outcome) can easily mask underlying criteria of social utility (for example, the parents are divorced and unemployed). Both forms of utility should be constrained by considerations of distributive justice, but this moral imperative does not disqualify either form of utility when their use is fair and relevant.

Judgments about medical need and probability of success are value-laden, and the operational criteria for patient screening and selection require careful institutional and public scrutiny to ensure that these values are defensible. For instance, debate continues about what will count as success in organ transplantation—length of graft survival, length of patient survival, quality of life, or rehabilitation—and about the factors that should influence judgments about the probability of success.

Final Selection of Patients

Standards proposed for final selection of patients have been more controversial than those for initial screening. Debate has centered on medical utility, social utility, and impersonal mechanisms such as lotteries and queuing. All have been used in the selection of patients. For example, in the days of scarce kidney dialysis equipment in the United States, centers providing dialysis all made judgments of medical suitability. But some centers also made judgments of social worth, some used queuing ("first come, first served"), and at least one used a lottery.[94] In addition, no center dropped patients from dialysis treatment once treatment had begun, even if someone of superior candidacy subsequently appeared.

Medical utility. We assume, as an unargued premise, that in rationing scarce medical resources, it is morally imperative to consider medical utility. Differences in patients' need and in their prospects for successful treatment are both relevant considerations. If the resource is not reusable, as in the case of transplanted organs, protection against waste is critical. Selection procedures should also be gauged to save as many lives as possible through the available resources. Hence, "medical utility" points to the effective and efficient use of scarce medical resources.

This approach does not violate principles of justice, but some difficulties already mentioned recur here. Both need and prospect of success are value-laden concepts, and uncertainty sometimes exists about likely outcomes and about the factors that contribute to success. For example, kidney transplant surgeons dispute the importance of having a good tissue match, because minor tissue mismatches can be managed by cyclosporine, a highly effective medication in reducing the body's tendency to reject transplanted organs. Insisting on the seemingly objective criterion of tissue type in distributing organs can have the effect of disadvantaging persons with a rare tissue type. Medical need and prospect of success also sometimes come into conflict. For example, in intensive care units, trying to save a patient whose need is medically urgent sometimes inappropriately consumes resources that could be used to save more people.[95] If an ICU reaches capacity, and other patients need admission, decisionmakers face a dilemmatic choice of whether to raise the headcount and thereby lower the standard of care or to examine the claims of all.[96] Giving priority to the sickest patients or those with the most urgent medical needs may itself be unfair, because it may be a poor use of resources.

Rationing schemes that altogether exclude considerations of medical utility in using resources are indefensible. However, judgments of medical utility are not solely sufficient if utility is roughly equal among candidates or if an unjust distribution occurs. This problem takes us to the subject of chance and queuing.

Impersonal mechanisms of chance and queuing. Chance and queuing are sometimes justified by considerations of equality and fair opportunity. We began this chapter by noting the oddity and unacceptability of using a lottery to distribute social positions. However, a lottery or other system of chance is not always odd and unacceptable. If medical resources are scarce and not divisible into portions, and if no major disparities exist in medical utility for patients (particularly when selection determines life or death), then considerations of fair opportunity, equal respect, and the equal evaluation of lives justify queuing, a lottery, or randomization—depending on which procedure is the more appropriate and feasible in the circumstances. A similar conclusion was reached by the Artificial Heart Assessment Panel of the National Heart and Lung Institute: "If the pool of patients with equal medical needs exceeds supply, procedures should be devised for some form of random selection. Social worth criteria should not be used."[97]

Some critics of random selection contend that use of impersonal mechanisms involves an irresponsible refusal to make a decision, but such procedures can be justified on several grounds. In addition to promoting fair opportunity and equal treatment, random methods make the selection with little investment of time and financial resources and thus provide utilitarian benefits. Lotteries can also be less stressful for all involved, including patients. In Seattle, members of a closely watched committee that selected patients for dialysis felt intense pressure and stress, often accompanied by guilt.[98] In a random system, decisions are made efficiently, and rejected candidates often feel less distress at being rejected by chance than by judgments of comparative social worth. When *perceived* as fair, random methods also tend to result in more agreement about the fairness of the outcomes of the selection process.

However, both theoretical and practical problems require attention. One question concerns the weight of the rule "first come, first served." Under some conditions a patient already receiving a particular treatment has a severely limited chance of survival, whereas other patients who need the treatment have a far better chance of survival. Does "first come, first served" imply that those already receiving treatment have absolute priority over those who arrive later but have either more urgent needs or better prospects of success?

Although admission to the ICU establishes a presumption in favor of continued treatment, it does not give a person a permanent or absolute claim for priority regardless of changing medical circumstances. An example appears in neonatal intensive care decisions about the use of extracorporeal membrane oxygenation (ECMO), a form of cardiopulmonary bypass used to support newborns with life-threatening respiratory failure. ECMO qualifies as a truly scarce resource, because it is not widely available and requires the full-time presence of well-trained personnel. Robert Truog argues, rightly in our judgment, that ECMO should be withdrawn from a newborn with a poor prognosis in favor of another with a good prognosis if a child who is more likely to benefit requires the therapy to survive and a transfer cannot safely be made to another facility.[99] Requirements of medical utility sometimes justify early discharge to make room for others who have a more urgent need or a higher probability of benefit. Such displacement from the ICU requires justification, but it does not constitute abandonment or injustice if other forms of care are provided.

Our arguments for the use of systems of chance or queuing in rationing heath care to patients applies only if no major disparities in medical utility exist. Which mechanism, queuing or chance, is then preferable will depend largely on practical considerations, but queuing appears to be more feasible in many health care settings, including emergency medicine, ICUs, and organ transplant lists. A complicating factor is that some people do not enter the queue (or the lottery) in time because of factors such as slowness in seeking help, inadequate or incompetent medical attention, delay in referral, or overt discrimination. For example, a person might be uninformed about options, or a person's limited funds might have prevented a search for medical care until it was too late to benefit from a particular therapy. A system is clearly unfair if some people gain an advantage in access over others because they are better educated, better connected, or have more money for frequent visits to physicians. A frequent lottery would overcome this problem but might introduce other forms of un-fairness unless carefully controlled for medical utility.

Social utility. The criterion of social utility is more controversial, but the comparative social value of potential recipients is, under some conditions, a relevant and decisive criterion. An analogy often used to show the importance of such judgments is giving priority to some sailors on a crowded lifeboat to increase the chances of saving more people than would otherwise be saved. Another familiar (though more disputed) example is taken from World War II, when the scarce resource of penicillin was distributed to U.S. soldiers suffering from venereal disease rather than to those suffering from battle wounds. The rationale was military need: The soldiers suffering from venereal disease could more quickly be restored to battle.[100]

An argument in favor of social-utilitarian selection is that medical institutions and personnel are trustees of society and must consider the probable future contributions of patients in need of scarce lifesaving resources. As Nicholas Rescher contends, "in its allocation . . . society 'invests' a scarce resource in one person as against another and is thus entitled to look to the probable prospective 'return' on its investment."[101] This argument has merit, but it can be criticized from several perspectives of fairness and utility. For example, one might resist judgments of social worth in order to protect the relationship of personal care and trust between patients and physicians, which would be threatened if physicians routinely looked beyond their patients' needs to society's needs. Other problems include difficulties in developing acceptable criteria of social worth in a pluralistic society with many different conceptions of the valuable life, reduction of persons to their social roles and functions, violation of equal respect for persons, and denial of fair equality of opportunity.[102] We acknowledge the merit of each of these criticisms. However, below we argue

that, in certain exceptional cases involving persons of critical social importance, criteria of social value rightly become overriding.

Triage. Defenders of social-utilitarian calculations in rationing health care
sometimes invoke the model of triage, which has become increasingly common
in health care facilities. The French term *triage* means "sorting," "picking,"
or "choosing." It has been applied to sorting items such as wool and coffee
beans according to their quality. In the delivery of health care, triage has been
practiced in war, in community disasters, and in emergency rooms where injured persons have been sorted for medical attention according to their needs
and prospects. Decisions to admit and to discharge patients from ICUs often
involve some form of triage. In all cases in health care the objective is to use
available medical resources as effectively and as efficiently as possible. The
traditional and contemporary rationale for triage is the utilitarian maxim "Do
the greatest good for the greatest number."[103]

Triage decisions often appeal to medical utility rather than social utility in
determining the maximal utilitarian outcome. In a typical situation, disaster
victims are sorted according to medical needs. Those who have major injuries
and will die without immediate help, but who can be salvaged, are ranked first;
those whose treatment might be delayed without immediate danger are ranked
second; those with minor injuries are ranked third; and those for whom no
treatment will be efficacious are ranked fourth. This medical-utility priority
scheme is fair and does not involve judgments about individuals' comparative
social worth.

However, judgments of comparative social worth are inescapable and are
acceptable in some situations. Suppose, for example, that after an earthquake
some injured survivors are medical personnel who suffer only minor injuries.
They are in some contexts justifiably given priority of treatment so that they
can then help others. Similarly, in an outbreak of infectious disease, it is justifiable to inoculate physicians first to enable them to care for others. In emergencies, communities and individuals need immediate protection against disaster.
Under such conditions, a person may be given priority for treatment on grounds
of social utility if and only if his or her contribution is indispensable to attaining a major social goal or function—for example, the president of a country
in wartime would justifiably be given priority. As in the analogous lifeboat
cases, judgments of comparative social value should be limited to the *specific*
qualities and skills that are essential to the community's protection. They
should not attempt to assess the *general* social worth of persons.

If exceptions based on social utility are limited to emergencies involving
necessity, they do not threaten the ordinary moral universe or imply the general
acceptability of social-utilitarian calculations in distributing health care. The

structure of justification in exceptional cases follows our usual pattern of seeking coherence: Presumptions are set by our considered moral judgments, including important principles that are prima facie binding; but in some cases of
conflict those presumptions are rebuttable. Arguments to rebut the presumptions should follow the procedures of reasoning outlined in Chapters 1 and 2.

Our contention, then, is that principles and rules of justice, in conjunction
with utility and other principles, mandate attention to medical utility followed
by the use of chance or queuing for scarce resources when medical utility is
roughly equal for eligible patients. This nexus of standards should prove to be
both coherent and stable despite appeals to both justice and utility. Our approach therefore does not demand equality of opportunity regardless of the
consequences. Nevertheless, the contrast between our proposals and a system
such as Rescher's is significant. His system relies on social utility until no
major disparities in social value among the candidates for a scarce resource
emerge. At this point, he resorts to chance. By contrast, our approach starts
with medical need and probability of successful treatment (i.e., medical utility), and then it uses chance and queuing as ways to express fairness and equality, unless major disparities exist in potential recipients' specific social responsibilities and probable social contributions in an emergency.

This range of ethical considerations needs to be kept in the foreground, because of evidence that various nonethical and perhaps unethical factors play
roles in rationing health care. For instance, it has been widely assumed on the
basis of prior studies that in ICUs the number of cases of severely ill patients
admitted and denied admission would increase as bed availability decreases.
To investigate this assumption, researchers used retrospective chart review to
determine the factors that influenced patient-selection decisions in a surgical
ICU. The study occurred during a temporary nursing shortage that resulted in
the closure of two to six of the unit's sixteen beds over a three-month period.
The researchers discovered that bed allocation was decisively influenced by
considerations other than medical suitability and severity of illness. According
to the researchers, "political power [in the institution], medical provincialism
[one service pitted against another], and income maximization overrode medical suitability in the provision of critical care services."[104]

Conclusion

In this chapter we have examined several philosophical approaches to justice,
including egalitarian, communitarian, libertarian, and utilitarian theories. We
have not maintained that a single theory of justice is essential for constructive
reflection on health policy, and we have not argued for a single type of theory.
The limitations of ethical theories have been evident in the discussion of theory
in earlier chapters, but those limitations are particularly prominent in debates

about what justice implies for allocation decisions. Considerable controversy persists regarding the theoretical basis of justice and ways to handle conflicts between principles and rules.

Each influential general theory of justice is a philosophical reconstruction of a valid perspective on the moral life, but one that only partially captures the range and diversity of that life. The richness of our moral practices, traditions, and theories helps explain why diverse theories of justice have all been skillfully defended in recent philosophy. Absent a social consensus about these competing theories of justice, we can expect that public policies will shift ground, now emphasizing one theory, later emphasizing another. Nevertheless, the piecemeal approach that the United States has taken to its health care system is not justified by the existence of rival theories. A piecemeal approach avoids asking larger questions of justice about what we as a nation should expect from the system and how we should address the needs of millions of people for increased insurance, long-term care, and the like.

Policies of access to and financing of health care, together with strategies of efficiency in health care institutions, dwarf in social importance every other issue considered in this book. Many barriers exist to achieving access to health care. For millions who encounter those barriers, a just health care system remains a distant ideal. Experience with conditions of scarcity suggests that we are not likely to be able to satisfy fully every facet of this ideal. Our society may, however, be able to close gaps in access more conscientiously than we have in the past.

We have suggested a general perspective from which these problems might be approached—namely, by recognizing an enforceable right to a decent minimum of health care within a framework for allocation that coherently incorporates utilitarian and egalitarian standards. In this conception, the justice of social institutions of health care is to be gauged by their tendency to counteract lack of opportunity caused by natural and social lotteries over which individuals lack substantial control and by their commitment to efficient and fair procedures in the allocation of health care resources.

Notes

1. Jorge Luis Borges, *Labyrinths* (New York: New Directions, 1962), pp. 30–35.
2. See Martin Golding's "Justice and Rights: A Study in Relationship," in *Justice and Health Care,* ed. Earl E. Shelp (Boston: D. Reidel, 1981), 23–35. See also Allen Buchanan, "Justice: A Philosophical Review," in the same volume, pp. 3–21.
3. *The Totally Implantable Artificial Heart: A Report of the Artificial Heart Assessment Panel of the National Heart and Lung Institute* (September 1973), DHEW Publication No. NIH 74-191.

4. *Campbell v. Mincey,* 413 F. Supp. 16 (1975), 16–23, aff'd 542 F.2d 573.

5. *Goesaert v. Cleary,* 335 U.S. 464, overruled in *Craig v. Boren,* 429 U.S. 190, at 210 n.23 (1976). See also *Whitney v. State Tax Commission,* 309 U.S. 530 (1940); *Campbell v. Mincey,* 413 F. Supp. at 22.

6. See, e.g., Nicholas Rescher, *Distributive Justice* (Indianapolis, IN: Bobbs-Merrill, 1966), ch. 4.

7. This case was reported by Robert E. Stevenson in *Hastings Center Report* 10 (December 1980): 25.

8. *International Union, UAW. v. Johnson Controls,* 111 S.Ct. 1196 (1991).

9. Audience Survey, Symposium on Death and Dying, Southeastern Dialysis and Transplantation Association Meetings, Miami, FL, August 1977 (unpublished).

10. John Stuart Mill, *Utilitarianism,* in vol. 10 of the *Collected Works of John Stuart Mill* (Toronto: University of Toronto Press, 1969), ch. 5.

11. *A Theory of Justice* (Cambridge, MA: Harvard University Press, 1971), pp. 307–10.

12. Robert Nozick, *Anarchy, State, and Utopia* (New York: Basic Books, 1974), esp. pp. 149–82.

13. See Alasdair MacIntyre, *Whose Justice? Which Rationality?* (Notre Dame, IN: University of Notre Dame Press, 1988), pp. 1, 390–403.

14. See James S. Todd et al., "Health Access America—Strengthening the US Health Care System," *Journal of the American Medical Association* 265 (May 15, 1991): 2503–6.

15. See Henk Ten Have and Helen Keasberry, "Equity and Solidarity: The Context of Health Care in the Netherlands," *Journal of Medicine and Philosophy* 17 (August 1992): 463–77, esp. 474–76.

16. Ezekiel J. Emanuel, *The Ends of Human Life: Medical Ethics in a Liberal Policy* (Cambridge, MA: Harvard University Press, 1991).

17. Michael Walzer, *Spheres of Justice: A Defense of Pluralism and Equality* (New York: Basic Books, 1983), esp. pp. 86–94.

18. See Ronald Dworkin's review of *Spheres of Justice* in *The New York Review of Books,* April 14, 1983, and his exchange with Walzer in *The New York Review of Books,* July 21, 1983.

19. Rawls, "Kantian Constructivism in Moral Theory" (The Dewey Lectures), *Journal of Philosophy* 77 (1980): 519. In his later writings, Rawls has progressively emphasized Kantian conceptions of rationality less and traditions in modern constitutional democracies more.

20. See Ronald M. Green, "Health Care and Justice in Contract Perspective," in *Ethics and Health Policy,* ed. Robert M. Veatch and Roy Branson (Cambridge, MA: Ballinger, 1976), pp. 111–26.

21. Daniels, *Just Health Care* (New York: Cambridge University Press, 1985), pp. 34–58.

22. Rawls, *A Theory of Justice,* pp. 73f (italics added).

23. See Bernard Williams, "The Idea of Equality," as reprinted in *Justice and Equality,* ed. Hugo Bedau (Englewood Cliffs, NJ: Prentice-Hall, 1971), p. 135.

24. H. Tristram Engelhardt, Jr., "Health Care Allocations: Responses to the Unjust, the Unfortunate, and the Undesirable," in *Justice and Health Care,* ed. Shelp, pp. 126–27, and *The Foundations of Bioethics* (New York: Oxford University Press, 1986), pp. 339–43.

25. See Judith Shklar, *The Faces of Injustice* (New Haven: Yale University Press, 1990), pp. 9ff.

26. Norman G. Levinsky and Richard A. Rettig, "The Medicare End-Stage Renal Disease Program: A Report from the Institute of Medicine," *Journal of the American Medical Association* 324 (April 18, 1991): 1143–48; Roger W. Evans, Christopher R. Blagg, and Fred A. Bryan, Jr., "Implications for Health Policy: A Social and Demographic Profile of Hemodialysis Patients in the United States," *Journal of the American Medical Association* 245 (February 6, 1981): 487–91.

27. Kenneth C. Goldberg, Arthur J. Hartz, Steven J. Jacobsen et al., "Racial and Community Factors Influencing Coronary Artery Bypass Graft Surgery Rates for All 1986 Medicare Patients," *Journal of the American Medical Association* 267 (March 18, 1992): 1473–77.

28. UNOS, "Heart Allocation Policy," *UNOS Update* 5 (1989): 1–2; see James F. Childress, "Fairness in the Allocation and Delivery of Health Care," in *A Time to Be Born and a Time to Die: The Ethics of Choice,* ed. Barry S. Kogan (New York: Aldine de Gruyter, 1991), ch. 11.

29. See Office of the Inspector General, *The Distribution of Organs for Transplantation: Expectations and Practices,* OEI-01-89-00550 (Washington, DC: U.S. Department of Health and Human Services, Office of Analysis and Inspection, 1991). Another study covering a slightly longer period found only a twenty-nine percent increase in waiting time for blacks and attributed the overall disparity in waiting time to various factors, including the fact that more whites were likely to be on multiple waiting lists. See Fred P. Sanfilippo et al., "Factors Affecting the Waiting Time of Cadaveric Kidney Transplant Candidates in the United States," *Journal of the American Medical Association* 267 (January 8, 1992): 247–52.

30. See Robert M. Veatch, "Allocating Organs by Utilitarianism Is Seen as Favoring Whites over Blacks," *Kennedy Institute of Ethics Newsletter* 3 (July 1989): Contrast Sanfilippo et al. "Factors Affecting the Waiting Time of Cadaveric Kidney Transplant Candidates in the United States," which found that the changes in UNOS policy to emphasize HLA match "did not worsen the disparity in waiting time for black or presensitized patients."

31. Council on Ethical and Judicial Affairs, American Medical Association, "Gender Disparities in Clinical Decision Making," *Journal of the American Medical Association* 266 (July 24, 1991): 559–662.

32. Richard M. Steingart et al., "Sex Differences in the Management of Coronary Artery Disease," *New England Journal of Medicine* 325 (July 25, 1991): 226–30. See also John Z. Ayanian and Arnold M. Epstein, "Differences in the Use of Procedures between Women and Men Hospitalized for Coronary Heart Disease," *New England Journal of Medicine* 325 (July 25, 1991): 221–25.

33. Bernadine Healy, "The Yentl Syndrome," *New England Journal of Medicine* 325 (July 25, 1991): 274–76.

34. Kenneth E. Thorpe, "Expanding Employment-Based Health Insurance: Is Small Group Reform the Answer?" *Inquiry* 29 (1992): 128–36; and Employee Benefit Research Institute, *Issue Brief* No. 104 (July, 1990).

35. R. R. Bovbjerg and C. F. Koller, "State Health Insurance Pools," *Inquiry* 23 (1986): 111–21.

36. See Norman Daniels, "Insurability and the HIV Epidemic: Ethical Issues in Underwriting," *The Milbank Quarterly* 68 (1990): 497–525; and Office of Technology

Assessment, U.S. Congress, *AIDS and Health Insurance* (Washington, DC: OTA, 1988).

37. These statistics are derived from: U. S. Bureau of the Census, *Current Population Reports,* Series P-70, No. 17 (Washington, DC: U.S. Government Printing Office, 1990); Alain Enthoven, "Universal Health Insurance Through Incentives Reform," *Journal of the American Medical Association* 265 (May 15, 1991): 2532–36; and Lawrence D. Brown, "The Medically Uninsured: Problems, Policies, and Politics," *Journal of Health Politics, Policy and Law* 15 (1990): 413–26.

38. This case was prepared by Bethany Spielman on the basis of Paul Taylor, "Ailing, Uninsured and Turned Away," *Washington Post,* June 30, 1985, pp. A1, A15.

39. Public Law 99-272, § 9121 (April 7, 1986).

40. For more detail regarding these and other arguments, see Tom L. Beauchamp, "The Right to Health Care in a Capitalistic Democracy," in *Rights to Health Care,* ed. T. J. Bole III and W. B. Bondeson (Boston: D. Reidel, 1992); and James F. Childress, "Rights to Health Care in a Democratic Society," in *Biomedical Ethics Reviews 1984,* ed. James Humber and Robert Almeder (Clifton, NJ: Humana Press, 1984), pp. 47–70.

41. As the U.S. Supreme Court held in *Youngberg v. Romeo,* 457 U.S. 307 (1982).

42. See Loren E. Lomasky, "Medical Progress and National Health Care," *Philosophy and Public Affairs* 10 (1980): 72–73; and Gary E. Jones, "The Right to Health Care and the State," *Philosophical Quarterly* 33 (1983): 278–87.

43. See Daniels, *Just Health Care,* ch. 3 and 4.

44. Engelhardt, *The Foundations of Bioethics,* p. 340.

45. Allen Buchanan, "Health-Care Delivery and Resource Allocation," in *Medical Ethics,* ed. Robert Veatch (Boston: Jones and Bartlett Publishers, 1989), esp. pp. 321–25, and "The Right to a Decent Minimum of Health Care," in President's Commission for the Study of Ethical Problems in Medicine and Biomedical and Behavioral Research, *Securing Access to Health Care* (Washington, DC: U.S. Government Printing Office, 1982), vol. 2, esp. p. 234.

46. President's Commission, *Securing Access to Health Care,* vol. 1, p. 4.

47. See Brown, "The Medically Uninsured;" Allen Buchanan, "Health-Care Delivery and Resource Allocation," ch. 11; and Gerald M. Oppenheimer and Robert A. Padgug, "AIDS: The Risks to Insurers, the Threat to Equity," *Hastings Center Report* 16 (October 1986): 18–22.

48. Robert M. Veatch, "Voluntary Risks to Health: The Ethical Issues," *Journal of the American Medical Association* 243 (January 4, 1980): 50–55.

49. Louise B. Russell, "Some of the Tough Decisions Required by a National Health Plan," *Science* 246 (Nov. 17, 1989): 892–96.

50. See, for example, Howard Leichter, "Public Policy and the British Experience," *Hastings Center Report* 11 (October 1981): 32–39, incorporated into his *Free to Be Foolish: Politics and Health Promotion in the United States and Great Britain* (Princeton, NJ: Princeton University Press, 1991), p. 38.

51. Robert J. Blendon and Karen Donelan, "The Public and the Emerging Debate over National Health Insurance," *New England Journal of Medicine* 323 (July 19, 1990): 208–12.

52. These data are from the United Network for Organ Sharing (UNOS), which is the source of other data about transplantation in this chapter unless otherwise indicated.

53. T. E. Starzl, D. Van Thiel, A. G. Tzakis, et al., "Orthotopic Liver Transplantation

for Alcoholic Cirrhosis,'' *Journal of the American Medical Association* 260 (November 4, 1988): 2542–44.

54. Alvin H. Moss and Mark Siegler, "Should Alcoholics Compete Equally for Liver Transplantation?" *Journal of the American Medical Association* 265 (March 13, 1991): 1295–98.

55. An argument based on justice against the total exclusion of alcoholics from liver transplantation appears in Carl Cohen, Martin Benjamin, and the Ethics and Social Impact Committee of the [Michigan] Transplant and Health Policy Center, "Alcoholics and Liver Transplantation," *Journal of the American Medical Association* 265 (March 13, 1991): 1299–1301.

56. Daniels, *Just Health Care,* p. 2.

57. See Paul Ramsey, *The Patient as Person* (New Haven: Yale University Press, 1970), chap. 7.

58. See Paul Starr, "The Politics of Therapeutic Nihilism," *Hastings Center Report* 6 (October 1976): 23–30.

59. A particularly illuminating discussion of this issue is found in Paul T. Menzel, *Medical Costs, Moral Choices* (New Haven: Yale University Press, 1983), ch. 7.

60. See Thomas C. Schelling, "The Life You Save May Be Your Own," in *Problems in Public Expenditure Analysis,* ed. Samuel B. Chase, Jr. (Washington, DC: Brookings Institution, 1966), pp. 127–76.

61. See Leslie Rothenberg et al., "That Which is Wanting . . . ," *Hastings Center Report* 18 (December 1988): 34–37.

62. Henry J. Aaron and William B. Schwartz, *The Painful Prescription: Rationing Hospital Care* (Washington, DC: The Brookings Institution, 1984); and "Rationing Hospital Care: Lessons from Britain." *New England Journal of Medicine* 330 (January 5, 1984): 52–56. For a critical response to their interpretation of the situation in Great Britain, see Frances H. Miller and Graham A. H. Miller, *"The Painful Prescription:* A Procrustean Perspective?" *New England Journal of Medicine* 314 (1986): 1383–86.

63. See Richard Zeckhauser, "Procedures for Valuing Lives," *Public Policy* 23 (Fall 1975): 447–48. Contrast Richard A. Rettig, "Valuing Lives: The Policy Debate on Patient Care Financing for Victims of End-Stage Renal Disease," *The Rand Paper Series* (Santa Monica, CA: Rand Corporation, 1976).

64. Oregon Senate Bill 27 (March 31, 1989). See also David M. Eddy, "What's Going on in Oregon?" *Journal of the American Medical Association* 266 (July 17, 1991): 417–20, and Arnold S. Relman, "Is Rationing Inevitable?" [editorial], *New England Journal of Medicine* 322 (June 21, 1990) 1809–10.

65. Oregon has a constitutional mandate for a balanced budget. An effort was made beginning in 1982 to develop public awareness and consensus on allocation issues through the involvement of local communities. The effort focused on two fundamental questions: (1) How does society value expensive curative medical care relative to preventive services being progressively curtailed in government budgets? (2) Can the present implicit rationing of health care be made explicit and congruent with community values? A series of approximately three hundred town meetings with more than five thousand citizens was followed by a statewide parliament in fall 1984, which produced a document, "Society Must Decide: Oregon Health Decisions Final Report." A major conclusion of that report was that "collective financing of health care should be accomplished by community responsibility for the

ethics of allocation and rationing policies." See H. Gilbert Welch and Eric B. Larson, "Dealing with Limited Resources: The Oregon Decision to Curtail Funding for Organ Transplantation," *New England Journal of Medicine* 319 (1988): 171–73.

66. See the analysis in David C. Hadorn, "The Oregon Priority-Setting Exercise," *Hastings Center Report* 21 (May-June 1991): 11–16, "Setting Health Care Priorities in Oregon," *Journal of the American Medical Association* 265 (May 1, 1991): 2218-25, and "The Problem of Discrimination in Health Care Priority Setting," *Journal of the American Medical Association* 268 (September 16, 1992): 1454–59.

67. For an analysis of "Oregon Health Priorities for the 1990s," see Ralph Crawshaw et al., "Developing Principles for Prudent Health Care Allocation: The Continuing Oregon Experiment," *The Western Journal of Medicine* 152 (April 1990): 441–48.

68. See Charles Dougherty, "Setting Health Care Priorities: Oregon's Next Steps," *Hastings Center Report* 21 (May–June 1991): S1–S10.

69. For this reason, the Bush administration refused to grant a federal waiver for the Oregon plan to implement changes in Medicaid; however, the Clinton administration granted the waiver, with attached conditions.

70. Norman Daniels, "Is the Oregon Rationing Plan Fair?" *Journal of the American Medical Association* 265 (May 1, 1991): 2232–35.

71. See A. J. Wing, "Why Don't the British Treat More Patients with Kidney Failure?" *British Medical Journal* 287 (1983): 1157; V. Parsons and P. Lock, "Triage and the Patient with Renal Failure," *Journal of Medical Ethics* 6 (1980): 173–76; and Aaron and Schwartz, *The Painful Prescription.*

72. See Roger Evans, "Advanced Medical Technology and Elderly People," in *Too Old for Health Care? Controversies in Medicine, Law, Economics, and Ethics,* ed. Robert H. Binstock and Stephen G. Post (Baltimore: The Johns Hopkins University Press, 1991), ch. 3.

73. See Binstock and Post, eds., *Too Old for Health Care?, passim;* and Organization for Economic Co-operation and Development, *Financing and Delivering Health Care* (Paris: OECD, 1987), esp. p. 90.

74. See especially Daniels, *Just Health Care,* ch. 5, and *Am I My Parents' Keeper?* (New York: Oxford University Press, 1988). Our discussion in the text will be drawn from the latter unless otherwise indicated.

75. The prudential life span account differs from another argument for age-based rationing that also appeals to fairness and equality. This argument holds that the young should have priority for life-extending medical care because the old have had an opportunity to live more years and, on grounds of fairness, the young deserve an equal chance. See, for example, Robert M. Veatch, ed., *Life Span: Values and Life-extending Technologies* (New York: Harper and Row, 1979).

76. See especially Daniel Callahan, *Setting Limits,* but also *What Kind of Life* (New York: Simon and Schuster, 1990). Most of our discussion has been drawn from the former.

77. Callahan, "Afterward," in *A Good Old Age? The Paradox of Setting Limits,* ed. Paul Homer and Martha Holstein (New York: Simon and Schuster, 1990), p. 301; "Old Age and New Policy," *Journal of the American Medical Association* 261 (February 10, 1989): 905–6.

78. For a comparison and modest criticism of both, see Dan W. Brock, "Justice, Health Care, and the Elderly," *Philosophy and Public Affairs* 18 (1989): 297–312.

79. See Dennis W. Jahnigen and Robert H. Binstock, "Economic and Clinical Realities: Health Care for Elderly People," in *Too Old For Health Care?*, ed., Binstock and Post, ch. 2.

80. For an overview of the developments into 1986, see U.S. Department of Health and Human Services, Report of Task Force on Organ Transplantation, *Organ Transplantation: Issues and Recommendations* (Washington, DC: DHHS, 1986).

81. For assessments supporting this conclusion, see Deborah Mathieu, ed., *Organ Substitution Technology: Ethical, Legal, and Public Policy Issues* (Boulder, CO: Westview Press, 1988).

82. Task Force, *Organ Transplantation*, pp. 105, 11.

83. Roger W. Evans et al., *The National Health Transplantation Study* (Seattle: Battelle Human Affairs Research Centers, 1984), vols. I–V, and Evans, *Executive Summary: The National Cooperative Transplantation Study*, BHARC-100-91-020 (Washington, DC: U.S. Department of Commerce, June 1991).

84. For one case, see Arthur Caplan, *If I Were a Rich Man Could I Buy a Pancreas?* (Bloomington, IN: Indiana University Press, 1992), p. 166.

85. See David M. Eddy, "The Individual vs. Society," *Journal of the American Medical Association* 265 (May 8, 1991): 2399–2401, 2405–6.

86. See Kevin Grumbach et al., "Liberal Benefits, Conservative Spending: The Physicians for a National Health Program Proposal," *Journal of the American Medical Association* 265 (May 15, 1991): 2549–54.

87. Examples of such plans include The Health Access America plan of the American Medical Association (See Todd references, note 14); the Kennedy-Waxman Bill, which emerged from the Senate Committee on Labor and Human Resources (See *Congressional Record*, April 12, 1989: 3763–75); The Report of the U.S. Bipartisan Commission on Comprehensive Health Care (The Pepper Commission, *A Call for Action: Final Report*, Washington, DC: U.S. Government Printing Office, 1990); and Alain Enthoven and Richard Kronick, "A Consumer-Choice Plan for the 1990s," *New England Journal of Medicine* 320 (January 5, 1989): 29–37, 94–101.

88. Nicholas Rescher, "The Allocation of Exotic Medical Lifesaving Therapy," *Ethics* 79 (1969): 173–86.

89. Task Force, *Organ Transplantation*.

90. Task Force, *Organ Transplantation*, p. 95. The task force recommended that hearts and livers not be allocated to nonimmigrant aliens unless it was clear that no U.S. citizen or resident could use the organs. The different recommendations for renal and for extrarenal organs were based in part on the fact that there is no alternative or back-up treatment for heart or liver failure, whereas dialysis is available for most cases of end-stage kidney failure.

91. See James Childress, "Triage in Neonatal Intensive Care: The Limitations of a Metaphor," *Virginia Law Review* 69 (1983): 547–61.

92. Task Force, *Organ Transplantation*, ch. 5.

93. See *Report of the Massachusetts Task Force on Organ Transplantation* (October 1984).

94. See "Scarce Medical Resources," *Columbia Law Review* 69 (1969): 621–92.

95. Contrast Robert M. Veatch, "The Ethics of Resource Allocation in Critical Care," *Critical Care Clinics* 2 (January 1986): 73–89. For fuller discussion see Gerald

Winslow, *Triage and Justice: The Ethics of Rationing Life-Saving Medical Resources* (Berkeley: University of California Press, 1982), and John Kilner, "Who Lives? Who Dies?" *Ethical Criteria in Patient Selection* (New Haven: Yale University Press, 1990).

96. H. Tristram Engelhardt, Jr. and Michael A. Rie, "Intensive Care Units, Scarce Resources, and Conflicting Principles of Justice," *Journal of the American Medical Association* 255 (March 7, 1986): 1159–64.
97. *The Totally Implantable Artificial Heart*, pp. 192–98.
98. See John Broome, "Selecting People Randomly," *Ethics* 95 (1984): 41.
99. Robert D. Truog, "Triage in the ICU," *Hastings Center Report* 22 (May–June 1992): 13–17.
100. See Ramsey, *The Patient as Person*, pp. 257–58. For the controversy about this example, see Robert Baker and Martin Strosberg, "Triage and Equality: An Historical Reassessment of Utilitarian Analyses of Triage," *Kennedy Institute of Ethics Journal* 2 (1992): 101–123.
101. Rescher, "The Allocation of Exotic Medical Lifesaving Therapy," p. 178.
102. See James F. Childress, "Who Shall Live When Not All Can Live?" *Soundings* 53 (1970): 339–55.
103. See Winslow, *Triage and Justice,* but contrast Baker and Strosberg, "Triage and Equality: An Historical Reassessment."
104. Mary Faith Marshall et al., "Influence of Political Power, Medical Provincialism and Economic Incentives on the Rationing of Surgical Intensive Care Unit Beds," *Critical Care Medicine* 20 (March 1992): 387–94.

7

Professional–Patient Relationships

In the previous four chapters we presented moral principles relevant to medicine, health care, and research with human subjects. In this chapter we further specify these principles in treating problems of veracity, privacy, confidentiality, and fidelity. Some proposals specify a single principle, and others specify several principles. We also examine several types of relationship between health care professionals or researchers and their patients or subjects. The discussions are framed in terms of virtue and character as well as principles and rules.

Veracity

Surprisingly, codes of medical ethics have traditionally ignored obligations and virtues of veracity. The Hippocratic oath does not recommend veracity, nor does the Declaration of Geneva of the World Medical Association. The Principles of Medical Ethics of the American Medical Association (AMA) in effect from its origins until 1980 made no mention of an obligation or virtue of veracity, giving physicians unrestricted discretion about what to divulge to patients. In its 1980 revision, the AMA recommends simply and without elaboration that physicians "deal honestly with patients and colleagues."[1] By contrast to this traditional disregard of veracity, virtues of candor and truthfulness are among the most widely praised character traits of health professionals in contemporary biomedical ethics.

In both traditional codes and current literature, significant uncertainties and ambiguities exist about the nature and status of norms of veracity. We can say now, as Henry Sidgwick observed in the nineteenth century, that "It does not seem clearly agreed whether Veracity is an absolute and independent obligation, or a special application of some higher principle."[2] One contemporary philosopher, G. J. Warnock, includes veracity as an independent principle (and virtue) that ranks in importance with beneficence, nonmaleficence, and justice.[3] Others maintain that rules of veracity derive from principles of respect for autonomy, fidelity, or utility. We will argue that obligations of veracity are best understood as specifications of several principles and that conscientious adherence to these specifications is vital for a successful patient–professional relationship.

Both *conceptual* problems and problems of *justification* need attention, and we begin with justification.

Arguments for Obligations of Veracity

Three arguments contribute to the justification of obligations of veracity. First, the obligation of veracity is based on respect owed to others. As we saw in Chapter 3, respect for autonomy provides the primary justificatory basis for rules of disclosure and consent. Consent cannot express autonomy unless it is informed; thus, when disclosures are made, valid consent depends on truthful communication. Even if consent is not the issue, the obligation of veracity still depends on respect owed to others. As Alan Donagan writes, "The respect owed to other human beings includes respect for their liberty to withhold their thoughts when it is not their duty to divulge them; but, if anybody chooses to divulge his thoughts, the respect he owes to his audience requires that the thoughts he communicates must really be his."[4]

Second, the obligation of veracity has a close connection to obligations of fidelity and promise-keeping.[5] When we communicate with others, we implicitly promise that we will speak truthfully and that we will not deceive our listeners. Voluntary participation in these social conventions engenders an obligation of veracity. In biomedical contexts, a specific, although implicit, contract or promise is often identifiable. By entering into a relationship in therapy or research, the patient or subject enters into a contract, thereby gaining a right to the truth regarding diagnosis, prognosis, procedures, and the like, just as the professional gains a right to truthful disclosures from patients and subjects.

Third, relationships of trust between persons are necessary for fruitful interaction and cooperation. At the core of these relationships is confidence in and reliance on others to be truthful. Relationships between health care professionals and their patients and between researchers and their subjects ultimately depend on trust, and adherence to rules of veracity is essential to foster trust.

Lying and inadequate disclosure, then, show disrespect for persons, violate implicit contracts, and threaten relationships of trust.

However, like other obligations in this volume, veracity is prima facie binding, not absolute. Nondisclosure, deception, and lying will all occasionally be justified when veracity conflicts with other obligations. Forms of deception that violate obligations of truth-telling include giving placebos and manipulating information, as described in Chapter 3. Although the weight of various obligations of veracity is difficult to determine outside specific contexts, some generalizations may be tendered: Deception that does not involve lying is generally less difficult to justify than lying, because it does not as deeply threaten the relationship of trust between deceiver and deceived. Underdisclosure and nondisclosure are typically still less difficult to justify. By contrast to obligations not to lie and deceive, the obligation to disclose usually depends on special relationships. For example, the patient entrusts care to the clinician and thereby gains a right to information that the clinician would not otherwise be obligated to provide. It is, then, advisable not to conflate the various obligations to disclose information, not to lie, and not to deceive, although much of the literature treats them as a single obligation.

Meaning, Scope, and Weight of Obligations of Veracity

As with informed consent, courts have typically assimilated obligations of *veracity* to obligations of *disclosure* about procedures that require consent or refusal. But this conception is too narrow for biomedical ethics, where veracity refers to comprehensive, accurate, and objective transmission of information, as well as to the way the professional fosters understanding in the relationship.

In one case, *Truman v. Thomas*,[6] an influential court permitted the children of a woman who died from cervical cancer to sue her doctor for failing to disclose the risks of *not* undergoing the Pap test, which she had repeatedly refused. The court held that the patient must be apprised of risks of "a decision *not* to undergo the treatment," as well as the "risks inherent in the procedure." This obligation to disclose the risks of no treatment resembles the well-established obligation to disclose alternatives to a proposed procedure. In many instances, no treatment is one alternative to the procedure proposed. Thus, the risks of doing nothing are likely to fall within the scope of the physician's obligation to disclose information about any proffered procedure.

Of interest in this case is the recognition of an obligation of disclosure even if the patient refuses a physician's recommendation and no bodily intrusion occurs. The court held that the importance of the right to make decisions about one's body is not diminished by the kind of decision one makes, because no other result is consistent with the fiduciary nature of the physician's obligation to present the proper information. We can generalize this conclusion in the moral context. Veracity in medical practice can pertain to any truthful and honest management of information that may affect a patient's understanding or decisionmaking. It is not limited to situations of informed consent.

Limited Disclosure and Deception

Withholding a diagnosis of cancer and a prognosis of imminent death is a widely discussed case of withholding information. In one case, Mr. X, a fifty-four-year-old patient, consented to surgery for probable malignancy in his thyroid gland. After the surgery, he was told that the diagnosis had been confirmed and that the tumor had been successfully removed, but he was not informed of the likelihood of lung metastases and death within a few months. His wife, son, and daughter-in-law were well informed by the physician about the consequences of surgery, but they and the physician agreed to conceal the diagnosis and prognosis from Mr. X. He was told only that he needed "preventive" treatment, and he then consented to irradiation and chemotherapy. He was also not informed of the probable causes of his subsequent shortness of breath and back pain. He was unaware of his impending death and died three months later.[7]

Mr. X was once a typical case, but over the last thirty years, a dramatic shift has occurred in physicians' stated policies of disclosure of the diagnosis of cancer to patients. In 1961, eighty-eight percent of the physicians surveyed indicated that they sought to avoid disclosing a diagnosis of cancer to the patient, but by 1979, ninety-eight percent of those surveyed reported a policy of telling the cancer patient. Although practices of disclosure may vary significantly, changes in physicians' stated policies for disclosing a diagnosis of cancer are well documented. The reasons for the changes include the availability of more treatment options for cancer (including experimental treatments), improved rates of survival from some forms of cancer, fear of malpractice suits, involvement of team members in hospitals, altered societal attitudes about cancer, increased attention to patients' rights, and physicians' increased recognition of communication as an effective means of enhancing the patient's understanding and compliance.[8]

In the 1979 survey, physicians identified the "four most frequent factors considered in the decision to tell the patient" as age (fifty-six percent), a relative's wishes regarding disclosure to the patient (fifty-one percent), emotional stability (forty-seven percent), and intelligence (forty-four percent).[9] From our standpoint, familial preferences are often unjustifiably influential in clinicians' decisions about disclosure of diagnosis and prognosis to patients. Critics of our position often contend that the family can help the physician determine whether the patient is autonomous, able to accept information about serious risk, and genuinely wants the information. Although true, this response begs an important question. By what right does a physician initially disclose information to a family without the patient's consent? The family provides desirable care and support for many patients, but the autonomous patient has the moral right to veto familial involvement. If veracity (and respect for the patient's autonomy) is a primary rule or virtue in the physician's moral orientation, it is difficult to understand why the physician would first disclose information to a family, even when the family requests it. The best policy is to ask the patient both at the outset and as the illness progresses about the extent to which he or she prefers to involve others.

In caring for nonautonomous or doubtfully autonomous patients, clinicians may have obligations to disclose appropriate diagnostic and prognostic information to the patients even when surrogates request nondisclosure. For example, in Case 3 (in the appendix), a man brought his father to a physician because of a suspicion of early Alzheimer's disease and requested that the physician not disclose a diagnosis of Alzheimer's to his father. Despite the son's request, the physician is not relieved of the obligation to inform the patient of the diagnosis.

In literature on the justification of limited disclosure and deception in therapeutic settings, three arguments deserve consideration. They assume that breaches of obligations of veracity are prima facie wrong, but can sometimes be justified. The first argument rests on what Henry Sidgwick and many after him called "benevolent deception." Such deception has long been a part of medical tradition. It holds that disclosure sometimes violates obligations of beneficence and nonmaleficence by causing the patient anxiety, by retarding or erasing a therapeutic outcome, by leading the patient to commit suicide, and the like. This line of argument—"What you don't know can't hurt and may help you"—is consequentialist. One objection to this argument is based on the uncertainty of predicting consequences, as we saw in examining Worthington Hooker's position (in Chapter 2). Samuel Johnson states this objection sharply: "I deny the lawfulness of telling a lie to a sick man for fear of alarming him. You have no business with consequences; you are to tell the truth. Besides, you are not sure what effects your telling him that he is in danger may have." [10]

Objections to benevolent deception often stress its negative consequences, particularly its long-term threat to the special relationship of trust between physicians and patients and to the physician's moral integrity. Deception may also have long-term negative effects on the patient's self-image. These are strong reasons for caution. Although it is sometimes sufficient to justify the use of deceptive means by its probable impact on the patient's health (see Chapter 5, pp. 278–284), alternative nondeceptive means are usually more satisfactory. The prima facie obligation of veracity demands a search for alternatives even when they require more time, energy, and financial resources. We accept benevolent deception in a narrow range of cases, but its use will be infrequently justified.

A second reason for nondisclosure and deception is that health care professionals cannot know the "whole truth," and if they could, many patients and subjects would not be able to comprehend and understand the scope and implications of the information. This reason, however, does not undermine the obligation of veracity. Disclosure of the "whole truth" about a complex circumstance is an ideal against which health care professionals can measure their performance, but it can only be approximated, never fully realized. We can best use this ideal to help formulate a standard of *substantial* completeness that is realistic and appropriate for health care professionals (as discussed in Chapter 3).

A third argument is that some patients, particularly the very sick and the dying, do not want to know the truth about their condition, despite opinion surveys that indicate they do want to know. According to this argument, neither the obligation of fidelity nor the obligation of respect for autonomy requires truth-telling, because patients indicate by various signals, if not by actual words, that they do not want the truth. To the rejoinder that many, and perhaps most, patients say they want relevant information disclosed, proponents of this third argument hold that the patients they have in mind do not want to know even when they say they do.

Claims about what patients genuinely want are inherently dubious when they contradict the patients' own reports, and this third argument sets dangerous precedents for paternalistic actions under the guise of respect for autonomy. The argument also improperly suggests that professionals' distrust of patients' communications is appropriate. However, more subtle versions of this third argument for incomplete disclosure appeal to the patient's implicit request not to be informed, sometimes combined with the claim that the patient already knows but does not want to confront in open discussion some truth about a diagnosis or prognosis.

One Italian oncologist reports that she tries to tell her patients "the complete truth," but sometimes the patient's family asks her not to use the word "cancer."[11] She then relies on nonverbal communication to establish truthful and therapeutic relationships with patients, listening to them and respecting their need for information. In the Italian cultural background, the emphasis placed on beneficence toward the patient is not accompanied by the same pronounced emphasis on autonomy that prevails in the United States. Surveys show that Italians are divided, roughly fifty-fifty, on whether they want truthful disclosures. In a 1991 study of 1171 breast cancer patients and their physicians and surgeons in general hospitals in Italy, only forty-seven percent of the women reported that they had been informed that they had cancer, whereas twenty-five percent of their physicians indicated that they had not given accurate information.[12] Although social practices in Italy reflect different ideals than U.S. practices, they do not necessarily fail to respect individual autonomy. We can affirm the physician's obligation to respect the patient's autonomy, while recognizing that the way patients exercise their autonomy will be shaped by sociocultural contexts, including religious and other beliefs. Autonomous patients may choose to delegate decisionmaking to others, as often occurs in some parts of Italy and among many ethnic groups in North America.

Edmund Pellegrino rightly argues that "To thrust the truth or the decision on a patient who expects to be buffered against news of impending death is a gratuitous and harmful misinterpretation of the moral foundations for respect for autonomy." [13] Care and sensitivity are required to respect a particular patient's autonomy by varying the information according to his or her preferences. Pervasive cultural ideals can only set presumptions about particular patients' preferences. It is still essential to determine whether particular patients authentically affirm or reject those ideals.

Disclosure of Unwanted Information

Some writers have suggested that patients have an obligation to seek and to accept the truth about their medical conditions, not merely a right to the truth. From this perspective, patients have a responsibility to ask questions and inquire into their conditions and the consequences of their decisions. [14] This view is sustainable, but it does not follow that we have a right to force unwanted information on patients for their benefit, an act that may violate patients' autonomy rights and disrespect them as autonomous agents. Imposing undesired information on an unreceptive patient can, on rare occasions, be justified—as when a person is acting on false beliefs. But persons have a right not to know if they are adequately informed about the risks of not knowing and do not place others at serious risk. How, then, should health care professionals handle such delicate situations?

Consider discussions of predictive testing for Huntington's disease and other late-onset disorders. Huntington's disease is a rare, incurable, debilitating, and fatal neurological disorder caused by a defective gene. It usually becomes manifest between ages thirty-five and fifty, producing a loss of muscle control and dementia. The current test for Huntington's involves closely linked markers for the gene rather than direct tests for the gene itself. Instead of providing definitive information, it provides the odds that the person will or will not develop Huntington's (at 95% reliability). No treatment is available. This test is burdensome and potentially involves losses of privacy and confidentiality, because several relatives must give blood for DNA analysis and undergo neurological examinations; yet the test cannot predict when the disease might occur or how severe its manifestations will be.

Some commentators argue that individuals at risk for Huntington's disease have a right to know and a right not to know, but also that the at-risk individual has a moral obligation to know whether he or she is a carrier in circumstances in which a third party might be harmed by the lack of knowledge.[15] These circumstances include choices about reproduction, based on moral obligations to prevent harm to spouse and offspring. In addition, because the current test requires testing relatives, they too would have a moral obligation of beneficence to participate. Studies indicate that the majority of people at risk want to undergo a simple, safe, and reliable predictive test,[16] but in one study only twelve percent of at-risk individuals were willing to participate in a trial.[17] Various reasons may account for these discrepancies. For example, some individuals at risk view a predictive test with ninety-five percent probability as insufficiently accurate, some do not want to involve other family members required for this genetic-linkage test, and some seek to avoid the hopelessness they feel sure to develop after testing positive.

In a Canadian study of one hundred thirty-five at-risk individuals, fifty-eight learned that they probably did not inherit the defective gene for Huntington's (the decreased-risk group); thirty-seven learned that they had a high probability of developing Huntington's disease (the increased-risk group); and forty decided not to undergo testing or received inconclusive test results (the no-change group). All groups received extensive pre-test and post-test counseling, as well baseline and three post-test psychological evaluations, including tests for distress and depression. The decreased-risk group made the best adjustment to the information, although ten percent of that group had "serious difficulties coping with their new status." The increased-risk group initially faced problems of adjustment and depression, and some needed additional counseling, but none attempted to commit suicide or needed psychiatric hospitalization. After a year, their psychological evaluations indicated only small declines from their baseline distress and depression. The group that refused the test or had inconclusive test results made the poorest adjustment over time. Even the increased-risk group reported less depression and a greater sense of psychological well-being after one year than the no-change group. The authors of this study conclude that predictive testing for Huntington's disease when accompanied by adequate counseling offers psychological benefits by reducing uncertainty and providing an opportunity for appropriate planning, even when the results indicate increased risk (from 50% to 95%) of getting the disease.[18]

The results of this study must be used with caution, in part because the study population was middle-aged, well educated, and perhaps unrepresentative, but also because the study's intensive counseling may have been as momentous as knowledge of the test results. The study presents information that could and should be provided to at-risk individuals considering the test, but it does not provide a basis for forcing or pressuring individuals to take the test. No evidence exists that any group would have been better off if the test and its results had been compulsory. Individuals at risk for Huntington's disease also need to consider the potential economic and social ramifications of such diagnostic information, because they may risk losing health insurance and life insurance.

Another test case for the ethics of imposing information has developed from the AIDS epidemic. The right not to know has appropriately been challenged when those donating blood have tested antibody-positive for HIV. The paternalistic case for disclosure of a positive HIV-antibody test to those who do not want to know and seek to avoid disclosure became stronger as physicians could do more to help people infected with HIV, including starting anti-retroviral treatment earlier. Disclosure also can play a pivotal role in changing behavior in order to reduce risks to others—an important consequentialist argument for unwanted disclosure. In one case, a thirty-five-year-old man who had engaged in homosexual activities went to a physician because of symptoms consistent with HIV infection and consented to have his blood tested for HIV antibodies. The next day the patient called to say that he had changed his mind and wanted to cancel the test. The test had already been completed, and the physician, who had been notified that the patient did not want to know the results, decided to tell the patient of his HIV infection to reduce the risks for sexual partners.[19] In light of the possible consequences, the disclosure was justified despite the fact that the patient did not want the information.

A related problem involves a health care professional's responsibility when a test undertaken for a specific purpose reveals information not specifically requested by the testee, who might nonetheless need or want the information. In one case a forty-one-year-old woman had unexpectedly become pregnant and was referred by her physician to the human genetics unit in order to determine whether her fetus might have Down syndrome.[20] Amniocentesis showed that the fetus did not have Down syndrome, but the sex chromosomes were abnormal. They were XYY rather than the normal patterns of XX for female or XY for male. The significance of the extra Y chromosome is debatable. Although some studies show that XYY males tend to commit more violent crimes, other studies reject those findings. What should the genetic counselor do?

The fact that the causal connection between the XYY chromosomes and antisocial behavior is disputed makes assessment of this disclosure more difficult. There are risks, because disclosure could lead the woman to choose an abortion, or, if the woman did not abort, the parents and others subsequently might treat the child as potentially antisocial. The question is whether the pregnant woman should have the right to make her decision about the significance of this information. If the obligation of veracity rests in part on the potential value of the information for others, a strong case can be made for disclosure, although the woman did not specifically request this information.

Managing Negative Information Affecting Colleagues and Patients

Incompetent or unscrupulous health care professionals present additional problems about veracity. The AMA Principles of Medical Ethics require disclosure of information in order to preserve trust between the public and the medical profession: "A physician shall deal honestly with patients and colleagues, and strive to expose those physicians deficient in character or competence, or who engage in fraud or deception." Exposés by fellow physicians are, however, uncommon. Bonds of professional loyalty, accented in the Hippocratic and collegial traditions of medical ethics, present a formidable barrier, but this sociological fact does not excuse failures to expose serious deficiencies. Often disclosures are essential to preserve institutional or public trust, as well as the confidence of professional colleagues. In some cases, the health professional has an obligation both to investigate and to ameliorate specific problems.

A wall of silence frequently surrounds medical malpractice, particularly when the patient is unaware of the malpractice and members of the treatment team or consultants are aware of it. In one case a boy, age three and a half, was taken by his parents to a medical center for treatment of a respiratory problem. After being placed in the adult intensive care unit, he was given ten times the normal dosage of muscle relaxant, after which the respirator tube slipped and pumped oxygen into his stomach for several minutes. He suffered cardiac arrest and permanent brain damage. The parents accidentally overheard a conversation that mentioned the overdose. The physician involved explained that he had decided not to inform the parents of the mistake because they "had enough on [their] minds already."[21]

To reduce such abuses, some commentators have suggested a legally imposed obligation on both the primary physician and observing members of the treatment team to report malpractice to the victim, not simply to organizations that determine physician competence.[22] Apart from questions of defensible public policy, silence in a circumstance of malpractice is morally indefensible. It is sometimes equally indefensible to fail to defend a colleague when his or her truthfulness eventuates in a malpractice suit or dismissal from a position. Health care professionals who disclose that their error placed a patient at risk deserve their colleagues' support, especially in the wake of overreactions. For example, a promising young physician in Chicago candidly reported that he had mistakenly used a swab on a patient that previously had been used on an HIV patient. Although no one was known to have been harmed, the physician's honesty earned him dismissal and collegial indifference to his plight.[23] The clear message imparted to younger physicians is that nondisclosure and deception are more prudent than veracity.

Beyond these problems of misplaced loyalty to and unjustified abandonment of colleagues, health professionals sometimes experience a conflict between the obligation of confidentiality and the obligation of veracity. For example, difficult cases appear in medical genetics when health care professionals discover nonpaternity. Suppose that following the birth of a child with a genetic problem, a married couple seeks counseling about whether to have another child, and tests indicate that the husband is not the child's biological father. In a cross-cultural study of geneticists in nineteen countries, ninety-six percent of respondents (and over 90% in all countries) indicated that they would not disclose false paternity to the husband. Eighty-one percent of respondents said they would tell the wife in private, away from the husband, and let her decide what to tell him, whereas thirteen percent would lie to the couple (for example, by telling them that both are genetically responsible), and two percent would indicate that the child's disorder is the result of a new mutation. Only four percent of respondents would tell both the wife and the husband. The reasons for nondisclosure to the husband include preserving the family unit (58%), honoring the wife's right to decide (30%), and respecting the wife's right to privacy (13%). Although there were no gender differences in the response to the situation, female geneticists (75% of female respondents) were more likely than male counterparts (57% of male respondents) to use potential marital conflict as a reason for their decisions.[24] Yet, refusing to disclose nonpaternity deprives the husband or sexual partner of potentially important information generated in a relationship with the genetic counselor based in part on materials he provided. Whether nondisclosure can be justified on the grounds indicated (confidentiality, privacy, and protection of family relationships) will finally depend on the circumstances.

A psychologically and ethically more complex case occurs when a physician has a patient, who, with her spouse, seeks help because she is infertile, and the counselor determines that she is an XY female—that is, genetically male but phenotypically female. One question is whether to provide the patient and the patient's husband an accurate biological explanation of testicular feminization syndrome. In the cross-cultural study mentioned in the previous paragraph, the vast majority of counselors selected nondisclosure on grounds that they wanted to avoid causing psychological harm to the patient. However, at least three premises feed an argument for disclosure: (1) the patient's infertility requires an explanation, and the genetic explanation may help relieve guilt; (2) surgical removal of the abdominal or inguinal testes is recommended to prevent cancer, but such surgery requires consent based on adequate information; and (3) the physician—patient relationship generally requires the disclosure of meaningful information to patients.[25]

Difficult problems emerge about the specific information that ought to be provided—to the wife and the husband—and how it might be provided in order to minimize the potential harm. What and how to disclose to the woman depends in part on the risks of disclosure (see our discussions of paternalism in

Chapter 6 and informed consent in Chapter 3). Regarding disclosure to the husband, this case is analogous to the nonpaternity case and may be decided on similar grounds. Because no risk of physical harm exists for the husband, it is difficult to defend a breach of medical confidentiality against the wife's wishes. Nevertheless, the information will likely be important to the husband, and he too has come to the counselor seeking help. Geneticists can encourage the wife to make disclosures to the husband, while offering assistance in counseling, and thus avoid a breach of confidentiality. We should not rule out full disclosure to both parties, under some circumstance, even if the wife resists disclosure to her husband and appeals to confidentiality.

We have seen in this section that obligations of veracity often conflict with obligations of confidentiality and privacy. We will first examine privacy and then confidentiality.

Privacy

When columnist Jack Anderson reported that lawyer Roy Cohn was being treated for AIDS in an experimental trial of the drug AZT at the National Institutes of Health, critics argued that some health care professionals had violated Cohn's rights of privacy and confidentiality by releasing information to Anderson, who in turn violated Cohn's right of privacy by publishing the report.[26] Many such claims about obligations of privacy and confidentiality have pervaded controversies about policies to control the spread of AIDS. Various proposals to screen individuals to determine whether they are antibody-positive for HIV threaten a loss of privacy, yet physicians question traditional obligations of confidentiality when patients with HIV infection refuse to inform or allow physicians to inform their spouses or lovers of their condition. These questions about privacy and confidentiality appear in several areas of biomedicine—for example, in biomedical research and in screening employees in the workplace for genetic diseases and use of illicit drugs.

These specific issues are parts of a much larger problem of data protection in the health care system. Although privacy and confidentiality are often closely linked—for example in federal regulations and in professional codes of ethics—they are distinct concepts that partially overlap.

History in the Law

In the history of moral and legal theory,[27] privacy received little explicit attention until late in the nineteenth century.[28] The U.S. Supreme Court early in the 1920s employed an expansive "liberty" interest to protect family decisionmaking about various issues, including child rearing and education.[29] It later switched to the term *privacy* and expanded the individual's and the family's protected interest in family life, child rearing, and other areas of personal choice.[30] The clearest expression of this privacy right appears in the Court's family-planning decisions. *Griswold v. Connecticut* (1965), a contraception case, was the first to construe the right of privacy not only as shielding information from others, but as protecting an area of individual freedom from governmental interference. According to this legal interpretation, the right to privacy protects liberty by delineating a zone of private life that by its nature is protected from state intrusion. The Court's decision in this case overturned state legislation that prohibited the use or dissemination of contraceptives, and in 1973 the Court expanded the scope of privacy rights to overturn restrictive abortion laws.[31]

Although not explicitly enumerated in the Bill of Rights, the right of privacy was held in *Griswold* and in some subsequent Supreme Court decisions to arise from the "penumbra" of the first, third, fourth, fifth, ninth, and fourteenth amendments to the Constitution. The argument is that a personal right to privacy exists because so many amendments imply it. An individual holds the right, like most other constitutional rights, only against the state and against parties acting on behalf of the state, not against other individuals or nongovernmental entities. It may seem inapposite to make this personal right one of privacy rather than liberty or autonomy, and increasingly the term *privacy* is being used as a synonym for *autonomy*. However, the right to privacy is a right of limited physical or informational inaccessibility, and it can be confusing to think of this right as reducible to a right to be free to do something or a right to act autonomously. We will later argue that the right to privacy is a specification of and is justified by the principle of respect for autonomy, but *privacy* and *autonomy* are not synonyms.

The constitutional right of privacy is still inchoate and controversial, and the current state of statutory and case law is chaotic. Further legal developments can be expected. Of special relevance to biomedical ethics are laws governing computerized patient record systems and appeals to the right to privacy as a legal and constitutional basis for termination of life-sustaining treatments. These issues in biomedical ethics are complicated by competing conceptions of privacy and by disagreements regarding the grounds, limits, and weight of a right to privacy.

The Concept of Privacy

Some definitions of *privacy* focus on the agent's control over access to himself or herself,[32] but these definitions confuse privacy, which is a state or condition of physical or informational inaccessibility, with control over privacy or a right to control privacy, which involves the agent's right to control access. These definitions focus on powers and rights rather than conditions of privacy. A person can have privacy without having any control over access by others. It occurs, for example, when others ignore a person. The state or condition of privacy thus often results from sheer indifference, a particularly significant moral problem in some long-term care facilities. Control-over-access definitions, then, provide neither a necessary nor a sufficient condition of privacy.

Definitions of privacy are too narrow if presented solely in terms of limited access to *information* about a person. A loss of privacy occurs if others use several forms of access to a person, including intervening in zones of intimacy, secrecy, anonymity, seclusion, or solitude.[33] Privacy as inaccessibility also extends to bodily products and objects intimately associated with the person, as well as to a person's intimate relationships with friends, lovers, spouses, physicians, and others. However, information about persons is an important part of privacy. The Institute of Medicine in the United States has identified thirty-three representative users of patient records in health care facilities and over fifty primary and secondary uses of these records, thereby indicating a robust need for privacy protection in the health care system.[34]

Defining *privacy* in terms of several types of inaccessibility or restricted access to a person may appear overly broad. If one could more precisely circumscribe the types of restricted access and the aspects of persons that count as private, one could develop a narrower definition. Much of the literature on privacy undertakes to restrict the concept in just this way, for example, narrowing the range of types of access to *knowledge of information* about persons, thereby disallowing as a loss of privacy the types of access to persons identified in the previous paragraph. The goal is to find precise necessary and sufficient conditions of privacy, instead of leaving the analysis at the apparently vague level of all forms of restricted access.[35]

We agree that the flexibility native to the concept of privacy makes it desirable to provide a tighter meaning. This objective is particularly germane for policies regarding which forms of access to which aspects of persons will constitute losses that are violations of privacy. We are, however, reluctant to castrate the concept to make it more serviceable for policy. Instead, we recommend that those who propose policies carefully specify conditions of restricted access that will and will not count as a loss or violation of privacy. The policy should accurately define the zones that are considered private and not to be invaded, and it should also state interests that may legitimately be balanced against privacy interests. Often the focus will be informational privacy and restricting modes of access to information about persons; but in other cases policies will govern privacy in making decisions, in intimate relationships, and the like.

Finally, a person's privacy (or loss of privacy) should not be confused with that person's sense of privacy (or sense of loss of privacy). A person may have privacy while wrongly believing that someone is eavesdropping, and a person may unknowingly have lost some measure of privacy when someone discovers a medical history or chart and discloses its contents to others. What counts as a loss of privacy and what affects an individual's sense of loss of privacy also can vary from society to society and individual to individual, in part because no particular item is intrinsically private.[36] The value we place on a condition of non-access explains how it comes to be categorized as private. A loss of privacy may also depend not only on the kind or amount of access but also on who has access through what means to which aspect of the person. As Charles Fried notes, "We may not mind that a person knows a general fact about us, and yet feel our privacy invaded if he knows the details. For instance, a casual acquaintance may comfortably know that I am sick, but it would violate my privacy if he knew the nature of the illness."[37]

Justifications of the Right to Privacy

In their celebrated article "The Right to Privacy,"[38] Warren and Brandeis argue that a legal right to privacy can be derived from fundamental rights to life, liberty, and property, but they derive it largely from "the right to enjoy life— the right to be let alone." In recent discussions, several alternative justifications of the right to privacy have been proposed, three of which deserve attention.

One approach reduces the right to privacy to a cluster of other rights from which the right to privacy is derivative. According to Judith Thomson, this cluster of personal and property rights includes rights not to be looked at, not to be listened to, not to be caused distress (for example, by the publication of certain information), not to be harmed, hurt, or tortured (for example, to obtain certain information), and so on. However, her argument rests on several allegedly foundational rights that themselves have an uncertain status, such as the right not to be looked at. We are not convinced that each of these alleged rights is a right, and, more importantly, some of these rights may have the right to privacy as their basis, rather than the converse.[39] These rights are not as easily divided into more basic units in the way Thomson suggests. One might plausibly argue that each violation of these "basic" rights is wrong because it involves wrongfully gaining access to a person—that is, because it violates a right to privacy.

Another and more promising approach emphasizes the instrumental value of privacy and the right to privacy by identifying various ends that are served by rules of privacy. Different consequentialist theories, including utilitarianism, justify rules of privacy according to their instrumental value for ends such as personal development, creating and maintaining intimate social relations, and expressing one's freedom.[40] Charles Fried argues that privacy is a necessary condition—"the necessary atmosphere"—for maintaining intimate relationships of respect, love, friendship and trust. Without privacy, he argues, these relationships are inconceivable.[41] Privacy certainly has such instrumental value. We grant others access to ourselves in order to have and maintain such relationships. Whether we grant someone else access to some aspect of our lives will depend on the kind of relationship we want in pursuit of our goals. For example, we allow physicians access to our bodies in order to protect our health. But is the instrumental value of privacy its only value? And is this value the only justification of rights and obligations of privacy?

Both of the above rationales merit serious consideration, but the primary justification resides in a third rationale based on the principle of respect for autonomy. For example, we often respect persons by respecting their autonomous wishes not to be observed, touched, or intruded upon. This thesis may seem odd in light of our claim above that the right to privacy is easily confused with the right to act autonomously; but our present thesis has to do with justifying the right to privacy and specifying the principle of respect for autonomy: Rights of privacy are valid claims against unauthorized access that have their basis in the right to authorize or decline access. These rights are justified by rights of autonomous choice that are correlative to the obligations expressed in the principle of respect for autonomy. In this respect, the justification of the right to privacy is parallel to the justification of the right to give an informed consent that was developed in Chapter 3.

Joel Feinberg has observed that historically the language of autonomy has functioned as a political metaphor for a domain or territory in which a state is sovereign. Personal autonomy carries over the idea of a region of sovereignty for the self and a right to protect it by restricting access, an idea closely linked to the concepts of privacy and the right to privacy. Using the spatial and territorial model, Feinberg interprets the personal domain to include "a certain amount of 'breathing space' around one's body."[42] Other metaphors expressing privacy in the personal domain include *zones* and *spheres* of privacy that protect autonomy. The principle of respect for autonomy therefore includes the right to decide insofar as possible what will happen to one's person—to one's body, to information about one's life, to one's secrets, etc.

The U.S. Supreme Court has argued that the protection of interests in privacy law incorporates the protection of personal interests in autonomous decisionmaking; the law does not merely protect interests in being inaccessible. The closer one models the right to privacy on the right to make such decisions, the closer one associates the right to privacy with the right to choose autonomously. The decisions of the Court have functioned by design to protect citizens from interference with autonomy in making decisions about abortion, contraception, the termination of life-prolonging treatments, and the like. The Court has often hinted that the right to privacy is primarily a right of self-determination in decisionmaking, on which certain clear boundaries must be placed.[43] This idea that certain forms of self-determination are immune from social control has made the legal right of privacy controversial throughout its history.

One possible objection to our claim that respect for autonomy is the main justificatory basis of obligations to respect privacy is the following: Suppose that a patient in a hospital leaves a sealed note for a night nurse. A physician who suspects a conspiracy between the two not to follow a prescribed regimen opens and reads the note while the patient is asleep. The patient's privacy has been violated, but has respect for autonomy violated? If no disrespect for autonomy occurs, then the right to privacy is not based on respect for autonomy. However, a violation does occur. Respect for the patient's autonomy requires that no one read the note without being authorized to do so by the patient. Reading the note without permission is as much a violation of rights of autonomy as proceeding to surgery without consent.

A second objection to our autonomy-based justification would focus on the incompetent patient who cannot exercise autonomy, such as the patient in a permanent vegetative state.[44] A nonautonomous patient still has the right of privacy. Some dimensions of this right flow from the incompetent patients's previous exercises of autonomy, but patients who have never been autonomous have rights of privacy, such as the rights not to be needlessly viewed or touched by others. It seems intuitively correct to say that it is a violation of privacy, not merely a tasteless act of negligence, to leave a comatose person undraped on a cart in the hospital corridor. One possibility, although not one that we pursue or defend here, is to emphasize a broader conception of respect for persons that includes both respect for their autonomy *and* respect for their dignity. Another possibility is to argue that, if comatose patients could express their wishes, they would reject needless exposure, just as autonomous patients do, and we should protect their interest.

When a person voluntarily grants others access, this act is an *exercise* of the right to privacy, not a *waiver* of the right. For example, a patient's decision to grant a physician access for diagnostic, prognostic, and therapeutic procedures is an exercise of a right to control access that includes the right to grant access as well as to exclude access. The different kinds of access do not alter this conclusion. For example, a physician may need to take a personal history of certain private activities, touch our bodies, observe or listen to our bodies directly or through various instruments, run tests on our blood, and so on. With a psychotherapist we expose our innermost thoughts, emotions, dreams, and fantasies. Here we exercise our right to privacy by reducing privacy in order to gain other goals.

We grant others access to ourselves through implicit as well as explicit consent. In voluntary admission to a hospital, a patient gives both explicit and implicit consent to limited losses of privacy, but the patient's decision to enter the hospital does not grant or imply unlimited access. However, the limits of access are often not well understood by the patients, professionals, or administrators in institutions. Few patients understand the extent of their potential loss of privacy when they enter a teaching hospital, where professionals in training often seek access to them for reasons that have nothing to do with their care. Relevant information about teaching hospitals therefore should be disclosed to patients as part of the consent process in admission, and patients should also have the right to limit some or all access of professionals and students not involved in their care.

Indefensible Paternalism

We are occasionally justified in overriding obligations to respect privacy in order to protect other moral objectives. However, some reasons offered for limiting or overriding the right of privacy in medicine are indefensibly paternalistic. An example is found in H. J. McCloskey's argument that

> respect for privacy would seem to be dictated by respect for persons only in that persons commonly wish their privacy to be respected, hence in so far as we ignore such wishes, without good reason, to that extent we show lack of respect. If we have good reason to ignore a person's wishes, for example, if we suspect that he is concealing a tumor which is now operable but will soon become inoperable and fatal, we are showing no lack of respect in intruding on his privacy in this matter.[45]

This intrusion does, in our judgment, deeply infringe obligations of respect for privacy as well as respect for autonomy (in the autonomous patient). In the sort of case envisioned by McCloskey, it is sometimes justified to override the person's right of privacy, at least temporarily, in order to make a better diagnosis or to determine whether the person is autonomous. But we invoke the wrong premises and justifying argument if we act as if there were no infringement of privacy and no disrespect for autonomy.

Specifying and Balancing Rules of Privacy for Public Policy

Two examples will indicate how we propose to fashion rules and rights of privacy, while also allowing some justified intrusions on privacy by balancing legitimate interests against privacy interests. These examples are concerned with privacy in screening and testing for HIV antibodies and in ensuring effective treatment for patients with active tuberculosis.

Compulsory and voluntary screening for HIV. Because policies of screening sometimes infringe rights of privacy and confidentiality, we need to ask first what society plans to do with information about a person who is antibody-positive. This question is vital because no evidence exists that the virus is spread through casual contact. Most transmission occurs between parties in consensual, intimate relations that are paradigmatic areas of protected privacy. It is customary to distinguish between testing individuals and screening groups for antibodies to HIV, but we will use the term *screening* to cover both. Screening that identifies the individual screened necessarily involves some loss of privacy, because some persons gain access to private information. If testing is anonymous, no loss of privacy occurs, and the moral and policy issues are less complex. The following chart depicts possible policies toward screening (with identifiers) for exposure to HIV.

		Form of Authorization	
		Voluntary	*Compulsory*
	Universal	1	2
Scope of Screening			
	Selective	3	4

No adequate justification has emerged for either of the first two types of screening policy. (1) voluntary (by choice of those screened) and universal (for all in the society), and (2) compulsory (mandatory) and universal. Voluntary-universal screening rests on encouragement rather than coercion and consequently does not violate any moral rights of privacy and autonomy. However, neither voluntary nor compulsory universal screening is justified by current evidence. Universal screening is not necessary to protect the public health; HIV infection is not widespread outside groups engaging in high-risk activities; screening in groups or areas with low prevalence of HIV infection produces a high rate of false-positives; and universal screening would be very costly and not cost-effective.

However, rejection of (1) and (2) is subject to reversal if various conditions change. For example, the disease could spread and make it far more difficult to identify classes of persons at risk; many more people might be harmed by the failure of their sexual partners to inform them of their infection; the false-positive and false-negative rates in testing might be substantially reduced by improved techniques; if an effective anti-AIDS drug is developed, a need would exist to contact affected parties; the cost-effectiveness of screening programs could improve substantially; and social policies could reduce the psychosocial risks to those identified as seropositive. Hence, our position is not opposed in principle to universal testing, but it cannot currently be justified for HIV infection.

Policy 3, voluntary-selective screening, can be justified, especially for people engaging in unsafe sexual practices and sharing needles in intravenous drug use. However, there are unresolved questions, including who should be encouraged to be tested, who should bear the costs, what sort of pre-test and post-test counseling should be provided, and what conditions make the decision to undergo the test reasonable. Reasoned choice is particularly important because HIV screening presents major benefits and harms that need to be understood and balanced.[46] If we assume the accuracy of the test results, the possible benefits of testing to those who test negative (seronegative) include reassurance, the opportunity of making future plans, and the motivation to make behavioral changes to prevent infection. Possible benefits to those who test positive (seropositive) include closer medical follow-up, earlier use of retroviral agents, prophylaxis or other treatment of associated diseases, protection of loved ones, and a clearer sense of the future.

No significant risks exist for seronegative individuals, but major risks are presented to seropositive individuals. These risks are both psychological and social, with interaction between the two. The psychological risks include anxiety and depression, followed by a higher rate of suicide than for the population at large. Social risks include stigmatization, discrimination, and breaches of confidentiality. These risks can be substantially reduced by societal decisions to establish firm rules to protect individuals against breaches of confidentiality and against discrimination in housing, employment, and insurance. Without societal support and protection, the risks may outweigh the benefits of the test for individuals. The recommendations for their conduct also will be the same— avoid unsafe sex and sharing IV needles and syringes—whether individuals are seropositive or seronegative.

Finally, under option 4, several policies of compulsory-selective screening have already been adopted, and others can be expected. It is inappropriate to refer to some of these practices as compulsory, because individuals often can choose whether to enter situations or institutions in which screening is mandatory, such as voluntary military service. However, screening is mandatory for individuals who enter those situations or institutions, and in this regard it is situationally or institutionally compulsory. Such mandatory screening is justifiable whenever persons are engaged in actions or involved in procedures that impose risks on others without their consent. Examples include blood donation, sperm donation, and organ donation.

Other selective mandatory screening policies are more controversial. A few years ago considerable interest developed in legally mandated HIV testing of applicants for marriage licenses in order to protect spouses and offspring. However, two state legislatures (Illinois and Louisiana) that passed statutes mandating premarital screening subsequently rescinded them because they were not cost-effective. For example, reports on the first six months of experience in Illinois indicated that only 8 of 70,846 applicants for marriage licenses were found to be seropositive, while the cost of the testing program for that period was estimated at $2.5 million, or $312,000 for each seropositive individual identified. Half of those identified as seropositive admitted engaging in risky behavior and could probably have been identified more efficiently through voluntary programs aimed at populations with higher rates of infection.[47] The policy of mandatory premarital screening also fails conditions of effectiveness and proportionality. No evidence exists that these screening programs prevent additional illnesses, and the public health objective of protecting spouses (and future offspring) can be pursued in other ways that will not compromise respect for personal autonomy and privacy and yet will probably be more productive and cost-effective. For example, information about HIV risks and voluntary testing with counseling could be provided to all applicants for marriage licenses.

Policies of screening pregnant women and newborns also raise complex ethical questions. The justification for mandatory HIV screening of newborns parallels the justification for mandatory newborn screening policies that are already in place in all states in the U.S. for several genetic diseases. The latter policies have been introduced for serious genetic conditions for which presymptomatic interventions can prevent harms at acceptable cost-benefit trade-offs.[48] Neonatal screening for HIV focuses on a serious condition and increasingly more can be done for infected newborns, although the long-term benefits appear to be limited.

In view of the risk of transmission of HIV infection from mother to offspring, in the range of twenty-five to thirty percent, debates have occurred about whether it is morally responsible for HIV-infected women to continue or to terminate pregnancy and about what counselors should recommend. Even if society could agree on the morally responsible choice, the legal enforcement of moral obligations presents additional problems. Efforts to mandate prenatal testing would probably be ineffective, and perhaps counterproductive. For example, mandatory prenatal screening of all pregnant women who appear at clinics in areas with a high rate of HIV infection would put them at social risk of being reported if they were seropositive. Mandated testing during pregnancy therefore gives this class of women a motive not to seek prenatal care.[49] The policy most respectful of pregnant women's autonomy and privacy, and also the most likely to produce desirable consequences, is to offer prenatal testing for HIV while providing adequate information and appropriate counseling and support services.

Related issues arise in institutional settings, which differ in the extent to which individuals are free to enter and leave and to control risky contacts within the institutions. For example, it is doubtful that current policies of mandatory screening can be morally justified for soldiers; for foreign service applicants, officers, and their dependents; or for young people entering the U.S. Job Corps. Mandatory screening of prospective immigrants at first glance has a more plausible justification, but it suffers from problems of consistency, especially in light of precedents. The two major grounds for excluding immigrants are public health and public expenditures for health care. However, from the standpoint of public health, HIV-infected immigrants are not a major threat, and screening them will have only a modest impact on the course of the AIDS epidemic in the United States. In addition, the screening program discourages travelers from being tested and prevents illegal aliens from seeking counseling and preventive care. The second argument for exclusion of HIV-infected individuals from entry into this country is to avoid the additional social costs of providing health care. It is not intrinsically unjust for a society to exclude immigrants on grounds of the costs of providing health care, but it is unjust to exclude people with HIV on grounds of cost when persons with equally costly diseases are admitted.[50]

These examples can be extended to other types of policy. For example, it is inappropriate to undertake mandatory screening in the workplace unless exposure to bodily fluids would transmit the virus. Concern has been raised about HIV-infected health care professionals, especially dentists and surgeons, who might transmit the virus to their patients during invasive procedures. But studies indicate that the risk of transmission in dentistry or surgery is very low for any particular patient receiving care. A higher risk exists in invasive procedures, such as vaginal hysterectomies or pelvic surgery, in which the "blind" (that is, not directly visualized) use of sharp surgical instruments may produce cuts and bleeding despite universal precautions. If adequate grounds exist for restricting the activities of surgeons or dentists known to be HIV infected, then probable grounds exist for mandatory testing to determine which ones are infected. This area and others require careful attention to the overall risks and benefits of screening.

Mandatory treatment and detention of patients with tuberculosis. By contrast to HIV infection, tuberculosis (TB) is spread by airborne transmission. In the 1980s, public health officials predicted that tuberculosis could be eliminated in the United States within 25 years. However, the incidence of TB has increased each year for the last decade, and an increasing proportion of these cases involve multidrug-resistant, often fatal forms of TB. Such TB is difficult and costly to treat, over $200,000 in some cases, with limited success. As in the past, poverty, homelessness, inadequate and crowded housing, and substance abuse are associated with the spread of TB, but new problems include the susceptibility to TB infection among those who are HIV infected.

One perennial moral problem concerns how to handle noncompliant patients who lack either the capacity or the will to complete the recommended treatments. Although treatment regimens vary, the initial phase often requires daily medications for one to two months, followed by twice-weekly medications for several months (a total of six to nine months). The incidence of multidrug-resistant TB is much higher among previous recipients of anti-TB therapy, mainly because of their failure to continue the prescribed treatment until cured, not merely until rendered noninfectious. Their noncompliance or partial compliance with prescribed treatment regimens is the major cause of multidrug-resistant TB.

Obligations to respect privacy and autonomy dictate a priority for policies of voluntary compliance to control the TB epidemic, as in the AIDS epidemic. However, TB's different mode of transmission makes it easier to justify infringements of both autonomy and privacy. Mandatory TB screening is readily justifiable if substantial risk of transmission exists—for example, in crowded workplaces or prisons—and coercive police powers are justified to protect the public from persons identified to have active TB. Quarantine, isolation, and mandatory, directly-observed treatment (DOT) may all be justified. DOT entails directly observing patients take their medication. It has been used until patients with active TB become *noncontagious,* but many health professionals now argue that it should be used until such patients are *cured.* The rationale is not primarily paternalistic—to benefit the patient—but rather to protect others over time from exposure to TB. If patients with TB do not continue their treatments until cured, they run the risk of developing multidrug-resistant forms that pose serious threats to those they infect, as well as to themselves.

According to some studies, about one-third of patients with TB fail to adhere to treatment. Their noncompliance stems from the conditions that foster TB as well as other social and psychological factors. Furthermore, professionals lack clear ways to identify noncompliant patients in advance. Critics of mandatory DOT contend that, because the majority of TB patients comply, it would be "wasteful, inefficient, and gratuitously annoying" to mandate DOT for all patients with TB, in addition to failing to select the least restrictive and intrusive intervention for particular patients.[51] However, the risks of not implementing DOT include the further spread of TB, particularly its multidrug-resistant forms, and the escalation of treatment costs, which are estimated to be approximately $400 per patient for the full DOT.[52] Several jurisdictions now invoke police powers to mandate DOT. Forcible detention can be justified under some circumstances, but respect for privacy and autonomy suggest giving primacy to various inducements and incentives, such as food and travel vouchers, to secure compliance with DOT. However, mandatory DOT is less restrictive than quarantine or isolation, and detention should be undertaken only when necessary, following due process.

Treatment until cure is often needed to provide adequate public health protections, and forcible detention can be justified if patients have active TB and pose a risk to others. However, as George Annas notes, legal standards may make it difficult to detain non-cured patients whose TB is not currently communicable.[53] Furthermore, most state laws do not permit forced treatment even of forcibly detained patients. Practical considerations also limit attempts at forced treatment of TB. Medications usually require oral administration daily or two to three times a week for several months. Lawrence Gostin rightly argues that in view of the level of force required and the danger to caregivers from exposure to the patient's microbacteria in the process, we should recognize the limits of coercion and instead attempt over time to persuade the detained person to accept treatment.[54]

In conclusion, an effective public health strategy in response to the TB epidemic should pay primary attention to conditions that cause TB and should give priority to policies that emphasize freedom of choice. However, coercive measures are justified when necessary to protect the public health if priority is assigned to the least restrictive and least intrusive measures—first, induced DOT, then mandatory DOT, and both with priority over detention.

Confidentiality

We necessarily surrender some measure of privacy when we grant others access to our personal histories or bodies, but we also in principle retain some control over information generated about us, at least in diagnostic and therapeutic contexts and in research. For example, physicians are obligated not to grant an insurance company or a prospective employer access to information about patients without their authorization.[55] When others gain access to protected information without our consent, we sometimes say that their access infringes our right to confidentiality and at other times that it infringes our right to privacy. The difference is this: An infringement of X's right to confidentiality occurs only if the person to whom X disclosed the information in confidence fails to protect the information or deliberately discloses it to someone without X's consent. By contrast, a person who without authorization enters a hospital record room or computer data-bank violates rights of privacy rather than rights of confidentiality. Only the person (or institution) to whom information is given in a confidential relationship can be charged with violating rights of confidentiality.

Traditional Rules and Contemporary Practices in Health Care

Rules of confidentiality have long been common in codes of medical ethics. Requirements of confidentiality appear as early as the Hippocratic oath and continue in the Code of Ethics of the AMA. For example, the code adopted in 1957 included this rule: "A physician may not reveal the confidences entrusted to him in the course of medical attendance, or the deficiencies he may observe in the character of patients, unless he is required to do so by law or unless it becomes necessary in order to protect the welfare of the individual or of the community." In 1980, the AMA revised this rule to hold that a physician "shall safeguard patient confidences within the constraints of the law." The World Medical Association has likewise affirmed rules of confidentiality. Its Declaration of Geneva asserts an obligation of "absolute secrecy" and includes the following pledge: "I will respect the secrets which are confided in me, even after the patient has died." Its International Code of Medical Ethics states the most stringent requirement of all: "A doctor shall preserve absolute secrecy on all he knows about his patient because of the confidence entrusted to him."

Some commentators suspect these official rules function as little more than a ritualistic formula or convenient fiction, publicly acknowledged by professionals but widely ignored and violated in practice. Mark Siegler has argued that "confidentiality in medicine" is a "decrepit concept," because what both physicians and patients have traditionally understood as medical confidentiality no longer exists. It is "compromised systematically in the course of routine medical care." To make his point graphic, Siegler presents the case of a patient who became concerned about the number of people in the hospital who appeared to have access to his record and threatened to leave prematurely unless the hospital would guarantee confidentiality. Upon inquiry, Siegler discovered that many more people than he had suspected had legitimate needs and responsibilities to examine the patient's chart. When he informed the patient of the number, approximately seventy-five, he assured the patient that "these people were all involved in providing or supporting his health-care services." The patient retorted, "I always believed that medical confidentiality was part of doctors' code of ethics. Perhaps you should tell me just what you people mean by 'confidentiality.' "[56]

This request is entirely reasonable in the setting of contemporary health care. When William Behringer tested positive for HIV at the medical center in New Jersey where he worked as an otolaryngologist and plastic surgeon, he received numerous phone calls of sympathy within a few hours from members of the medical staff. Within a few days he received similar calls from his patients, and shortly thereafter his surgical privileges at the medical center were suspended and his practice ruined. Despite his expectation of and request for confidentiality, the medical center took no serious precautions to protect his medical records.[57] If physicians as patients cannot protect themselves in the system, it is not likely that the system will adequately protect other patients.

In a survey of patients, medical students, and house staff about expectations and practices of confidentiality, Barry D. Weiss reports that "patients expect a more rigorous standard of confidentiality than actually exists." According to one Harris poll, only seventeen percent of the patients surveyed were dissatisfied with the way physicians handled confidential information, but, according to Weiss's study, many more would be dissatisfied if they knew what actually occurs. Virtually all patients (ninety-six percent) recognized the common practice of informally discussing patients' cases for second opinions; most (sixty-nine percent) expected cases to be discussed openly in professional settings in order to receive other opinions; a majority (fifty-one percent) expected cases to be discussed in professional settings simply because they were medically interesting, and half of the patients expected cases to be discussed with office nursing staff. However, they generally did not expect cases to be discussed in other settings, such as in medical journals, at parties, or with spouses or friends. Yet, to take two examples, house staff and medical students reported that cases were frequently discussed with physicians' spouses (fifty-seven percent) and at parties (seventy percent).[58]

Threats to confidentiality are also present in many institutions with a capacity to store and disseminate confidential medical information such as medical records on file, drugs prescribed, medical tests administered, and reimbursement records. In occupational medicine, for example, computerized records in corporations are growing rapidly, and data in these records can be searched quickly and comprehensively. If the company routinely offers medical examinations by a corporate physician, records are computerized and merged with all claims filed by an employee's private physician for reimbursement under corporate insurance policies. Many employees (especially in industries with hazardous work environments) are concerned that this extensive, two-track set of records presenting a medical history will be used against them if a question of continued employment arises. This risk is reducible by severely limiting access to computerized information, but generally at least one physician and at least one employee in data-processing will have access to the full set of records, and access may also be granted to company epidemiologists, union officials, and the like.

It may be possible to alter current practices in the delivery of care to approximate more closely the traditional ideal of confidentiality, but a gulf will remain because of the need for information in medicine.

The Nature of Medical Confidentiality

Confidentiality is present when one person discloses information to another, whether through words or an examination, and the person to whom the information is disclosed pledges not to divulge that information to a third party without the confider's permission. In schematic terms, information I is confidential if and only if A discloses I to B, and B pledges to refrain from disclosing I to any other party C without A's consent. By definition, confidential information is both private and voluntarily imparted in confidence and trust. If a patient or subject authorizes release of the information to others, then no violation of rights of confidentiality occurs, although a loss of both confidentiality and privacy may occur.

A detailed rule or policy of confidentiality prohibits (some) disclosures of (some) information gained in certain relationships to (some) third parties without the consent of the original source of the information. A typical example is the following (taken from a recent epidemiological study):

> Strict rules of confidentiality will be followed. Individual data will not be reported. Only aggregate and summary results will be communicated. The identity of the individual will remain obscured, and no information will be linked to him or her or affect his or her employment or use of health care. . . . All parties will be assured of the confidentiality of the collected data. Moreover, the access to information will be limited to the principal investigators.

Acknowledged and justifiable exceptions exist to the kind of information that can be considered confidential in policy and practice. For example, external limits to confidentiality may be set by legal obligations, as when practitioners are required to report gunshot wounds and venereal diseases. Some disclosures of information to third parties that are resisted by patients may not be breaches of confidentiality because of the context in which the information was originally gathered. For example, IBM-physician Martha Nugent, informed her employer about her belief that an employee, Robert Bratt, had a problem of paranoia relevant to behavior on the job.[59] Bratt knew that Nugent had been retained by IBM to examine him, but he expected that conventional medical confidentiality would be maintained. The company held that the facts disclosed by Nugent were necessary for evaluating Bratt's request for transfer and, under law, were a legitimate business communication. In our view, it is a reasonable conclusion that such information is not confidential by the relevant standards of medical confidentiality and that Nugent was not bound by obligations of confidentiality in the same way as a private physician.

This is not to say that a physician employed by a corporation is free to disclose everything to the corporation, but valid contracts for at least limited disclosures are not illegitimate as long as employees are aware of provisions in the contract. A similar point applies to military physicians who have a dual responsibility, to the soldier as patient and to the military. Nevertheless, the company and the military, along with the physicians in each context, do have a moral responsibility to ensure that employee-patients and soldier-patients understand at the outset that traditional rules of confidentiality do not apply.

The Justification of Obligations of Confidentiality

It is not inherently or intrinsically wrong for one person to disclose information received from another in a special relationship. We can easily imagine a society that by consensus does not recognize any obligations of confidentiality. Many of the goods of medicine, and perhaps of research, could also be realized with-

422   PRINCIPLES OF BIOMEDICAL ETHICS

out rules of confidentiality. Can we, then, justify a system of expensive protections of confidentiality? We believe that three types of argument support (prima facie) rules to protect confidentiality: (1) consequentialist-based arguments, (2) rights-based autonomy and privacy arguments, and (3) fidelity-based arguments.

Consequentialist arguments. If patients could not trust physicians to conceal some information from third parties, patients would be reluctant to disclose full and forthright information or to authorize a complete examination and a full battery of tests. Without such information, physicians would not be able to make accurate diagnoses and prognoses or to recommend the best course of treatment. Although such consequentialist arguments clearly establish a need for some rule of confidentiality, consequentialists disagree about which rule of confidentiality should be adopted, and about the rule's scope and weight.

In *Tarasoff* (Case 1), both the majority opinion, which affirmed that therapists have an obligation to warn third parties of their patients' threatened violence, and the dissenting opinion, which denied such an obligation, used consequentialist arguments to justify their interpretation of the rule of confidentiality and its exceptions. Their debate hinged on different predictions and assessments of the consequences of (1) a rule that *required* therapists to breach confidentiality by warning intended victims of a client's threatened violence, and (2) a rule that *allowed* therapists to exercise their discretion and to maintain confidentiality in the face of some peril to a member of the public.

The majority opinion pointed to the victims who would be saved, such as the young woman who had been killed in this case, and contended that a professional's obligation to disclose information to third parties could be justified by the need to protect such potential victims. By contrast, the minority opinion contended that if it were common practice to override obligations of confidentiality, the fiduciary relation between the patient and the doctor would soon erode and collapse. Patients would lose confidence in psychotherapists and would refrain from disclosing information crucial to effective therapy. As a result, violent assaults would increase because dangerous persons would refuse to seek psychiatric aid or to disclose relevant information, such as their violent fantasies. Hence, the debate about different rules of confidentiality hinges in part on empirical claims about which rule would be more effective in achieving the desired objective of protecting others.

Consequentialist arguments for a strict obligation of confidentiality depend on the premise that the absence of confidentiality will prevent people who need medical and psychiatric treatment from seeking and fully participating in it. Although empirical, these claims have not been adequately tested. The few available studies appear to support a strong obligation of confidentiality. One study examined the responses of thirty psychiatric inpatients to hypothetical questions about confidentiality. Eighty percent of those surveyed indicated that an assurance of confidentiality improved their relationship with the staff; sixty-seven percent said they would be upset or angry at the release of verbal information without their permission; seventeen percent indicated that they would leave treatment if verbal information were released without their permission; and ninety-five percent said they would be upset if their charts were shared without their consent.[60] A subsequent study focused on fifty-eight outpatients, who indicated that they would take vigorous actions, such as complaints or legal suits, in cases of breaches of confidentiality.[61] While these studies support a strong rule of confidentiality, they do not support an absolute rule of nondisclosure and do not address the question of whether the absence of a promise of confidentiality deters some people from seeking treatment.

In the case of other legally accepted and mandated exceptions to confidentiality—such as reporting contagious disease, child abuse, and gunshot wounds—no substantial evidence exists that these requirements have reduced prospective patients' willingness to seek treatment and to cooperate with physicians, or have significantly impaired the physician–patient relationship.[62] Even in the aggregate, such reports are relatively isolated events with little effect on others' conduct.

A consequentialist justification for nonabsolute rules of confidentiality therefore is well supported. At the same time, a consequentialist will not overlook the fact that when medical confidentiality is breached, the rights of the physician's patients are infringed if a promise had been made to keep confidentiality and the relationship had been cemented by trust and the shared goal of therapy. The confider will almost certainly feel deeply disappointed and betrayed, and will perhaps be harmed. These negative consequences for confiders can be outweighed only by substantial threats to others, to the public interest, or to the patient. Nor can a physician who breaks confidence ignore the potential for eroding the system of medical confidentiality, trust, and fidelity. A consequentialist justification for breaching confidentiality can meet its own high standards only if all such consequences are considered.

Arguments from autonomy and privacy rights. A second approach to the justification of rules and rights of confidentiality does not ground them exclusively in goals or consequences, but looks to moral principles or rules such as respect for autonomy and privacy. The argument for privacy in the previous section can here be extended to confidentiality, where breaches have often been viewed as primarily violations of privacy and personal integrity. Such breaches take on a special importance when disclosures of information subject a patient to legal jeopardy, loss of friends and lovers, emotional devastation, discrimination, loss of employment, and the like. However, an argument that uses a privacy rationale does not appeal to these consequences, but purely to rights of privacy.

The principal thesis is that the value of privacy gives considerable weight to the rules of confidentiality that protect it. Common-law, statutory-law, and constitutional-law recognitions of protected privacy interests feed this argument, but it is primarily a moral rather than a legal thesis.

Fidelity-based arguments. Another obligation explored later in this chapter is fidelity in the physician–patient relationship, especially fidelity to implicit and explicit promises. The physician's obligation to live up to the patient's reasonable expectations of privacy and to the patient's trust that confidentiality will be maintained is one way to specify the general obligation of fidelity. The context of medical practice requires disclosure of private and sensitive information, and therefore a failure of fidelity tears at a significant dimension of the patient–physician relationship. Part of the binding force of confidentiality derives from an implicit or explicit promise by the health care professional to the person seeking help. For example, if the public oath taken by the professional or the accepted code of professional ethics pledges confidentiality, and if the professional does not expressly disavow confidentiality to the patient, the patient has a right to expect it.

None of these three arguments supports absolute rules of confidentiality. Whatever their basis, these rules are prima facie, not absolute—in ethics as in law.[63] These three arguments jointly provide a compelling justification for a strict rule of medical confidentiality, and they help explain why codes and oaths have typically expressed obligations of confidentiality in absolutist or near-absolutist terms. However, rules of confidentiality used as absolute shields can eventuate in outrageous circumstances of preventable injury and loss.[64] We therefore need a proper understanding of ways in which obligations of confidentiality are validly overridden by more compelling obligations.

Justified Infringements of Rules of Confidentiality

Health care professionals have a right to disclose confidential information in circumstances in which a person is not, all things considered, entitled to the confidence. For example, a person may confide ongoing child abuse or a serious intent to murder someone. In some cases, this lack of entitlement to a confidence makes disclosure *permissible,* but in other cases health care professionals have an *obligation* to breach confidentiality. Legal and moral obligations to divulge confidential information exist if serious dangers are present for third parties. The court correctly held in *Tarasoff* that therapists have a duty, not an option, to warn third parties of their patient's serious intention to kill or harm them. (We do not deny that in some circumstances a health care professional does have an option rather than a duty to disclose confidential information and is legally protected if he or she does so.)

Current AMA Principles of Medical Ethics appear to limit justified breaches of confidentiality to disclosures required by law, but, as we will see, the AMA interpretation of this principle is broader. Some legal obligations, such as the requirement to report epileptic seizures to the division of motor vehicles, are established to protect the patient as well as the society. Other obligations, such as the requirement to report child abuse, primarily protect the child. These legal obligations to break confidentiality sometimes pose difficult choices. In a just political system a moral obligation to obey the law is present, but this obligation, like the obligation of confidentiality, is prima facie; and sometimes the health care professional is justified in breaking the law in order to fulfill a responsibility to a patient. Obedience to law sometimes results in medical neglect of the patient and persecution or loss of employment for morally irrelevant or morally unjustifiable reasons. This frequently happens when psychiatric information is disclosed in contexts such as military service, in which knowledge of sexual preference has led to persecution and discharge. The point is that difficult moral dilemmas cannot be resolved merely because a law requires disclosure, and if a code of medical ethics were formulated only by reference to legal rules, that code would be inadequate.

In assessing which risks to others, if any, outweigh the rule of confidentiality, both the probability that a harm will materialize and the magnitude of harm should be balanced against the obligation of confidentiality. The chart of risk assessment introduced in Chapter 5 supplies the basic categories:

		Magnitude of Harm	
		Major	*Minor*
	High	1	2
Proba- bility of Harm			
	Low	3	4

As health professionals' assessments of a situation approach a high probability of a major harm (1 above), the weight of the obligation to breach confidentiality increases. As the situation approaches 4, the weight decreases, and typically no moral obligation to breach confidentiality exists; usually it would be wrong to do so. Many particularities of the case will determine whether one is justified in breaching confidentiality in 2 and 3, which are more complicated borderline categories. These particularities include the foreseeability of a harm, the preventability of the harm through intervention by a health care professional, and the potential impact on policies and laws regarding confidentiality.

We generally cannot have a high degree of confidence in our attempts to measure probability and magnitude of harm, and uncertainty will surround diagnoses and prognoses, as well as assessments of the likelihood of harmful outcomes. In one case a psychiatrist used hypnotic techniques to help a pilot recall suppressed information about his responsibility for the crash of a commercial plane. The information obtained indicated that it would be risky for the pilot to fly again, at least for the immediate future, but the risks were not precisely measurable and the therapist was unable to convince the pilot that he should not fly until he could solve his problems. Confidentiality was strictly maintained. Six months after returning to the cockpit, the pilot made an error of judgment that led to the crash of a jet on a transatlantic flight and many deaths.[65] Such cases involve difficult judgments about the probability and magnitude of a harm (or benefit), and even conscientious risk–benefit assessments usually leave a residue of uncertainty.

Health care professionals are usually under an obligation to seek alternative ways of realizing benefit or preventing harm before disclosing confidential information. For example, widespread controversy surrounds the question whether physicians and other health care professionals should notify spouses and lovers that a patient has tested positive for exposure to HIV and consequently has the potential to infect others through sexual intercourse or other exchanges of body fluids, particularly sharing needles in intravenous drug use. In one case, after several weeks of dry persistent coughing and night sweats, a bisexual man visited his family physician, who arranged for a test to determine whether he had antibodies to HIV. The physician informed the patient of a positive test, of the risk of infection for his wife, and of the risk that their children might lose both parents. The patient refused to tell his wife and insisted that the physician maintain absolute confidentiality. The physician reluctantly yielded to this demand. Only in the last few weeks of his life did the patient allow his wife to be informed of the nature of his illness, and a test then showed that she too was antibody-positive for HIV. When symptoms appeared a year later, she angrily, and we think appropriately, accused the physician of violating his moral responsibilities to her and to her children.[66] Here we have a case of a definite and severe harm presented to an identifiable individual, the paradigm case of a justified breach of confidentiality.

Legal and moral rules of confidentiality are still evolving in response to the AIDS epidemic, based in part on how relevantly similar cases were handled previously. Many well-grounded reasons support the practice of informing spouses and sexual partners (past and present) that a particular person has tested positive for exposure to the AIDS virus. For example, if people are at risk of serious harms, and the disclosure is necessary to prevent—and probably would prevent—the harms (to spouses or lovers or, if they are already infected, to their partners), disclosure is usually justified. Variations on these conditions appear in several recent statements of professional ethics by medical associations.

According to the American Psychiatric Association (APA), if the physician has "convincing clinical information" that the patient is infected with HIV and also has "good reason to believe" that the patient's actions place others at ongoing risk of exposure, then "it is ethically permissible for the physician to notify an identifiable person who the physician believes is in danger of contracting the virus." However, a breach of confidentiality is categorized as a "last resort," to be used only following "scrupulous attention . . . to all other alternatives," which include "the patient's agreement to terminate behavior that places other persons at risk of infection or to notify identifiable individuals who may be at continuing risk of exposure."[67]

Various ambiguities and gaps in this statement point to difficulties in specifying the nature and scope of the clinician's ethical obligation to protect third parties. We will use these guidelines as a case study in contemporary problems to conclude our discussion of confidentiality. First, which actions will discharge the physician's moral obligation to protect third parties? The guidelines do not hold that the physician has an obligation to determine whether the patient has in fact carried out the "agreement" to terminate the risky conduct or to warn those endangered, and it is not clear how far the physician should go in monitoring compliance or whether such monitoring requires the patient's consent. One study concludes that it is ineffective, however convenient, to leave partner notification to patients.[68] Perhaps the only responsible strategy is the one proposed by the AMA's Council on Ethical and Judicial Affairs: A physician who "knows that a seropositive individual is endangering a third party . . . should (1) attempt to persuade the infected patient to cease endangering the third party; (2) if persuasion fails, notify authorities; and (3) if the authorities take no action, notify the endangered third parties."[69]

Second, how are we to interpret the patient's "agreement to terminate behavior that places others at risk of infection or to notify [them]"? In particular, how far must the risk of transmission of HIV be reduced? Suppose the patient refuses to notify his or her sexual partner and refuses to abstain completely from sexual intercourse, but indicates that he or she will insist on the use of a condom. Would the patient's agreement to practice safe sex at all times be sufficient? This promise is usually not sufficient to release the physician from an obligation of disclosure. Consider the following case. A 35-year-old single, bisexual man tested positive for HIV about a year ago and has abstained from sexual activity during that period. Now he tells his psychotherapist, whom he has been seeing for about four months, that he has been dating a woman in her mid-thirties, that they just started having sexual intercourse with condoms and foam for contraception, and that they are considering marriage and having a family because he would like to have children. He has not told her that he is seropositive for HIV because he fears it would destroy their relationship, and he believes that the risk of transmission of the virus is very low. If the psychotherapist is unable to convince his patient to abstain from sexual intercourse or

428 PRINCIPLES OF BIOMEDICAL ETHICS

to inform his partner, risks to the third party will then set the terms of the psychiatrist's obligation. According to some studies, using a condom in a single act of heterosexual intercourse reduces the risk of transmission from 1 in 500 to 1 in 5000. After 500 sexual encounters with an HIV-infected person, the estimated risk of infection of partners is 2 in 3 without condoms and 1 in 11 with condoms. A good case can be made, assuming the accuracy of this information, that the psychotherapist has an obligation to warn the patient's sexual partner, because the woman should have the right to decide whether to accept the risks indicated by the above statistics.[70]

Third, the APA guidelines mention justifiable disclosure (and breach of confidentiality) only to "an identifiable person" with a "continuing risk of exposure." We agree that the physician is responsible only to protect identifiable third parties at continuing risk. No obligation exists to track down the patient's prior sexual or needle-sharing contacts. (However, public health officials often do have such a moral and legal responsibility.) Disclosure to other parties, including family members who are not sexual partners, is typically not necessary to protect them, although there are exceptions. In one case a nurse in an emergency room told a woman that her elderly father had AIDS as a result of a blood transfusion years before. The disclosure was made because the daughter was functioning as a care-giver in the home and needed to take appropriate precautions.

Fourth, the APA guidelines propose that physicians inform their patients in advance of the limits placed on confidentiality in their relationship. However, the guidelines are unclear regarding appropriate use of information about the patient's antibody-positive status that emerged prior to the physician's disclosure of the limits of confidentiality. Prior notification should not be considered an absolute condition for justified disclosures to third parties, but the physician should seek the patient's permission to warn a third party if the patient is unwilling to do so. If the patient has understood in advance that certain information will not be kept confidential and the physician then discloses that information to a third party, no breach of confidentiality occurs.

Fifth, how are physicians' obligations altered if they have some evidence that the third parties already know, or should already know, that they are engaging in high-risk activities, such as unprotected sexual intercourse or sharing IV needles? Physicians do not have an obligation to warn third parties who know, but when the evidence of knowledge is less than conclusive, the physician can and should underscore the dangers for third parties of nondisclosure.[71]

Sixth, the APA guidelines stress the ethical *permissibility* of the physician's disclosure, rather than its obligatoriness, whereas the Council on Ethical and Judicial Affairs of the AMA focuses on the physician's obligation. Permissibility is too weak, for reasons mentioned earlier. The primary justification for disclosure is that health professionals are *obligated* to reduce the risk of death.

Public officials need to consider carefully which societal rule of confidentiality would save more lives in the long run in these circumstances: One that permits or perhaps requires notification of sexual or needle-sharing partners or one that guarantees confidentiality. Answers to this question hinge in part on disputed claims about the importance of voluntary testing in changing behavior and reducing risky conduct over time. One consequentialist argument is that people who have been exposed to the AIDS virus but do not yet have symptoms will be reluctant to seek testing unless confidentiality is protected. They will consequently fail to obtain valuable information that could lead them reduce risks to others. A counterargument is that carefully limited breaches of confidentiality—namely, disclosure only to sexual partners or needle-sharing partners who are at reasonable risk of harm—would not deter people from seeking testing and medical attention. People would still seek testing if they were informed that confidentiality would be breached only under strictly limited conditions and then only to identifiable people who are at risk of serious harm.[72]

Insufficient evidence presently exists to resolve this debate. However, successful notification of partners, whether by physicians to identifiable third parties or by public health officials, depends on cooperation by patients in providing information, and a policy should be carefully hedged to gain such cooperation. Public health programs of contact tracing for those exposed to HIV pose fewer ethical problems because they typically do not disclose the index patient's name. The problem is that for diseases like syphilis and AIDS with long latency periods, it is often difficult and even impossible to locate previous sexual or needle-sharing partners, especially if they have been numerous and anonymous. Contact tracing is labor intensive and expensive, and it must compete with other programs for limited funds to reduce the spread of HIV infection.[73]

In conclusion, we have argued that obligations of medical confidentiality are not at present well delineated and need restructuring. On the one hand, if we are to honor obligations of respect for autonomy, patients often should be told more about practices of confidentiality and threats to confidentiality, such as computerized record-keeping. They should be able to consent to the inclusion of information in their records, and should have access to those records, as well as retaining considerable control over others' access. On the other hand, moral obligations to protect confidentiality sometimes must be overridden in the face of moral demands, such as protection of the rights and interests of third parties.

Fidelity

We earlier noted the importance of fidelity in medical care. Paul Ramsey has argued that the fundamental ethical question in research, medicine, and health care is, "What is the meaning of the faithfulness of one human being to another?"[74] Few today would agree that fidelity is the fundamental moral norm, but many would accept it as an essential norm.

The Nature and Place of Fidelity

Obligations of fidelity are best understood as norms that specify the moral principles discussed in previous chapters, especially respect for autonomy, justice, and utility.[75] These principles justify the obligation to act in good faith to keep vows and promises, fulfill agreements, and maintain relationships and fiduciary responsibilities. Fidelity in ethical theory has often been modeled on fidelity to voluntary promises, commitments, and oaths. A disposition to be true to one's word is the primary condition in this model. However, some obligations of fidelity are not captured by this model of voluntary agreements and promises. Both law and medical tradition distinguish the practice of medicine from business practices that rest on contracts and marketplace relationships. The patient–physician relationship is a fiduciary relationship—that is, founded on trust or confidence; and the physician is therefore necessarily a trustee for the patient's medical welfare. This model of fidelity relies more on values of loyalty and trust than on being true to one's word. Whether or not the physician makes a pledge or takes an oath upon entry into the profession, obligations of fidelity are present in this second model whenever the physician establishes a relationship with the patient. Similarly, the physician is obligated not to "withdraw from the case without giving notice to the patient, the relatives, or responsible friends sufficiently long in advance of withdrawal to permit another medical attendant to be secured."[76] Abandonment is a breach of fidelity, an infidelity amounting to disloyalty. Whether or not a promise was made, such infidelity undermines trustworthiness (as well as other virtues discussed in Chapter 8).

Fiduciary relationships sometimes encounter competing moral obligations that limit and override obligations of fidelity. Determinations of obligations often require a careful interpretation of the weight of special relationships and explicit or implicit promises. For example, in an epidemiological study of what happens to people who are antibody-positive for HIV but do not yet have signs of AIDS, some investigators indicated that they would use the information gathered exclusively for epidemiological purposes. But this assurance came into question when a researcher discovered that an antibody-positive subject had not informed his lover and continued to practice unprotected sex. In considering whether to warn the lover, this researcher had to weigh his specific promise of confidentiality against the obligation to prevent harm.[77] Here fidelity to a very specific promise suggests a different course than we earlier proposed in discussing HIV patients and their sexual partners, but we still would not rule out an obligation to notify the endangered third party.

Conflicts of Fidelity and Divided Loyalties

Several moral problems about the meaning and strength of obligations of fidelity arise because of conflicts of fidelity, which often produce divided loyalties. The phrase "conflicts of fidelity" is less familiar than "conflicts of loyalty" and "conflicts of interest," and we need first to analyze the meaning of these terms. Some writers treat loyalty, in the relevant sense of fidelity, as implying obligations that persons have as the result of familial, institutional, and national relationships that contribute to their self-understanding.[78] As such, loyalty emanates from self-identity and fundamental commitments, rather than from a series of specific and discrete contracts, promises, vows, oaths, and the like. However, this analysis does not adequately capture the meaning of *professional loyalty,* used in reference, for example, to what physicians owe their patients and what lawyers owe their clients.

Professional fidelity or loyalty has been traditionally conceived as giving the patient's interests priority in two essential respects: (1) the professional effaces self-interest in any conflict with the patient's interests, and (2) the patient's interests take priority over others' interests.[79] In practice, of course, fidelity has never been so unadulterated. For instance, caring for patients in epidemics has usually been considered praiseworthy and virtuous rather than obligatory fidelity,[80] and physicians have never been expected to care for all patients free of charge. Nevertheless, the rhetoric of the primacy of the patient's interests was once more plausible than it is now, because of major changes in the structure of health care and its social context that have produced divided loyalties in many areas of medical practice, nursing, and clinical research.

These divided loyalties derive from the structure of authority in medical institutions. The issuing of orders and the assignment of duties create some forms of divided loyalty, but divided loyalty also occurs when fidelity to patients, subjects, or clients conflicts with allegiance to colleagues, institutions, funding agencies, corporations, or the state. In these cases, two or more roles and associated loyalties have become incompatible and irreconcilable, forcing a moral choice between them. If the two loyalties were reconcilable in a morally satisfactory way, the situation would not be *divided* loyalty, which in compelling a moral choice alters the landscape of one's commitments.[81] A divided loyalty can be reconciled only by giving up or seriously modifying one or more of the conflicting loyalties.

In other cases dual loyalties are not as starkly opposed, and the main commitments can be framed and specified so that neither loyalty has to be yielded or seriously modified. Dual loyalties are often sustainable, and indeterminate loyalties can often be specified to overcome problems of incompatibility. Ideally, all conflicting loyalties can be either specified or balanced in a way that eliminates both moral problems and divided loyalties. However, as we will now see, this ideal is often very difficult to implement.

Third-party interests. Physicians, nurses, and hospital administrators sometimes find some aspects of their role-obligations in conflict with obligations to
patients. For example, they may have a therapeutic contract with a party other
than the patient, and the contractor may not be the direct beneficiary in the
relationship. When parents bring a child to a physician for treatment, the physician's primary responsibility is to serve the child's interests, although the parents made the contract and the physician has obligations of fidelity to the parents. The latter obligations are sometimes easily and validly overridden, as
occurs when physicians go to court to oppose irresponsible parental decisions.
For example, courts have often allowed adult Jehovah's Witnesses to reject
blood transfusions for themselves, while rightly refusing to allow them to reject
medically necessary blood transfusions for their children. Parents are also
sometimes charged with child neglect when they fail to seek or permit highly
beneficial medical treatment recommended by physicians.[82]

A physician has a fundamental responsibility to the patient even if a third
party establishes the initial contract for services. This loyalty to the patient
should almost never be yielded when loyalties become divided, even if a court
order must be obtained to authorize surgery, a blood transfusion, or the like.
Ideally, familial interests such as avoiding the depletion of financial resources
would not be viewed as relevant considerations. However, familial interests
cannot simply be dismissed, because families themselves are not obligated to
do everything possible to save the lives or promote the health of their members.
There may be serious disagreements not only about what would be in the patient's best interests, but also about how to balance those interests against the
family's wider interests. (See Chapter 4, pp. 244–249)

Maternal–fetal relations have recently become more complex and open to
conflicts because of the diagnosis and treatment of some maladies in utero—
for example, treatment of hydrocephalus through intrauterine surgery. The fetus
typically becomes a patient because of the pregnant woman's decision to enter
the health care system, but once both patients, the pregnant woman and the
fetus, are under care, conflicting obligations of fidelity and divided loyalties
may develop. For example, the possibility of cesarean sections late in pregnancy sometimes presents a conflict between the survival and health of the
fetus and the wishes of the pregnant woman. Rules of privacy and informed
consent have usually allowed the pregnant woman's interests to prevail in the
legal arena in cases of conflict. Since *Roe v. Wade* in 1973, the U.S. Supreme
Court has consistently allowed states to place some restrictions on abortion, but
it is a matter of ongoing debate whether a pregnant woman's decision to forgo
a legal abortion increases the professional's and the court's, as well as the
pregnant woman's, responsibility to act to ensure the survival and well-being
of the fetus.

The sensational case of Angela Carder illustrates some of these issues. This

27-year-old patient—referred to as A.C.—was terminally ill with cancer and twenty-six weeks pregnant. She was ordered by a court to undergo a cesarean section against her wishes, in part because doubt existed about her competence and about her stable preferences. Attorneys for the hospital had sought a declaratory judgment to determine whether the hospital had a duty to attempt to save the baby's life through a cesarean section when it appeared that the woman's death was imminent. A superior court judge held a three-hour emergency hearing at the hospital. The judge never entered A.C.'s room, but ordered the cesarean section after being informed of a neonatologist's estimate that the baby had perhaps a fifty to sixty percent chance of surviving the operation but that the operation could hasten the woman's death, which was already considered imminent. A three-judge panel of the District of Columbia Court of Appeals denied the request by A.C.'s counsel for a stay of the order. After the cesarean section was performed, the baby was named and a birth certificate was issued; but she died within two and one-half hours, and the mother died two days later. They were buried together. The panel's opinion, filed five months later, noted that the pregnant woman was predicted, at best, to have only two days left of sedated life. The panel relied on previous court holdings that the state's interest in protecting innocent third parties from an adult's decision to refuse medical treatment may validly override the patient's interest in bodily integrity.[83]

Following major public controversy over this opinion, involving several medical and legal associations, the full District of Columbia Court of Appeals reheard the case and vacated and remanded the trial court's order.[84] The majority opinion focused on the right of competent adults to make an informed choice to accept or forgo medical treatment. It noted that courts have consistently refused to compel someone to donate bodily tissue to benefit someone else through transplantation. According to this opinion, the trial court erred in balancing A.C.'s rights against the interests of the fetus without a prior effort to determine her informed choices—or, if she were incompetent, through substituted judgment (that is, ascertainment of "what the patient would do if faced with the particular treatment question"). The court held that the pregnant woman's wishes "will control in virtually all cases." The court viewed the cesarean section as a "massive intrusion" comparable to organ or tissue donation. Hence, the court established a strong presumption against court-ordered cesarean sections, based on analogy with practices and policies that govern organ and tissue donation.

We accept the majority opinion's argument as morally and legally defensible, despite several unresolved problems about how to balance interests and how to specify the factors that could make a case exceptional. However, the important matters for our purposes are that (1) courts continue to order cesarean sections, (2) new standards of care, fiduciary responsibility, and fidelity could easily emerge,[85] and (3) physicians could then be sued for   to seek a court order.

Institutional interests. In other types of conflict, it is still less clear what the health care professional owes the "patient." The institutions involved often are not health care institutions, but to discharge their primary and legitimate functions they may need medical information about individuals and may provide some care for those individuals. Examples include a physician's contract to provide medical examinations for applicants seeking employment positions in a company or to determine whether applicants for insurance policies are good risks. The health care professional may rightly not regard the person examined as his or her patient, but the professional still has certain responsibilities of due care—for example, care in examinations so as not to injure the individual.

In some jurisdictions the health care professional does not have a legal obligation to disclose the discovery of a disease to the examinee, although nondisclosure is clearly a morally dubious practice. For example, in one pre-employment physical examination, x-ray films indicated that a woman who was subsequently hired had tuberculosis, yet the physician and the employer did not disclose these findings to her. After three years, the employee became ill with tuberculosis and was hospitalized for a prolonged period. The court held that the woman's only recourse was worker's compensation. It disallowed her suit against her employer and the physician who examined her, on grounds that there was no established patient–physician relationship and hence no legal obligation to disclose the information to her.[86] However, from a moral standpoint, both the employer and the physician had an obligation to disclose the information. The examinee had a legitimate expectation of disclosure in the absence of a specific disavowal of that responsibility. At a minimum, health care professionals have a moral responsibility to oppose, avoid, and withdraw from contracts that would require them to withhold information of significant benefit to examinees.

Physicians similarly owe "due care" to individuals who become their patients under a third-party contract in an institutional arrangement. Examples include health care professionals in industries, prisons, and the armed services. However, care of the patient sometimes conflicts with institutional objectives and policies, and the patient's needs may or may not take precedence even when they are owed due care. For example, in 1966, an Air Force newsletter reported that a twenty-six-year-old sergeant who had been on active duty in Vietnam for seven months and had flown more than one hundred missions developed a fear of flying because several of his acquaintances had been killed. The diagnosis was gross stress reaction, "manifested by anxiety, tenseness, a fear of death expressed in the form of rationalizations, and inability to function. His problem was 'worked through' and insight . . . was gained to the extent that he was returned to full flying duty in less than six weeks."[87] This case raises questions about the point at which health care professionals should refuse to engage in military or other services if they cannot combine fidelity to patients with fidelity to the institution. The military physician must accept a different set of obligations than the nonmilitary physician, in particular, to place the military's interests above both the patient's and the physician's interests.

For example, the physician's primary responsibility is to advise a commander regarding a patient's fitness for duty, not to care for the patient. However, some actions grossly violate canons of medical ethics. They thereby warrant disobedience of orders and defiance of superiors, rather than loyalty and compliance. An example is a commander's order for a physician to help torture a prisoner of war in order to gain information or to verify the efficacy of the techniques being used.[88] Despite borderline cases, physicians and psychotherapists can in principle remain loyal to military commitments and can render valuable care to wounded soldiers, even in an unjust war, without violating moral obligations. They render service to the soldier as a human being rather than to the soldier as a soldier, and thereby honor the values of the medical profession.

Medical assistance in prisons also presents explosive moral problems, in part because obligations of fidelity to the patient are limited by the institutional mandate to punish. Medical values are sometimes made subordinate to the correctional institution's functions, and yet the physician is expected to be loyal to both. The correctional institution usually expects physicians and other health care professionals to participate in the administration of justice and of punishment. Examples include surgical removal of a bullet for evidence when it is not a hazard to the inmate and can be safely left in place, forced examinations of inmates' body cavities for evidence of contraband drugs, and participation in corporal or capital punishment—for example, by administering a lethal injection.[89]

Related questions arise about medical assessments of prisoners' physical conditions to determine whether they can endure punishments, and about medical monitoring of these prisoners during punishment. Medical supervision can prevent extreme or unintended injury or harm, but participation in the administration of punishment, whether corporal or capital, represents a compromise of the profession's commitments of fidelity.[90] For similar reasons, the Council on Ethical and Judicial Affairs of the AMA has held for several years that physician participation in capital punishment through administration of a lethal injection is unethical. In 1992 it further defined unethical participation to include a physician's administration of tranquilizers or other medications as part of an execution, monitoring of a condemned prisoner's vital signs, professional witnessing of an execution, or rendering technical advice for an execution.[91] The premise is that in these acts a physician's conflicts of fidelity are unjustifiably resolved in favor of institutional needs.

Nursing. Perhaps in no area of health care are conflicts among obligations of fidelity more pervasive and morally troubling than in nursing, in part because of the structure of health care institutions: "Traditionally, nurses have been discouraged from developing and acting on their own ethical judgments. Although the institutions of nursing and medicine developed separately until the late eighteenth century, the increasing importance of the hospital in health care brought nursing under the dual command of physicians and hospital administrators."[92] Recent codes of nursing ethics define the moral responsibility of nurses in sharply different ways from the codes of two or three decades ago. For example, in 1950, the first code of the American Nurses' Association stressed the nurse's obligation to carry out the physician's orders, but the 1976 revision stressed the nurse's obligation to the client. Whereas the original code emphasized the nurse's obligation to protect the reputation of associates, the later code emphasized the obligation to safeguard the client and the public from the "incompetent, unethical or illegal" practices of any person. Many nurses today conceive their role to be, in part, that of "client advocate" or "patient advocate."[93]

Alterations in these codes reflect changes in the profession of nursing, but their implications have not been fully clarified or implemented in institutions. Consequently, nurses may have to choose between obligations of fidelity to the physician and to the institution, on the one hand, and to the patient, on the other.[94] Consider the following case. Mrs. R., who is approximately forty-five years old, divorced, and the mother of teenage daughters who live with her, suffers from multiple sclerosis. She often comes to the emergency room of the local community hospital for treatment of acute episodes of asthma. The physician has ordered "no code" (no cardiopulmonary resuscitation—CPR) should Mrs. R. suffer a cardiac arrest. The nurses believe that the physician made the decision without discussing it with Mrs. R. or the family, and they are not sure what Mrs. R. would want because she is often depressed when she comes to the emergency room and has not expressed her wishes.[95]

A conscientious nurse will first ascertain in these circumstances whether the patient's wishes are known and are being respected.[96] If Mrs. R. competently and voluntarily requested or consented to the "no code" order, and if Mrs. R. and the physician are in agreement, the "no code" order should be followed. But if Mrs. R. enters the emergency room and suffers a cardiac arrest before this information can be obtained, the nurse and others may legitimately ignore the "no code" and provide the treatment ordinarily indicated in such cases. Should the nurse discover that the physician has ordered "no code" against the express wishes of Mrs. R., the nurse should refuse to follow the order. (We return to conscientious refusals in Chapter 8.) But refusing to carry out the "no code" order will not be sufficient. The nurse has pledged, by accepting nursing codes, to seek to have the physician's order countermanded in order to protect the patient's best interest and wishes. The nurse may also have a responsibility to pressure the hospital into developing clearer and more satisfactory policies governing CPR.

Political as well as moral problems will persist in nursing as long as some professionals make the decisions and order their implementation by other professionals who have not participated in the decisionmaking. In several cases nurses have blown the whistle on parents and physicians who decided not to treat newborns with serious disabilities and who required nurses and others to implement their decisions. Such conflicts are largely avoidable, but in the rush of health care they are not always anticipated and prevented. In a study of relationships in health care, investigators examined different perceptions of ethical problems by nurses and doctors. In structured interviews with twenty-six nurses and twenty-four physicians who work in acute care units, both groups said they frequently encountered ethical problems. Most of the physicians (21 of 24) and most of the nurses (25 of 26) recognized differences of opinion or ethical conflicts within the health care team. However, in twenty-one of the twenty-five cases reported by nurses, the ethical conflict was between a nurse and a physician, whereas only one physician reported a conflict with a nurse rather than with another physician. The authors of the study believe it likely that conflicts with nurses were present in cases the physicians presented but that the physicians "were not aware of them, or did not see conflict with a nurse as forming an *ethical* problem."[97]

These findings may be explainable by several features of the working relationship between physicians and nurses. Physicians write orders; nurses carry them out. By virtue of their close, sustained relationships with patients, nurses often experience the problems that arise from medical decisions more immediately than physicians. These common features of nursing roles sharpen obligations of fidelity to patients but also open avenues of conflict with colleagues.

Clinical teaching. Conflicts of fidelity also emerge in health care institutions that serve multiple functions, such as institutions that educate health professionals through the care of patients or that engage in clinical research. The use of patients in the teaching of physicians and nurses need not violate the prohibition against treating persons merely as means if patients understand the divided loyalties of teaching hospitals, are not subjected to undue risks, and are protected in other ways (for example, by meaningful rules of privacy and confidentiality). Some studies indicate that many patients find bedside rounds (a declining practice) to be a positive and educational experience.[98] However, one study indicates that only thirty-seven to fifty-one percent of teaching hospitals provide information to patients about the role of students in medical care,[99] although fidelity to the patient suggests consent upon admission, as well as specific disclosures. For example, the patient should be told who will be on the surgical team and who will be in charge, and patients should be able to consent to the use of students in their care. Justice also requires that any burdens of participation, even if only inconveniences, not be inequitably assigned to poorer and less educated patients, especially when the patients remain ignorant of the students' participation.

Conflicts of interest. Over the last several years, new or at least more serious conflicts have further weakened traditional rules of fidelity. In particular, third-party payers and institutional providers have imposed constraints on medical decisions about diagnostic and therapeutic procedures. These economic interests form a part of the daily life of physicians. Loyalties are formed to these different parties as well as to patients.[100] Various mechanisms have been established to control the escalating costs of health care, including prospective payment and diagnosis related groups, utilization review, preferred provider arrangements, and various forms of managed care. These mechanisms often function to limit and constrict the physician's fidelity to the patient through a mixture of incentives and disincentives, some of which place the physician's self-interest in conflict with the patient's best interest, thereby producing serious ethical conflicts of interest in addition to conflicts of fidelity.

Some constraints are imposed through efforts to standardize care by means of practice guidelines. Such standards of care can be helpful to both clinicians and patients, but their limitations are evident. Directives often do not match a particular patient's individual needs, particularly at the point of reducing diagnostic and therapeutic uncertainty through procedures of marginal (but nevertheless some) value. At a minimum, fidelity to the patient, requires efforts to meet the patient's needs as completely as possible within the guidelines, as well as disclosure to the patient of why a potentially useful diagnostic or therapeutic procedure is not being provided. A clinician's fidelity to patients also may require efforts to change professional and institutional constraints that are inconsistent with patients' interests. The clinician may have to assess whether fidelity to the patient's interests requires manipulation of the system for the patient's benefit, even though this practice may involve deception and violations of fidelity to contracts and promises to third parties. We discussed such a strategy and its problems earlier in the case of the physician who wrote ''rule out cancer'' rather than ''screening mammography'' in order to manipulate an insurance company.

Financial and other incentives to motivate the clinician to consider the economic effects of particular clinical decisions are ubiquitous in modern medicine. For example, most Health Maintenance Organizations (HMOs) keep part of the primary physician's income—ten to thirty percent (the higher figures appearing in for-profit HMOs). Part or all of that income is returned at the end of the year, depending on the overall financial condition of the HMO and, in some cases, the physician's productivity and frugality. Such an arrangement creates an incentive for physicians to limit their care to patients—a worrisome conflict of interest. The patient is in a very different position when the physician has incentives to *restrict* needed treatment than when the physician has incentives to provide *unnecessary* treatment. In the latter situation, patients can obtain another opinion. In the former situation, patients may never be aware of a needed treatment because no one has recommended it.[101]

Widespread self-referral—that is, referral of patients to medical facilities or services that physicians themselves own or in which they have a financial investment—has also threatened fidelity to patients' interests by extending the temptation inherent in fee-for-service to provide unnecessary care or unnecessarily expensive care. Physicians create such economic conflicts of interest by owning or investing in various medical facilities or services, such as diagnostic imaging centers, laboratories, or physical therapy services to which they refer patients. Recent evidence indicates that physician ownership of radiation therapy and physical therapy services, for instance, substantially increases both use and costs, without compensatory benefit such as increased access. Such practices are now widespread. Ten percent of physicians in the United States (forty percent in Florida) who are involved in direct patient care have an investment interest in a health care business to which they may refer patients for services.[102]

Fee-for-service is often less problematic than self-referral, because the patient can more easily recognize the physician's economic gain in providing additional procedures and can exercise caution accordingly—for example, by seeking a second opinion. For this reason some contend that the physician has an obligation to disclose economic conflicts of interest in instances of self-referral. This disclosure is an ethical minimum of fidelity and honesty, but it rarely occurs, and it may only function to protect physicians by reducing their risk of liability.[103] A strong case can be made that fidelity to patients requires a far stricter rule prohibiting self-referral, as has now been recognized by the AMA.

Within a period of twelve months the AMA twice reversed its position on the ethics of self-referral. Its earlier view (1986) held that physicians could be trusted to handle the conflicts. Then, in December 1991, the Council on Ethical and Judicial Affairs of the AMA noted "inherent problems with the practice." It stressed that "physicians am not simply businesspeople with high standards. Physicians are engaged in the special calling of healing, and, in that calling, they are the fiduciaries of their patients. They have different and higher duties than even the most ethical businessperson." The council then altered its policy

on self-referral, finding "the practice presumptively inconsistent with the physician's fiduciary duty when adequate alternative facilities exist." It recommended that "in general, physicians should not refer patients to a health care
facility outside their office practice at which they do not directly provide care
or services when they have an investment interest in the facility." [104]

The council's report was accepted by the AMA House of Delegates, but in
June 1992, this same body reversed itself and declared that self-referral arrangements could be ethical if referring physicians disclosed to patients their
investment interests and informed them of alternate facilities or services. For a
few months the AMA had no clear-cut policy on self-referral because of the
discrepancy between the council report and the new position. In December
1992, however, the AMA again shifted, reaffirming the council report. These
shifts over a short period reflect moral ambivalence and a lack of consensus in
the medical profession. The prohibition of self-referral, allowing exceptions for
disclosure when self-referral is necessary because of a lack of other facilities
or services, is the most appropriate expression and protection of fidelity to
patients. Avoidance of self-referral should not be considered an option, but
rather a firm obligation of fidelity and a necessary condition of moral integrity.

Some relationships encountered in clinical research involve similar problems
of conflict of interest. For example, many clinical trials are financially supported by the pharmaceutical industry, which is willing to assume the financial
risk because the returns from a successful trial can be extremely high. The
financial advantages for physician-investigators and corporations promote a relationship with a consistent flow of funding.[105] A subtle desire is sometimes
created to arrange another and better contract or grant by producing research
results that are favorable from a funding source's perspective. In some cases
personal financial interests of the physician-investigator are at stake. Medical
centers, both inside and outside university research facilities, increasingly are
staffed with physicians who have a financial interest in the drugs, medical devices, and technologies they prescribe or recommend to their patients.[106] For
example, some physicians have stock or stock options in companies that manu-
facture the products they recommend. In a few cases investigators have advance knowledge of a medical device because of their research, and they purchase stock in the belief its price will rise.

A conflict of interest is present whenever the researcher's role-obligation or
personal interest in accommodating an institution, in job security, in personal
goals, and the like compromises or threatens to compromise obligations to others who have a right to expect objectivity and fairness. For example, any investigators who accelerate research beyond methodological acceptability in order
to attract or retain funding have a conflict of interest. Financial interests in
particular stand to compromise both the quality of the research and the objectivity of recommendations to patients. Having clinician-investigators with an eco-

nomic interest in products they are evaluating for safety and efficacy threatens both honesty and quality of care. Yet this arrangement is largely unchecked and growing.

The Dual Roles of Physician and Investigator

The Declaration of Geneva of the World Medical Association affirms that "the health of my patient will be my first consideration," and the Physician's oath of the same association demands that "Concern for the interests of the subject [of research] must always prevail over the interests of science and society." But can these obligations be consistently honored in research involving patients and other subjects? The dual roles of research scientist and clinical practitioner pull in different directions and present both conflicting obligations and conflicting interests. As an investigator, the physician acts to generate scientific knowledge anticipated to benefit individual patients in the future. As a clinical practitioner, contracts and responsibilities for care require acting in the best interests of present patients. Both roles are intended to benefit the sick, but the scientific role is directed at unknown, future patients, whereas the clinical role is tailored for known, current patients. Accordingly, responsibility to future generations may conflict with due care for particular current patients.

Research involving human subjects is both important for society and morally perilous because subjects are exposed to some risk for the advancement of science. Ethically justified research must satisfy several conditions, including the pursuit of knowledge, a reasonable prospect that the research will generate the knowledge that is sought, a favorable balance of benefits to the subject and the society over risks to the subject, fair selection of subjects, and the necessity of using human subjects.[107] Only after these conditions have been met, as certified by investigators and by an institutional review board, is it appropriate to request subjects to participate. Consent is necessary, but consent alone is insufficient to justify the research.

Limiting contracts between potential subjects and investigators to research that passes the above conditions has been criticized as a paternalistic interference with free choice.[108] However, because society encourages extensive research, and because investigators and subjects are unequal in knowledge and vulnerability—especially if sick patients are involved—public policy and review committees must act to prevent potentially exploitative contracts, to protect privacy and confidentiality, and the like. In some cases a straightforward paternalistic decision is warranted. For example, if healthy persons with no heart disease volunteer as subjects in a protocol to have an artificial heart transplanted, as occurred at the University of Utah,[109] an institutional review board (IRB) should declare that the risk relative to benefit for a healthy subject is too substantial to permit the research, although the risk relative to benefit for a patient with a seriously diseased heart may be acceptable.

These observations apply to both *nontherapeutic* research, which offers no prospect of medical benefit to the subject, and *therapeutic* research, which offers some prospect of medical benefit to the patient-subject and is usually conducted as a part of the care of the patient. This use of the term *therapeutic* can deflect attention from the fact that *research* is being conducted. As a systematic scientific effort, therapeutic research is distinguishable from both routine therapy and experimental or innovative therapy, which are directed at particular patients. Attaching the favorable term *therapeutic* to research can be dangerous, because it suggests "justified intervention" in the care of particular patients. Yet sick patients may be heavily dependent on a physician, and they may believe that anything the physician recommends will be beneficial. The conditions of justified research therefore must be satisfied for therapeutic research as well as for nontherapeutic research.

Conflicts in Clinical Trials

Controlled clinical trials are sometimes needed in order to confirm that an observed effect, such as reduced mortality from a particular disease, is the result of a particular intervention rather than the result of an unknown variable in the patient population. The evidence supporting many available treatments is tenuous and in need of validation, and some have never been adequately tested for either safety or efficacy. If doubt surrounds the efficacy or safety of a treatment, or its relative merits in comparison to another treatment, scientific research that can resolve the doubt is clearly in order. Controlled trials are scientific instruments intended to protect current and future patients against medical enthusiasm and hunches, replacing them with validated treatments.

In such research one group receives the experimental therapy, while a "control group" receives either no treatment, a standard therapy, or a placebo (that is, a procedure or substance, such as a sugar pill, that the investigator believes is pharmacologically or biomedically inert for the patient's condition) in order to allow investigators to determine whether an experimental therapy is more effective and safer than a standard therapy or a placebo. A standard procedure in research design is to assign subjects to control and experimental groups randomly in order to avoid intentional or unintentional bias. Randomization is designed to keep variables other than the particular treatments under examination from distorting study results. Most controlled trials are randomized clinical trials (RCTs), which are generally preferred to observational or retrospective studies on grounds that their results have a higher degree of validity.

Blinding certain persons to some information about the RCT provides an additional protection against bias. RCTs may be single-blind (the subject does not know whether he or she is in the control group or the experimental group), double-blind (neither the subject nor the investigator knows), or unblinded (all parties know). Double-blind studies are designed specifically to reduce bias in observations and interpretations by subjects and physicians. Blinding the physician-investigator, according to some interpretations, also serves an ethical function, because it obviates any conflict of interest for those who both provide therapy and conduct research.

Problems of consent. Although RCTs are generally sound ways to generate knowledge, they present moral problems and require justification. One problem and its solution follow from the analysis of informed consent in Chapter 3. In the specific case of randomized clinical trials, no justification exists for failure to disclose to potential subjects the full set of methods, treatments, and placebos (if any) that will be used, their known risks and benefits, and any known uncertainties. There is also no justification for failure to disclose the fact of randomization and the reason for it. If all this information is supplied, potential subjects should have an adequate informational base for deciding whether to participate, even though they lack knowledge of which treatment or placebo they personally will receive.

Here the question arises whether potential subjects who understand that they are being kept partially ignorant about a particular intervention or research project can give an informed consent, especially if new information generated during the research will not be disclosed to the subject. A satisfactory answer depends on a subject's ability to judge the materiality of the undisclosed information. Subjects are not always in a good position to make such a judgment, and it is sometimes too difficult to determine whether unknown information will be pivotal. The research will not be justified if there is significant doubt about the materiality of undisclosed information or if scientifically sound alternative research designs are available. Placebos present a special problem: Telling subjects that they are receiving a placebo undermines the very purpose of using it. But again the only acceptable solution seems to be to disclose that the research involves use of a placebo whose identity and distribution must remain undisclosed. Subjects would then have to accept or decline participation in the research based on this information.

Because patients commonly assume that decisions about their treatment are made in their best interests, rather than in the interests of a research design or of future patients, the physician-researcher should disclose all significant alternatives to patient-subjects. One relevant item of information is the method used to determine who receives a particular treatment. Some investigators contend that disclosure of the allocation system would cause distress to the patient or would lead some patients to refuse to participate in the research. They also argue that disclosure of the allocation system is not necessary because patients do not need to know how the allocation is made between two treatments that appear to be equally effective and equally risky. However, because the physician-researcher has dual responsibilities, he or she has a fiduciary obligation to inform patient-subjects of every matter directly relevant to their decisions, including conditions that might involve the physician-researcher in a conflict of interest.[110]

This obligation of disclosure is not always met. In Denmark a randomized clinical trial was conducted to assess the value of intestinal bypass in the treatment of gross obesity. One hundred thirty patients received surgery and were compared with sixty-six patients who received medical treatment. The subjects, at least the ones receiving medical treatment, did not give informed consent, because the researchers withheld relevant information and used deception. As the researchers reported, "We did not ask for informed consent for randomization. Patients allocated to medical treatment were told that surgery had to be postponed for an undetermined period primarily because liver-biopsy findings showed fatty infiltration," an untrue statement.[111]

Several moral problems in addition to those of consent also appear in randomized clinical trials. For example, are RCTs as essential as their proponents say? Can they be used without compromising acknowledged responsibilities to patients?[112] The increased certainty of the results in RCTs is only a matter of degree, and we may have grounds to prefer a less conclusive method if it would more adequately fulfill obligations to current patients. It seems inconsistent with serving the patient's best interests to select a treatment randomly in order to promote social goals of accumulating knowledge and benefiting future patients. No two patients are alike, and it is essential that a physician be able to modify the course of therapy as required by the patient's best interests. But is this axiom of medical ethics consistent with controlled trials?

The problem of clinical equipoise. Proponents argue that RCTs do not violate moral obligations to patients because they are used only in circumstances in which justifiable doubt exists about the merits of existing, standard, or new therapies. No one knows prior to conducting the research whether it is more advantageous to be in the control group or in the experimental group (sometimes called the "null hypothesis"[113]). Reasonable physicians are therefore in a state of "clinical equipoise"[114]: On the basis of the available evidence, members of the relevant expert medical community are equally poised between the treatment strategies being tested in the RCT, because they are equally uncertain about and equally comfortable with the known advantages and disadvantages of the treatments to be tested. No patient, then, will receive a treatment known to be less effective or more dangerous than an available alternative. Because current patients are not asked to sacrifice a superior treatment and may benefit from the experiment, the use of RCTs seems justifiable, especially in light of the promise of benefit to future patients. No reasonable person could have objective grounds before the trial for preferring to be in one group or another, although he or she may prefer one over the other on the basis of hunches or intuitions about effectiveness and safety or on the basis of factors not being studied in the trial. For example, if two treatments for breast cancer are in veritable clinical equipoise, a woman may prefer the less disfiguring treatment (see below).

Whether these justifying conditions are satisfied in particular trials is often the central issue. If some cooperating physicians believe prior to the trial that one therapy is more beneficial or safer, they should not simply suspend this belief in the interests of scientific objectivity. It is not sufficient to argue that the trial provides a corrective to the physician's hunches, because this claim evades questions about whether the physician has an obligation not to participate or to inform patients about a hunch or belief. Physicians clearly are obligated to communicate their beliefs about risks and benefits together with an overall assessment of what is in the patient's best interest, and an honest communication will not conceal any of the physician's relevant beliefs and will disclose what will happen as the trial proceeds if the physician forms new or altered opinions.

Before an RCT is begun, some evidence often exists about a treatment's safety or efficacy relative to other treatments, and physicians often have beliefs about treatments based on clinical experience or anecdotal evidence. RCTs demand that these beliefs or suspicions be set aside as guesswork unworthy of science. Having knowledge *means* having scientific knowledge based on the results of a statistical test. The standard of statistical significance that is widely used—probability of at least 0.05, which means that less than a 5% chance exists both that there is no difference in effects and that the difference results from a variable other than the tested treatments—is reasonable and well established, but the convention involves a range of normative choices as to which cutoff establishes significance.[115] The convention has also been criticized as arbitrary, although it is well entrenched and widely believed to define "knowledge."

Two examples illustrate ways in which RCTs are controversial. According to one report, a controlled double-blind experiment on a new drug, adenine arabinoside (ara-A), indicated that it is an effective treatment for herpes simplex encephalitis, a virus-caused inflammation of the brain that is fatal to approximately seventy percent of those who contract it. Of the ten people given a placebo, seven died, one suffered severe damage, and two recovered to lead reasonably normal lives. Of the eighteen who received ara-A, five died, six had serious brain or nerve damage, and seven recovered to lead reasonably normal lives. The ten who received the placebo were given standard care, which mainly consisted of palliative care because no treatment prior to ara-A had been found to be effective.

Critics charge that it was not necessary to have a placebo group instead of historical controls. Because ara-A had already been shown to be effective and nontoxic in some localized herpes simplex hominis infections, and because no other treatment was available to prevent mortality or serious brain and nerve damage, moral questions have been raised about the rationale for using an RCT and for administering the placebo in this case. Whenever no satisfactory therapy for a disease exists, the control group by definition must be given a non-treatment or placebo even if some hope exists for the experimental therapy (otherwise the trial would not be justified). Physicians are then placed in the awkward position of recommending randomization when they believe the new agent may possess therapeutic value. However, the new agent also may have side effects that are serious enough to outweigh its possible benefits.

Defenders of RCTs respond that the mortality rate of herpes simplex encephalitis was not known prior to the research. Historical controls were inadequate because the disease is difficult to diagnose apart from brain biopsies, and it was not known whether ara-A would be toxic when administered with large amounts of fluid to such patients. The research was stopped when the above-mentioned statistics emerged, but several scientists contend that it was stopped prematurely, before statistically significant evidence had emerged about effectiveness and toxicity. They note that, because of the small groups involved, it is misleading to say that 20 percent of the placebo recipients and 38.8 percent of ara-A recipients had reasonable recovery. If only one person, the next placebo-recipient, had had reasonably normal recovery, the figures would have been much closer.[116]

Second, a similar conflict erupted over placebo-controlled trials of AZT (azidothymidine) in the treatment of AIDS. After it had proved to be ineffective in the treatment of cancer, AZT was shelved for several years by its manufacturer, Burroughs Wellcome, only to be pulled off the shelves in the massive search for an effective agent against HIV, the retrovirus that causes AIDS. Promising laboratory tests were followed by a trial (phase I) to determine the safety of AZT among AIDS patients. Several patients showed clinical improvement during the trial. Because AIDS is invariably fatal, many people argued that compassion dictated making AZT immediately available to all AIDS patients and perhaps to those who are antibody-positive to the AIDS virus.

For several reasons, the drug was not made generally available. The company did not have an adequate supply of AZT to supply all AIDS patients. As required by federal regulations, it used a placebo-controlled trial of AZT to determine its effectiveness for several groups of AIDS patients. A computer randomly assigned some AIDS patients to AZT and others to a placebo. For several months, no major differences emerged in effectiveness, but then patients receiving the placebo began to die at a significantly higher rate. Of the 137 patients on the placebo, 16 died. Of the 145 patients on AZT, only 1 died. In view of these results, the trial was terminated on the advice of a data and safety monitoring board. Subjects who had received the placebo in the trial were, as promised, the first to receive the drug.

As a result of this trial, later research on anti-retroviral treatments for AIDS will have to compare new treatments with AZT (or other subsequently approved therapies), and placebo-controlled trials must be considered unethical, at least for certain groups of patients.

Later data have shown that AZT is not effective over a long period for most patients (it does not cure the underlying disease) and that many patients stop AZT because of its toxicity. Beginning in early 1987, the drug was distributed according to strict criteria because the supply was so limited, because there was inadequate evidence about its effectiveness for some groups of patients, and because there was uncertainty about whether the risks of the drug (for example, its toxicity) would outweigh its benefits to patients at earlier stages of the disease. Proponents of compassion for present patients have raised questions about starting such a placebo-controlled trial when a disease appears to be universally fatal and no promising alternative to the new treatment exists. They also raise questions about when to stop a trial and how broadly to distribute a new treatment.[117]

Even in the face of *objective* scientific evidence that two proposed treatments are roughly equal in safety and efficacy, patients may have strong *subjective* preferences for one treatment or group over another. Suppose two surgical procedures for treating the same disease appear to have the same survival rate (say, an average of fifteen years), and suppose we test their effectiveness by an RCT. The patient might have a preference if treatment A has little risk of death during the operation but a high rate of death after ten years, while treatment B has a high risk of death during the operation or postoperative recovery but a low rate of death after recovery (say, for thirty years). A patient's age, family responsibilities, and other circumstances might lead to a preference for one over the other.[118] If no known difference exists in the rates of survival, patients may have a strong preference for a particular form of intervention—for example, high-risk surgery rather than high radiation dosage—or for a less invasive or less disfiguring procedure, as they did in trials of treatments for breast cancer.[119] Some patients will prefer the lowest risk procedure, whereas others will gamble on risk for a potentially greater benefit.

The Use of Prerandomization

The use of prerandomization, or pre-consent randomization, is another controversial development. In conventional RCTs, a patient is screened for eligibility and is then informed about the study, the different arms of treatment or placebo (if one is used), the risks and benefits, and the method of assignment to the different arms. If the patient consents to participate, he or she is then randomized to one arm of the study. In prerandomization a shift occurs in the time of randomization, because it occurs prior to consent to participate.

The National Surgical Adjuvant Project for Breast and Bowel Cancers designed a study of treatments of breast cancer to determine whether survival rates differed among patients randomly assigned to simple mastectomy versus lumpectomy with or without radiation. This RCT had a low rate of patient participation, and researchers thought it might have to be discontinued because the small number of subjects threatened the canons of statistical significance. Two statisticians associated with the project describe the problem:

A major problem with the protocol appeared to be the lack of acceptability of the randomization. Physicians were reluctant to approach patients at the time of the operation about chance assignment to surgical therapies that involved either removal or cosmetic preservation of the breast. Patients also had difficulty dealing with randomization. In many cases, patients were not even certain whether or not they had a breast cancer and yet they were being asked to consider quite dissimilar surgical procedures if cancer was found at the time of the surgery. Further, even when the patient knew the diagnosis, it was disquieting not to know which surgery would be performed, i.e., whether she would wake up with or without a breast.[120]

For this RCT to be ethically justified, it had to be reasonable to assume that neither treatment was superior in survival rate. If conditions of clinical equipoise regarding survival are satisfied, considerations of quality of life become central in decisions to participate, and in this case many women preferred the less invasive and disfiguring surgery. A survey of physicians who decided not to enter patients in this nationwide RCT identified several other perceived difficulties:

(1) concern that the doctor–patient relationship would be affected by a randomized clinical trial (73 percent), (2) difficulty with informed consent (38 percent), (3) dislike of open discussions involving uncertainty [including uncertainty about the superior treatment and about which treatment patients would receive through randomization] (22 percent), (4) perceived conflicts between the roles of scientist and clinician (18 percent), (5) practical difficulties in following procedures (9 percent), and (6) feelings of personal responsibility if the treatments were found to be unequal (8 percent).[121]

However, after a policy of prerandomization was adopted, the accrual rate increased sixfold and the trial was salvaged, producing sound evidence that the survival rates are as good with the less disfiguring surgery for early breast cancer.[122]

Critics raise several moral questions about prerandomization. A central problem is how the mere shift in time from randomization to prerandomization could result in increased patient accrual without some distortion in the information patients received, particularly in view of the physicians' stated reasons for their reluctance to enroll all of their eligible patients. Even if they had no preference for one treatment over the other, some patients may have refused conventional randomization because of its uncertainty—that is, because of their lack of knowledge about which treatment they would receive. But no evidence supports this hypothesis.[123] It would be odd if rational behavior under randomization could shift so dramatically under prerandomization.[124] Many suspect that disclosure of information becomes distorted, perhaps unconsciously, when the physician knows the assigned treatment in advance.[125] Clearly the process of obtaining informed consent under prerandomization merits unusually careful scrutiny to ensure adequate disclosure. In practice, consent forms must be approved by an IRB, but rarely is the consent process monitored.

Another problem arises with a version of prerandomization that solicits consent only from patients who receive the experimental treatment, not from those who receive the standard treatment, although those receiving the standard treatment are followed through chart review. In addition to problems of scientific validity caused by one group having more knowledge than the other group, ethical problems arise because the physician only discusses the experimental therapy with the patient and does not mention that a random process determined the therapy.[126] A justified RCT does involve something akin to tossing a coin, and the physician-researcher should not hide that relevant fact from the patient.

Early Termination of and Withdrawal from Clinical Trials

Physician-researchers sometimes face difficult questions about whether to stop an experiment before its planned completion, occasionally before they have sufficient data to support final conclusions. During clinical trials access to data is limited in order to protect the integrity of the research. Consequently, physicians are excluded from access to information about trends. If they were aware of trends prior to the point of statistical significance, they might pull their patients from the trial, thereby invalidating the research. As noted earlier, some researchers contend that the trial of ara-A was stopped before the evidence became statistically convincing, precluding a definitive determination that ara-A is superior to standard, palliative care.

If a physician determines that a patient's condition is deteriorating and that the patient's interests dictate withdrawal from the research, then that physician should be free to act on behalf of the patient, assuming the patient concurs. In an RCT it may be difficult to determine whether the experiment as a whole should be stopped even if some physician-researchers insist that they are satisfied by the preliminary evidence regarding trends. One procedural way to handle this ethical conflict is to differentiate roles. We can distinguish between individual physicians who must make decisions regarding their own patients and a data-monitoring committee established to determine whether to continue or stop a trial. Unlike the physicians, a committee is charged to consider the impact of its decision on treatments for future patients, as well as for current patient-subjects. A major function of data-monitoring committees is to stop a trial if accumulated data indicate that the circumstance of equipoise has shifted and uncertainty no longer prevails. Accordingly, any RCT needs a well-functioning data-monitoring committee to determine if and when clinical equipoise no longer exists.

This differentiation of roles by using a data-monitoring committee, particularly in a double-blind RCT, is procedurally sound, but it relocates rather than resolves some central ethical questions. The committee still must determine when, if ever, it is legitimate to impose risks on current patients in order to benefit future ones by establishing with a high degree of certainty the superiority of one treatment over another or over a placebo. A committee will likely take the perspective that clinical equipoise must have been eliminated *for the expert medical community*.[127] But the individual physician and his or her patient may be concerned primarily with whether clinical uncertainty has been eliminated *for them*.

Consent forms typically indicate that subjects may withdraw at any time, without detriment to their care.[128] However, many questions are relevant to a patient-subject's decision to withdraw from an RCT, including questions about interim data and early trends. Trends are often misleading and are sometimes later shown to be temporary aberrations. However, they might be relevant at a given point to a patient-subject's decision about whether to continue to participate, despite the fact that the evidence would not satisfy statisticians working on the project or the expert medical community. As a rule, information about trends is not released prior to the completion or early termination of the RCT, and this rule is justifiable as long as prospective subjects understand and accept it as a condition for participating in the RCT.

Some hold that the research physician's commitment to the welfare of his or her patients is their best protection, exceeding other forms of protection such as those afforded by an IRB and a data-monitoring committee. Others contend that we should differentiate roles so that physicians do not use their patients in research. The point is not that a person cannot be both an investigator and a clinician but that a person should not assume both roles for the same patient-subject, at least without a clear priority of roles (and full disclosure to the patient-subject).[129]

Justifying Conditions for Randomized Clinical Trials

These moral problems about RCTs express the tension between utilitarian theories and Kantian theories as well as theories oriented toward individual rights
that we have been examining since Chapter 2. Utilitarianism is concerned
broadly with maximizing human welfare, for future generations as well as the
present one. The commitment of the research scientist is to eliminate inferior
and dangerous therapies and provide proven therapies, for both present and
future patients. The risks to some are justified by the far greater benefits anticipated for others. This goal of proving therapies, rather than operating with a
patchwork of hunches or guesswork, merits society's support. Nonetheless,
Kantians and those concerned about rights fear that this research will treat patients as means to scientific ends, without due regard for their rights and interests. Some critics therefore hold that patients in RCTs do, in the end, sacrifice
their interests for the sake of the interests of others.[130]

Although we have now considered several problems with RCTs, we believe
they are justified if (and only if) the following conditions are satisfied:

1. True clinical equipoise is present in the group of relevant medical experts.
2. The trial is designed as a crucial experiment between therapeutic alternatives
   and shows scientific promise of achieving this result.
3. An IRB has approved the protocol and certified that no physician has a
   conflict of interest or incentive that would threaten the patient—physician relationship.
4. Comprehensive informed consent (as specified in Chapter 3) has been obtained.
5. Placebos cannot be used if evidence exists of an adequate treatment.
6. A data-monitoring committee will either end the trial when clinical equipoise is displaced by statistically significant data or will supply physicians
   and patients with significant safety and therapeutic information that is, in
   the committee's judgment, relevant to a reasonable person's decision to remain in or to withdraw from the trial.
7. The right of physicians to recommend withdrawal and the right of patients
   to withdraw at any time are protected.

The first condition is worth stressing. Equipoise is essential for clinical research, because without it the superior treatment must be provided. In trials
with several arms, every arm must exhibit equipoise. A shift in data that dis-
turbs equipoise destroys the rationale for using the patients involved, because
a treatment preference has emerged. Equipoise is also a necessary condition of
all clinical research, not of randomized clinical trials alone.

Beyond these conditions, we take the view that medical knowledge and scientific progress are vital goals, but that particular research protocols are often optional. Our obligations to future patients are strong enough that we should permit, encourage, and support research that can generate knowledge, but without violating the rights and interests of current patients. The obligation of beneficence to future generations of patients is generally less stringent than the obligation to benefit the sick, who already have a relationship with clinicians.

RCTs should not become indispensable rituals or necessary canons of valid research. As we have noted, historical controls may sometimes be sufficient. In some cases prospective studies can be conducted without randomization, with evaluations performed by other parties not involved in the research in order to eliminate bias. In a few cases it may be morally appropriate and scientifically advantageous to use a blinded, randomized clinical trial only for subjects who consent to all aspects of the arrangement (perhaps a small number), at the same time also studying the progress of all persons who refuse randomization but who, nonetheless, receive the experimental treatment.[131] Many such alternatives are now under consideration. Some research designs take advantage of emerging evidence to alter the protocol; and some play the winner by using what appear to be the best therapies until they fail.[132]

In the last half-century scientific research has transformed medicine from a caretaking role with little power to cure serious disease to a robust practice capable of remarkable forms of cure, palliation, and risk reduction. This transformation has been so complete that we forget how profoundly the modern world has been shaped by biomedical research. Nonetheless, this research can present serious risks to its subjects, and for that reason, among others, it requires constant scrutiny in light of the demands of fidelity and the fundamental moral commitments of the medical enterprise.

Conclusion

In this chapter we have further interpreted and specified principles of respect for autonomy, nonmaleficence, beneficence, and justice for relationships in research and health care. We have concentrated on obligations that express these principles—obligations of veracity, privacy, confidentiality, and fidelity—and their conflicts. In each instance, we have explored the basis, meaning, limits, and stringency of these obligations in the context of professional and patient or subject relationships. Our analysis has indicated some conditions under which these obligations can be overridden when they cannot be sufficiently specified to dissolve the conflicts.

Morality includes more than obligations. When moral conflicts occur, we often recognize that the character traits of persons who must make judgments are no less important than obligations expressed in principles and rules. Several times in this chapter we have noted the importance of virtues such as truthfulness, trustworthiness, and fidelity. Any adequate ethical theory must attend to these virtues as well as to moral ideals. We turn to these topics in the final chapter.

Notes

1. *Current Opinions of the Judicial Council of the American Medical Association* (Chicago: AMA, 1981), p. ix; but see also p. 30 on informed consent.
2. Henry Sidgwick, *The Methods of Ethics,* 7th Ed. (Indianapolis, IN: Hackett Publishing Company, 1907), pp. 315–16.
3. G. J. Warnock, *The Object of Morality* (London: Methuen, 1971), pp. 85–86.
4. Alan Donagan, *The Theory of Morality* (Chicago: University of Chicago Press, 1977), p. 88; and see Charles Fried, *Right and Wrong* (Cambridge, MA: Harvard University Press, 1978), ch. 3.
5. See W. D. Ross, *The Right and the Good* (Oxford: Clarendon Press, 1930), ch. 2.
6. *Truman v. Thomas,* 611 P.2d 902, 906 (Cal. 1980), citing *Cobbs v. Grant,* 502 P.2d 1, 10 (1972). See also a subsequent Canadian case that required physicians to explain the consequences of leaving an ailment untreated: *Haughian v. Pain,* 37 D.L.R. (4th) (April 2, 1987): 624–49.
7. This case is discussed in Bettina Schöne-Seifert and James F. Childress, "How Much Should the Cancer Patient Know and Decide?" *CA—A Cancer Journal for Physicians* 36 (March–April 1986): 85–94.
8. See Donald Oken, "What to Tell Cancer Patients: A Study of Medical Attitudes," *Journal of the American Medical Association* 175 (1961): 1120–28; Dennis H. Novack et al., "Changes in Physicians' Attitudes toward Telling the Cancer Patient," *Journal of the American Medical Association* 241 (March 2, 1979): 897–900; Saul S. Radovsky, "Bearing the News," *New England Journal of Medicine* 313 (August 29, 1985): 586–88.
9. Novack et al., "Changes in Physicians' Attitudes."
10. James Boswell, *Life of Johnson,* vol. IV, p. 306, as quoted in Donagan, *The Theory of Morality,* p. 89.
11. Antonella Surbone, "Truth Telling to the Patient," *Journal of the American Medical Association,* 268 (October 7, 1992): 1661–62, which is the source of other points about the Italian situation.
12. See P. Mosconi, B. E. Meyerowitz, M. C. Liberati, et al., "Disclosure of Breast Cancer Diagnosis: and Physician Reports," *Annals of Oncology* 2 (1991): 273–280, as discussed in Surbone, "Truth Telling to the Patient."
13. Edmund D. Pellegrino, "Is Truth Telling to the Patient a Cultural Artifact?" *Journal of the American Medical Association* 268 (October 7, 1992): 1734–35.
14. See Robert Veatch, *Death, Dying, and the Biological Revolution,* Rev. Ed. (New Haven, CT: Yale University Press, 1989), chap. 7.
15. Margery W. Shaw, "Testing for the Huntington Gene: A Right to Know, a Right Not to Know, or a Duty to Know?" *American Journal of Medical Genetics* 26 (February 1987): 243–46. Emphasis added.

16. See several studies in the *American Journal of Medical Genetics* 26 (1987), esp. C. Mastromauro, R. H. Myers, and B. Berkman, "Attitudes toward Presymptomatic Testing in Huntington's Disease," pp. 271–82.

17. Kimberly A. Quaid et al., "The Decision to Be Tested for Huntington's Disease," *Journal of the American Medical Association* 257 (June 26, 1987): 3362.

18. Sandi Wiggins et al., "The Psychological Consequences of Predictive Testing for Huntington's Disease," *New England Journal of Medicine* 327 (November 12, 1992): 1401–5. For a more cautious perspective, see Nancy S. Wexler, "The Tiresias Complex: Huntington's Disease as a Paradigm of Testing for Late-Onset Disorders," *The FASEB Journal* 6 (July 1992): 2820–25.

19. Perry L. Bartelt and Marjorie A. Bowman, letter to the editor, *Journal of the American Medical Association* 258 (September 25, 1987): 1604.

20. See Robert Veatch, *Case Studies in Medical Ethics* (Cambridge, MA: Harvard University Press, 1977), pp. 137–39.

21. Joan Vogel and Richard Delgado, "To Tell the Truth: Physician's Duty to Disclose Medical Mistakes," *UCLA Law Review* 28 (1980): 55.

22. Ibid., pp. 52–94, esp. p. 61, *n.* 55.

23. See Michael A. Greenberg, "The Consequences of Truth Telling," *Journal of the American Medical Association* 266 (July 3, 1991): 66.

24. Dorothy C. Wertz, "The 19-Nation Survey: Genetics and Ethics Around the World," and John C. Fletcher, "Ethics and Human Genetics: A Cross-Cultural Perspective," in *Ethics and Human Genetics: A Cross-Cultural Perspective,* ed. Wertz and Fletcher (New York: Springer-Verlag, 1989), pp. 13–17.

25. See Fletcher, "Ethics and Human Genetics: A Cross-Cultural Perspective," p. 482.

26. See Jonathan Alter with Peter McKillop, "AIDS and the Right to Know: A Question of Privacy," *Newsweek,* August 18, 1986, pp. 46–47.

27. A useful history of privacy in American law, including original sources, is presented in Richard C. Turkington, George B. Trubow, and Anita L. Allen, eds, *Privacy: Cases and Materials* (Houston: John Marshall Publishing Co., 1992), ch. 1.

28. See James Fitzjames Stephen, *Liberty, Equality and Fraternity* (New York: Henry Holt, 1873); Samuel Warren and Louis Brandeis, "The Right to Privacy," *Harvard Law Review* 4 (1890): 193–220. The latter is reprinted in Ferdinand D. Schoeman, ed. *Philosophical Dimensions of Privacy: An Anthology* (New York: Cambridge University Press, 1984), pp. 75–103. Our analysis of privacy has benefited from an unpublished paper by and from discussion with Michael Duffy.

29. *Pierce v. Society of Sisters,* 268 U.S. 510 (1925); *Meyer v. Nebraska,* 262 U.S. 390 (1923). But see *Parham v. J.R.,* 442 U.S. 584 (1979).

30. For example, see *Wisconsin v. Yoder,* 406 U.S. 205 (1972); *Stanley v. Georgia,* 394 U.S. 557 (1969); *Loving v. Virginia,* 388 U.S. 1 (1967); *Skinner v. Oklahoma,* 316 U.S. 535 (1942).

31. *Griswold v. Connecticut,* 381 U.S. 479 (1965); *Roe v. Wade,* 410 U.S. 113 (1973); a critical intervening case is *Eisenstadt v. Baird,* 405 U.S. 438 (1972), esp. at 453, and a later case giving shape to the doctrine is *Planned Parenthood of Southeastern Pennsylvania v. Casey,* 112 S.Ct. 2791 (1992). See also *Bowers v. Hardwick,* 478 U.S. 186 (1986), which upholds Georgia's right to forbid sodomy in the privacy of the bedroom and limits the protected zone of privacy. Justice William O. Douglas, writing the majority opinion for the Court in *Griswold,* rested his decision on pri-

vacy, but four separate opinions by members of the majority cited different grounds to justify their concurrence in the result.

32. See Alan F. Westin, *Privacy and Freedom* (New York: Athenaeum, 1967), and the critique by Schoeman, "Privacy: Philosophical Dimensions of the Literature," in *Philosophical Dimensions of Privacy,* pp. 3–4.

33. Ruth Gavison, "Privacy and the Limits of Law," *The Yale Law Journal* 89 (January 1980): 428; reprinted in Schoeman, ed., *Philosophical Dimensions of Privacy,* pp. 346–402.

34. Richard Dick and Elaine Steen, eds., *The Computer-Based Patient Record* (Washington, DC: National Academy of Sciences, I.O.M., 1991), pp. 32ff.

35. See Anita Allen, *Uneasy Access: Privacy for Women in a Free Society* (Totowa, NJ: Rowman and Allanheld, 1987): 11–17; and W. A. Parent, "Privacy, Morality, and the Law," *Philosophy and Public Affairs* 12 (Fall 1983): 269–88.

36. Richard Wasserstrom, "Privacy: Some Arguments and Assumptions," *Philosophical Law,* ed. Richard Bronaugh (Westport, CT: Greenwood Press, 1978); reprinted in Schoeman, ed., *Philosophical Dimensions of Privacy.*

37. Charles Fried, "Privacy: A Rational Context," *The Yale Law Journal* 77 (1968): 475–93; reprinted in Schoeman, ed., *Philosophical Dimensions of Privacy,* pp. 203–22.

38. Warren and Brandeis, "The Right to Privacy."

39. Thomson, "The Right to Privacy," *Philosophy and Public Affairs* 4 (Summer 1975): 295–314, reprinted in Schoeman, ed., *Philosophical Dimensions of Privacy,* pp. 272–89; esp. 280–87.

40. James Rachels, "Why Privacy is Important," p. 292, and Bloustein, "Privacy as an Aspect of Human Dignity," both in Schoeman, ed., *Philosophical Dimension of Privacy;* see also Jeffrey Reiman, "Privacy, Intimacy, and Personhood," *Philosophy and Public Affairs* 6 (1976): 26–44, esp. 38f.

41. Fried, "Privacy: A Rational Context."

42. Joel Feinberg, *Harm to Self,* vol. III in *The Moral Limits of the Criminal Law* (New York: Oxford University Press, 1986), ch. 19.

43. See *Whalen v. Roe,* 429 U.S. 589, 599–600 (1977). In *Roe v. Wade,* 410 U.S. 113 (1974), the court held that the right to privacy is "founded in" the Fourteenth Amendment's protection of "personal liberty and restrictions upon state action." These rights were held to be "fundamental" and "implicit in the concept of ordered liberty." Such language has led commentators on the Court's opinions to speak of the "zone of autonomy-privacy" and of "privacy rights protecting autonomy interests." See Louis Henkin, "Privacy and Autonomy," *Columbia Law Review* 74 (1974), esp. 1419–31; and Howard B. Radest, "The Public and the Private," *Ethics* 89 (1979): 280–91.

44. W. A. Parent, "Recent Work on the Concept of Privacy," *American Philosophical Quarterly* 20 (October 1983): 343.

45. H. J. McCloskey, "Privacy and the Right to Privacy," *Philosophy* 55 (January 1980): 36.

46. Bernard Lo, Robert L. Steinbrook, Moly Cooke, et al., "Voluntary Screening for Human Immunodeficiency Virus (HIV) Infection: Weighing the Benefits and Harms," *Annals of Internal Medicine* 110 (May 1989): 730. Our account of risks and benefits relies in part on this account.

47. See Bernard J. Turnock and Chester J. Kelly, "Mandatory Premarital Testing for

Human Immunodeficiency Virus: The Illinois Experience," *Journal of the American Medical Association* 261 (June 16, 1989): 3415–18, and Jack McKillip, "The Effect of Mandatory Premarital HIV Testing on Marriage: The Case of Illinois," *American Journal of Public Health* 18 (May 1991): 650–53.

48. See Kathleen Nolan, "Ethical Issues in Caring for Pregnant Women and Newborns at Risk for Human Immunodeficiency Virus Infection," *Seminars in Perinatology* 13 (February 1989): 55–65. See also Carol Levine and Ronald Bayer, "The Ethics of Screening for Early Intervention in HIV Disease," *American Journal of Public Health* 79 (December 1989): 1661–67, and several essays in Ruth Faden, Gail Geller, and Madison Powers, eds., *AIDS, Women and the Next Generation* (New York: Oxford University Press, 1991).

49. Nolan, "Ethical Issues in Caring for Pregnant Women and Newborns," p. 64. See also LeRoy Walters, "Ethical Issues in HIV Testing During Pregnancy," in *AIDS, Women and the Next Generation,* ch. 4.

50. Lawrence O. Gostin, Paul D. Cleary, Kenneth H. Mayer, et al., "Screening Immigrants and International Travelers for the Human Immunodeficiency Virus," *New England Journal of Medicine* 322 (June 14, 1990): 1745–46, from which several points in this paragraph have been drawn. See also Margaret Sommerville, "The Case Against HIV Antibody Testing of Refugees and Immigrants," *Canadian Medical Association Journal* 141 (November 1, 1989): 869–94.

51. George J. Annas, "Control of Tuberculosis—The Law and the Public's Health," *New England Journal of Medicine* 328 (February 25, 1993): 585–88.

52. Michael D. Iseman, David L. Cohn, and John A. Sbarbaro, "Directly Observed Treatment of Tuberculosis: We Can't Afford Not to Try It," *New England Journal of Medicine* 328 (February 25, 1993): 576–78.

53. George J. Annas, "Control of Tuberculosis."

54. Lawrence O. Gostin, "Controlling the Resurgent Tuberculosis Epidemic," *Journal of the American Medical Association* 269 (January 13, 1993): 255–61; and see United Hospital Fund of New York, *The Tuberculosis Revival: Individual Rights and Societal Obligation in a Time of AIDS: A Special Report* (New York: United Hospital Fund, 1992).

55. However, this obligation is not recognized or is routinely breached in some countries. See Robert E. Lorge, "How Informed Is Patients' Consent to Release of Medical Information to Insurance Companies?" *British Medical Journal* 298 (1989): 1495–96.

56. Mark Siegler, "Confidentiality in Medicine—A Decrepit Concept," *New England Journal of Medicine* 307 (1982): 1518–21.

57. Superior Court of New Jersey, Law Division, Mercer County, Docket No. L88–2550 (April 25, 1991).

58. Barry D. Weiss, "Confidentiality Expectations of Patients, Physicians, and Medical Students," *Journal of the American Medical Association* 247 (1982): 2695–97.

59. *Bratt v. IBM,* 467 N.E.2d 126 (1984).

60. Donald Schmid et al., "Confidentiality in Psychiatry: A Study of the Patient's View," *Hospital and Community Psychiatry* 34 (April 1983): 353–55.

61. Paul S. Appelbaum et al., "Confidentiality: An Empirical Test of the Utilitarian Perspective," *Bulletin of the American Academy of Psychiatry and the Law* 12 (1984): 109–16.

62. See Kenneth Appelbaum and Paul S. Appelbaum, "The HIV Antibody-Positive Patient," in *Confidentiality Versus the Duty to Protect: Foreseeable Harm in the*

Practice of Psychiatry, ed. James C. Beck (Washington, DC: American Psychiatry Press, Inc., 1990), pp. 127–28.

63. For views to the contrary that propose absolute or near-absolute rules, see Michael H. Kottow, "Medical Confidentiality: An Intransigent and Absolute Obligation," *Journal of Medical Ethics* 12 (1986): 117–22; and H. T. Engelhardt, Jr., *The Foundations of Bioethics* (New York: Oxford University Press, 1986), pp. 297–301.

64. See Sissela Bok, *Secrets* (New York: Pantheon Books, 1982), ch. 9.

65. Bernard B. Raginsky, "Hypnotic Recall of Aircrash Cause," *International Journal of Clinical and Experimental Hypnosis* 17 (1969): 1–19.

66. For a discussion of this case, see Grant Gillett, "AIDS and Confidentiality," *Journal of Applied Philosophy* 4 (1987): 15–20, from which this case study has been adapted.

67. Ad Hoc Committee on AIDS Policy, subsequently approved by Board of Trustees, APA, "AIDS Policy: Confidentiality and Disclosure," *American Journal of Psychiatry* 145 (April 1988): 541. See also APA, "Guidelines on Confidentiality," *American Journal of Psychiatry* 144 (November 1987): 1522–26.

68. See Susanne E. Landis, Victor J. Schoenbach, David J. Weber, et al., "Results of a Randomized Trial of Partner Notification in Cases of HIV Infection in North Carolina," *New England Journal of Medicine* 326 (January 9, 1992): 101–106.

69. Council on Ethical and Judicial Affairs, "Ethical Issues Involved in the Growing AIDS Crisis," *Journal of the American Medical Association* 259 (March 4, 1988): 1360–61.

70. See Appelbaum and Appelbaum, "The HIV Antibody-Positive Patient."

71. See Appelbaum and Appelbaum, "The HIV Antibody-Positive Patient," and William J. Winslade, "AIDS and the Duty to Inform Others," in *The Meaning of AIDS,* ed. Juengst, ch. 12.

72. See Gillett, "AIDS and Confidentiality," and Case Studies, "AIDS and a Duty to Protect," *Hastings Center Report* 17 (February 1987): 22–23, with commentaries by Morton Winston and Sheldon H. Landesman.

73. See Ronald Bayer and Kathleen E. Toomey, "HIV Prevention and the Two Faces of Partner Notification," *American Journal of Public Health* 82 (August 1992): 1158–64.

74. Paul Ramsey, *The Patient as Person* (New Haven: Yale University Press, 1970), p. xii. While Ramsey interprets faithfulness along theological lines as covenant fidelity, it is often expressed in philosophy in terms of fidelity or promise-keeping and in law in terms of contracts, trust, or fiduciary relations.

75. For example, Rawls has plausibly contended that "the principle of fidelity" is only a special case of the principle of fairness applied to social practices of promising; see *A Theory of Justice* (Cambridge, MA: The Belknap Press of Harvard University Press, 1971), p. 344. And Charles Fried has grounded the obligation of promise-keeping in respect for autonomy; see *Contract as Promise: A Theory of Contractual Obligation* (Cambridge, MA: Harvard University Press, 1981), p. 16.

76. Council on Ethical and Judicial Affairs of the American Medical Association, *Current Opinions—1992* (Chicago: American Medical Association, 1992), 8.11.

77. This case was prepared by John Fletcher.

78. See George P. Fletcher, *Loyalty: An Essay on the Morality of Relationships* (New York: Oxford University Press, 1993), p. 21.

79. On professional self-effacement, see Edmund Pellegrino, "Altruism, Self-Interest, and Medical Ethics," *Journal of the American Medical Association* 258 (October

9, 1987): 1939–40. We consider some limits on obligatory self-effacement, by contrast to supererogatory self-effacement, in Chapter 8.

80. See Abigail Zuger and Steven Miles, "Physicians, AIDS, and Occupational Risk: Historic Traditions and Ethical Obligations," *Journal of the American Medical Association* 258 (October 9, 1987): 1924–28.

81. Our formulation is indebted to Stephen Toulmin, "Divided Loyalties and Ambiguous Relationships," *Social Science and Medicine* 23 (1986): 784.

82. *In re Sampson,* 317 N.Y.S.2d (1970).

83. *In re A.C.,* 533 A.2d 611 (D.C. App. 1987), vacated and reh'g granted 539 A.2d 203 (1988).

84. *In re A.C.,* 573 A.2d 1235 (D.C. App. 1990).

85. See the recommendations for change in Frank A. Chervenak and Laurence B. McCullough, "Inadequacies with the ACOG and AAP Statements on Managing Ethical Conflict During the Intrapartum Period," *Journal of Clinical Ethics* 2 (1991): 23–24.

86. Angela Roddey Holder, *Medical Malpractice Law,* 2d Ed. (New York: John Wiley and Sons, Inc., 1978), p. 19 [a summary of *Lotspeich v. Chance Vought Aircraft Corporation,* 369 S.W.2d Tex. (1963)].

87. *PACAF Surgeon's Newsletter* 7 (December 1966): 5, as in Veatch, *Case Studies in Medical Ethics,* p. 245 (a selection from the *Hastings Center Report*).

88. See Leonard A. Sagan and Albert Jonsen, "Medical Ethics and Torture," *New England Journal of Medicine* 294 (1976): 1428. See also *Medicine Betrayed: The Participation of Doctors in Human Rights Violations,* Report of a Working Party, British Medical Association (London: Zed Books, 1992).

89. See Curtis Prout and Robert N. Ross, *Care and Punishment: The Dilemmas of Prison Medicine* (Pittsburgh, PA: University of Pittsburgh Press, 1988).

90. Richard J. Bonnie, "The Death Penalty: When Doctors Must Say No," *British Medical Journal* 305 (August 15, 1992): 381–82.

91. Brian McCormick, "Ethics Panel Spells Out Physician Role in Executions," *American Medical News,* December 28, 1992, p. 6.

92. Martin Benjamin and Joy Curtis, "Ethical Autonomy in Nursing," in *Health Care Ethics,* ed. Donald VanDeVeer and Tom Regan (Philadelphia: Temple University Press, 1987), p. 394.

93. See Gerald Winslow, "From Loyalty to Advocacy: A New Metaphor for Nursing," *Hastings Center Report* 14 (June 1984): 32–40.

94. For helpful discussions of these conflicts, see Benjamin and Curtis, "Ethical Autonomy in Nursing," and their *Ethics in Nursing,* 3d Ed. (New York: Oxford University Press, 1992).

95. This case has been adapted from Anne J. Davis and Mila A. Aroskar, *Ethical Dilemmas and Nursing Practice,* 1st Ed. (New York: Appleton-Century-Crofts, 1978), pp. 207–8.

96. See Mila Aroskar, Josephine M. Flaherty, and James M. Smith, "The Nurse and Orders Not to Resuscitate," *Hastings Center Report* 7 (August 1977): 27–28; and R. R. Yarling and B. J. McElmurry, "Rethinking the Nurse's Role in 'Do Not Resuscitate Orders,' " *Advances in Nursing Science* 5 (1983): 1–12.

97. Gregory F. Gramelspacher, Joel D. Howell, and Mark J. Young, "Perceptions of Ethical Problems by Nurses and Doctors," *Archives of Internal Medicine* 146 (March 1986): 577–78.

98. Eugene W. Linfors and Francis A. Neelson, "The Case for Bedside Rounds," *New England Journal of Medicine* 303 (November 20, 1980): 1231.

99. Daniel L. Cohen et al., "Informed Consent Policies Governing Medical Students' Interactions with Patients," *Journal of Medical Education* 62 (October 1987): 789–98.

100. See E. Haavi Morreim, *Balancing Act: The New Medical Ethics of Medicine's New Economics* (Boston: Kluwer Academic Publishers, 1991), which has influenced the following paragraphs.

101. Morreim, *Balancing Act,* p. 37.

102. See Jean M. Mitchell and Elton Scott, "Physician Ownership of Physical Therapy Services: Effects on Charges, Utilization, Profits, and Service Characteristics," *Journal of the American Medical Association* 268 (October 21, 1992): 2055–59; Jean M. Mitchell and Jonathan H. Sunshine, "Consequences of Physicians' Ownership of Health Care Facilities—Joint Ventures in Radiation Therapy," *New England Journal of Medicine* 327 (November 19, 1992): 1497–1501; Alex Swedlow, Gregory Johnson, Neil Smithline, and Arnold Milstein, "Increased Costs and Rate of Use in the California Workers' Compensation System as a Result of Self-Referral by Physicians," *New England Journal of Medicine* 327 (November 19, 1992): 1502–6; Arnold S. Relman, " 'Self-Referral'—What's At Stake?" *New England Journal of Medicine* 327 (November 19, 1992): 1522–24.

103. Marc A. Rodwin, "Physicians' Conflicts of Interest: The Limitations of Disclosure," *New England Journal of Medicine* 321 (November 16, 1989): 1405–8.

104. Council on Ethical and Judicial Affairs, AMA, "Conflicts of Interest: Physician Ownership of Medical Facilities," *Journal of the American Medical Association* 267 (May 6, 1992): 2366–69.

105. See David Blumenthal et al., "University-Industry Research Relationships in Biotechnology: Implications for the University," *Science* 232 (June 13, 1986): 1361–66.

106. See Arnold S. Relman, "Economic Incentives in Clinical Investigation" [editorial], *New England Journal of Medicine* 320 (April 6, 1989): 933–34.

107. See the Nuremberg Code and *The Belmont Report* of the National Commission for the Protection of Human Subjects. See also Alexander M. Capron, "Human Experimentation," in *Medical Ethics,* ed. Robert M. Veatch (Boston: Jones and Bartlett Publishers, 1989), ch. 6; James F. Childress, *Priorities in Biomedical Ethics* (Philadelphia: Westminster Press, 1981), ch. 3; and Robert M. Veatch, *The Patient as Partner: A Theory of Human-Experimentation Ethics* (Bloomington: Indiana University Press, 1987).

108. E. L. Pattullo, "Institutional Review Boards and the Freedom to Take Risks," *New England Journal of Medicine* 307 (October 28, 1982): 1156–59.

109. Disclosed by surgeon William DeVries, as reported in Denise Grady, "Summary of Discussion on Ethical Perspectives," in *After Barney Clark: Reflections on the Utah Artificial Heart Program,* ed. Margery W. Shaw (Austin: University of Texas Press, 1984), p. 49. DeVries and his colleagues at the University of Utah implanted the first artificial heart with the intention that it be permanent in December 1982; the patient, Barney Clark, survived 112 days. Dr. Denton Cooley implanted the first artificial heart in a human being in 1969 (and then again in 1981) as a bridge to cardiac transplantation.

110. See Fried, *Medical Experimentation,* p. 71.

111. See the Danish Obesity Project, "Randomised Trial of Jejunoileal Bypass versus Medical Treatment in Morbid Obesity," *Lancet* (1979): 1255.

112. See the essays in *Journal of Medicine and Philosophy* 11 (November 1986), devoted to "Ethical Issues in the Use of Clinical Controls"; and Bruce Miller, "Experimentation on Human Subjects: The Ethics of Random Clinical Trials," in *Health Care Ethics,* ed. Donald VanDeVeer and Tom Regan (Philadelphia: Temple University Press, 1987).

113. See Robert J. Levine, *Ethics and Regulation of Clinical Research,* 2d Ed. (New Haven, CT: Yale University Press, 1988), pp. 187–89, 203.

114. See Charles Fried, *Medical Experimentation* (New York: American Elsevier, 1974), and the specific proposals by Benjamin Freedman, "Equipoise and the Ethics of Clinical Research," *New England Journal of Medicine* 317 (July 16, 1987): 141–45, and Eugene Passamani, "Clinical Trials—Are They Ethical?," *New England Journal of Medicine* 324 (May 30, 1991): 1590–91.

115. See Michael Ruse, "At What Level of Statistical Certainty Ought a Random Clinical Trial to Be Interrupted?" in *The Use of Human Beings in Research,* ed. S. F. Spicker et al. (Boston: Kluwer Academic Publishers, 1988): 189–222; and Loretta Kopelman, "Consent and Randomized Clinical Trials: Are There Moral or Design Problems?" *Journal of Medicine and Philosophy* 11 (November 1986): 322.

116. The case of Ara-A and the discussion are based on information in the following sources: Richard J. Whitley et al., "Adenine Arabinoside Therapy of Biopsy-Proved Herpes Simplex Encephalitis," *New England Journal of Medicine* 297 (August 11, 1977): 289–94; correspondence, *New England Journal of Medicine* 297 (December 8, 1977): 1288–90; James J. McCartney, "Encephalitis and Ara-A: An Ethical Case Study," *Hastings Center Report* 8 (December 1978): 5–7; R. J. Whitley and C. A. Alford, "Encephalitis and Adenine Arabinoside: An Indictment without Fact," *Hastings Center Report* 9 (August 1979): 4, 44–47.

117. See M. A. Fischl et al., "The Efficacy of Azidothymidine (AZT) in the Treatment of Patients with AIDS-Related Complex: A Double-Blind, Placebo-Controlled Trial," *New England Journal of Medicine* 317 (1987): 185–91; D. D. Richman et al., "The Toxicity of Azidothymidine (AZT) in the Treatment of Patients with AIDS and AIDS-Related Complex: A Double-Blind, Placebo-Controlled Trial," *New England Journal of Medicine* 317 (1987): 192–97.

118. See Weinstein, "Allocation of Subjects in Medical Experiments," p. 1280.

119. See the discussion below, and also Cancer Research Campaign Working Party in Breast Conservation, "Informed Consent: Ethical, Legal, and Medical Implications for Doctors and Patients Who Participate in Randomised Clinical Trials," *British Medical Journal* 286 (April 2, 1983): 1117–21; and C. R. Brewin and C. Bradly, "Patient Preferences and Randomised Clinical Trials," *British Medical Journal* 299 (July 29, 1989): 313–15.

120. C. Redmond and M. Bauer, "Statisticians' Report on Prerandomization," *NSABP Progress Report* (Pittsburgh, PA: National Surgical Adjuvant Project for Breast and Bowel Cancers, 1979), as quoted in Kenneth F. Schaffner, "Ethical Problems in Clinical Trials," *Journal of Medicine and Philosophy* 11 (November 1986): 306.

121. Kathryn M. Taylor, Richard Margolese, and Colin L. Soskolne, "Physicians' Reasons for Not Entering Eligible Patients in a Randomized Clinical Trial of Surgery for Breast Cancer," *New England Journal of Medicine* 310 (May 4, 1984): 1363.

122. Bernard Fischer et al., "Five-Year Results of a Randomized Clinical Trial Comparing Total Mastectomy and Segmental Mastectomy with or without Radiation in the Treatment of Breast Cancer," *New England Journal of Medicine* 312 (1985): 665–73.

123. See Don Marquis, "An Argument that All Prerandomized Clinical Trials Are Unethical," *Journal of Medicine and Philosophy* 11 (November 1986): 380.

124. Marcia Angell, "Patient Preferences in Randomized Clinical Trials," *New England Journal of Medicine* 310 (May 24, 1984): 1385–87.

125. See Susan S. Ellenberg, "Randomization Designs in Comparative Clinical Trials," *New England Journal of Medicine* 310 (May 24, 1984): 1404–08; Marquis, "Prerandomized Clinical Trials Are Unethical," p. 377. Contrast Kopelman, "Consent and Randomized Clinical Trials," pp. 334–36.

126. See Marvin Zelen, "A New Design for Randomized Trials," *New England Journal of Medicine* 300 (May 31, 1979): 1243–45.

127. This was Freedman's proposal in "Equipoise and the Ethics of Clinical Research."

128. There are experiments in which a subject appropriately must agree not to withdraw after a certain time. For example, in a bone marrow transplant experiment, total-body irradiation is used to prepare the recipient to receive the bone marrow. At that point the recipient would die if the subject-donor were permitted to withdraw.

129. See Fried, *Medical Experimentation,* pp. 160–61.

130. For a demanding but problematic critique, see Samuel Hellman and Deborah S. Hellman, "Of Mice but Not Men—Problems of the Randomized Clinical Trial," *New England Journal of Medicine* 324 (May 30, 1991): 1585–89.

131. See the proposal for a "semi-randomized clinical trial" in Robert Veatch, *The Patient as Partner,* ch. 9.

132. See Schaffner, "Ethical Problems in Clinical Trials." Joseph B. Kadane has proposed a substitute version of adaptive designs in "Progress Towards a More Ethical Method for Clinical Trials," *Journal of Medicine and Philosophy* 11 (November 1986): 385–404.

8

Virtues and Ideals in Professional Life

Throughout this book we have concentrated primarily on the analysis and justification of acts and policies, using the language of ethical principles, rules, obligations, and rights. In this final chapter we examine other aspects of morality, especially virtues and moral ideals. These categories complement our earlier analyses of principles and continue the discussion of character and virtue commenced in Chapter 2. As we have seen in several chapters, principles do not provide precise or specific guidelines for every conceivable set of circumstances. Principles require judgment, which in turn depends on character, moral discernment, and a person's sense of responsibility and accountability.

Often what counts most in the moral life is not consistent adherence to principles and rules, but reliable character, moral good sense, and emotional responsiveness. Principles and rules cannot fully encompass what occurs when parents lovingly play with and nurture their children, or when physicians and nurses provide palliative care for a dying patient and comfort to the patient's distressed spouse. Our feelings and concerns for others lead us to actions that cannot be reduced to the following of principles and rules, and we all recognize that morality would be a cold and uninspiring practice without various traits of character, emotional responses, and ideals that reach beyond principles and rules.

Virtues in Professional Roles

Character is comprised of a set of stable traits that affect a person's judgment and action. Although we have different character traits, all normal persons have the capacity to cultivate the traits that are centrally important in morality. Each such trait incorporates a complex structure of beliefs, motives, and emotions. In professional life, the character traits that deserve to be encouraged and admired often derive from role responsibilities. Accordingly, we begin with an analysis of virtues in institutional roles and practices.

Virtues in Roles and Practices

Professional roles are often tied to institutional expectations and professional practices. These roles incorporate virtues as well as obligations. Roles internalize conventions, customs, and procedures of teaching, nursing, doctoring, and the like. Each organized body of professional practices has a history that sustains a tradition and requires professionals to cultivate certain virtues. These standards of virtue incorporate criteria of professional merit and distinction, and possession of these virtues disposes a person to act in accordance with the objectives of the practices.[1]

Roles and practices in medicine and nursing embody *social* expectations as well as standards and ideals internal to these professions, but the traditional virtues of the health professional derive largely from health care relationships.[2] Virtues in practice are habituated character traits that dispose persons to act in accordance with the worthy goals and role expectations of health care institutions. The particular virtues we analyze below are compassion, discernment, trustworthiness, and integrity. Other key virtues—such as respectfulness, nonmalevolence, benevolence, justice, truthfulness, and faithfulness—appeared in previous chapters in discussions of corresponding principles and rules, and they will be minimally treated here. We cannot attend to the whole range of virtues that are important—even indispensable—for morality and professional practice, but they would include classical virtues such as courage and temperance (self-control).

Virtues in practices should be distinguished from role-related technical skills. To exhibit the difference between moral standards of character and standards that define technical skills, we begin with an instructive study of surgical error. Charles L. Bosk's *Forgive and Remember: Managing Medical Failure* provides an ethnographic study of the way two different surgical services in "Pacific Hospital" handle medical failure, especially failures by surgical residents.[3] Bosk found that these surgical services distinguish, at least implicitly, between several different forms of error or mistake. The first is *technical:* The professional discharges role responsibilities conscientiously, but his or her technical training or information falls short of what the task requires. Every surgeon can be expected to make this sort of mistake occasionally. The second sort of error is *judgmental:* A conscientious professional develops and follows an incorrect strategy. These errors are also to be expected. Attending surgeons forgive momentary technical and judgmental errors but remember them in case a pattern develops indicating that a person lacks the technical and judgmental skills to be a competent surgeon.

The third sort of error is *normative:* This error violates standards of conduct, particularly by failing to discharge moral obligations conscientiously. At this point a moral judgment about the person enters. Bosk contends that technical and judgmental errors are subordinated in importance to these moral errors, because every conscientious person can be expected to make "honest errors" or "good faith errors." However, moral errors are especially serious because a pattern indicates a defect of moral character.

Bosk's study and related examples in medicine, nursing, and research help us appreciate how persons of high moral character acquire a reservoir of good will in assessments of the praiseworthiness or blameworthiness of their actions. If a conscientious surgeon and another surgeon who is defective in conscientiousness make the same technical or judgmental error, the conscientious surgeon is not likely to be subjected to moral blame in the same way as the other surgeon.

The Virtues in Alternative Professional Models

In previous eras professional virtues were often integrated with professional obligations and ideals in codes of health care. Insisting that the medical profession's "prime objective" is to render service to humanity, an American Medical Association (AMA) code in effect from 1957 to 1980 urged the physician to be "upright" and "pure in character and . . . diligent and conscientious in caring for the sick." It also endorsed the virtues that Hippocrates commended: modesty, sobriety, patience, promptness, and piety. However, in contrast to its first code in 1847, the AMA over the years has deemphasized virtues in its codes. The references that remained in the 1957 version were perfunctory and marginal, and the 1980 version eliminated all traces of the virtues except for the admonition to "expose those physicians deficient in character or competence."

Different models of the role of health care professionals suggest different primary virtues. For example, if medicine is conceived in paternalistic terms, the physician's virtues will differ from those drawn from a conception of medicine as a contract. In a paternalistic model, virtues of benevolence, care, and compassion are dominant. In other models, especially an autonomy model, virtues of respectfulness for autonomy, privacy, and the like are more prominent. In one paternalistic conception of the physician's role, *arrogance* is seen as a virtue, and as preferable to the virtue of humility.[4]

A classic example of an attempt to establish the proper set of virtues in medicine is found in Thomas Percival, who wrote the most influential treatise on medical ethics in the last two centuries—a work that formed the substantive basis of the first AMA code. Percival assumed that the patient's best medical interest is the proper goal of medicine, and on this basis reached conclusions about the physician's proper traits of character. Recognizing the dependence of patients, he counseled physicians that professional authority should direct medicine's understanding of its virtues, which, for Percival, are invariably tied to responsibility for the patient's medical welfare. For example, Percival attempted to balance truthfulness and benevolence in a defense of benevolent deception:

> To a patient, therefore, perhaps the father of a numerous family, or one whose life is of the highest importance to the community, who makes inquiries which, if faithfully answered, might prove fatal to him, it would be a gross and unfeeling wrong to reveal the truth. His right to it is suspended, and even annihilated; because, its beneficial nature being reversed, it would be deeply injurious to himself, to his family, and to the public. And he has the strongest claim, from the trust reposed in his physician, as well as from the common principles of humanity, to be guarded against whatever would be detrimental to him. The only point at issue is, whether the practitioner shall sacrifice that delicate sense of veracity, which is so ornamental to, and indeed forms a characteristic excellence of the virtuous man, to this claim of professional justice and social duty.[5]

Virtues of nurses similarly reflect different models of the nursing profession and its role-responsibilities. In the traditional model, the nurse, as "handmaiden" of the physician, is counseled to cultivate the passive virtues of obedience and submission. In contemporary models, active virtues are more prominent. For example, if the nurse's role is viewed as advocacy for patients, prominent virtues will include respect for autonomy, justice, persistence, and courage.[6] Obedience to rules is demanded in the traditional model, but constant attention to patients' rights and preservation of the nurse's integrity are emphasized in contemporary autonomy models, especially those that call on the nurse to be the patient's advocate. Even if the same virtue—conscientiousness, for example—is accepted in competing models, its content may be specified differently.

Controversies also arise regarding the conditions under which certain virtues eventuate in unworthy and condemnable actions. Everyone would agree that virtues such as loyalty, courage, kindness, and benevolence at times lead persons to act inappropriately and unacceptably. As we saw in Chapter 7, the physician who acts kindly and loyally by not reporting the incompetence of a fellow physician acts improperly. These human failures do not suggest that loyalty and kindness are not virtues, but only that virtuous acts require appropriate judgment. The virtues need to be accompanied by an understanding of what is right, good, and deserving of our kindness, generosity, and the like. Aristotle attempted to avoid this problem by suggesting that right action arising from moral virtue requires practical wisdom (phronesis)—an intellectual virtue that unifies judgment and moral disposition. The moral virtues direct us to the right ends, and practical wisdom directs us to the right means to those ends.

Caution is particularly warranted with regard to virtues such as loyalty, courage, respectfulness, fondness, tenderness, generosity, and patriotism, because these human traits can easily be misdirected by zealousness, obedience, commitment, devotion, and the like—again pointing to the importance of sound judgment and moral perspective. We should also resist the view that a person who acts wrongly but from virtue is excusable. Loyalty, patriotism, and even generosity and kindness can eventuate in fiendish and thoroughly inexcusable acts.

Four Focal Virtues

One or two virtuous traits do not amount to a virtuous person. A virtuous person has a virtuous *character*. However, some virtues are more pivotal than others in characterizing a virtuous person. We cannot now assess each of the many other virtues that are important to the virtuous professional, but we can isolate and analyze a few central virtues, with an emphasis on compassion, discernment, trustworthiness, and integrity. They may not be the cardinal virtues (an idea that has never been made very clear in moral writings), but they are widely acknowledged in biomedical ethics and they help us focus on the character of health professionals.

Compassion

The virtue of compassion is a trait combining an attitude of active regard for another's welfare with an imaginative awareness and emotional response of deep sympathy, tenderness, and discomfort at the other person's (or animal's) misfortune or suffering.[7] Both "fellow-feeling" and "sympathy" were once widely used terms in ethical theory to refer to the importance of compassion in the moral life. Compassion presupposes sympathy, has affinities with mercy, and is expressed in acts of beneficence that attempt to alleviate the misfortune or suffering of the other person. Unlike integrity, which is inwardly focused on the self, compassion is outwardly focused on other selves. The trait of compassion therefore resembles the moral sentiment of care, as discussed in Chapter 2, and reflects benevolence, as sketched in Chapter 5.

Compassion need not be restricted to others' pain, suffering, disability, and misery, but in health care these conditions are the typical sources of compassionate responses. Using the language of sympathy, eighteenth-century philosopher David Hume pointed to a typical circumstance of feeling compassion in health care, together with a psychological explanation of how it arises:

> Were I present at any of the more terrible operations of surgery, 'tis certain, that even before it begun, the preparation of the instruments, the laying of the bandages in order, the heating of the irons, with all the signs of anxiety and concern in the patient and assistants, wou'd have a great effect upon my mind, and excite the strongest sentiments of pity and terror. No passion of another discovers itself immediately to the mind. We are only sensible of its causes or effects. From *these* we infer the passion: And consequently *these* give rise to our sympathy.[8]

In many contexts, within and without health care, the expression of compassion makes a critical moral difference. People feel reassured and cared for by a person of compassion. The emotional tone displayed in the interaction is part of the assistance rendered. The physician or nurse lacking altogether in the appropriate display of compassion is morally defective, although he or she may also display other important moral qualities, including integrity, trustworthiness, and discernment. Physicians and nurses who express no emotion in their behavior, but only professional skill, often fail to provide what patients most need even if they feel compassion for patients. Emotional engagement and communication are important parts of human relationships in general and health care in particular.

However, compassion may also cloud judgment and preclude rational and effective responses. For example, in one reported case, a long-alienated son wanted to continue indefinitely a futile and apparently painful treatment in an ICU for his near-comatose father in order to have time to "make his peace" with his father. Although the son understood that his alienated father had no cognitive capacity, the son wanted to work through his sense of regret. Some hospital staff argued that the patient's grim prognosis and pain, combined with the needs of others waiting to receive care in the ICU, justified stopping the treatment (as had been requested by the patient's close cousin and informal guardian). But another group in the unit viewed this case almost entirely as an appropriate act of compassion toward the son, who they thought should have time to express his farewells and regrets in order to make himself feel better about his father's death. The first group viewed such compassion as misplaced because of the patient's prolonged agony and dying. In effect, they thought compassion prevented clear-headed thinking about primary obligations to the patient.[9]

Many writers in ethical theory, most notably Spinoza and Kant, have maintained that a passionate (even a compassionate) engagement with others frequently blinds reason and renders partial what should be impartial reflection. Health care professionals understand and appreciate this phenomenon. Constant contact with suffering can overwhelm and sometimes paralyze a compassionate physician or nurse. Impartial judgment gives way to impassioned decision; emotion distorts prudence, and emotional burnout sometimes occurs. For these reasons, in part, medical and nursing education is designed to inculcate detachment as well as compassion. The language of *detached concern* and *compassionate detachment* occasionally appears in health care ethics expressly to identify a characteristic of the good physician or good nurse.

Still, the fact that compassion and emotional involvement are sometimes misplaced and excessive should serve only as a warning, not as grounds for emotional withdrawal. Emotional responses are not necessarily irrational or impulsive. They are often controlled and voluntary. When compassion appropriately motivates and expresses good character, it has a role in ethics alongside impartial reason and dispassionate judgment.

Discernment

The virtue of discernment rests on sensitive insight involving acute judgment and understanding, and it eventuates in decisive action. Discernment includes the ability to make judgments and reach decisions without being unduly influenced by extraneous considerations, fears, or personal attachments. Resistance to these influences when making controversial decisions brings the virtue of discernment into contact with the virtue of courage.

Discernment has been closely associated in some analyses with practical wisdom *(phronesis,* or classical *prudence)*. A person of practical wisdom knows which ends should be chosen and knows how to realize them in particular circumstances, while keeping emotions within proper bounds and carefully selecting from among the range of possible actions. In Aristotle's model, the practically wise person understands how to act with the right intensity of feeling, in just the right way, at just the right time, with a right balance of reason and desire.[10]

More generally, the person of discernment is disposed to identify what a circumstance calls for in the way of human responsiveness. For example, a discerning physician will see when a despairing patient needs comfort rather than privacy, and vice versa. If comfort is the right choice, the discerning physician will find the right type and level of consolation in order to be helpful rather than intrusive. If a rule guides the behavior, seeing *how* to follow the rule involves a form of discernment that is independent of seeing *that* the rule applies. Sizing up a situation and fitting the rule to it flow from a person's character, commitments, and sensitivity. Such discernment is usually a necessary condition of a good decision.

Different forms of discernment, as well as different virtues, are needed to address the variety of patients in health care. Vulnerable and dependent patients need forms of sensitivity that other patients, do not need. For example, in dealing with depressed and suicidal patients, psychiatrists need special forms of discernment that cannot reasonably be expected of those lacking such specialized training and experience. Some writers in biomedical ethics maintain that persons of discernment (when they are also conscientious, compassionate, etc.) afford greater protection against moral wrongdoing in medicine than do frameworks of rules and regulations.[11]

A more balanced perspective, we suggest, is that the virtue of discernment involves understanding both *that* and *how* principles and rules are relevant in a variety of circumstances. Principles and virtues are similar in this respect. They require attention and sensitivity attuned to the demands of a particular context. Respect for autonomy and beneficence will be as different in different contexts as compassion and discernment, and the ways in which health professionals manifest these principles and virtues in the care of patients will be as different as the ways in which devoted parents care for their children. Understanding that one's action should be in conformity with a balance of moral principles itself exhibits a complex form of discernment. In addition to understanding that a principle rightly applies, discernment appears in understanding how to employ a principle. Furthermore, there are considerations of how to manifest virtues in caring for patients. It would be mistaken to try to reduce discernment to the following of norms, but it would be no less mistaken to suppose that discernment has nothing to do with following general guidelines. Discernment is often manifest through a creative response in meeting responsibilities.

The ability to understand what needs to be done for patients, understanding how to do it, and then acting with sensitive and caring responses are moral qualities of character, not merely forms of practical intelligence and judgment. Forms of caring sometimes themselves open up discerning insights into what is at stake, what counts the most, and what needs to be done.

Trustworthiness

Another prominent virtue in health care is trustworthiness. Trust is a confident belief in and reliance upon the ability and moral character of another person. Trust entails a confidence that another will act with the right motives in accord with moral norms.[12] Such trust is often the most important ingredient in our choice of one physician rather than another, and a physician's perceived lack of trustworthiness may be the primary reason for a patient's decision to switch to another physician.

Our most celebrated ethical theories have typically not exalted trustworthiness. However, Aristotle took note of one aspect of trust and trustworthiness. He argued that when relationships are voluntary and among intimates, by contrast to legal relationships among strangers, it is appropriate for the law to forbid lawsuits for harms that occur. Aristotle reasoned that in intimate relationships "dealings with one another as good and trustworthy" rather than "bonds of justice" hold persons together. The former bond he regarded as strictly a matter of character.[13]

It is hard to fault this assessment. At the same time, it is a fading ideal in contemporary health care institutions, especially the part about lawsuits. For centuries health care professionals managed to keep trust at center stage, even when they had far less scientific understanding to offer patients than today's professionals. But recently the centrality of trust has declined, as is evidenced by the dramatic rise in medical malpractice suits and adversarial relations between health care professionals and the public. Talk has increased of the need for ombudsmen, patient advocates, advance "directives," and the like.

Among the contributing causes of the erosion of trust are the loss of intimate contact between physicians and patients, the increased use of specialists, high charges for health care, conflicts of interest in referrals and investments in clinical centers, and the growth of large, impersonal, and bureaucratic medical institutions. These factors have undermined interactions that over time would foster knowledge of the professional's or the patient's character and would provide an adequate basis for trust. Physicians now wonder whether they can trust many of their patients, especially if an injury occurs and litigation looms as a possibility. As a consequence, many physicians and patients welcome mutually agreed-upon rules and require signed documentation of mutual decisions; and many physicians practice defensive medicine.

In a close doctor–patient relationship, virtues and character are likely to be all-important, whereas rules, especially institutional or governmental rules, are likely to be seen as unhelpful and intrusive. However, when strangers interact in health care, character will generally play a less significant role than principles and rules that are backed by sanctions.[14]

Integrity

Some writers claim that the first or primary virtue is integrity, because it plays such a central role in health care ethics.[15] We justify many of our actions on grounds that we would sacrifice our integrity if we acted otherwise. Health care professionals sometimes refuse to comply with the requests of patients or with the decisions of their colleagues on grounds that beliefs very close to their sense of themselves would be compromised in unacceptable ways. Such problems arise from an individual's perception that what another party asks would require a sacrifice of the individual's core beliefs. Later we will analyze these appeals to integrity as they appear in appeals to conscience; now we will analyze the virtue of integrity.

Problems in the maintenance of integrity sometimes arise not from *moral* conflict, but from demands that persons abandon some of their *personal* goals and projects. Such persons feel violated by having to abandon the projects and commitments that they care most deeply about in order to realize goals set by others. This loss of integrity is not a loss of *moral* integrity if the projects and commitments are not governed by moral norms; it is rather a loss of *personal* integrity. However, conflicts produced by personal projects are significant for ethical theory.[16] Sometimes very demanding moral principles, such as the principle of utility, constrain our personal undertakings, because the welfare of other persons constantly makes a moral claim on how we live our lives. Morality, so conceived, may deprive us of the liberty to structure and integrate our lives as we see fit. If one has structured one's life around personal goals, forms of relationship, and educational strategies that are ripped away by the agendas of others, a loss of personal integrity occurs just as certainly as if one's moral fiber were ripped away by others' coercive actions. One can feel alienated from one's sense of self and one's deepest attachments—those values with which one is most intimately identified. Here personal integrity is threatened by wrenching moral demands.

The *value* of moral integrity is beyond serious dispute, but what we *mean* by the term is not entirely clear. In its most general sense, *moral integrity* means soundness, reliability, wholeness, and integration of moral character. In a more restricted sense, and the one we will primarily use, *moral integrity* means fidelity in adherence to moral norms. Accordingly, the virtue of integrity represents two aspects of a person's character. The first is a coherent integration of aspects of the self—emotions, aspirations, knowledge, etc.—so that each complements and does not frustrate the others. The second is the character trait of being faithful to moral values and standing up in their defense when they are threatened or under attack. This second sense of integrity cannot be reduced to merely personal commitments and projects, because it would then not be a *moral* virtue. A person of integrity in the first sense is not necessarily morally admirable or virtuous. Indeed integrity in the first sense is compatible with being morally evil, whereas integrity in the second sense is not.

However, moral integrity is compatible with a wide range of moral convictions. Our argument is that moral integrity in science, medicine, and health care should be understood primarily in terms of the principles, rules, and virtues that we have identified in the common morality. These represent what should be core convictions in biomedical ethics, although they are indeterminate and require specification and balancing. Of course, ours is not the only substantive moral framework for integrity in biomedical ethics, and we cannot wave away all other approaches. However, we have provided arguments for this framework.

Persons can lack moral integrity in several respects. Most lists of deficiencies in moral integrity include hypocrisy, insincerity, bad faith, and self-deception, among other vices. These vices all represent some break in the connections among a person's moral convictions, actions, and emotions. Perhaps the most obvious deficiency is the lack of core moral convictions. However, vices such as self-deception and hypocrisy incorporate false claims about the presence or function of those convictions. Critically important for our purposes in this chapter is the failure to act on fundamental moral beliefs that are held and professed, a failure that compromises integrity. In many disputes about integrity, it may be unclear whether persons' actions against their professed moral principles indicate that they never had integrity or that they have lost their integrity.

Disputes about the ascription of integrity may also center on whether a particular action represents a breach of a person's fundamental moral convictions. C. Everett Koop, a pioneering pediatric surgeon who was appointed U.S. Surgeon General by President Ronald Reagan, provides an interesting example. Conservatives praised his appointment as Surgeon General because they were impressed by his strong religious and moral convictions about the sanctity of human life. By contrast, liberals, who generally conceded that Koop is a person of integrity, sharply criticized his appointment because they viewed his integrity as too narrowly focused on conservative moral positions such as the sanctity of human life. As an opponent of both abortion and euthanasia, Koop was instrumental in the Reagan administration's formulation of the Baby Doe rules to prevent withholding or withdrawing life-sustaining treatment from handicapped newborns. He also played an increasingly active role in opposing smoking on health grounds and in combating the emerging AIDS epidemic as a medical and public health problem. Even though he strongly disapproved of many behavioral patterns that led to HIV transmission, he was committed to saving human lives and reducing human suffering. This compassion, combined with the best available scientific evidence, led him to promote the use of condoms, while still giving priority to abstinence and monogamous relations.

Suddenly, he later noted, "I found myself praised by my former liberal adversaries and condemned by my former conservative allies." Both groups insisted that Koop had abandoned his previous moral core. His former adversaries praised the change as evidence of moral development, while his former allies condemned the change as an unacceptable moral and political compromise reflecting a loss of integrity. However, Koop's own interpretation is plausible. Rather than compromising his moral core, his dominant "pro-life" commitment led him to do what was necessary to save human lives under a broad range of circumstances, including the AIDS epidemic. Because of his religious and moral convictions, he insisted, "my course was clear: to do all I could to halt the spread of AIDS by educating the American people, accurately and completely." He advised people to use condoms if they could not or would not follow what he considered the safer and morally preferable alternatives of abstinence and monogamy. Thus, he supported very explicit public-school sex education, even at an early age, "because if kids are sexually active in the age of AIDS, they could die." On a plausible interpretation, Koop maintained his moral integrity because he sought to do the best he could to protect human life in every circumstance. He was faithful to his fundamental moral conviction about the sanctity of human life, and that conviction required different actions in different circumstances.[17]

This case points to another dimension of integrity that is often neglected in ethical theory: Integrity is a matter of coherent, personal integration over time, not merely a present integration. Both integrity and, more generally, character are evaluated in terms of a person's sustained moral effort and accomplishment. Some philosophers have attempted to explicate integrity almost exclusively in terms of a person's life story, narrative unity, life as a whole, or life as a quest.[18] This approach is, by itself, too narrow, because it cannot account for the impersonal and social dimensions of integrity as a moral virtue.[19] However, integrity cannot be adequately understood without attending to a person's actions and character in the context of the person's history of commitments, stability and coherence of values, and sense of personal accountability.

Moral integrity, then, is the character trait of a coherent integration of reasonably stable, justifiable moral values, together with active fidelity to those values in judgment and action. A person of moral integrity will meet what morality demands but may also accept higher standards than the moral minimum (what we discuss below as moral ideals). The exemplary person of moral integrity is not disordered or disoriented by moral conflict and is faithful to the standards of the common morality as well as to personal moral ideals. This virtue of integrity can only be approximated, but it is still both worthy and practicable.

This analysis of integrity has the additional benefit of further integrating an ethics of character and an ethics of principles and rules. A vital aspect of moral integrity is faithfulness to basic norms of obligation, and the person who violates those norms is likely to be disqualified as a person of moral integrity. Although consistent fidelity to norms does not necessarily produce integrity,[20] conscientious and consistent attentiveness to *impersonal* action-guides should play a role in any account of moral integrity. Conscientiousness is often appropriately understood in terms of strictness in following principles or rules in the face of temptations to set them aside. However, individual conscience and *personal* commitments also have a clear role in an account of integrity.

For example, some medical practitioners with religious commitments to the sanctity of life find it morally difficult to participate in decisions not to do everything possible to prolong life. To them, participating in removing ventilators and IV fluids from patients, even with an advance directive, would violate their integrity. To do less than what the health care system can do to extend life violates their integrity, even though others do not share their commitments. Their integrity is attacked if a superior determines that a procedure is futile and then demands that subordinates agree that the procedure is futile, when in fact they believe the procedure is warranted and perhaps even morally obligatory. If a health professional is under the dictate of an authority who commands rather than consults and rules rather than negotiates, problems of integrity are inevitable in moral conflicts. Such conflicts are not rare in health care institutions and can erupt at almost any time at any level—for example, where deep differences exist among health care professionals regarding patients' rights. Highly authoritarian settings, then, can impair or destroy integrity.[21]

The undisputed fact that persons have different evaluative commitments creates morally difficult situations in which one party must either compromise on commitments or resign. Yet compromise seems, by definition, to be what a person of integrity cannot do. At least the person cannot sacrifice his or her deep moral commitments. Does this mean that behavior involving compromise is inconsistent with the maintenance of integrity? Will it turn out on close inspection that moral integrity is little more than a dogmatic insistence that one's cherished values are higher than others' values?[22]

Staff disagreements in modern health care facilities cannot always be overcome even by reasonable and conscientious persons. Integrity is sometimes unavoidably compromised in conflict situations. This problem cannot be eradicated, but it can be ameliorated by persons with the virtues of patience, humility, and tolerance. Situations that compromise integrity can usually be avoided if participants recognize the indeterminateness and fallibility of their own moral views and respect others' perspectives and if a consultative institutional process, such as a hospital ethics committee, is available. A moral climate of mutual respect together with channels of reasoned recourse in institutions usually prevent people from feeling that their integrity has been compromised. In the absence of this climate and these channels, threats to integrity can become serious.

However, it would be morally bad advice to conclude that the person of integrity should always negotiate and compromise in a circumstance of institutional confrontation. There is something ennobling and admirable about the person who refuses to compromise beyond a certain moral threshold, another reason why integrity has a legitimate claim to being a primary or first virtue. To compromise below the threshold of integrity is simply to lose it.

Conscientiousness

We can now develop these themes about integrity and compromise with regard to conscientious refusal, withdrawal, and disassociation from the wrongdoing of others. In examining Bosk's study of "Pacific Hospital," we noted that we often evaluate ourselves and others in terms of conscientiousness, a virtue needed both to establish trustworthiness and to maintain moral integrity. Roughly speaking, an individual acts conscientiously if he or she has tried with due diligence to determine what is right, intends to do what is right, exerts an appropriate level of effort, and is motivated to do what is right because it is right. Like other virtues, conscientiousness is significant for both ordinary morality and moral ideals.

The virtue of conscientiousness is sometimes said to be particularly congenial to Kantian theories, but it is also recognized in utilitarian theories. A utilitarian views conscientiousness as a settled and serious commitment to follow the principle of utility. In almost all ethical theories, conscientiousness is at work in carefully interpreting moral situations, specifying the norms relevant to the situation, determining whether one norm outweighs or overrules another when they conflict, seeking alternatives to infringing norms, and minimizing any infringement.

The Nature of Conscience

The analysis to this point may seem to have neglected what many people have in mind when they view conscience as a faculty of or authority for moral decisionmaking. Slogans such as "Let your conscience be your guide" and "Just follow your conscience" suggest that conscience is the final authority in moral justification. However, such an account fails to capture the nature of conscience and conscientiousness. We can see why by examining the following case: Having recently completed his Ph.D. in chemistry, George has not been able to find a job. His family has suffered from his failure: They are short of money, his wife has had to take additional work, and their small children have been subjected to considerable strain, uncertainty, and instability. An established chemist can get George a position in a laboratory that pursues research in chemical and biological warfare. Despite his perilous financial and familial circumstances, George feels that he cannot accept this position because of his conscientious opposition to chemical and biological warfare. The older chemist notes that although he is not enthusiastic about this project, the research will continue no matter what George decides. Furthermore, if George does not take this position, it will be offered to another young man who would probably pursue the research with great vigor. Indeed, the older chemist confides, his concern about this other candidate's nationalistic fervor and uncritical zeal for research in chemical and biological warfare in part led him to recommend George for the job. George's wife is puzzled and hurt by George's reaction, since she sees nothing wrong with the research. She is mainly concerned about the instability of their family and their children's problems.[23] Nonetheless, George forgoes

this opportunity to help his family and prevent a destructive fanatic from obtaining the position, because his conscience stands in the way.

Conscience in this example is not a special moral or psychological faculty.
Rather, it is a form of self-reflection on and judgment about whether one's acts
are obligatory or prohibited, right or wrong, good or bad. It is an internal
sanction calling attention to the actual or potential loss of a sense of integrity
and wholeness in the self. This sanction comes into play in critical reflection
and judgment on acts. This sanction often appears as a bad conscience—in the
form of painful feelings of remorse, guilt, shame, disunity, or disharmony—as
the individual recognizes his or her acts as wrong. The experience of a bad
conscience does not, however, signify bad moral character. In truth, this experience is likely to occur in its most admirable forms in persons of cultivated
moral character. Only people who affirm moral standards and strive to live up
to them will be troubled by their failures to do so. Only they will experience a
bad conscience and the need to maintain moral self-esteem.[24] A good conscience, by contrast, is associated with *integrity, psychological wholeness,* and
peacefulness and is often described using the adjectives *quiet, clear,* and
easy.[25]

A violation of conscience can result in unpleasant feelings of guilt or shame,
as well as a loss of integrity, peacefulness, and harmony. Conscientious agents
who feel these consequences acutely sometimes make predictive appeals in dramatic language: "I couldn't live with myself if I did that." "I would hate
myself." "I could not look at myself in the mirror." As kidney donors have
been known to say, "I had to do it. I couldn't have backed out, not that I had
the feeling of being trapped, because the doctors offered to get me out. I just
had to do it."[26] Such poignant statements indicate that for the individuals in
question some ethical standards are sufficiently fundamental and powerful that
violating them would diminish their integrity and result in guilt or shame.[27]
Individuals who make such statements also believe that they will not be able to
forget their deed or shift responsibility for it to others. Such claims appear to
be at work in the case of George.

Conscience is personal because it involves an individual's awareness of and
reflection on his or her acts in relation to his or her own standards. Agents may
or may not apply those standards to the conduct of others. They may hold only
themselves (or only persons with the same commitments) to such standards.
Even if they view their standards as applicable to everyone, it would be odd
and even absurd to say, "My conscience indicates that you should not do
that." We may say that someone else ought not to engage in some conduct;
but we cannot justify this admonition by saying, "I would have a guilty conscience if he did that."

When people claim that their actions are conscientious, they sometimes feel
compelled by conscience to resist demands made by others. They may claim

that if they were to perform the act in question—for example, providing an illegal drug to a patient or torturing a prisoner—they would violate their conscience and compromise their integrity. In one case, a nurse changed her mind about assisting with abortions and "refused in conscience" to assist, although she had no problem giving care to and supporting patients who came to the unit for abortions. She was aware that her own sense of moral conflict deepened the experience of moral conflict within the nursing staff, but, even though she wanted to avoid this conflict, her conscience and sense of integrity were unyielding.

In particularly troublesome cases, agents act out of character in order to perform what they judge to be the morally most appropriate action. For example, a normally cooperative and cheerful person may angrily protest another's decision. Such behavior sometimes produces a personal conflict, because the person's character and the expectations of others dispose the person one way, whereas the person's moral judgment in this situation suggests a different course. But a conscientious and discerning person will not attempt to justify actions merely because they are in character or because other persons expect them to act characteristically. In cases involving serious wrongdoing, the conscientious agent will resist the temptation to set aside what he or she believes to be right. Moral indignation and outrage are sometimes warranted.

Other interesting examples include military physicians who believe they have to answer first to their consciences and cannot plead "superior orders" when commanded by a superior officer to commit what they believe to be a moral wrong. When Capt. Howard B. Levy, a military physician, refused to obey his commander's order to establish and operate a program in dermatology, he argued that to obey the order would implicate him in war crimes committed by Special Forces in Vietnam and would—for him, as a physician—be a violation of medical ethics.[28] Any person who makes such claims might be a victim of self-deception, might later be able to forget the act or change his views, or might later find a legitimate reason to shift the responsibility to someone else. But for this physician, at this time, his conscience would not allow performance of the act.

Appeals to Conscience in Moral Justification

Thomas Hobbes thought the opinions of conscience, though not doubted by the agent, yet "may be erroneous" and can never be accepted on their face as demonstrating knowledge or truth.[29] Clearly persons can perform bad acts in good conscience and good acts in bad conscience. When individuals appeal to conscience to explain and justify to others their actions or refusals to act, they need more than an opinion about the correctness of their views; they need a further justification. Conscience is not self-certifying from the moral point of view, and we sometimes experience remorse of conscience when we begin to doubt that what we at one time did conscientiously was right or good.

When people "consult" their consciences, they presumably examine their moral convictions to determine what, upon reflection, they judge to be the best course of action. By definition, a person cannot act against conscience without believing that he or she has acted wrongly. Consulting conscience can yield only one answer: Do what you believe you ought to do, or suffer the consequences. Consulting conscience is thus only one step in the examination of one's moral convictions and is not sufficient for justification. Despite a long tradition to the contrary,[30] conscience is formal and empty if left exclusively to its own workings. Insofar as it provides its own content and level of devotion without any constraint of external justification, conscience is morally blind and dangerous.[31]

Reflective persons seeking justification for a course of action sometimes experience serious internal conflicts. A *conflict of conscience* occurs when a person faces two conflicting moral demands, neither of which can be met without a partial rejection of the other. The dilemma is particularly painful when both courses of action are firmly required from the perspective of conscience. Occasionally a person confronts "dirty hands," because all available courses of action in the pursuit of a vital goal involve a serious moral violation. In the case discussed above, George's conscience may direct him both to refuse the position because it involves unethical research on chemical and biological warfare and to accept the position because it will prevent the research from being pursued by fanatics and will also benefit his family. It might be argued that George has misconstrued his situation and that his apparent conflict of conscience is an instance of an ambivalent or unsure judgment about the relevant standards, their specifications, and their weights in the situation. Perhaps, however, George believes with sound reason that he faces a genuine moral tragedy.

Those who defend the maxims "Let your conscience be your guide" or "Just follow your conscience" need not and should not hold that conscience is either a sufficient or an infallible guide. They can and typically do recognize the possibility of an erroneous conscience. Several theologians and philosophers across the centuries have held that it is blameworthy to act against conscience even if it is erroneous.[32] They hold an individual morally blameless for a wrongful action done out of conscience; and they believe that an action done against conscience is necessarily morally culpable. That is, individuals are always morally culpable if they fail to follow conscience, because they intend to violate what they believe to be binding moral standards. To intend what is *subjectively* wrong is morally blameworthy, even if the action is not *objectively* wrong. The point is simple and important: People should do everything possible to ensure that their consciences are properly informed by relevant moral principles and rules, but in the end they must make a judgment and act in a way that protects their moral integrity. To act against one's best moral judgment would be to intend to do what one conscientiously believes to be morally wrong.

These observations are not meant to suggest that we should acquiesce to the demands of conscience, whatever its content and justification. Conscientious judgments may be seriously mistaken, and claims of conscience may be rationalizations for immoral acts. Furthermore, as a procedural virtue, conscientiousness requires agents to searchingly examine their personal convictions by external moral standards and thorough evidence about the facts of the situation. Nothing less will stand the test of justification.

Conscientious Objection

As we saw in discussing integrity, conscience sometimes requires resistance to the demands of other persons or situations in the form of conscientious objection or refusal. Suppose a nurse believes that a doctor's order to turn off a ventilator for a patient is unethical. The nurse may judge the doctor's order a sufficiently grave matter that it should be reported immediately to the proper authority in an effort to countermand it. Alternatively, the nurse may believe that his or her cooperation in the doctor's order would involve complicity in a moral wrong, but may not believe that reporting the matter to others is necessary. In effect, the nurse says to the physician, "I see that the arguments you give are sufficient for you to judge that you are doing the right thing by switching off the machine. I do not doubt that *you* are acting according to your conscience, but *my* conscience instructs me differently."[33]

Conflicts of conscience—within a person or between persons—sometimes emerge in health care because people regard as unethical some role-obligation or official order that descends from a hierarchical structure of authority. In many cases of refusals, the individual does not rebuke others or obstruct them from performing an act, but only says "Not through me."[34] Occasionally this situation arises when a patient refuses a procedure in a context the physician views as medically unconscionable or requests a procedure the physician finds morally objectionable, such as amniocentesis for sex selection or an untested cancer therapy. In a case introduced in Chapter 5, a young unmarried intern requested a sterilization procedure because she did not like available contraceptives and did not want children. Her gynecologist could not in good conscience perform the procedure because she thought it was not in the young woman's best interests to preclude the possibility of having children later. However, the gynecologist did not try to prevent the woman from getting someone else to perform the operation.[35] In such cases, the physician usually has a moral obligation to refer or to transfer the patient to another physician. This obligation is written into many recent natural death acts, which do not mandate coercion of physicians' consciences in carrying out a patient's directive, but do require physicians to make a reasonable effort to transfer the patient to another physician.

If a physician wishes to withdraw because the patient's requests or refusals seem morally repugnant, the physician's conscientious convictions should be respected, and he or she should be free to withdraw—assuming that the requested actions are not among the responsibilities one generally accepts in agreeing to be someone's physician. A patient's right of autonomy should not be purchased at the price of the physician's parallel right. In some situations, professionals question the degree of participation that is required of them in what they take to be a morally wrong action by others.

Moral theologians have sometimes distinguished different degrees of cooperation: In *formal* cooperation, the individual consents to and actively participates in morally wrong actions, whereas in *material* cooperation the individual does not consent, but his or her actions are involved in the wrongdoing. Material cooperation in wrongdoing can be justified in some traditions only if the agent's actions are not morally wrong and if there are compelling reasons for participation. For example, Roman Catholic moral theology has allowed an assistant to a surgeon performing an "evil operation" of abortion or sterilization to cooperate, in order to prevent additional harms, by sterilizing instruments, preparing the patient, and administering the anesthesia.[36]

These guidelines attempt to deal with the reality that individuals are in some complex circumstances unable to detach themselves without unacceptable losses from morally evil acts and outcomes. Conscientious individuals must decide how far they can cooperate, for example, while in military service in an unjust war, in a bureaucratic health care institution with unjust policies, and in unjustified research. In a striking example, some physicians and hospitals attempted to disassociate themselves from evil by refusing to participate in medical preparedness programs that could be part of plans for nuclear war or that could increase the likelihood of nuclear war. Sixty physicians at Contra Costa Hospital in San Francisco refused a Defense Department request to pledge at least fifty civilian beds for the care of military casualties who would be airlifted from overseas in the event of a large-scale war. A year earlier the Defense Department had established the Civilian-Military Contingency Hospital System (CMCHS), a voluntary planning program, to obtain fifty-thousand beds in civilian hospitals for military casualties in the event of "a future large-scale conflict overseas [that] could begin very rapidly and produce casualties at a higher rate than any other war in history." Although this plan was supported by the American Medical Association and the American Hospital Association, it was opposed by Physicians for Social Responsibility, who agreed with the medical staff at Contra Costa—and several other hospitals—that participation "would offer tacit approval for the planning of a nuclear war."

Physician Jack Geiger argued that it is "precisely the professional commitment to the protection and preservation of human life that would make it unethical for any physician to participate in either civilian or military 'disaster' plans specifically designed to attempt to cope with the consequences of nuclear war." In contrast to ordinary medical disaster plans, he argued, nuclear war disaster plans may increase the likelihood of the disaster occurring, because they provide false assurance that medical care can enable the society to survive and win a nuclear war. Steven Goodman, a physician, describes the dilemma: "On the one side there is the perception of unnecessarily lost lives if we do not adopt the CMCHS, and on the other a possible increased risk of nuclear war if we do. . . . If there is even a grain of truth in either of the two sides, a physician pledged to 'do no harm' is faced with a profoundly difficult moral choice."[37]

Conscientious refusal, withdrawal, or disassociation may not be sufficient moral responses if an individual believes that others are violating fundamental obligations, such as nonmaleficence and justice. For instance, nurses may believe that such obligations are violated in a case in which a physician refuses to inform a patient that she has cancer, or in a case in which an order not to resuscitate has apparently been written without the patient's informed consent. In these cases, individuals often believe they must try to ensure or prevent certain actions. After unsuccessful appeals to appropriate officials in the hierarchy of authority, they may decide that it is warranted to blow the whistle in order to direct public attention to the actions in question.[38]

The rules for justified interference with autonomous actions, discussed in Chapter 3, are equally applicable to conscientious actions. A person's conscientious action can be overridden if it, for example, imposes serious risks on others, invades the autonomy of others, or treats others unjustly. However, society can, under some circumstances, respect an individual's conscientious refusals while requiring alternative actions or forms of service. For example, it may fairly require hospital service in lieu of military service. Society occasionally can protect a person's conscience by performing the act for that person, who only objects to performing it himself or herself. For example, some Jehovah's Witnesses believe that the prohibition against taking blood forbids them to consent to blood transfusions but that court-ordered transfusions free them of responsibility, because the transfusion is imposed by law. In one case, Judge J. Skelly Wright granted a hospital the right to give medically necessary blood transfusions to a woman without her consent or her husband's consent. Among his several reasons, Wright determined that neither the woman nor her husband could conscientiously consent to the transfusions, and by granting a court order he thought he could adequately protect their consciences while saving her life.[39] However, removal of responsibility is not a strategy that works for all Jehovah's Witnesses, and certainly not for all conscientious refusers of medical treatments. For instance, some Jehovah's Witnesses hold that blood transfusions contaminate the recipients, irrespective of who makes the decision.

Often health care professionals and the state can accommodate conscientious objection without undermining important societal rules and policies. However, serious tensions sometimes emerge between policies to accommodate claims of conscience and efforts to promote equality and fairness. The following example is illustrative. Throughout the United States a person can be declared dead when his or her whole brain has irreversibly ceased to function, as measured by neurological tests, or when the heart and lungs have irreversibly ceased to function (the traditional cardiopulmonary standard). Even though a patient's heart and lungs still function because of life-support systems, physicians may determine that the patient is dead by neurological standards. States have sought *uniform* legal rules for the determination of death. However, some groups and individuals—for instance, many Orthodox Jews, some citizens of Japanese descent, and some native Americans—have religious and philosophical reservations about whole-brain death and conscientiously object to the use of neurological criteria to determine when they are dead.

Should the state and health care professionals attempt to accommodate such conscientious objections? New Jersey law, to take one example, allows conscientious objection to its brain-death statute.[40] It allows conscientious objectors to the neurological standard to be declared dead by the cardiopulmonary standard, but it does not allow totally free conscientious choice among a wide variety of standards. At first glance, the New Jersey statute appears to accommodate conscientious objectors without serious problems. However, challenges can be raised, based on claims of equality and fairness. For instance, should health insurance cover the medical care provided to a "patient" who is dead according to neurological criteria but not yet dead according to cardiopulmonary criteria, and should a brain-dead "patient" have equal access to scarce life-extending technologies, such as space in intensive care units? The New Jersey statute addresses the first question by holding that in the case of recognized conscientious objection the "patient" is not dead until the cardiopulmonary standard has been met and that insurance payments for medical care must continue during the period. The statute does not specifically address the microallocation question, but, following the arguments we presented in Chapter 6, sound ethical reasons exist for giving brain-dead "patients" lower priority based on improbability of success.

In conclusion, when we encounter serious conflicts of conscience in health care and elsewhere, we may legitimately rely on procedures of resolution and on virtues such as conscientiousness. As John Rawls notes, "In times of social doubt and loss of faith in long established values, there is a tendency to fall back on the virtues of integrity: truthfulness and sincerity, lucidity and commitment, or, as some say, authenticity."[41] The maintenance of mutual trust often depends on the willingness of parties to preserve virtues of integrity and to acknowledge fair procedures. If conflicts are too serious or too profound to permit mutual trust, conscientiousness in taking further steps would still involve a willingness to reconsider the basis of one's position, especially if it involves the refusal to accept another's position.

Moral Ideals

Two levels of moral standards were mentioned earlier—ordinary moral standards and extraordinary moral standards—and they need now to be analytically distinguished. The first level is limited to standards in the common morality that pertain to everyone, a moral minimum. It includes obligations specified in moral principles and rules, as well as the virtues that we expect all moral agents to possess—for example, virtues of faithfulness, trustworthiness, and honesty. The second level is a morality of aspiration in which individuals adopt moral ideals that do not hold for everyone. These standards are adopted by some agents, but others are not bound by them. Those who fulfill these ideals can be praised and admired, whereas those who fall short cannot be rightly blamed or condemned by others.

With the addition of moral ideals, four categories of moral action can be distinguished: (1) actions that are right and obligatory (such as truth-telling); (2) actions that are wrong and prohibited (such as murder); (3) actions that are optional and morally neutral (neither wrong nor obligatory); and (4) actions that are optional in terms of the moral minimum, but morally meritorious and praiseworthy. We concentrated in previous chapters on 1 and 2, occasionally mentioning 3. Now we will be concerned exclusively with 4. Later we will turn to the closely related idea of moral excellence in character and performance.

Supererogatory Actions

We begin with supererogation, a category of moral ideals pertaining principally to *actions* (category 4), rather than to *virtues, motives, or emotions.*[42] The etymological root of *supererogation* means paying or performing beyond what is owed—that is, doing more than is required. It has four defining conditions, which specify category (4) above. The first two conditions presume a threshold of obligations in the common morality (the level of ordinary standards). First, a supererogatory act is optional, neither required nor forbidden by common-morality standards. Second, supererogatory acts exceed what is expected or demanded by the common morality. Third, supererogatory acts are intentionally undertaken for the welfare of others. Fourth, supererogatory acts are morally good and praiseworthy (not merely undertaken from good intentions).

Despite the first condition, individuals may not *consider* their actions (or their characters) to be morally optional. Many heroes and saints describe their actions in the language of *ought, duty,* and *necessity:* "I had to do it." "I had no choice." "It was my duty." The point of this language is to express a personal sense of obligation. At the end of Albert Camus's *The Plague*, Dr. Rieux decides to make a record of those who fought the pestilence. It is to be a record, he says, of "what *had to be done* . . . despite their personal afflictions, by all who, while unable to be saints but refusing to bow down to pestilences, strive their utmost to be healers."[43] These healers accept major risks and thereby exceed both the obligations in the common morality and the obligations traditionally associated with the role of healer.

Some accounts therefore deny the literal appropriateness of the language of obligation in such cases, interpreting it as a form of moral modesty designed to deflect merit or praise from the agent.[44] A more sympathetic interpretation is that the agent accepts a personal norm as laying down what ought and must be done. It is a pledge or assignment of personal responsibility, despite the fact that it is not obligatory in the common morality or in a professional tradition. Supererogatory acts typically *would be required* were it not for some abnormal adversity or risk present in the particular circumstances, but the individual elects not to invoke an exemption from acting based on the abnormal adversity or risk.[45] If persons have the strength of character that enables them to resist extreme adversity or assume additional risk in order to fulfill their own conception of their obligations, why not simply accept their account that they are under a self-imposed obligation? The hero who says, "I was only doing my duty," is, from this perspective, speaking correctly, as a person who accepts standards of moral excellence. The individual does not make a mistake in regarding the action as personally required, and can view failure as grounds for guilt, although no one else is free to view the act as obligatory or the failure to act as an occasion for moral blame.

Not all supererogatory acts are exceptionally arduous, costly, or risky in the way this analysis may suggest. Examples of less demanding forms of supererogation include generous gift-giving, volunteering for public service, forgiving another's costly error, exceptional kindness, and complying with requests made by other persons when these exceed the obligatory requirements of the common morality. Many everyday actions exceed obligation without being at the highest level of supererogation. For example, a nurse may put in extra hours of work and return to the hospital to visit patients without being saintly or heroic.

Often we are uncertain whether an action exceeds obligation, because the boundaries are ill-defined. For example, what is a nurse's obligation to desperate, terminally ill patients who cling to the nurse for comfort in their few remaining days? If the obligation is that of spending, say, forty hours a week in conscientious satisfaction of a job description, then the nurse exceeds that obligation by a few off-duty visits to patients for an extra hour after work. If the obligation is to help patients overcome burdens and meet a series of challenges, then a nurse who displays exceptional patience, fortitude, and friendliness also exceeds the demands of obligation. There are, in addition, many cases of health care professionals living up to what would ordinarily be an obligation (for example, standard care of a patient), but where a sacrifice or risk exceeds that ordinarily faced in such care (for example, in risky care for HIV patients).

In some special relationships between parties—involving, for example, debts of gratitude, close kinship, and commitments of loyalty—acts that would otherwise be optional can become obligatory. This is not surprising because, as we will now see, the distinction between the obligatory and the nonobligatory is not as sharp as many in ethical theory have suggested.

The Continuum from Ordinary Standards to Supererogation

We have distinguished two levels of normative standards—obligatory and supererogatory—but some actions straddle these two levels. They are strongly recommended, but neither obligatory nor supererogatory. The problem is that the two "levels" are continuous and lack sharp boundaries; some territory does not belong clearly to either category. Each level also has many sublevels, and there is a continuum both internal to each level and ranging across their boundaries. This continuum requires analysis.

Contemporary ethical theory tends to classify anything in the domain of morality as either an obligation or beyond obligation, thereby omitting anything bridging the two. However, as we saw in Chapters 2 and 5, we often distinguish between strong and weak demands of the moral life, and between principles such as beneficence that express obligations and other forms of beneficence that are continuous with the principle of beneficence, but nonetheless on the borderline between what is obligatory and not obligatory. A continuum runs from strong obligation (the core demands in the common morality) through weaker forms of obligation (the periphery of ordinary expectations in the common morality) and on to the domain of morally optional *ideals*. The territory of ideals starts with low-level supererogation (for example, generously assisting a visitor lost in a hospital's corridors) and ends with high-level supererogation (for example, heroic acts of self-experimentation).

The continuum, then, moves from the strictest obligation to the most arduous form of supererogation.

Obligation		Beyond Obligation (Supererogation)	
Strong Obligation [1]	Weak Obligation [2]	Low-Level Supererogation [3]	High-Level Supererogation [4]

The horizontal line in this chart represents a continuum with only rough rather than sharply defined categories, connecting both the four lower categories and action within each of those categories. Many points on the continuum are not captured by the abstract labels placed on the four categories below the line. For example, as noted previously, some ideals are far more demanding than others. Later we will discuss some of the differences by distinguishing increasingly demanding ideals.

Joel Feinberg argues that supererogatory acts are "located on an altogether different scale than" obligations.[46] The above chart suggests that this comment is correct in one respect and misleading in another. The right half of the chart is not scaled by obligation at all, whereas the left half is. In this respect Feinberg's comment is correct. However, the full horizontal line is connected by a single scale of moral value in which the right is continuous with the left. For example, obligatory acts of beneficence and supererogatory acts of beneficence are on the same scale by being morally of the same kind. The domain of the supererogatory is continuous with the domain of principles of obligation by exceeding those demands in accordance with the several defining conditions of supererogation listed previously.

Many beneficent and caring actions by health care professionals straddle the territory in the above chart between obligations and ideals (that is, between [2] and [3]). Here matters become more complicated than the chart indicates, because we need to distinguish professional obligations and common-morality obligations. Many moral *obligations* in health care are moral *ideals* from the perspective of the common morality. For example, the Code of Ethics of the International Council on Nurses makes it a professional responsibility of the nurse to initiate action to meet the health and social needs of the public, and various medical codes state that a physician should neither pay nor receive a commission for referral of patients. Many such expected obligations in medicine and nursing are profession-imposed, rather than obligations either in the common morality or in other forms of professional practice. (They may or may not be parts of the legal code applying to physicians and nurses.) Some are role-obligations, even when not formally stated in professional codes. For example, the expectation that physicians and nurses will encourage and cheer patients, giving them hope, is a profession-imposed obligation (though not every health professional will recognize it as obligatory).

Some customs are more ambiguous and occasionally generate controversy. Consider again the belief that physicians and nurses have an obligation to efface self-interest and take risks in attending to patients. Is this dimension of professional practice a matter of supererogation, a role-obligation, or somewhere between? One frequently discussed topic is the nature of "obligations" to care for patients with HIV when the risk of transmission is significant. All answers to this question have been controversial, and professional codes and medical association pronouncements have varied extensively.[47] One explanation of the uncertainty, ambivalence, and controversy surrounding this issue is that it is unclear in medical ethics (as well as in ethical theory and the common morality) whether the risky care of patients with HIV is obligatory or optional. Neither the health care professions nor the society has decided whether to accept traditional obligations of setting aside some self-interest to care for patients or to accept a model of behavior that allows for a wider framework of optional treatment in which ideals displace obligations.[48] These issues probably cannot be resolved without specifically considering the level of risk that health care workers are expected to assume and setting a threshold beyond which the level of risk is so high as to be optional rather than obligatory.

The unresolved character of this problem should help us appreciate why some medical associations urge their members to exhibit the *virtue of courage* and treat HIV-infected patients, why other associations advise their members that treatment is *optional* (category 3, rather than 1 or 4, in our list above, p. 483),[49] and why still others with particularly high expectations for medicine insist that both virtue and obligation converge to the conclusion that health care professionals should set aside self-interest to care for such patients and that the health care professions should take actions to ensure that such patients receive appropriate care.[50]

The last position coheres with many traditional beliefs in the health care professions, but it also assigns the health care professions more role-obligations and more demanding role-obligations than perhaps any other profession. To ask health care professionals to set aside substantial self-interest by requiring actions that elsewhere are considered supererogatory is, paradoxically, to do what traditional morality has avoided by distinguishing the supererogatory from the obligatory: Refrain from holding people to standards that are arduous, risky, and frightening. It is doubtful that health care professionals fail to discharge moral obligations when they fall short of such standards, even if obligations are measured exclusively by role-obligations. On the one hand, it is ill-advised to distance medical morality from the common morality, as if they are separate worlds with separate standards—medical morality being fixed only by the profession itself, without public input, advice, or consent. On the other hand, when individuals voluntarily assume professional role-responsibilities, they do engender uncommon expectations, encourage special forms of reliance, and acquire more specific obligations of fidelity.

It may be supererogatory to promise to perform an inconvenient and risky act, but, because of the promise, the performance of the promised act is not itself supererogatory. It is, rather, the discharge of a prima facie obligation.[51] However, the promises made in entering the medical profession (or another health care profession) are not very specific, and debates emerge as a result about the line between obligatory and optional (but praiseworthy) risk-taking. One effort to specify physicians' obligations to engage in risky conduct places them in the context of societal expectations about risky actions in other occupations. Society expects law enforcement officials, firefighters, and life-guards, among others, to take some personal risks in pursuit of the aims of their occupations. These societal expectations rest in part on the agents' acceptance of these occupational roles. In medicine, society's expectations are usually based not on a specific contract but on the nature of the profession and its commitments.

Can an analysis of societal expectations about risk-taking in various occupations help determine whether physicians caring for HIV-infected patients are discharging their role-obligations or acting heroically from a supererogatory ideal? Ezekiel Emanuel notes that there are predictably 1 to 9 deaths each year among the 1,600 or so active firefighters in Boston. These firefighters thus face a risk of death of approximately 0.5 percent in each of the worst years and 0.2 percent in each of the best years. Emanuel contends that this risk is comparable to the risk faced by an internist from needle sticks in caring for patients with HIV infection—high but not excessive. However, the risks are much higher and perhaps even excessive for surgeons who operate on a large number of patients with HIV infection because of frequent and unavoidable punctures. In such cases, it may be appropriate to disperse such patients among several surgeons, to ask for volunteers, to offer increased compensation for risk-taking, and the like. And it may even be justifiable for surgeons to decline to perform some elective procedures on grounds of the risks involved. Judgments about obligatory and supererogatory levels of risky care depend on the best available scientific evidence about transmission, but also on societal judgments about reasonable and excessive risks in various professions and occupations.[52]

Confusion arises because of vagueness and indeterminateness regarding obligations in the common morality and in the community of health professionals. Unfortunately, we may not be able to reduce this indeterminateness substantially. Just as we could not in Chapter 5 distinguish obligatory and nonobligatory beneficence with precision (or determine specific levels of risk that must be undertaken to discharge professional duty), so we can only make rough distinctions across many other areas of the moral life. An absence of charitableness, a failure of friendship, and an insufficiency of generosity are clearly defects in the moral life, but they are not necessarily failures of either ordinary obligation or role-obligation.

A related complication is that the category of *obligation* (or duty) does not exhaust what we *ought* to do in our encounters with others, as various interpretations of the general form "X ought to do it" indicate. *Ought* in this schema might mean that (1) X ought to do it because of a strong moral obligation, (2) X ought to do it because of a weak moral obligation, (3) X ought to do it because of a self-imposed requirement such as a moral ideal or a rule of charity, (4) X ought to do it in accordance with one or more standards of virtue, or (5) X ought to do it because it is what exemplary, saintly, or heroic persons do. The term *ought,* then, operates across the boundaries separating obligation, that which is virtuous, and that which exceeds both obligation and ordinary virtue.

Many ethical theories have been criticized for failures to accommodate some part or all of this moral terrain. It has been argued, for example, that Kantians cannot accept supererogation because they leave no room for action that is beyond obligation (or at least no grounds for saying that such an action is morally good). Kantian theory seems exhausted by (1) an all-embracing account of obligation that sweeps into its territory what others classify as supererogatory and (2) an account of what is morally indifferent.[53] Some people likewise claim that utilitarians cannot account for the category of supererogation, because every act that is maximally good is obligatory in utilitarian theory. If an act would produce more good than any alternative act for all affected parties, it is obligatory. If it would not maximize good outcomes, it is deficient or wrong.[54] As we have seen on several occasions, utilitarians seem to demand both more impartiality and more sacrifice than does the common sense morality from which the obligatory-supererogatory distinction springs. In their purest forms, then, both Kantian and utilitarian theories tend to be anti-supererogationist.[55]

However, there may be room in both types of ethical theory for a modest area of supererogation. For example, utilitarians can support supererogatory acts by recognizing that if we allow some acts to be optional but praiseworthy, this classification will produce better results than would be produced by making the acts obligatory. For utilitarians of this persuasion, acts should be categorized as supererogatory whenever adoption of a rule making them obligatory would turn out not to have the best or even good consequences, although the performance of these acts through the autonomous choices of agents would have extremely good consequences. However, this solution places utilitarians in the uncomfortable position of undermining the strict demands of the principle of utility. They seem to be offering consequentialist reasons based on practicability for restraining (or perhaps even rejecting) the principle of utility in favor of the very commonsense demands that the principle of utility supposedly corrects.

Like pure utilitarian and Kantian theories, classical theories of virtue do not in their purest forms suggest a clear distinction between (1) ideals that surpass, supersede, or rise above ordinary morality and (2) virtues that everyone is expected to manifest. It might be argued that a virtue-based theory has no need for such distinctions, because the virtues do not inherently require, command, or compel actions. However, the difference between ordinary and extraordinary morality (both of which are within the common morality) affects virtue theory no less than theories of obligation. A primary virtue standard is a norm of the moral life for everyone, not a target only for the person of saintly, heroic, or excellent character. Virtues such as respectfulness, benevolence, and fairness, for example, are not exclusively optional. These virtues establish communal expectations for good and decent human relationships. Persons who violate these standards violate ordinary canons of morality, not extraordinary canons.

We conclude that distinctions between what is obligatory, what is beyond obligation, and also what is virtuous have often been overplayed in contemporary ethical theory. The distinctions are not as sharp as some theories suggest, do not exhaust the relevant alternatives, and obscure the rich variety of the moral life.

Moral Excellence

Aristotelian ethical theory has long insisted that moral excellence is a supremely important topic and one closely connected to both virtues and moral ideals: A virtue *is* an excellence of character displaying appropriate desires for right actions, and ethics is centrally concerned with self-cultivated excellences. We will consult and draw on this Aristotelian tradition for an account of moral excellence relevant to health care that builds on our prior analysis of moral ideals and supererogation. However, we do not claim to be presenting a distinctively Aristotelian theory, and we are motivated by objectives that contemporary Aristotelians may or may not share. We begin with four reasons that motivate us to attend to moral excellence in contemporary ethics.

The Value and Place of Moral Excellence

Our first motive is to overcome an undue emphasis and imbalance in contemporary ethical theory, which focuses on the moral minimum of obligations while largely ignoring supererogation and moral ideals.[56] This concentration on a set of minimal obligations has diluted our conception of the moral life, including our expectations for ourselves, our close associates, and our institutional contexts. If we expect only the moral minimum, we will lose a sense of excellence in both character and performance. We aspire, then, to rectify this bias toward minimal obligations.

The second motivating reason is connected to the first. We seek to overcome a certain skepticism in contemporary ethical theory about high ideals in the moral life. This skepticism is found in some of our best writers, including some who have profoundly influenced the present authors (for example, Bernard Williams and Thomas Nagel), as well as some who have provided influential works in character ethics (for example, Susan Wolf and Philippa Foot).[57] We cannot develop their arguments here, but the thrust of their skepticism is the following: High moral ideals must compete with many other goals and responsibilities in life, and these ideals may demand too much of persons or may lead them to neglect matters worthy of attention, including personal projects, family relationships, personal friendships, and experiences that broaden one's outlook.

We do not wholly reject this view, and we agree that some skeptical reservations are warranted. Nonetheless, the cumulative impact of these writings suggests that high moral ideals are, in the end, only one of life's major considerations and that moral excellence is no more valuable or worthwhile than hobbies, recreation, and other "agent-relative" projects. Lost is the Aristotelian goal of aspiring to an admirable life of moral achievement. As a result, their model of a moral person is uninspiring and devoid of moral challenge for earnest and reflective persons. As Mill once noted, "The contented man, or the contented family, who have no ambition to make any one else happier, to promote the good of their country or their neighborhood, or to improve themselves in moral excellence, excite in us neither admiration nor approval."[58] Some writers in contemporary ethical theory thus subtly undermine moral excellence, and their views need to be countered by an appropriate model of high merit and worthiness in the moral life.

Our third motive recalls the criterion of comprehensiveness in an ethical theory, as discussed in Chapter 2. A theory of moral excellence will allow us to incorporate moral virtues and forms of supererogation beyond the obligations and virtues that comprise ordinary morality. Virtues such as tactfulness, courage, patience, hospitality, and occasionally what Aristotle called "greatness of soul" can be included without maintaining that these virtues are conditions of morality that everyone is somehow required to meet or that there are principles of patience, hospitality, courage, and the like. These vital aspects of the moral life merit inclusion in a comprehensive account.

Finally, a model of moral excellence is worth examining because it indicates what is worthy of our aspiration. Morally paradigmatic lives provide developed ideals of exemplary character that help guide and inspire us to higher goals and morally better lives. Such models give some depth to the idea that high moral aspiration and achievement are important in the moral life, alongside moral principle and virtue.

Aristotelian Ideals

Aristotle maintained that human virtues are dispositions to act, feel, and judge that are developed from an innate capacity by proper training and exercise. We acquire virtues much as we do skills such as carpentry, playing a musical instrument, or cooking. Right action deriving from good moral character presupposes intelligent judgment, which is itself a form of virtue, including the virtue of discernment. This model is one of excellence in both performance and character. To love what is morally superior and to act from practical intelligence *(phronesis)* with appropriate motives from a stable and well-developed character are of the highest importance.

Obligations play a less central role in this account, because the theory turns on motive, effort, commitment, action from virtue, and development of character. Consider, for example, a person who undertakes to expose scientific fraud in an academic institution. It is easy to frame this action as a matter of obligation, especially if the institution has a policy on fraud. But suppose this person's reports to superiors are ignored, and eventually her job is in jeopardy and her family receives threats. Her efforts to bring about institutional reform then take on heroic dimensions. At some point we likely would say that she has fulfilled her obligations and is not morally required to pursue the matter further, although it would be commendable to pursue it. But in an Aristotelian theory this situation might be framed and evaluated differently. A person's fight against fraud in an institution might be gauged primarily by the person's level of commitment, the perseverance and endurance shown, the resourcefulness and discernment in marshalling evidence, the courage but also the decency and diplomacy displayed in confronting superiors, etc.

An analogy to educational goals helps explain why setting higher than ordinary goals is central to the Aristotelian framework. Most of us are trained to aspire to an ideal of education. We are taught to prepare ourselves as best we can. No educational aspirations are too high unless they exceed our abilities and cannot be attained. If we reach only an ordinary educational level, this achievement is considered a matter of disappointment and regret. In the midst of fulfilling our aspirations, we sometimes expand our goals beyond what we had originally planned. We think of getting another degree, learning another language, or reading widely beyond our specialized training. We do not say, however, that we have an *obligation* to achieve as high a level of education as we can achieve.

The Aristotelian model for ethics is analogous. Moral character and moral achievement are functions of education, self-cultivation, and habituation. Each individual should aspire to a level as elevated as his or her ability permits. This "should" is not construed as a moral obligation to become as virtuous as possible (although some writers in ethical theory do defend precisely this duty[59]). To achieve only the moral minimum of socially imposed obligations is a moral disappointment, though not a failure of moral obligation. Persons vary in the quality of their performances in athletics, in medical practice, in lecturing, etc.; and in the moral life, too, some persons are more able than others. For this reason they deserve more acknowledgment, praise, and admiration.

Persons who are serious about their educational goals typically do not aim only at high grades, degrees, and good jobs. They think in terms of personal achievement and character development. In learning a second language, for example, the most able students think not about a grade achieved in a course, but about whether they are learning to use the language properly, whether they can conduct a sustained conversation, and whether their knowledge and accent are conducive to meaningful communication with native-speakers. They think about personal development and levels of achievement in the way an Aristotelian thinks about moral development and achievement.

Some persons are so advanced morally that what they believe they must do or achieve is different from what those who are less morally developed must do or can expect to achieve. Here we encounter a new continuum. One's goals of moral excellence enlarge as moral development advances. This Aristotelian continuum implies that every person who has already achieved a certain level of virtue has the opportunity to strive for a higher level of virtue, in accordance with an ideal of excellence. It is both simplistic and morally undesirable to distinguish sharply between ordinary moral requirements and extraordinary ideals. What persons should strive to achieve when at lower levels of moral development is different from what they should attempt at more advanced levels of development. But, wherever one is on the continuum of development, there will be a goal of moral excellence that exceeds what has already been achieved. What we ought to do, then, is to follow a moving target of moral excellence.

We can thus see why, in Aristotelian ethics, ideals rather than principles of obligation take center stage. This account is suited for persons with the will to aspire, not for persons who merely want to know what social obligations require. For example, the investigator who uses human subjects of research might ask (as is typical in protocol review), "What am I obligated to do to protect human subjects?" The presumption is that once this question has been addressed, the researcher can then accept a burden of moral obligation and proceed with the research. But on the Aristotelian model, this question and answer are only starting points. The more important question is, "How could I conduct this research so that subjects are maximally protected and minimally inconvenienced, commensurate with achieving the objectives of the research?" Not to address this latter question at all, but only to ask the question about basic obligations indicates that one is morally less serious than one could be.

The Aristotelian model does not expect perfection, only that one strive toward perfection. Although this model might be viewed as scoring low on the criterion of practicability developed in Chapter 2, a fairer assessment is that moral ideals *are* practical instruments. As *our* ideals, they motivate us in a way that obligations likely will not, and they also set out a path that can be climbed in stages, with a renewable sense of growth and achievement. Just as parental goals and ideals guide parents in directing a child's moral development, moral ideals help direct our moral development.

Elevated Moral Excellence: Saints and Heroes

Exceptional persons often function as models of excellence whose examples we aspire to follow. For instance, all college teachers can think of one or more of their teachers who inspired them to pedagogical ideals and who have in some measure served as professional models. Morally exceptional individuals have a similar capacity to guide others. Among the many types of models, the moral hero and the moral saint (here used in a secular sense) are the most prominent, and deservedly so. We will concentrate below on saints and heroes, but we also note from the outset that many persons who serve as our moral models, or from whom we draw moral inspiration, are not so advanced morally that they can be correctly described as either saints or heroes (although we sometimes incorrectly think of them as saints and heroes).

A person typically becomes morally exceptional by possessing an abundance of well-developed virtues, displayed in appropriate actions. But we also learn about virtuous conduct from persons with a limited repertoire of exceptional virtues, such as exceedingly conscientious health professionals. We learn about moral excellence wherever we find it, and many who are neither saints nor heroes may be the most important influences we ever experience. The fact that we concentrate in this section on the most exceptional persons, saints and heroes, should not cause us to lose sight of other moral exemplars.

Consider, for example, John Berger's biography of an English physician, John Sassall, who chose to practice medicine in a poverty-ridden, culturally deprived country village in a remote region of Northern England. Under the influence of the books of Joseph Conrad, Sassall chose this village from an "ideal of service" that reached beyond "the average petty life of self-seeking advancement." Sassall was aware that he would have almost no social life and that the villagers had few resources with which to pay him, to develop their community, and to attract better medicine, but he focused on their needs rather than his own. Progressively, Sassall grew morally as he interacted with members of the community. He developed a deep understanding of and profound respect for the members of the village and learned how to attend to them as whole human beings. He became a person of exceptional caring, devotion, discernment, conscientiousness, and patience when taking care of the villagers. His moral character increased and deepened year after year in caring for them. They, in turn, trusted him under the most adverse and personally difficult circumstances.[60]

From the exemplary life of John Sassall and from our previous analysis, we can now extract four criteria as general conditions of moral excellence and then test these criteria against our experience of other exceptional persons.[61] First, Sassall is faithful to a worthy *moral ideal* that he keeps constantly before him in making judgments and performing actions. In his case, the ideal is unusually devoted service to a poor and needy community. Second, he has a *motivational structure* that conforms closely to our description of the motivational patterns of virtuous persons (primarily in Chapter 2). Third, he has an *exceptional moral character;* that is, he possesses moral virtues and performs supererogatory actions to an exceptional extent.[62] Fourth, he is a *person of integrity*—both of moral integrity and of a deep personal integrity—and thus is not overwhelmed by distracting conflicts or personal desires in making judgments and performing actions. These four conditions do not suggest that a morally excellent person possesses all possible virtues. One can be morally excellent, and even a moral exemplar, while lacking various virtues that also qualify as morally excellent.

These four conditions appear to be sufficient conditions of moral excellence; they are also relevant (but not sufficient) conditions of moral saintliness and moral heroism. John Sassall, exceptional as he is, is neither a saint nor a hero. To achieve this elevated status, he would have to satisfy additional conditions. Sassall is not a person who faces either deep adversity (though he faces modest adversity), very difficult tasks, or a high level of risk, and these are typically the sorts of conditions that contribute to making a person a saint (or a hero). As is true for moral excellence in general, many factors, especially motives, can affect our evaluation. If, for example, a physician went to a plague-stricken city motivated primarily by a desire to gain public recognition or to have experiences that could serve as the basis of a profitable book, we would likely not judge his or her acts to be heroic. Evaluations are similar but not identical for saints. One who acts in a manner normally deserving the tribute "saintly," but who acts purely for public recognition, does not qualify as a saint.

Examples of prominent moral saints include St. Francis, Mother Theresa, and Albert Schweitzer. Examples of prominent moral heroes include soldiers, political prisoners, and ambassadors who take substantial risks to save endangered persons by acts such as falling on hand grenades and resisting political tyrants. Scientists and physicians who experiment on themselves in order to generate knowledge that can benefit others are also significant heroes. There are many famous examples: Daniel Carrion injected blood into his arm from a patient with verruga peruana (an unusual disease marked by many vascular eruptions of the skin and mucous membranes as well as fever and severe rheumatic pains), only to discover that it had given him a fatal disease (Oroya fever). Werner Forssman performed the first heart catheterization on himself, walking to the radiological room with the catheter sticking into his heart.[63] More recently, a French researcher, Dr. Daniel Zagury, injected himself with an experimental AIDS vaccine, maintaining that his act was "the only ethical line of conduct."[64]

A person can qualify as a moral hero or a moral saint, we suggest, only if he or she meets some combination of the above-listed four conditions of moral excellence. These four conditions are neither individually necessary nor jointly sufficient for moral heroism; and they are probably not sufficient for moral sainthood, although they do seem to be necessary. Thus, all four conditions need not be satisfied to be a moral hero, but all must be satisfied to be a moral saint. We will not attempt an argued defense of this claim here, but by a gradual ascent of examples and argument we will give reasons to think that this conclusion is approximately correct.

We begin with a seminal article on moral saints and heroes by J. O. Urmson that in 1958 reinvigorated a long tradition of reflection on supererogation. Urmson objected to the way in which the dominant ethical theories classify acts as either obligatory, permissible, or prohibited, because this classification scheme fails to capture the special quality of saintly and heroic acts and the way these acts surpass the threshold of obligation. He distinguished between saints and heroes primarily in terms of the self-control and sacrifice made by saints and the control of fear and level of risk assumed by heroes.[65] His thesis that a hero faces significant personal risk is, we believe, more successful than his account of the saint. Many saints, by their own reports as well as those of their biographers, endure and combat adversity or confront very difficult tasks for the sake of others, but they do not necessarily suffer large costs or make major sacrifices.[66] From the saint's perspective there may be no cost or sacrifice at all, but almost all saints know that adversity is present; it is unlikely that anyone qualifies as a saint without successfully meeting a condition on the scale of adversity, hardship, difficulty, or misfortune. A fifth relevant condition of moral sainthood, then, is striving to overcome such a condition—though perhaps a particularly spotless person might be a saint without satisfying this condition—and an added condition of being a moral hero is assuming extraordinary risk for the sake of others.

Urmson distinguishes in a different way between minor and major saints and heroes. He claims that minor saints and heroes live up to obligations when others generally would not, whereas major saints and heroes surpass their obligations when others generally would not.[67] He proposes that heroes act when others would succumb to fear, whereas saints act when others would yield to other interests. Some of this analysis coheres well with our earlier continuum between obligations and ideals, but Urmson's claim that minor saints and heroes typically live up to moral *obligations* when lesser persons would not is inconsistent with our previous analysis. A more plausible thesis is that minor saints and heroes live up to what *would have been* an obligation were it not for some additional and substantial adversity, difficulty, or risk they faced. But this thesis too is flawed. Heroism and saintliness can occur at any level if no obligation is present and would not be present in the absence of additional risk, adversity, or difficulty.

We can now return to the conditions that must be satisfied to qualify as saints and heroes. We said that a saint must meet all four of the above-listed conditions plus a condition of meeting adversity, hardship, difficulty, or misfortune, whereas heroes need only meet some subset of the four conditions plus a condition of accepting extraordinary risk. This formulation entails that the conditions of moral saintliness are more fixed than the conditions of moral heroism. Although risks may be lower for a saint by comparison to a hero, we otherwise expect a higher level of moral excellence from saints: more noble ideals, a purer motivational structure, a fuller-bodied mixture of moral virtues, and a stronger measure of moral integrity. This higher standard of character, together with successfully meeting adversity or difficulty, is distinctive of the moral saint.

Saintliness also requires consistent fulfillment of and transcendence of obligation over time, while living up to (not merely aspiring to) moral ideals. A final judgment about a person's saintliness cannot be made until his or her record is substantially complete, and a saint's character cannot change dramatically over time without losing its distinctive quality as saintly. Even a gradual deterioration in moral qualities of excellence counts against saintliness. A physician or nurse who works long days at low pay for several years in a poverty-stricken area could easily qualify as a moral saint. If his or her actions are required by a role, such as a position in a clinic in the slums, acceptance of that role with its responsibilities under conditions of adversity or difficulty is still beyond the demands of moral obligation. By contrast, regardless of past conduct, a person may become a hero instantly, through a single action, such as taking a major risk while trying to save someone's life or, as in an aforementioned case, overcoming fear to serve in a plague-ridden city. Radical moral change after an act of heroism can change a person's character, but will not disqualify the act(s) as heroic.

One might argue, simplifying Urmson, that we have made matters unduly complicated and that there are only two necessary conditions of being a hero: (1) assuming extraordinary risk, while (2) acting for the welfare of others. This analysis may be adequate for heroes in general (exceptional bravery and beneficence being the most general conditions of heroism), but it is not adequate as an analysis of *moral* heroes. Occasionally morally disgraceful persons satisfy conditions (1) and (2)—for example, bloodthirsty military commanders sometimes act heroically to protect their troops. Some persons who act on morally worthy motives for morally worthy goals under exceptional risk often do not have deep moral convictions or exemplary characters. At the next opportunity, they may lose their courage and retreat. For this reason, some subset of our four conditions, evidencing deep and worthy motivation, commitment, or character seems essential for moral heroism.

We can test this thesis by again considering health professionals who care for AIDS patients. Many have insisted that heroism is not involved in their work, on grounds that the risks are not extraordinary. However, in the early 1980s before solid evidence existed about the transmission of the disease, those who cared for AIDS patients often were moral heroes; and some types of care of HIV-infected patients still qualify as heroic. However, these health professionals do not become moral heroes merely by assuming extraordinary risk. Their moral character, their motives, and their role as healers combine to tip the balance from generic heroism to moral heroism.

Moral saintliness has typically been recognized as a still more difficult level of moral excellence because of the demands it places on human beings across an extended period of time. A major moral saint is as close to a morally good and worthy person as circumstances permit. Such a person's life is dominated by a commitment to benefit others or to a moral ideal, sometimes at significant inconvenience. This commitment can involve striving for moral excellence that approximates moral perfection.[68]

However, as noted previously, caveats about such perfectionist goals are sometimes appropriate. A perfectionist ideal, joined with an overwhelming commitment in one dimension of life, may lead the agent to neglect other dimensions of human life or to devalue the personal projects of others. Following Susan Wolf's influential analysis, one might challenge the saint's apparent assumption that it is always better to be morally superior by reaching ever higher levels of moral excellence in accordance with one's ideals.[69] Even saints have sometimes fallen short in human dimensions such as education, friendship, or family life by sacrificing too many nonmoral interests to a central all-consuming moral project. From this perspective a saint can be personally defective while striving for moral perfection. Similar points may hold for moral heroes who act at substantial sacrifice.

Ill-advised and unduly risky acts of beneficence can be similarly criticized for their failure to consider competing moral obligations. To return to our previous example, imagine that a physician volunteers to take a grave risk by serving in a plague-stricken city that has attracted the world's sympathy, and imagine that there are no other physicians or medical services in the small town he leaves unprotected in his absence. His apparently heroic action might deserve criticism as an exercise of poor moral judgment, especially on grounds of abandoning a community that relies on him for medical care. Related issues of questionable judgment emerge when physicians, courts, guardians, and society at large receive offers of supererogatory and sometimes heroic actions that exceed ordinary obligations.

Heroic Offers of Organ Donation

We have focused on supererogatory acts by physicians, nurses, and other health care professionals. These professionals also function as moral gatekeepers to determine who will be allowed to make sacrifices and take risks for others, particularly through live donations of kidneys and other organs and tissues for transplantation. Transplant teams not only remove, transfer, and implant the donated organ, but they also select the donors, often searching for them in a family of a needy patient, screening prospective donors for compatibility and suitability, offering them an uncommon opportunity to help others, advising them about courses of action, estimating the risks involved, and evaluating those risks as "reasonable," "excessive," and so forth. They frequently assess the potential donor's understanding, voluntariness, and motives, as well as determining whether the risks are "acceptable." They may even give medical excuses for potential donors who choose not to donate. An example appears in Case 2 (discussed at length in Chapter 2), in which a father was reluctant to donate a kidney to his dying daughter and asked the physician to lie. Finally, physicians and other health-care professionals decide, within societal and institutional limits, when to offer people the opportunity to donate organs or tissues for experimental transplants, such as transplants of portions of livers and lungs from living donors.

Does the language of "moral gatekeeping" appropriately describe these activities? Gatekeeping is evident in the transplant team's selection of living donors, allowing some but not others to perform supererogatory acts, but many health care professionals view the process of selection as medical and clinical, rather than moral. According to two commentators, transplant "physicians are in the position of having to make *clinical judgments* about whether, for a particular person [a potential donor], the risk of harm outweighs the likelihood of benefit."[70] However, the judgments involved are not merely clinical, in the usual sense; they are fundamentally moral. Living organ donation raises complex ethical issues because the transplant team subjects a healthy person to a risky surgical procedure, with no medical benefit to him or her, in order to provide a medical benefit to someone else. Some commentators urge a system in which the competent prospective donor should decide whether donation is worth the risks involved.[71] However, simply letting prospective donors decide or letting transplant teams decide (assuming the potential donor's willingness to donate) is inadequate. Both parties should be involved as responsible moral agents in the donation process.

The scarcity of cadaveric kidneys persists, and living kidney donors are still needed, despite the development and extension of renal dialysis and cadaveric kidney transplantation. Kidney transplantation also saves society money when patients are removed from dialysis. In this context, transplant teams use various criteria to select living donors of a gift of life or at least of a higher quality of life. Genetically related living kidney donors have been preferred, in part because of the greater likelihood of successful outcomes. Transplant teams have generally been suspicious of living genetically unrelated donors, not only strangers and acquaintances but spouses and friends, in part because of suspicion of their motives and their competence to decide, as if supererogatory action signals immorality or incompetence. However, opinion surveys indicate that a strong majority of the public holds that the gift of a kidney to a stranger is reasonable and proper and that it should be accepted by the transplant team.[72]

This dispute hinges in part on conceptions of reasonable risk. Researchers report that at least seventeen perioperative deaths of living kidney donors have occurred in the United States and Canada. They conclude that the risk of perioperative mortality is low (estimated at 0.03%). In addition, they found no evidence of progressive renal deterioration or other serious disorders among a group of living kidney donors twenty or more years after their donations, but other studies have identified some risk of less serious long-term morbidity.[73] In view of these data, it is doubtful that transplant teams can view a level of risk as excessive for genetically unrelated living donors, such as friends, acquaintances, and strangers, but low and acceptable for genetically related living donors. The offer to donate a kidney by a friend, acquaintance, or stranger typically does not involve such high risks to the donor that questions should automatically emerge about his or her competence to decide. Some opponents of a policy of accepting donations by acquaintances and strangers argue that such volunteers, pursuing heroic ideals, are emotionally unstable. Proponents, by contrast, contend that kidney donation entails low risks and enhances the donor's self-esteem as well as benefiting another person; thus, it is neither irrational nor unreasonable.

Some heroic offers of organs should be declined by transplant teams, even when the donors' decisions are informed and voluntary and their moral excellence is beyond question. For instance, transplant teams would rightly decline a mother's offer to donate a heart to save her dying child, because the removal of her heart would be fatal, even though we praise a mother's sacrifice of her life in other settings—for example, to try to save her drowning child. Cases of risk, in contrast to certain death, are more controversial. Suppose a woman wants to donate her only remaining kidney for transplantation to her son who is not doing well on dialysis, faces a long wait for a cadaveric kidney, and appears to be at imminent risk of suicide because of his medical problems. Any decision about acceptable levels of sacrifice must carefully and discerningly weigh the factual circumstances—for instance, whether the mother is doomed to die shortly because of some other illness that would not preclude kidney donation, or whether she could do well on dialysis. Under some circumstances it could be justifiable to accept the offer of the kidney, while under other circumstances there could be sufficient reasons to reject it. We are not invariably obligated to help even morally excellent persons realize their heroic ideals.

No consensus exists about the selection or rejection of potential kidney donors who are at additional or elevated risk. If the potential donor has a medical condition that would make the donation extremely dangerous, medical practitioners may justifiably decline the gift—desired by the potential recipient. In other circumstances, if the donor's act would increase the risks for others, the transplant team might again have adequate grounds for declining the gift—for example, if a widow with three small children wants to donate a kidney to a cousin or friend. However, these refusals to accept donations of kidneys should be tempered by an appreciation that the reasonableness of a risk is generally difficult to assess; that, within limits, potential donors should have the final say after receiving all the relevant information; and that the transplant team's refusal to accept the gift may jeopardize some patient's life or quality of life.

One important question is whether physicians and other health care professionals should inquire into the quality of and the motivation behind the decision to donate a kidney for transplantation. The decision to donate may be voluntary, but also could be manipulated or coerced by others. In addition, because the transfer of organs for valuable consideration is illegal, transplant teams should decline any offer of an organ that is based on receiving valuable consideration from the recipient or another party. However, we need to distinguish the provision of financial incentives from the removal of financial disincentives to living donation (for example, reimbursement for lost wages), the latter of which is justifiable. Even if there are sufficient reasons—such as the avoidance of exploitation and commodification—to prohibit the sale of organs, many forms of "rewarded gifting" need not be excluded as an expression of the society's or the recipient's gratitude for the gift of a kidney.

Some significant differences have emerged in the way men and women respond to the opportunity to donate a kidney. First, of the 2,264 living donations of kidneys in 1991, 1,265 (55.8%) donors were women and 999 (44.1%) were men. More research is needed to determine the reasons for this disparity. Second, women and men tend to interpret their acts of kidney donation differently. For men, the decision to donate is more momentous, involves more questioning and ambivalence, and produces more dramatic post-donation reactions of regret or elevated self-esteem, expressed in the evaluation of themselves as "better persons." By contrast, for women, the donation is more taken for granted, with less regret and less perception of the act as "an extraordinary one on her part, as an act that proves her to be a greater person." As Roberta Simmons suggests, living organ donation typically appears to the female as "a simple extension of her usual family obligations, while for the male it is an unusual type of gift." Perhaps these differences emerge because society has traditionally expected the female role to involve altruism and sacrifice within the family, and giving a family member a second chance at life is close psychologically to the experience of giving birth.[74] This interpretation fits with an ethic of care focusing on personal relationships (see Chapter 2). However, feminists would rightly challenge the operative psychosocial norms of obligatory female donation and supererogatory male donation, because these norms appear to reflect differential social power and are in tension with relevant principles of justice.

From the standpoint of the society and of health care professionals, living organ donation must be construed as optional but praiseworthy, even if donors interpret their acts in different terms. Transplant teams need to subject their criteria for living donor selection to careful and public scrutiny to make sure that their own values are not inappropriately incorporated into moral gatekeeping for acts of live organ donation. Within reasonable limits, transplant teams should allow superogatory donations that they previously have excluded.

We can now conclude this discussion of saints, heroes, and moral excellence. We have not said, and do not maintain, that moral saints are more valued or more admirable than moral heroes; but we have proposed some conditions of moral excellence that are typically more stringent for saints than for heroes. We have not considered whether these conditions might point to another and still higher form of moral excellence: the combination of saint and hero in one person. There certainly have been such extraordinary persons, and we could make a case, in light of our continuum analysis, that some of these extraordinary figures are *more excellent* than others. But at this level of exemplariness, such fine distinctions are unhelpful.

Conclusion

In this final chapter we have moved beyond principles, rules, obligations, and rights. Virtues, ideals, and aspirations for moral excellence support and enrich the moral framework developed in the previous chapters. Ideals transcend obligations and rights, and many virtues dispose persons to act in accordance with principles and rules as well as their ideals.

In Chapter 2 we argued that diverse ethical theories often converge to a similar set of principles and rules. It deserves notice at the conclusion of this book that diverse accounts of character ethics often display a similar pattern of convergence and that appeals to principles are often intertwined in these accounts with appeals to the virtues. Aristotle and Hume, for example, often agree in their appeals to and accounts of the virtues; and, although both are primarily virtue theorists, they acknowledge the importance of general normative principles. Kant and Mill, too, exhibit a deep concern with what Mill calls "the general cultivation of nobleness of character."[75] Almost all great ethical theories converge to the conclusion that the most important ingredient in a person's moral life is a developed character that provides the inner motivation and strength to do what is right and good.

Notes

1. This analysis is influenced by Alasdair MacIntyre, *After Virtue: A Study in Moral Theory*, 2d Ed. (Notre Dame, IN: University of Notre Dame Press, 1984), esp. pp. 175–80, and Dorothy Emmet, *Rules, Roles, and Relations* (New York: St. Martin's Press, 1966).

2. A similar thesis is defended in dissimilar ways in Edmund D. Pellegrino, "The Virtuous Physician and the Ethics of Medicine," in *Virtue and Medicine*, ed. Earl Shelp (Dordrecht, the Netherlands: D. Reidel, 1985), pp. 237–56. This volume contains a diverse set of assessments of the virtues in biomedical ethics.

3. Charles L. Bosk, *Forgive and Remember: Managing Medical Failure* (Chicago: University of Chicago Press, 1979). Bosk recognizes a fourth type of error: "quasi-normative errors" based on the attending's special protocols.

4. See Franz J. Ingelfinger, "Arrogance," *New England Journal of Medicine* 303 (December 25, 1980): 1507–11.

5. Thomas Percival, *Medical Ethics; or a Code of Institutes and Precepts, Adapted to the Professional Conduct of Physicians and Surgeons* (Manchester, England: S. Russell, 1803), pp. 165–66.

6. For models of nursing, see Dan W. Brock, "The Nurse–Patient Relation: Some Rights and Duties," in *Nursing: Images and Ideals*, ed. Stuart F. Spicker and Sally Gadow (New York: Spring Publishing Company, 1980), pp. 102–24, and Gerald Winslow, "From Loyalty to Advocacy: A New Metaphor for Nursing," *Hastings Center Report* 14 (June 1984): 32–40. See also Betty J. Winslow and Gerald Winslow, "Integrity and Compromise in Nursing Ethics," *Journal of Medicine and Philosophy* 16 (1991): 307–23.

7. See Lawrence Blum, "Compassion," in *Explaining Emotions*, ed. Amélie Oksenberg Rorty (Berkeley: University of California Press, 1980), and David Hume, *A Dissertation on the Passions*, Sect. III, §§ 4–5 (London, 1772), pp. 208–9.

8. David Hume, *A Treatise of Human Nature*, 2nd Ed., ed. L. A. Selby-Bigge and P. H. Nidditch (Oxford: Clarendon Press, 1978), p. 576.

9. Baruch Brody, "Case No. 25. 'Who is the patient, anyway,': The difficulties of compassion," in *Life and Death Decision Making* (New York: Oxford University Press, 1988), pp. 185–88.

10. Aristotle, *Nicomachean Ethics*, trans. Terence Irwin (Indianapolis, IN: Hackett Publishing Company, 1985), 1106^b15–29, 1141^a15–1144^b17.

11. Leon R. Kass, "Ethical Dilemmas in the Care of the Ill," *Journal of the American Medical Association* 244 (October 17, 1980): 1811; Henry K. Beecher, "Ethics and Clinical Research," *New England Journal of Medicine* 274 (1966): 1354–60.

12. See the instructive analyses in Annette Baier, "Trust and Antitrust," *Ethics* 96 (1986): 231–60; H. J. N. Horsburgh, "Trust and Collective Security," *Ethics* 72 (July, 1962): 252–65, and "The Ethics of Trust," *Philosophical Quarterly* 10 (October 1960): 343–54; and Bernard Barber, *The Logic and Limits of Trust* (New Brunswick, NJ: Rutgers University Press, 1983).

13. Aristotle, *Eudemian Ethics*, 1242^b23–1243^a13, in *The Complete Works of Aristotle*, ed. Jonathan Barnes (Princeton, NJ: Princeton University Press, 1984).

14. See Robert M. Veatch, "Against Virtue: A Deontological Critique of Virtue Theory in Medical Ethics," in *Virtue and Medicine*, ed. Shelp, pp. 329–45.

15. Brody, *Life and Death Decision Making*, p. 35.

16. Thomas Nagel's *The View from Nowhere* (New York: Oxford University Press, 1986) and Bernard Williams's "A Critique of Utilitarianism," in J. J. C. Smart and Williams, *Utilitarianism: For and Against* (Cambridge: Cambridge University Press, 1973), esp. p. 117, have been especially influential. See also Susan Wolf's "Moral Saints," *Journal of Philosophy* 79 (August 1982): 419–39, as discussed below.

17. See C. Everett Koop and Timothy Johnson, *Let's Talk* (Grand Rapids, MI: Zondervan Publishing House, 1992), ch. 3, from which the quotations in the text have been drawn; and C. Everett Koop, *Koop: The Memoirs of America's Family Doctor* (New York: Random House, 1991).

18. See MacIntyre, *After Virtue,* pp. 225ff, and Martin Benjamin, *Splitting the Difference: Compromise and Integrity in Ethics and Politics* (Lawrence: University Press of Kansas, 1990), pp. 59–72.

19. See Jerome B. Schneewind, "Virtue, Narrative, and Community: MacIntyre and Morality," *Journal of Philosophy* 79 (1982): 653–63.

20. A detailed argument to this conclusion is found in Mark S. Halfon, *Integrity: A Philosophical Inquiry* (Philadelphia: Temple University Press, 1989), pts. I–II.

21. Adam Smith argued that a true slave—as distinct from a hired servant—could never possess the virtue of integrity, because the slave's lack of liberty allows no room to set and maintain projects. *An Inquiry into the Nature and Causes of the Wealth of Nations* (Oxford: Clarendon Press, 1979), bk. 4, ch. 7, pt. 2, p. 587.

22. For useful discussions of this question, see Martin Benjamin and Joy Curtis, *Ethics in Nursing,* 3d Ed. (New York: Oxford University Press, 1992), pp. 105–8; and Betty J. Winslow and Gerald R. Winslow, "Integrity and Compromise in Nursing Ethics," pp. 307–23.

23. Adapted from Bernard Williams, "A Critique of Utilitarianism," pp. 97–98.

24. We have here drawn on two sources: Hannah Arendt, *Crises of the Republic* (New York: Harcourt, Brace, Jovanovich, Inc., 1972), p. 62; and John Stuart Mill, *Utilitarianism,* ch. 3, pp. 228–29, and *On Liberty,* ch. 3, p. 263, in *Collected Works of John Stuart Mill,* vols. 10, 18 (Toronto: University of Toronto Press, 1969, 1977).

25. For a discussion of these themes, see Peter Winch, *Moral Integrity* (Oxford: Basil Blackwell, 1968); Bernard Williams, "A Critique of Utilitarianism," esp. pp. 108–18; and Bernard Williams, *Moral Luck: Philosophical Papers 1973–1980* (Cambridge: Cambridge University Press, 1981), esp. pp. 40–53. See also James F. Childress, "Appeals to Conscience," *Ethics* 89 (July 1979): 315–35, from which several of the following points are drawn.

26. Carl H. Fellner, "Organ Donation: For Whose Sake?," *Annals of Internal Medicine* 79 (October 1973): 591.

27. See Larry May, "On Conscience," *American Philosophical Quarterly* 20 (January 1983): 57–67. See also C. D. Broad, "Conscience and Conscientious Action," in *Moral Concepts,* ed. Joel Feinberg (Oxford: Oxford University Press, 1970), pp. 74–79, and Childress, "Appeals to Conscience."

28. See Robert M. Veatch's discussion of this case, *Case Studies in Medical Ethics* (Cambridge, MA: Harvard University Press, 1977), pp. 61–64.

29. Hobbes, *Elements of Law,* ed. Ferdinand Tonnies (London: Simpkin, Marshall and Co., 1889), pt. 1, ch. 6, p. 27; *Leviathan,* ed. William Molesworth (London: J. Bohn, 1837), pt. 2, ch. 29, p. 311.

30. In a celebrated analysis of conscience, Joseph Butler argued in the eighteenth century that insofar as the supreme moral faculty of conscience governs, one lives in

accordance with the dictates of human nature. Obligation is erected on the law of nature in this theory: "Your obligation to obey this law is its being the law of your nature. . . . Conscience does not only offer itself to show us the way we should walk in, but it likewise carries its own authority with it." *Sermons,* in *The Works of Joseph Butler,* ed. W. E. Gladstone (Oxford: Clarendon Press, 1896), vol. II, p. 71. More recently, see the similar doctrine in H. A. Prichard, *Moral Obligation* (Oxford: Clarendon Press, 1949), ch. 1–2.

31. As Jeremy Bentham noted, "Fanaticism never sleeps: . . . it is never stopped by *conscience;* for it has pressed *conscience* into its service." Bentham, *Introduction to the Principles of Morals and Legislation,* ed. J. H. Burns and H. L. A. Hart (London: Athlone Press, 1970), ch. 12, p. 156*n.*

32. See Alan Donagan, *The Theory of Morality* (Chicago: University of Chicago Press, 1977), pp. 131–38.

33. Alastair V. Campbell, *Moral Dilemmas in Medicine,* 2d Ed. (Edinburgh: Churchill Livingstone, 1975), p. 25 (italics added).

34. See Williams, *Moral Luck,* esp. p. 50.

35. See ch. 5, p. 288, and Marc D. Basson, ed., *Rights and Responsibilities in Modern Medicine* (New York: Alan R. Liss, 1981), pp. 135–36.

36. Daniel C. Maguire, "Cooperation with Evil," *Dictionary of Christian Ethics,* 2d Ed., ed. James F. Childress and John Macquarrie (Philadelphia: Westminster Press, 1986), p. 129.

37. *CMCHS: In Combat, In the Community, Saving Lives . . . Together,* available from the Office of the Assistant Secretary of Defense (Health Affairs) at the Pentagon; John F. Beary, Jay C. Bisgard, and Philip C. Armstrong, "The Civilian Military Contingency Hospital System," *New England Journal of Medicine* 306 (September 16, 1982): 738–40; Physicians for Social Responsibility, Executive Committee, "Medical Care in Modern Warfare: A Look at the Pentagon Plan for the Civilian Sector," *New England Journal of Medicine* 306 (1982): 741–42; letters to the editor, *New England Journal of Medicine* 307 (1982): 751–53, 1578; Jay C. Bisgard, "The Obligation to Care for Casualties"; H. Jack Geiger, "Why Survival Plans Are Meaningless"; and James T. Johnson, "The Moral Bases of Contingency Planning," *Hastings Center Report* 12 (April 1982): 15–21. See also *Medical Ethics for the Physician* 1 (October 1986): 6–7, 10.

38. See Natalie Abrams, "Moral Responsibility in Nursing," in *Nursing,* ed. Spicker and Gadow, pp. 148–59.

39. *Application of President and Directors of Georgetown College,* 331 F. 2d 1000 (D.C. Cir.), certiorari denied, 377 U.S. 978 (1964).

40. Even though the New Jersey Bioethics Commission had recommended exemptions for objectors who appeal to "personal religious beliefs and moral convictions," the law enacted only recognizes religiously based conscientious objections. However, in decisions relating to conscientious objectors to military service, the U.S. Supreme Court has broadly interpreted religious beliefs to include beliefs that are not normally considered religious, and it is likely that such a broad interpretation would prevail in a constitutional challenge to the New Jersey statute. See Robert Olick, "Brain Death, Religious Freedom, and Public Policy: New Jersey's Landmark Legislative Initiative," *Kennedy Institute of Ethics Journal* 1 (1991): 275–88, to which we are indebted in our discussion of the New Jersey statute.

41. John Rawls, *A Theory of Justice* (Cambridge, MA: Harvard University Press, 1971), p. 519.

42. Our analysis is indebted to David Heyd, *Supererogation: Its Status in Ethical Theory* (Cambridge: Cambridge University Press, 1982), and to J. O. Urmson, "Saints and Heroes," *Essays in Moral Philosophy,* ed. A. I. Melden (Seattle: University of Washington Press, 1958), pp. 198–216. Other analyses that have influenced our views include John Rawls, *A Theory of Justice,* pp. 116–17, 438–39, 478–85; Joel Feinberg, "Supererogation and Rules," in *Ethics,* ed. Judith J. Thomson and Gerald Dworkin (New York: Harper & Row, 1968), pp. 391–411; Roderick M. Chisholm, "Supererogation and Offense: A Conceptual Scheme for Ethics," *Ratio* 5 (June 1963): 1–14; and Millard Schumaker, *Supererogation: An Analysis and Bibliography* (Edmonton, Alberta: St. Stephen's College, 1977).

43. Albert Camus, *The Plague,* trans. Stuart Gilbert (New York: Alfred A. Knopf, Inc., 1988), p. 278.

44. See Heyd, *Supererogation,* pp. 138–39.

45. The formulation in this sentence relies in part on Rawls, *A Theory of Justice,* p. 117.

46. Feinberg, "Supererogation and Rules," p. 397.

47. See, for example, Bernard Lo, "Obligations to Care for Persons with Human Immunodeficiency Virus," *Issues in Law & Medicine* 4 (1988): 367–81; John Arras, "The Fragile Web of Responsibility: AIDS and the Duty to Treat," *Hastings Center Report* 18 (April/May 1988): S10–S20; Raanan Gillon, "Do Doctors Owe a Special Duty of Beneficence to their Patients?," *Journal of Medical Ethics* 12 (1986): 171–73.

48. Abigail Zuger and Steven Miles record a long history of ambiguity regarding the level of care owed to patients with contagious epidemic diseases. "Physicians, AIDS, and Occupational Risk: Historic Traditions and Ethical Obligations," *Journal of the American Medical Association* 258 (October 9, 1987): 1924–1928.

49. See George J. Annas, "Legal Risks and Responsibilities of Physicians in the AIDS Epidemic," *Hastings Center Report* 18 (April–May 1988): 26S–32S; American Medical Association, Council on Ethical and Judicial Affairs, "Ethical Issues Involved in the Growing AIDS Crisis," *Journal of the American Medical Association* 259 (March 4, 1988): 1360–61.

50. Health and Public Policy Committee, American College of Physicians and Infectious Diseases Society of America, "The Acquired Immunodeficiency Syndrome (AIDS) and Infection with the Human Immunodeficiency Virus (HIV)," *Annals of Internal Medicine* 108 (1988): 460–61; Norman Daniels, "Duty to Treat or Right to Refuse?," *Hastings Center Report* 21 (March–April 1991): 36–46; Edmund Pellegrino, "Altruism, Self-interest, and Medical Ethics," *Journal of the American Medical Association* 258 (1987): 1939; and Pellegrino, "Character, Virtue, and Self-Interest in the Ethics of the Professions," *Journal of Contemporary Health Law and Policy* 5 (1989): 53–73, esp. 70–71.

51. See Gregory Mellema, *Beyond the Call of Duty: Supererogation, Obligation, and Offence* (Albany: State University of New York Press, 1991), pp. 7, 38, 177–78.

52. See Ezekiel Emanuel, "Do Physicians Have An Obligation to Treat Patients with AIDS?" *New England Journal of Medicine* 318 (June 23, 1988): 1686–90.

53. Heyd, *Supererogation,* ch. 3; Marcia Baron, "Kantian Ethics and Supererogation," *Journal of Philosophy* 84 (1987): 237–62.

54. Alan Donagan, "Is There a Credible Form of Utilitarianism?," in *Contemporary Utilitarianism,* ed. Michael D. Bayles (Garden City, NY: Anchor Books, and Doubleday Company, Inc., 1968), pp. 187–202. Donagan's *objection* appears to be

accepted as a point in *favor* of utilitarianism by Christopher New, who finds saintly and heroic acts obligatory. "Saints, Heroes, and Utilitarians," *Philosophy* 49 (1974): 179–89, esp. 183–84.

55. Heyd, *Supererogation,* pp. 74, 88, 105. Heyd offers some speculative ways out of Kant's problems on pp. 61–72, esp. 68–71.

56. Urmson recognized part of this problem in "Saints and Heroes," pp. 206, 214. A telling sign of such imbalance is found in contemporary utilitarianism, which as much as any ethical theory makes exceedingly strong demands. Despite some brilliant passages on moral excellence in Mill, there has never been a systematic or even sustained utilitarian treatise on supererogation or conceptions of moral excellence.

57. Several of these sources are cited and criticized in Richard B. Brandt, "Morality and Its Critics," chap. 5 in his *Morality, Utilitarianism, and Rights* (Cambridge: Cambridge University Press, 1992). Brandt develops a different line of criticism than we present below.

58. John Stuart Mill, *Considerations on Representative Government,* in *The Collected Works of John Stuart Mill,* vol. 19 (Toronto: University of Toronto Press, 1977), ch. 3, p. 409.

59. See Elizabeth Pybus, "Saints and Heroes," *Philosophy* 57 (1982): 193–200; and Christopher New, "Saints, Heroes, and Utilitarians."

60. John Berger (and Jean Mohr, photographer), *A Fortunate Man: The Story of a Country Doctor* (London: Allen Lane, the Penguin Press, 1967), esp. pp. 48, 74, 82f, 93f, 123–25, 135. Lawrence Blum directed us to this book.

61. Our conditions of moral excellence are indebted to Lawrence A. Blum, "Moral Exemplars," *Midwest Studies in Philosophy* 13 (1988): 204.

62. Our second and third conditions are influenced by the characterization of a saint in Wolf's "Moral Saints," pp. 420–23.

63. Jay Katz, ed., *Experimentation with Human Beings* (New York: Russell Sage Foundation, 1972), pp. 136–40.

64. Philip J. Hilts, "French Doctor Testing AIDS Vaccine on Self," *Washington Post,* March 10, 1987, p. A7. For a thorough discussion of self-experimentation in medicine, see Lawrence K. Altman, *Who Goes First?: The Story of Self-Experimentation in Medicine* (New York: Random House, 1987).

65. Urmson, "Saints and Heroes," pp. 200–201.

66. Substantially this point is made against Urmson by Blum, "Moral Exemplars," p. 207.

67. Urmson, "Saints and Heroes," pp. 201–2.

68. In a discussion of nonreligious saints, Edith Wyschogrod defines a "saintly life . . . as one in which compassion for the Other, irrespective of cost to the saint, is the primary trait." She contends that a postmodernist ethic must look not to moral theory but to the life narratives of saints for guidance. *Saints and Postmodernism: Revisioning Moral Philosophy* (Chicago: University of Chicago Press, 1990), p. xxiii.

69. Susan Wolf, "Moral Saints," esp. pp. 419–27. For critical responses to Wolf's argument, see Robert Merrihew Adams, "Saints," *Journal of Philosophy* 81 (July 1984): 392–401; and Blum, "Moral Exemplars," pp. 212–15.

70. John Lantos and Mark Siegler, "Re-evaluating Donor Criteria: Live Donors," in *The Surgeon General's Workshop on Increasing Organ Donation: Background Pa-*

pers, U.S. Department of Health & Human Services, Public Health Service (July 8–10, 1991), p. 280, emphasis added.

71. See Aaron Spital, "Living Organ Donation: Shifting Responsibility," *Archives of Internal Medicine* 151 (February 1991): 234.

72. See Aaron Spital and Max Spital, "Living Kidney Donation: Attitudes Outside the Transplant Center," *Archives of Internal Medicine* 148 (May 1988): 1077–80, and Carl H. Fellner and Shalom H. Schwartz, "Altruism in Disrepute," *New England Journal of Medicine* 284 (March 18, 1971): 582–85.

73. John S. Najarian et al., "20 Years or More of Follow-up of Living Kidney Donors," *The Lancet* 340 (October 3, 1992): 807–10.

74. Roberta G. Simmons, "Psychological Reactions to Giving a Kidney," in *Psychonephrology* 1, ed. Norman B. Levy (New York: Plenum Publishing Co., 1981), p. 235.

75. Mill, *Utilitarianism,* ch. 2, p. 213.

Appendix

Cases in Biomedical Ethics

Case 1: The Tarasoff Case

Facts in the Case

On October 27, 1969, Prosenjit Poddar killed Tatiana Tarasoff. Plaintiffs, Tatiana's parents, allege that two months earlier Poddar confided his intention to kill Tatiana to Dr. Lawrence Moore, a psychologist employed by the Cowell Memorial Hospital at the University of California at Berkeley. They allege that on Moore's request, the campus police briefly detained Poddar, but released him when he appeared rational. They further claim that Dr. Harvey Powelson, Moore's superior, then directed that no further action be taken to detain Poddar. No one warned plaintiffs of Tatiana's peril.

Plaintiffs, Tatiana's mother and father, . . . [allege] that on August 20, 1969, Poddar was a voluntary outpatient receiving therapy at Cowell Memorial Hospital. Poddar informed Moore, his therapist, that he was going to kill an unnamed girl, readily identifiable as Tatiana, when she returned home from spending the summer in Brazil. Moore, with the concurrence of Dr. Gold, who had initially examined Poddar, and Dr. Yandell, assistant to the director of the

This case is edited from *Tarasoff v. Regents of the University of California,* 17 Cal.3d 425 (1976); 131 California Reporter 14 (July 1, 1976). The language is that of the court. The facts and majority opinion are written by Justice Tobriner. The dissenting opinion is written by Justice Clark.

department of psychiatry, decided that Poddar should be committed for observation in a mental hospital. Moore orally notified Officers Atkinson and Teel of the campus police that he would request commitment. He then sent a letter to Police Chief William Beall requesting the assistance of the police department in securing Poddar's confinement.

Officers Atkinson, Brownrigg, and Halleran took Poddar into custody, but, satisfied that Poddar was rational, released him on his promise to stay away from Tatiana. Powelson, director of the department of psychiatry at Cowell Memorial Hospital, then asked the police to return Moore's letter, directed that all copies of the letter and notes that Moore had taken as therapist be destroyed, and "ordered no action to place Prosenjit Poddar in a 72-hour treatment and evaluation facility."

Plaintiff's second cause of action, entitled "Failure to Warn of a Dangerous Patient," . . . adds the assertion that defendants negligently permitted Poddar to be released from police custody without "notifying the parents of Tatiana Tarasoff that their daughter was in grave danger from Prosenjit Poddar." Poddar persuaded Tatiana's brother to share an apartment with him near Tatiana's residence; shortly after her return from Brazil, Poddar went to her residence and killed her.

Majority Opinion in the Case   TOBRINER, Justice

We shall explain that defendant therapists cannot escape liability merely because Tatiana herself was not their patient. When a therapist determines, or pursuant to the standards of his profession should determine, that his patient presents a serious danger of violence to another, he incurs an obligation to use reasonable care to protect the intended victim against such danger. The discharge of this duty may require the therapist to take one or more of various steps, depending upon the nature of the case. Thus it may call for him to warn the intended victim or others likely to apprise the victim of the danger, to notify the police, or to take whatever other steps are reasonably necessary under the circumstances. . . .

In each instance the adequacy of the therapist's conduct must be measured against the traditional negligence standard of the rendition of reasonable care under the circumstances. . . . In sum, the therapist owes a legal duty not only to his patient, but also to his patient's would-be victim and is subject in both respects to scrutiny by judge and jury. . . . Some of the alternatives open to the therapist, such as warning the victim, will not result in the drastic consequences of depriving the patient of his liberty. Weighing the uncertain and conjectural character of the alleged damage done the patient by such a warning against the peril to the victim's life, we conclude that professional inaccuracy in predicting violence cannot negate the therapist's duty to protect the threatened victim. . . .

We recognize the public interest in supporting effective treatment of mental illness and in protecting the rights of patients to privacy. . . . and the consequent public importance of safeguarding the confidential character of psychotherapeutic communication. Against this interest, however, we must weigh the public interest in safety from violent assault.

The revelation of a communication under the above circumstances is not a breach of trust or a violation of professional ethics; as stated in the Principles of Medical Ethics of the American Medical Association (1957), section 9: ''A physician may not reveal the confidence entrusted to him in the course of medical attendance . . . unless he is required to do so by law or unless it becomes necessary in order to protect the welfare of the individual or of the community.'' We conclude that the public policy favoring protection of the confidential character of patient–psychotherapist communications must yield to the extent to which disclosure is essential to avert danger to others. The protective privilege ends where the public peril begins.

Dissenting Opinion in the Case   CLARK, Justice (dissenting)

Until today's majority opinion, both legal and medical authorities have agreed that confidentiality is essential to effectively treat the mentally ill, and that imposing a duty on doctors to disclose patient threats to potential victims would greatly impair treatment. . . .

Policy generally determines duty. Principal policy considerations include foreseeability of harm, certainty of the plaintiff's injury, proximity of the defendant's conduct to the plaintiff's injury, moral blame attributable to defendant's conduct, prevention of future harm, burden on the defendant, and consequences to the community.

Overwhelming policy considerations weigh against imposing a duty on psychotherapists to warn a potential victim against harm. While offering virtually no benefit to society, such a duty will frustrate psychiatric treatment, invade fundamental patient rights and increase violence.

The importance of psychiatric treatment and its need for confidentiality have been recognized by this court. ''It is clearly recognized that the very practice of psychiatry vitally depends upon the reputation in the community that the psychiatrist will not tell. . . . ''

Assurance of confidentiality is important for three reasons.

DETERRENCE FROM TREATMENT. First, without substantial assurance of confidentiality, those requiring treatment will be deterred from seeking assistance. It remains an unfortunate fact in our society that people seeking psychiatric guidance tend to become stigmatized. Apprehension of such stigma—apparently increased by the propensity of people considering treatment to see themselves in the worst possible light—creates a well-recognized reluctance to seek aid. This reluctance is alleviated by the psychiatrist's assurance of confidentiality.

FULL DISCLOSURE. Second, the guarantee of confidentiality is essential in eliciting the full disclosure necessary for effective treatment. The psychiatric patient approaches treatment with conscious and unconscious inhibitions against revealing his innermost thoughts. . . .

SUCCESSFUL TREATMENT. Third, even if the patient fully discloses his thoughts, assurance that the confidential relationship will not be breached is necessary to maintain his trust in his psychiatrist—the very means by which treatment is effected. . . .

Given the importance of confidentiality to the practice of psychiatry, it becomes clear the duty to warn imposed by the majority will cripple the use and effectiveness of psychiatry. Many people, potentially violent—yet susceptible to treatment—will be deterred from seeking it; those seeking it will be inhibited from making revelations necessary to effective treatment; and, forcing the psychiatrist to violate the patient's trust will destroy the interpersonal relationship by which treatment is effected.

VIOLENCE AND CIVIL COMMITMENT. By imposing a duty to warn, the majority contributes to the danger to society of violence by the mentally ill and greatly increases the risk of civil commitment—the total deprivation of liberty—of those who should not be confined. The impairment of treatment and risk of improper commitment resulting from the new duty to warn will not be limited to a few patients but will extend to a large number of the mentally ill. Although under existing psychiatric procedures only a relatively few receiving treatment will ever present a risk of violence, the number making threats is huge, and it is the latter group—not just the former—whose treatment will be impaired and whose risk of commitment will be increased.

Case 2: Nondisclosure of Prostate Cancer

A sixty-nine-year-old man, estranged from his children and with no other living relatives, underwent a routine physical examination in preparation for a brief and much anticipated trip to Australia. The physician suspected a serious problem and ordered more extensive testing, including further blood analysis (detailing an acid phosphatase), a bone scan, and a prostate biopsy. The results were conclusive: The man had an inoperable, incurable carcinoma—a small

This case was prepared especially for this volume. David Bloom, M.D., was a contributing consultant.

prostate nodule commonly referred to as cancer of the prostate. The carcinoma was not yet advanced and was relatively slow growing. Later, after the disease had progressed, it would be possible to provide good palliative treatment. Blood tests and x-ray films showed the patient's renal function to be normal. (The physician consulted with the urologist who had performed the prostate biopsy in order to confirm the diagnosis.)

The physician had treated this patient for many years and knew that he was fragile in several respects. The man was neurotic and had an established history of psychiatric disease—although he functioned well in society and clearly was capable of rational thought and decisionmaking. He had recently suffered a severe depressive reaction, during which he behaved irrationally and attempted suicide. This episode immediately followed the death of his wife, who died after a difficult and protracted battle with cancer. It was clear that he had not been equipped to deal with his wife's death, and he had been hospitalized for a short period before the suicide attempt. Just as he was getting back on his feet, the opportunity to go to Australia materialized, and it was the first excitement he had experienced in several years.

This patient had a history of suffering prolonged and serious depression whenever informed of serious health problems. He worried excessively and often could not exercise rational control over his deliberations and decisions. His physician thought that disclosure of the carcinoma under his present fragile state would almost certainly cause further irrational behavior and render the patient incapable of thinking clearly about his medical situation.

When the testing had been completed and the results were known, the patient returned to his physician. He asked nervously, ``Am I OK?'' Without waiting for a response, he asked, ``I don't have cancer, do I?'' Believing his patient would not suffer from or even be aware of his problem while in Australia, the physician answered, ``You're as good as you were ten years ago.'' He was worried about telling such a bald lie but firmly believed that it was justified.

Case 3: A Son's Request for Nondisclosure

Mr. Johnson, a man in his late sixties, is brought to his physician by his son who is concerned about his father's apparent problems in interpreting and dealing with what used to be normal day-to-day activities. He worries that his father may have Alzheimer's disease, but he asks the physician not to tell his father if Alzheimer's disease is confirmed as the diagnosis. After the appro-

This case has been formulated on the basis of and incorporates language from Margaret A. Drickamer and Mark S. Lachs, ``Should Patients with Alzheimer's Disease Be Told Their Diagnosis?'' *New England Journal of Medicine* 326 (April 2, 1992): 947–51.

priate tests, the physician believes that she has a firm diagnosis of Alzheimer's disease and discusses with a nurse and a social worker the son's "impassioned plea" not to tell his father the diagnosis. The nurse notes that a strong consensus has developed over the last twenty-five years about disclosing the diagnosis of cancer to patients and wonders whether the same reasoning applies to disclosure to patients with Alzheimer's disease.

The physician responds that "many of the arguments that support telling the patient with cancer assume the relative accuracy of diagnosis, an array of therapeutic options, a predictable natural history, and a fully competent patient." She is not sure that these arguments apply to patients with Alzheimer's disease because the diagnosis is made on the basis of clinical criteria and diagnostic algorithms (documented through autopsies to be as high as 92 percent), the prognosis is "unusually imprecise," life expectancy varies greatly, therapeutic options are limited, and patients with Alzheimer's disease "inevitably have an erosion of decision-making capacity and competency" and may also have limited coping mechanisms.

The social worker adds that, although there is empirical evidence that most patients now want to know if they have cancer, there is less evidence about the preferences of patients with Alzheimer's disease. Nevertheless, the nurse responds, "It is important to maximize individual autonomy whenever possible. We can be truthful with our patients about what we think is happening and our degree of certainty, whatever it is. Mr. Johnson may be able to make an advance directive about treatment and nontreatment. At the very least, he may be able to express his feelings and fears." "But wait," the physician responds, "Mr. Johnson will lose his ability to change his mind once he loses his ability to make decisions." "That's true," the nurse agrees, "but still the best indication we could have of what he would want under those circumstances would be his advance directive." The physician, nurse, and social worker agree to discuss the case tomorrow before deciding what to do.

Case 4: A Family of Potential Kidney Donors

A forty-year-old widow with chronic glomerulonephritis has been on maintenance hemodialysis for ten years. Over the past two years she has been progressively deteriorating from multiple complications, including severe renal osteodystrophy, inability to obtain adequate blood access, and malnutrition from intermittent depression. Peritoneal dialysis cannot be accomplished because of multiple abdominal surgical procedures with adhesions. Her physician has recommended transplantation because he feels she will not survive over four to six months on dialysis.

A case history at St. Francis Hospital, Honolulu, written by Arnold W. Siemsen, M.D., Institute of Renal Diseases.

The patient has four children (ages eleven to fourteen years) and wants a transplant to allow her to live and provide for the future well-being of her children.

The patient's forty-four-year-old brother is a farmer with eight children. He refused to donate or be tissue typed. The patient has a forty-two-year-old sister who was willing to donate but was not tissue typed because she has been an insulin-requiring diabetic for ten years.

The patient also has a thirty-five-year-old mentally retarded brother who has been institutionalized since age eight. This brother is an A match with four antigens being identified; his ABO blood type is compatible. He is so severely retarded that he cannot comprehend or understand any of the risks of nephrectomy. He is able to take care of his own personal needs and ambulate with guidance. He neither recognizes his own family members nor interacts with medical staff. The patient would regularly drive three hundred miles to see her brother four times per year until twelve years ago, when her own personal and family needs reduced the frequency to one to two times per year. She has not seen her brother for three years, because of her own medical illnesses. At the present time she feels she has an obligation to her brother, but there is no particular closeness.

Her fourteen-year-old daughter would like to donate a kidney, even though she is a two-antigen mismatch. Her ABO blood type is compatible. The daughter has demonstrated a perceptive, thorough, and reasonably unemotional grasp of her mother's situation and needs, and of the seriousness of her own potential donation.

The patient's older brother and sister feel the donor should be the younger, mentally retarded brother. The diabetic sister is the legal guardian of the retarded brother. Both parents are dead. The patient has been on the cadaveric transplant waiting list for two years.

The following statements are reasonable projections based on known data:

	2–yr. kidney survival (%)	2–yr. patient survival (%)
Retarded brother to patient	70	85
Minor child to patient	60	75
Cadaveric to patient	40	65

Case 5: The Spring Case

In November 1977, seventy-eight-year-old Earle Spring suffered a mild scratch on the instep of his foot. A fiercely independent outdoorsman, he left the cut

This case was prepared by John J. Paris, S.J. It derives from his "Death, Dying, and the Courts: The Travesty and Tragedy of the Earle Spring Case," *Linacre Quarterly* 49 (February 1982): 26–41.

unattended until his foot finally became gangrenous. Hospitalization was followed by pneumonia and then a diagnosis of kidney failure. After undergoing three five-hour dialysis sessions a week, Spring soon improved enough to return home. Meanwhile, his mental deterioration, which had been diagnosed before his injury as "chronic organic brain syndrome," became pronounced.

After more than a year of treatment, the nephrologist informed Spring's son, Robert, that his father was not benefiting from dialysis. He suggested it may have been a mistake to have initiated it on a man his age and that it might be best if the treatments were ended. The son and the wife agreed with the physician and requested that the treatments be stopped. However, because of the Massachusetts Supreme Judicial Court's 1977 *Saikewicz* ruling, decisions of such significance in that state had to be made by courts rather than by families and physicians.

On January 25, 1979, Robert Spring, who had been appointed temporary guardian, petitioned the Franklin County Probate Court for an order to terminate the hemodialysis treatments. A guardian *ad litem,* an attorney appointed by the court to represent the best interests of the patient, was given the responsibility for presenting "all reasonable arguments in favor of administering treatment to prolong the life of the individual involved."

Mark I. Berson, Spring's guardian *ad litem,* insisted (contrary to *Saikewicz*) that the court not render a "substituted judgment" (a statement of what Spring himself would have wanted) without some evidence from Spring's lucid moments on that subject. On May 15, 1979, Judge Keedy entered a judgment permitting the temporary guardian, Robert Spring, "to refrain from authorizing further life-prolonging medical treatment" for his father. Attorney Berson was not satisfied that there was sufficient evidence that Spring would have wanted to terminate the treatments, and he appealed. Judge Keedy vacated his original order and on July 2 entered a new one to the effect that Spring's wife and son, together with the attending physician, were to make the decision. Again Berson appealed.

The court of appeals upheld the probate court's action. It rejected Berson's position on the need for an express statement of intent to withhold treatment. In its words, "Such a contention would largely stifle the very rights of privacy and personal dignity which the *Saikewicz* case sought to secure for incompetent persons." Berson appealed.

On January 10, the supreme judicial court heard the case. It concluded that the trial judge's finding that Earle Spring "would, if competent, choose not to receive the life-prolonging treatment" was correct. But, unlike the trial judge and the court of appeals, the supreme judicial court found that the facts "bring the case within the rule of *Saikewicz.*" It therefore held "it was an error to delegate the decision to the attending physician and the ward's wife and son."

Once again, Spring's guardian was directed by the probate court to "refrain from authorizing any further life-prolonging treatment" for his father.

Meanwhile, it was becoming clear that the staff of the Holyoke Geriatric Center were, in their own words, "appalled over the decision to stop the dialysis treatment." Two nurses on the three p.m. to eleven p.m. shift asked Spring if he wanted to die. Reportedly, he replied, "No." Although a psychiatrist had previously evaluated Spring as "incompetent," the nurses taking his statement as proof of Spring's desires brought their story to a local newspaper, which used it as headline news. Berson responded immediately. On the basis of an affidavit filed by a right-to-life group, he petitioned Judge Keedy to reinstate the dialysis treatments until new evidence of Spring's competence could be gathered. The right-to-life activists hired a lawyer to petition the probate court to admit them as parties to the case. In the sixth judicial determination on Spring's case, Judge Keedy denied the petition to reinstate dialysis treatment. Berson appealed once more.

This appeal was granted by the supreme judicial court, which then appointed five psychiatrists and geriatric specialists to determine Spring's mental status. During that time, Spring had been admitted to the hospital, suffering from an infection and pneumonia. He responded to medical treatment and returned to the nursing home on March 25, but in an extremely weakened condition. The following Sunday, the day before the competency hearing was scheduled, Earle Spring died. The next day, the five court-appointed physicians filed their report: Spring "was suffering from such profound mental impairment that he had no idea where he was or what was going on. The dementia was not related to the kidney failure, was untreatable, and irreversible." Had he not died the day before, the responsibility for deciding to stop the dialysis treatments would have rested where it had fourteen months previously—with the court.

Case 6: The Wanglie Case

Mrs. Helga Wanglie, an eighty-five year old resident of a nursing home, was taken to Hennepin County Medical Center on January 1, 1990, to receive emergency treatment for her dyspnea that resulted from chronic bronchiectasis. Emergency intubation was provided, and Mrs. Wanglie was placed on a respirator. During the period that followed, she was not able to communicate clearly, but she did occasionally acknowledge discomfort, and she recognized

Sources: Steven H. Miles, "Informed Demand for Non-Beneficial Medical Treatment," *New England Journal of Medicine* 325 (August 15, 1991): 512–515, with additional information from Ronald E. Cranford, "Helga Wanglie's Ventilator," *Hastings Center Report* 21 (July/August 1991): 23–24; "Brain-Damaged Woman at Center of Lawsuit Over Life-Support Dies," *New York Times* (July 6, 1991), p. 8; and Edward Walsh, "Recasting 'Right to Die'," *Washington Post* (May 29, 1991), pp. A1, A6.

her family members who visited. The staff was unable to wean her from the respirator, and in May she was transferred to a chronic care hospital. A week later, during another effort to wean her from the respirator, her heart stopped. She was resuscitated and then taken to another hospital for intensive care. When she did not regain consciousness, a physician indicated to the family that it would be appropriate to consider withdrawing the life-support systems. The family responded by transferring her to the Hennepin County Medical Center on May 31. Tests over the next two weeks convinced the medical staff that she was in a persistent vegetative state (PVS) as a result of severe anoxic encephalopathy. Her care included maintenance on the respirator, with repeated courses of antibiotics, frequent airway suctioning, tube feedings, an air flotation bed, and biochemical monitoring.

During June and July 1990, physicians indicated to the family that the life-sustaining treatment was not benefiting the patient and recommended that it be withdrawn. However, Mrs. Wanglie's husband, daughter, and son insisted on continued treatment. As reported by Dr. Steven Miles, the family stated that "physicians should not play God, that the patient would not be better off dead, that removing her life support showed moral decay in our civilization, and that a miracle could occur." According to her husband, Mrs. Wanglie had never indicated her preferences about life-sustaining treatment. Nevertheless, with reluctance, the family did accept a do-not-resuscitate (DNR) order because of the improbability that Mrs. Wanglie would survive a cardiac arrest. The family declined the counseling recommended by an ethics committee consultant and asked in late July that the question of removal of the respirator not be raised again.

In August the nurses involved in Mrs. Wanglie's care expressed their consensus view that continued life support was inappropriate. In October 1990, a new attending physician in consultation with specialists confirmed that the patient's cerebral and pulmonary conditions were permanent and concluded that she was "at the end of her life and that the respirator was 'non-beneficial,' in that it could not heal her lungs, palliate her suffering, or enable this unconscious and permanently respirator-dependent woman to experience the benefit of the life afforded by respirator support." He did not characterize the respirator as "futile," because it could prolong her life.

In November, the physician, with the concurrence of Steven Miles, the ethics consultant for the hospital since August, informed the family that he was unwilling to continue the respirator. When the husband rejected this option and also refused to transfer the patient to another facility or to seek a court order to require this exceptional treatment, the hospital indicated that it would seek a court determination about its obligation to continue treatment. A follow-up conference two weeks later indicated that neither party had budged. The family had hired an attorney, and the husband indicated that the patient had consistently indicated her desire for respirator support under such conditions.

The Hennepin County Board of Commissioners, who serve as the medical center's board of directors, by a 4-to-3 vote authorized the hospital to go to court to try to resolve the dispute. Despite their efforts during the first several months of 1991, the family could not locate another facility that would accept Mrs. Wanglie. Even those with space declined because of her poor prognosis for rehabilitation.

The hospital first asked the court to appoint an independent conservator to determine whether the respirator was benefiting the patient. Then the hospital intended to seek a second hearing to determine whether it was obligated to continue the respirator if the conservator held that it was nonbeneficial. The trial court held a hearing in late May and on July 1, 1991, appointed Mr. Wanglie as the conservator, as he had requested, on the grounds that he could best represent his wife's interests. The court did not address the speculative question about whether a request to stop treatment would have been granted, because no request had been made, and the hospital indicated that it would continue the respirator because of the uncertainty about its legal obligation to provide it.

However, the patient died three days later (on July 4) of multisystem organ failure as a result of septicemia. The family did not want an autopsy and affirmed that the patient's care had been excellent, but, as the daughter put it, "we just had a disagreement on ethics." In the words of Mr. Wanglie, "We felt that when she was ready to go that the good Lord would call her, and I would say that's what happened."

The hospital and the county had no financial interest in withdrawing treatment to allow Mrs. Wanglie to die, because Medicare paid most of the $200,000 bill for the first hospitalization, and a private insurer paid the $500,000 bill for the second hospitalization.

Case 7: Willowbrook

The Willowbrook State School was an institution for mentally retarded children on Staten Island, New York. The number of its residents increased from two

Sources: Saul Krugman and Joan P. Giles, "Viral Hepatitis: New Light on an Old Disease," *Journal of the American Medical Association* 212 (May 10, 1970): 1019–29; Henry Beecher, *Research and the Individual* (Boston: Little, Brown, 1970); letters to the editor of *Lancet:* by Stephen Goldby (April 10, 1971), Saul Krugman (May 8, 1971), Edward N. Willey (May 22, 1971), Benjamin Pasamanick (May 22, 1971), Joan Giles (May 29, 1971), M. H. Pappworth (June 5, 1971), Geoffrey Edsall (July 10, 1971); F. J. Ingelfinger, "Ethics of Experiments on Children," *New England Journal*

hundred in 1949 to more than six thousand in 1963. Hepatitis was first noticed among the children in 1949, and in 1954 Dr. Saul Krugman and his associates, including Dr. Joan Giles and Dr. Jack Hammond, began to study the disease in the institution. Of the fifty-two hundred residents at Willowbrook during one part of their study, thirty-eight hundred were severely retarded, with IQs of less than 20. In addition, at least three thousand of the children were not toilet-trained. Because infectious hepatitis is transmitted via the fecal-oral route, and because susceptible children were constantly admitted to the institution, contagious hepatitis was persistent and endemic.

As Dr. Krugman (1971) describes the situation, "viral hepatitis is so prevalent that newly admitted susceptible children become infected within 6 to 12 months after entry in the institution. These children are a source of infection for the personnel who care for them and for their families if they visit with them. We were convinced that the solution of the hepatitis problem in this institution was dependent on the acquisition of new knowledge leading to the development of an effective immunizing agent. The achievements with small pox, diphtheria, poliomyelitis, and more recently measles represent dramatic illustrations of this approach."

Krugman continues, "It is well known that viral hepatitis in children is milder and more benign than the same disease in adults. Experience has revealed that hepatitis in institutionalized, mentally retarded children is also mild, in contrast to measles which is a more severe disease when it occurs in institutional epidemics involving the mentally retarded. Our proposal to expose a small number of newly admitted children [ultimately 750 to 800 children were involved altogether] to the Willowbrook strains of hepatitis virus was justified in our opinion for the following reasons: (1) they were bound to be exposed to the same strains under the natural conditions existing in the institution; (2) they would be admitted to a special, well-equipped, and well-staffed unit where they would be isolated from exposure to other infectious diseases which were prevalent in the institution—namely, shigellosis, parasitic infections, and respiratory infections—thus, their exposure in the hepatitis unit would be associated with less risk than the type of institutional exposure where multiple infections could occur; (3) they were likely to have a subclinical infection followed by immunity to the particular hepatitis virus; and (4) only children with parents who gave informed consent would be included."

Critics have leveled several charges against the Willowbrook hepatitis studies. First, some contend that it is "indefensible to give potentially dangerous

of Medicine 288 (April 12, 1973): 791–92; Saul Krugman, "The Willowbrook Hepatitis Studies Revisited: Ethical Aspects," *Reviews of Infectious Diseases* 8 (January–February 1986): 157–62.

infected material to children, particularly those who were mentally retarded, with or without parental consent, when no benefit to the child could conceivably result'' (Goldby). Hence, these critics reject the claim by Krugman and Giles that "the artificial induction of hepatitis implies a 'therapeutic' effect because of the immunity which is conferred.'' The ground for rejecting this claim is that most of the children would have become infected anyway and that this therapeutic effect is not different from what the natural environment would have bestowed. Thus, one major question is whether this experiment offered some therapeutic benefit to the subjects themselves or only to others. The aim of the study was to determine the period of infectivity of infectious hepatitis. Even if the experiment produced good results, as it did (see Krugman, 1986), critics contend that an experiment is justified not by its results but "is ethical or not at its inception'' (Beecher). In this case, "immunization was not the purpose of these Willowbrook experiments but merely a by-product that incidentally proved beneficial to the victims'' (Pappworth).

Second, critics contend that there were alternative ways to control hepatitis in the institution. According to the head of the State Department of Mental Hygiene in New York, for much of the period of the experiment a gamma-globulin inoculation program had already reduced the incidence of viral hepatitis in Willowbrook by eighty to eighty-five percent (Beecher). And the pediatrician's duty is to improve the situation, not to take advantage of it for experimental purposes (Goldby).

Third, questions have been raised about whether the parents' consent for their children to participate in the research was informed and voluntary. Originally, information was conveyed to individual parents by letter or personal interview, but later information was disclosed through a detailed discussion of the project with groups of six to eight parents who were invited to enroll their children in the research. Krugman and Giles contend that the "group method'' enabled them "to obtain more thorough informed consent.'' In either setting, "it was not clear whether any or all parents were told that hepatitis sometimes progresses to fatal liver destruction or that there is a possibility that cirrhosis developing later in life may have had its origin in earlier hepatitis'' (Beecher). Serious questions emerged about the voluntariness of parental consent when parents of prospective residents of Willowbrook were told in late 1964 that overcrowding prevented further admissions but were subsequently informed, often within a week or so, that there were some vacancies in the hepatitis unit and that if the parents wanted to volunteer their children for the research project the children could be admitted to Willowbrook.

Defenders of Willowbrook reject most of these criticisms and ask "is it not proper and ethical to carry out experiments in children, which would apparently incur no greater risk than the children were likely to run by nature, in which the children generally receive better medical care when artificially infected than if they had been naturally infected, and in which the parents as well as the physician feel that a significant contribution to the future well-being of similar children is likely to result from the studies?'' (Edsall).

Case 8: The Saikewicz case

By 1976, sixty-seven-year-old Joseph Saikewicz had lived in state institutions for more than forty years. His IQ was ten, and his mental age was approximately two years and eight months. He could communicate only by gestures and grunts, and he responded only to gestures or physical contacts. He appeared to be unaware of dangers and became disoriented when removed from familiar surroundings.

His health was generally good until April 1976, when he was diagnosed as having acute myeloblastic monocytic leukemia, which is invariably fatal. In approximately thirty to fifty percent of cases of this type of leukemia, chemotherapy can bring about temporary remission, which usually lasts between two and thirteen months. The results are poorer for patients older than sixty. In addition, chemotherapy often has serious side effects, including anemia and infections.

At the petition of the Belchertown State School, where Saikewicz was located, the probate court appointed a guardian *ad litem* with authority to make the necessary decisions concerning the patient's care and treatment. The guardian *ad litem* noted that Saikewicz's illness was incurable, that chemotherapy had significant adverse side effects and discomfort, and that Saikewicz could not understand the treatment or the resulting pain. For all these reasons, he concluded ''that not treating Mr. Saikewicz would be in his best interests.'' The Supreme Judicial Court of Massachusetts upheld this decision on July 9, 1976 (although its opinion was not issued until November 28, 1977). Mr. Saikewicz died on September 4, 1976.

This case is drawn from *Superintendent of Belchertown v. Saikewicz*, Mass. 370 N.E. 2d 417 (1977).

Case 9: The Brophy Case

Paul E. Brophy, Sr., a firefighter and emergency medical technician in Easton, Massachusetts, suffered a ruptured brain artery on March 22, 1983. Surgery was performed in April, but it was unsuccessful, and Brophy never regained consciousness. He was transferred to the New England Sinai Hospital in a

This case summary has been drawn from *Brophy v. New England Sinai Hospital, Inc.*, 497 N.E. 2d 626 (Mass. 1986), and Robert Steinbrook and Bernard Lo, ''Artificial Feeding—Solid Ground, Not Slippery Slope,'' *New England Journal of Medicine* 286 (February 4, 1988): 286–90.

persistent vegetative state. When he developed pneumonia in August, both his physicians and Patricia Brophy, his wife and legal guardian, concurred in an order not to resuscitate him if he suffered a cardiac arrest. In December 1983, Mrs. Brophy gave the physicians permission for a surgical procedure to insert a feeding tube into his stomach. He received seven and a half hours of nursing care each day, consisting of bathing, shaving, turning, and so on. Brophy's medical bills, approximately ten thousand dollars per month, were paid entirely by Blue Cross/Blue Shield.

Brophy had often told family members that he did not want to be kept alive if he ever became comatose. In a discussion of the Karen Ann Quinlan case, he had indicated to his wife that "I don't ever want to be on a life-support system. No way do I want to live like that; that's just not living." Several years earlier, the town of Easton had given Brophy and his partner a commendation for bravery after they had pulled a man from a burning truck. When he learned that the victim had suffered a great deal before dying several months after being saved, Brophy threw his commendation into the wastebasket, exclaiming to his wife, "I should have been five minutes later. It would have been all over for him." He told his brother, Leo, "If I'm ever like that, just shoot me, pull the plug." And prior to his own neurosurgery, he told one of his daughters, "If I can't sit up to kiss one of my beautiful daughters, I may as well be six feet under."

Mrs. Brophy, a devout Catholic and a nurse who worked part time with the mentally retarded, decided to question the continuation of artificial feeding when her husband's condition remained unchanged through the next year. There was no hope that he would regain consciousness, and, though he had never expressed a specific judgment about artificial feeding, she recalled his previously expressed wishes about "pulling the plug." She consulted with clergy, ethicists, and a lawyer before requesting withdrawal of artificial nutrition with the understanding that her husband would die in one to two weeks. Her decision received the unanimous support of their five children and other family members, including Brophy's seven brothers and sisters and his elderly mother, who was in her nineties. However, the physicians and the hospital administration refused to act on this request.

In February 1985, Mrs. Brophy asked a probate court for a declaratory judgment ordering the hospital to act affirmatively on her request. The New England Sinai Hospital responded that the physician-in-chief of the hospital could not "in good conscience, consistent with the ethical codes of the medical profession, participate in the discontinuation of all nutrition and hydration." And it requested that Brophy be transferred to another facility if the court ordered discontinuation of artificial nutrition and hydration.

The court-appointed guardian *ad litem* (a person appointed by the court to protect the interests of a ward in a legal proceeding) found that "removal of the G [gastrostomy] tube is not comparable to cessation of dialysis or removal of a respirator because removal of the aforesaid artificial mechanisms permits the illness or injury to run its natural course. Nutrition, however, is not a need required by Mr. Brophy as a result of his illness, but rather, it is a need common to all human beings.'' Furthermore, the guardian *ad litem* continued, ''Brophy is a chronically ill patient, but is not terminally ill. He is entitled to the same fundamentals of comfort, i.e., food, shelter and bedding, as is any other chronically ill patient, and it is the duty of the medical facility to provide him with the aforesaid care.'' The probate judge ruled that the feeding tube must be continued, even though he found that Brophy would have preferred to be dead than to have his life prolonged in a persistent vegetative state and that if competent he would reject artificial nutrition. Mrs. Brophy appealed this verdict.

In September 1986, in a split decision (4 to 3), the Supreme Judicial Court of Massachusetts held that Brophy's feeding tube could be removed. Three U.S. Supreme Court justices declined to review the decision. The Massachusetts court did not require the hospital to compromise its principles by terminating feeding, but it did require the hospital's cooperation in transferring Brophy to Emerson Hospital in Concord, which was willing to honor Mrs. Brophy's request.

In October 1986, Brophy was transferred to Emerson Hospital under the care of a neurologist who had earlier testified that Brophy was in a persistent vegetative state. Many of the hospital staff volunteered to help care for Brophy by providing supportive care, including anticonvulsants and antacids, while he died. Brophy, age forty-nine, died of pneumonia on October 23, 1986, eight days after the feeding tube was removed. He was surrounded by his wife, who had remained with him around the clock, their children, and a grandchild. According to the attending physician, Brophy's death was an ''amazing, peaceful, quiet time.''

Case 10: The case of Baby M

Mrs. Mary Beth Whitehead, a twenty-nine-year-old housewife from Brick Township, New Jersey, signed a contract on February 6, 1985, to bear a child for William and Elizabeth Stern. As part of the sixteen-page contract, arranged by the Infertility Center of New York, Mrs. Whitehead agreed ''that in the best interests of the child, she will not form or attempt to form a parent-child relationship with any child . . . she may conceive . . . and shall freely surrender custody to William Stern, Natural Father, immediately upon birth of the child; and terminate all parental right to said child pursuant to this agreement.'' Mrs.

In the Matter of Baby M, 109 N.J. 396, 537 A. 2d. 1227 (1988).

Whitehead was to receive ten thousand dollars for "compensation for services and expenses" from the Infertility Center as part of the total of approximately twenty-five thousand dollars Mr. Stern agreed to pay the center. Of the remainder, five thousand dollars went to Mrs. Whitehead's medical, legal and insurance costs during pregnancy, and seventy-five hundred to ten thousand dollars went to the center as its fee.

When the child, conceived through artificial insemination with Mr. Stern's sperm, was born on March 27, 1986, Mrs. Whitehead and her husband, who already had two children, were reluctant to part with the child. They turned her over to the Sterns on March 30, but Mrs. Whitehead would not accept the ten thousand, and within a few days she went to the Stern residence and begged to be allowed to take the child for a week. The Sterns agreed. But by early May, it was clear that Mrs. Whitehead would not willingly return the child, and the Sterns filed a successful petition for temporary custody with the family court. Mrs. Whitehead managed to hand the baby out a bedroom window to her husband when six policemen arrived to take the baby. The husband left with the baby, and Mrs. Whitehead was able to join them later without detection. The Whiteheads were able to elude law enforcement officials in Florida for three months. When the infant, known in the court records as "Baby M," was finally located, she was turned over to the Sterns, and Family Judge Harvey R. Sorkow's temporary custody order was extended, along with limited visitation rights to Mrs. Whitehead.

A court-ordered paternity test established that Mrs. Whitehead's husband, Richard Whitehead, who had had a vasectomy, could not have fathered the child. After a thirty-two-day trial, Judge Sorkow declared the surrogacy contract valid and enforceable, terminated Mrs. Whitehead's parental rights, and awarded sole custody of Baby M to Mr. Stern. Judge Sorkow required specific performance of the surrogate contract on the grounds that it was in Baby M's best interests. He also immediately granted Mrs. Stern an order of adoption.

Upon appeal, the New Jersey Supreme Court (February 3, 1988) held that a surrogacy contract that provides money to the surrogate mother and requires her irrevocable agreement to surrender her child at birth is invalid and unenforceable. The surrogacy contract in the case of Baby M violates New Jersey statutes that prohibit the use of money in connection with adoptions, that limit termination of parental rights to situations in which there has been a valid showing of parental unfitness or abandonment of the child, and that allow a mother to revoke her consent to surrender her child in private placement adoption. In addition, the surrogacy contract conflicts with New Jersey's public policy that custody be determined on the basis of the child's best interests (the surrogacy contract makes a determination of custody prior to the child's birth), that children be brought up by their natural parents (the surrogacy contract guarantees the separation of the child from its natural mother), that the rights of the natural father and the natural mother are equal (the surrogacy contract elevates the natural father's right by destroying the natural mother's right), that a natural mother receive counseling before agreeing to surrender her child (the surrogacy contract in this case did not have such a provision), and that adoptions not be influenced by the payment of money (the surrogacy contract was based on such a payment).

Regarding the point that Mrs. Whitehead "agreed to the surrogacy arrangement, supposedly fully understanding the consequences," the court responded: "Putting aside the issue of how compelling her need for money may have been, and how significant her understanding of the consequences, we suggest that her consent is irrelevant. There are, in a civilized society, some things that money cannot buy. In America, we decided long ago that merely because conduct purchased by money was 'voluntary' did not mean that it was good or beyond regulation and prohibition." In addition, the court expressed concern about the unknown long-term effects of surrogacy contracts on various parties: "Potential victims include the surrogate mother and her family, the natural father and his wife, and most importantly, the child." However, the court did not find any legal prohibition of surrogacy "when the surrogate mother volunteers, without any payment, to act as a surrogate and is given the right to change her mind and to assert her parental rights."

The New Jersey Supreme Court affirmed the lower court's grant of custody to the natural father, but reversed the lower court's termination of the natural mother's parental rights and required the lower court to determine the terms of the natural mother's visitation with Baby M.

Index

Aaron, Henry J., 391–92

Abandonment, 51, 164, 198, 219, 245, 383, 404, 430, 525

Abeloff, M.D., 185

Abortion, 10–11, 15–17, 25, 42, 73, 124, 207, 252, 319, 403, 407, 410, 432, 472, 480

Abrams, Natalie, 505

Absolute norms, 32–34, 42, 52, 60–61, 72, 78, 94, 100–101, 104–5, 118, 126–27, 194, 205, 260, 272–73, 315–17, 338, 383, 396–97, 419, 423–28, 457

Abstinence, 360, 472–73

A.C., In re, 432–33, 458

Access to health care, 9, 54, 70, 128, 154, 197, 214, 234, 301–3, 305, 311, 316, 326, 329, 332–41, 345–56, 364–68, 371–79, 384, 387–90, 393, 407–13, 418–21, 429, 439, 449, 455, 482, 514. *See also* Allocation of biomedical resources; Justice

Accountability, 238, 246, 462, 473

Acquired Immunodeficiency Syndrome (AIDS), 36, 43, 102, 129, 182, 201, 259, 286–87, 299–302, 305, 314, 321–23, 349, 358, 390, 403, 406, 413, 416–17, 426–30, 446–47, 454–60, 472–73, 495–97, 506–7

Active-passive distinction, 196ff, 219ff

Adams, Robert Merrihew, 507

Addiction, 122, 152–53, 164, 233–34, 277

Adherence, 51, 54, 91, 396, 462, 471

Adkins, Janet, 237–38

Adkins v. Ropp, 195

Advance-directives, 9, 39, 131–32, 174–79, 204, 214, 230, 241–44 256, 261, 473, 514

Ageism. *See* Discrimination

Aiken, Will, 318

Albert, Martin P., 251

Alcohol-related problems, and alcoholism, 135, 299, 358–61, 391

Alderson, Priscilla, 182

Alexander, Leo, 231, 255

Alfidi, Ralph J., 187

Alford, C. A., 460

Allen, Anita L., 454–55

Allen, Robert W., 185

527